1 MONTH OF
FREE
READING

at

www.ForgottenBooks.com

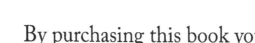

By purchasing this book you are eligible for one month membership to ForgottenBooks.com, giving you unlimited access to our entire collection of over 1,000,000 titles via our web site and mobile apps.

To claim your free month visit:
www.forgottenbooks.com/free693200

ISBN 978-0-428-98598-1
PIBN 10693200

THE BOSTON

MEDICAL AND SURGICAL

JOURNAL

J. COLLINS WARREN, M. D., ⎰
THOMAS DWIGHT, JR., M. D., ⎱ EDITORS

F. W. DRAPER, M. D., ASSISTANT EDITOR

VOLUME XCIII.

JULY—DECEMBER, 1875

BOSTON

H. O. HOUGHTON AND COMPANY

NEW YORK: HURD AND HOUGHTON

The Riverside Press, Cambridge

1875

CONTRIBUTORS TO VOLUME XCIII.

ROBERT AMORY, M. D.
F. K. BAILEY, M. D.
WILLIAM H. BAKER, M. D.
HENRY H. A. BEACH, M. D.
GEORGE H. BIXBY, M. D.
J. T. BOUTELLE, M. D.
H. P. BOWDITCH, M. D.
BUCKMINSTER BROWN, M. D.
FRANCIS F. BROWN, M. D.
C. E. BROWN-SÉQUARD, M. D.
CHARLES E. BUCKINGHAM, M. D.
GEORGE J. BULL, M. D.
GEORGE CAHILL, M. D.
PETER A. CALLAN, M. D.
JAMES R. CHADWICK, M. D.
D. W. CHEEVER, M. D.
DAVID CHOATE, M. D.
EDWARD H. CLARKE, M. D.
HALL CURTIS, M. D.
THOMAS B. CURTIS, M. D.
E. G. CUTLER, M. D.
F. W. DRAPER, M. D.
THOMAS DWIGHT, JR., M. D.
R. T. EDES, M. D.
T. W. FISHER, M. D.
R. H. FITZ, M. D.
CHARLES F. FOLSOM, M. D.
EDWARD J. FORSTER, M. D.
GEORGE E. FRANCIS, M. D.
J. F. GALLOUPE, M. D.
G. W. GARLAND, M. D.
GEORGE W. GAY, M. D.
J. ORNE GREEN, M. D.
F. B. GREENOUGH, M. D.

CARL GUSSENBAUER, M. D.
WILLIAM A. HAMMOND, M. D.
D. H. HAYDEN, M. D.
JOHN HOMANS, M. D.
C. L. HUBBELL, M. D.
B. JOY JEFFRIES, M. D.
F. I. KNIGHT, M. D.
H. LASSING, M. D.
F. B. A. LEWIS, M. D.
D. F. LINCOLN, M. D.
J. O. MARBLE, M. D.
CHARLES N. MILLER, M. D.
F. GORDON MORRILL, M. D.
CHARLES O'LEARY, M. D.
J. P. OLIVER, M. D.
CHARLES L. PIERCE, M. D.
C. B. PORTER, M. D.
JAMES J. PUTNAM, M. D.
W. L. RICHARDSON, M. D.
G. W. SARGENT, M. D.
B. F. SEABURY, M. D.
C. ELLERY STEDMAN, M. D.
GEORGE G. TARBELL, M. D.
O. F. WADSWORTH, M. D.
J. COLLINS WARREN, M. D.
S. G. WEBBER, M. D.
DAVID W. WEBSTER, M. D.
FRANK WELLS, M. D.
LEONARD WHEELER, M. D.
JAMES C. WHITE, M. D.
WILLIAM F. WHITNEY, M. D.
E. N. WHITTIER, M. D.
E. S. WOOD, M. D.
MORRILL WYMAN, M. D.

INDEX TO VOLUME XCIII.

THE BOSTON
MEDICAL AND SURGICAL JOURNAL.

VOL. XCIII. — THURSDAY, JULY 1, 1875. — NO. 1.

—————•—————

THE OBSTETRIC FORCEPS AS A TIME-SAVER.[1]

BY GEORGE E. FRANCIS, M. D., OF WORCESTER.

About twenty-five years ago Professor Simpson, of Edinburgh, asserted that "the mortality attendant upon parturition increases in a ratio progressive with the increased duration of the labor."

In 1829, Dr. John Beatty, of Dublin, having then attended more than five thousand labors in private practice, gave this testimony: "With respect to the ill effects said to follow the use of the forceps, I am bold to say that though I have read and heard of such, I have never witnessed any, when the instrument was used in time, or with proper discrimination and dexterity, and when the patient was not already too much exhausted; and from the success that has attended the use of the forceps in my hands, I might also assert that no unpleasant consequences can occur, provided the proper time be selected."

To look into the truth of these two propositions, and to study the results of combining them, are the objects of this brief paper.

The law proclaimed by Simpson was reached by analyzing the reports given by Dr. Collins of nearly sixteen thousand deliveries in the Dublin Lying-in Hospital. When these cases were tabulated according to the length of the labor, it at once appeared that the death-rate was lowest in the column of shortest labors, and that it steadily increased until its maximum was reached in the longest ones.

Ten years afterwards Mr. Harper made similar use of Johnston and Sinclair's reports of later cases in the same hospital, but treating only the *natural* labors, about twelve thousand in number. His results are to be found in the first volume of the Transactions of the London Obstetrical Society, and in their briefest form are as follows : —

Length of Labor.	Maternal Deaths.	Still-Births.
6 hours or under	1 in 470	1 in 71
7 to 12 hours	1 in 214	1 in 64
13 to 24 hours	1 in 145	1 in 31
Above 24 hours	1 in 21	1 in 5

It should be said that in forming this table the maternal deaths from

[1] Read at the Annual Meeting of the Massachusetts Medical Society.

non-puerperal causes have not been counted. It happens, however, that the general results are the same if we reckon *all* the deaths among the mothers.

"These results," Mr. Harper says, "are drawn from all those labors which are perfectly natural and uncomplicated with any secondary peculiarity which would modify or in any way alter their character. None of them were instrumental, but all were begun and finished by natural efforts alone. All foot, breech, arm, and placental presentations, as well as forceps and craniotomy cases, are thus excluded; the main object being to prove that mere duration alone, without any additional or abnormal circumstance, is the great element in rendering labor dangerous." "In proportion to increased duration is there a rapidly increasing rate of danger and mortality," to both mothers and children.

The deduction made by Simpson and Harper seems to be well drawn, since all of the cases were sufficiently alike to be compared, and were exposed to identical influences, — length of labor being, so far as we can see, the one condition which varied.

However true this law, it is of little use to us without an essential qualification which Simpson seems to have overlooked. In the words of Churchill, "delay in the first stage" (up to the passage of the head through the os uteri), "involves *per se* very little if any danger, no matter how tedious it may be; but delay in the second stage, beyond a comparatively short time, is always of serious import." This point is agreed upon by obstetric authorities, and needs no discussion.

Then Simpson's law of the relation between time and the death-rate applies especially to the second stage of labor: therefore, after the os is dilated, and the head begins to descend, it is our duty to save all the time we can, in order to lessen the danger.

The obstetric forceps being the most efficient means of shortening this second stage of labor, we have next to see whether or not it is a *safe* instrument, in order to learn whether we may properly use it to lessen danger by saving time.

In opposition to Dr. Beatty's very favorable testimony already quoted, listen to his contemporary, Dr. Clarke, an equally famous obstetrician: "It is certain that a labor really tedious under the best management is not without danger both to mother and child. I am, however, fully convinced that this danger is seldom lessened by the common expedient of extracting instruments" (meaning forceps). "Cases of convulsions excepted, I have rarely had reason to be pleased with the effects of extracting instruments, and not unfrequently have I had much reason to deprecate their evil consequences."

Here are two representative opinions, as wide apart as they well can be; without doubt they are both well founded. The simple fact is, that these eminent men had in view two distinct operations, the early and the late application of the forceps, — operations so different in their nature and results that just estimates of them must widely differ. Dr. Clarke used the forceps only after hours of delay, or even impaction, as the last resource which left the child a chance of living; the mischief which he and plenty more have found to follow such forceps deliveries is ascribed by them to the instrument rather than to the conditions which the instrument relieved. You will observe that the only reservation in Dr. Clarke's sweeping condemnation is in cases of convulsions, when the early operation was forced upon him.

Dr. Beatty, who used his forceps to prevent the evils of delay, found it a harmless instrument. To use his own language once more : "In no instance of the one hundred and eleven cases did any unpleasant result follow; none of the mothers died, none of them had the perinæum lacerated, nor any of those evils which are set forth as the effects of the forceps; and still more, all of the children that we had reason to think were alive at the commencement, were born living, and none of the whole number had any injury or mark whatever inflicted by the instrument."

This must be allowed to be strong evidence as to the harmlessness of the forceps when used early, before the mother's strength is exhausted, and especially before the soft parts have become swollen and devitalized by long pressure.

So far as I know, all the testimony against the forceps comes from those who have used them late ; while all who report the results of the early operation agree in substance with Dr. Beatty.

Dr. Churchill's treatment of this subject is somewhat curious : having collected statistics of forceps operations from every available source, he shows that they have, on the whole, been attended with decidedly less mortality than is found in tedious labors left to nature ; and he goes on to point out the obvious fact, that those who have used the forceps most freely have saved the most lives. In his own mild words, "to those who, like myself, regard the wider employment of the forceps as the best mode of diminishing the frequency of the employment of craniotomy, it is a matter of rejoicing to find this instrument increasingly employed, and that with each enlargement of our statistics the death-rate for mother and child has diminished." As he had already shown the danger of delay in the second stage of labor, it seems strange enough for so acute a writer to forthwith lay down the rule, that "in no case is the forceps to be applied until we are perfectly satisfied that the obstacle cannot be overcome by the natural powers with safety to the mother and child ;" which is practically the same as to say, "run the risks of tedious labor rather than the lesser risks of the forceps."

It seems to me that Dr. Churchill's premises logically lead to this very different conclusion: *the presumption is decidedly in favor of the early and frequent use of the forceps.*

Just how early or how often the instrument may be most successfully used can only be learned by studying the results of practice based upon this presumption.

Here we are indebted to Dr. Hamilton, of Falkirk, who has published his views and experience in various journals, particularly in the *Medico-Chirurgical Review* for April, 1853, and October, 1871, and in the *Edinburgh Medical Journal* for May, 1855, and October, 1861. The distinctive features of his practice are, to interfere very little until the os is well dilated; to make sure that the anterior lip of the uterus is not pushed down by the advancing head; then if the labor is not over within two hours, to deliver by the forceps.

The results which he reports are in brief these: the forceps were used in one seventh of the cases; the death-rate among the children was small beyond all precedent; for instance, he tells us of one series of seven hundred and thirty-one successive births of living children; the maternal mortality is nowhere definitely stated, but is said to be " very satisfactory." During thirty years he had not once to use the catheter in his own midwifery practice. He found the parts of the mother never to be more injured than in an easy, natural labor; rupture of the perinæum never once occurred in his whole experience, which in this respect is so unlike that reported by most good authorities as to throw a shade of doubt, not upon his honesty, but upon the accuracy of his observation; but this is a point concerning which error and oversight are easy and common. I am aware of no other published statistics of cases treated as his were, and this is my excuse for bringing before you a very short analysis of the last three hundred cases of head presentation occurring under my own care.

There were three hundred and one children, all born alive but four; of these one was believed to be dead when labor set in; one was a monstrosity, and one owed its death to prolapse of the cord. One child, born a month too soon, died in twelve hours; the remaining two hundred and ninety-six lived at least a week. In the last one hundred and thirty-eight cases there have been no still-births.

Three of the mothers died; one of them was at the point of death when first seen, probably from pulmonary thrombosis, and the child being nearly born was safely extracted at the very moment its mother died; another had erysipelas when labor set in, and died of blood-poisoning; the third was apparently exhausted by a very long first stage in which no interference was permitted; by the time the os was dilated she was in high fever. There have been no deaths in the one hundred and seventy-nine women last delivered. While it is true that the forceps was used in all three fatal cases, I see no reason to think that the operation affected the result in either of them.

After delivery the perinæum was always examined, and in but one case, which by the way was not instrumental, was there found sufficient tearing to need a stitch.

Almost all of these three hundred labors were completed within two hours after dilatation of the os; and to secure this end the forceps were used fifty-one times, once in six cases.

The application of the instrument rarely gave any more pain than the previous digital examination, and never required anæsthesia.

The catheter was not once required either during or after the confinement.

These statistics, as you will observe, are based upon the arbitrary limit of two hours for the second stage of labor; if a *standard* limit is ever found, it will only be through the study of many such reports. Meanwhile one result should not be overlooked, — the great and obvious saving of suffering and anxiety to the parturient woman and all about her.

I have tried to give you an outline sketch of the facts which go to show, first, that lapse of time in the second stage of labor brings increasing danger; second, that the forceps are not necessarily a dangerous instrument; and finally, that the experience of those who have used the forceps freely, to save time and avoid danger, is by no means unsatisfactory.

My purpose has been not so much to convince as to stimulate to thought and study upon an important practical question, and I have not hesitated to pass over many points of interest and importance for the sake of brevity and of keeping the main question clearly in view. Should it happen that a single hearer is led by this essay to use his forceps oftener than he did before, I should regret the fact without feeling any responsibility for it, since no man has a right to form or change his views upon a weighty matter without a much more thorough consideration than is possible within the limits of such a paper. A man so easily turned is by nature unfit for the practice of medicine, least of all fit for midwifery, which demands a well-stored and steadfast mind in a healthy and serviceable body, and above and ruling them both, a lively conscience; a conscience that never allows him to approach a woman in childbed without the feeling that two lives are trusted in his hands; a conscience that keeps this sense of responsibility always so close to him that there is no room for small and selfish motives to enter.   .

Conscience should hold us never more firmly than when we decide upon the use of a powerful instrument or remedy; we cannot shirk responsibilities for misusing it through carelessness or ignorance; neither are we blameless if we fear its power and fail to use it in the hour of need.

THE CLIMATE AND WEATHER OF NORTH AMERICA.

BY DR. JOHANN DAVID SCHOEPFF,

Surgeon of the Anspach-Bayreuth Troops in America.

TRANSLATED AND EDITED BY JAMES R. CHADWICK, M. D., OF BOSTON.

NEW YORK, *December* 20, 1780.

I REGRET not having seen the southern colonies, yet I am satisfied that in this part of the country and in the middle colonies there is field enough for new observations. The few Europeans who have traveled through these regions have, I hope, not been so impolite as to leave nothing for their successors, — and against discoveries on the part of the native-born Americans we are assured for many years to come. Making money and procuring luxuries are still their sole aims, and the sciences are only cultivated with reference to these dominant ideas.

The first and most striking comment of all travelers, not only in the northern but also in the southern half of America, may be summed up in this statement; that all the experience as to climate and weather acquired on the three old continents cannot be in the least applied to the new one. Cold has here the upper hand. As I, however, have only had a chance to see a very insignificant portion of the whole country, — namely, that along the coast from Delaware Bay to Rhod-Eyland and a small part of the adjoining provinces of Pennsylvania, East and West Jersey, New York, Connecticut, and Rhod-Eyland, I must confine my remarks chiefly to this section.

When we were first approaching the coast of New York,[1] I foolishly flattered myself that I should find a mild, fertile, and agreeable climate, such as those countries in Europe enjoy which lie in the same latitude. I was however soon convinced that the difference between the two was very considerable. A part of the States of the Church, the northern part of Naples, the southern provinces of France and Spain, and the equally delightful countries in the East, have the same solar elevation as the above-mentioned provinces in America. But all the agreeable features, all the advantages which have earned for Italy the name of the Garden of Europe, all the delicate wines, the excellent cereals, the multitude of delicious fruits which abound under the same parallel in Europe, and even much farther to the north, are here wanting. Instead of the moderate summers and mild winters of Naples, we have here heat and cold of extraordinary severity in both seasons, and no products which can be compared with those of that region. The two Carolinas and Floridas, although the most southerly colonies and exposed to the hottest summers, experience nevertheless for a longer or shorter period every year, all the effects of a winter, often severe. These comparisons are still more striking when applied to the northern

[1] In January, 1779.

regions of America. In the latitude of 48°, 49°, and 50°, we enjoy in
our fatherland a mild, temperate climate, sufficiently warm to produce
good wines, cereals, and delicious fruits. A land of almost eternal ice
and snow occupies the same parallels in North America. New Scotland,[1] Newfoundland, Canada, and New Britain[2] are as much unlike
the countries lying parallel to them in Europe as winter is to summer.
These provinces, as well as Labrador and the country about Hudson's
Bay, are enveloped in ice and snow for rather more than half the year,
so that Europeans living in the same latitude have not yet ventured to
settle there. The same cereals and fruits which are cultivated in Europe far above the fiftieth degree, here cease to grow at about the fortieth
degree. Wheat, for instance, hardly ripens any farther north. Alba-
nia and New England produce but little, and that of inferior quality.
The author of the Recierces Philosophiques sur les Americains
estimates the difference of warmth between the Old and New World at
twelve degrees.

New York and Philadelphia languish in the summer months, often
for many successive days, under a heat which, according to the sensations and testimony of travelers as well as the height of the thermometer, is as great as in the West Indies and the most southerly portions
of the terra firma ; it does not, however, persist so uninterruptedly and
for so many months as there. Almost every summer the Fahrenheit
thermometer has been observed repeatedly to stand at 95°, 96°, and 97°.
At the end of June and in July, 1778, while the British army was re-
treating from Philadelphia to Jersey, it remained for eight successive
days between 91° and 96°, and on the 28th of June, the day on which
the battle near Monmouth Court House took place, the thermometer
was at 96°. In Rhod-Eyland, which, owing to its exposed position on
the sea, has a temperate summer, I have frequently seen the mercury
in June, July, and August, between 84° and 90° ; in this last summer
we had an unusually persistent drought and heat in July and August. The height of the Fahrenheit thermometer at midday in the shade
was 84°, 88°, 90°, 92°, and 96°, on successive days. Uncovered and exposed to the sun it rose to 106°, 110°, 115°, etc. In the sun, but covered
with a thin, black silk ribbon to prevent refraction of the sun's rays, the
mercury in my thermometer filled the whole length of the glass, but
this only extended to 123°. On the other hand we have seen Dr.
Nooth's thermometers, which are prepared with great exactitude and
are marked to above the boiling point of water, stand between 128° and
135°, and once, on the 24th of August, at 146°, when covered as above
and exposed to the sun, or laid upon a stone which was warmed by the
solar rays. In the night mine has stood at 79°, 82°, 88°, and 90°, during the hottest weather.

---

[1] Nova Scotia.   [2] New England.

More unexpected, however, is the extreme cold of the winter when taken in connection with the latitude of the position and the heat of the summer. To judge from the variations of the weather, one would think that this stretch of territory was transported every year from under the line up to the north pole. The credulous Americans have long flattered themselves that, by the great progress of cultivation and by the destruction of the forests of the country, their climate has for some years been rendered much milder, and the severity of their winters been moderated. The past winter, however, has disappointed these premature anticipations. Few of the inhabitants can remember a similar one in respect to the severity or persistence of the cold and frost, and to the amount of the snow-fall. Even as early as the end of November and first weeks of December a steady frost set in ; snow fell frequently and remained everywhere upon the ground; in ordinary winters this is not wont to occur until four to six weeks later. Back in the country such an amount fell in various snow-storms that sleighs were driven over all the fences. In January the severest cold was experienced ; the North and East rivers froze so thick that loaded sleds were driven over both. All excursions towards Powles Hook, expeditions, all kinds of provisions and even twelve-pound cannon were carried to and fro upon the ice for nearly four weeks. Sleighs passed from here to Staaten-Eyland and Long-Eyland, and from one to the other of these islands. Between East Bay and Westchester people went for twenty miles upon the ice. In Philadelphia the usual oxen feast was held upon the Delaware, the river being frozen down to the bay. The position of the southern provinces protected them this time as little as ever from the inclemency of the winter. The James and York rivers, in latitude 37°, were frozen hard, and Chesapeake Bay was full of ice. The streams in Georgia and Carolina, in latitudes 32° and 33°, were covered with ice an inch thick. Instances of the extraordinary effects of cold in former years throughout the southern provinces are constantly recalled. "On February 7, 1747, it froze so hard in Charleston that two bottles, which some one had taken into bed, were found in the morning burst, and the water changed into a lump of ice. In one kitchen were a fire was kept up, the water, nevertheless, in an earthen vessel, which contained a live eel, froze to the bottom. On January 3, 1765, Mr. Bertram experienced such extraordinary cold in St. Augustine in latitude 30°, that in one night the ground along St. John's River was frozen an inch thick and all the lemon and banana trees about St. Augustine succumbed to the cold."[1] The famous winter of 1740, and perhaps a few others may, judging from the accounts and sensations of the inhabitants, be compared with this one for cold. According to observations which were taken before the war by gentlemen at the New York college, the

[1] Robertson's History of America, vol. ii., page 331.

mercury had often been seen under 6° below zero, 38° beneath the freezing point; in the last one this was a common occurrence. My thermometer only extends to zero, so that I have not been able to take any observations about the extreme fall of the mercury, though I have several times seen the tube quite empty. I doubt if so striking a contrast between heat and cold has been experienced in any other part of the inhabited globe as in this place whose climate has been so extolled by Franklin. From 13° below zero to a warmth of 96° in the shade, the difference is 109°, and to the greatest heat of the sun, 136°, amounts to 159°; the climate of England, on the other hand, though in a northerly situation, is so tempered that the variation from the greatest heat to the greatest cold does not exceed 65° in the shade.[1]

It is not enough that the extremes of heat and cold are so far apart; it is not enough that in the uninterrupted cycle of ages, the effect of one or other is reduced to nought, and that the land, which is exposed to all the discomforts of the torrid and frigid zones, yet does not enjoy the advantages of either. Rapid variations from heat to cold constantly take place every four or five days in these regions. In the north the weather appears to be somewhat more stable; yet very warm days often occur in the months of February and March, and alternate with frost and snow. It freezes in the middle of April, and often even in May. In the winter of 1789 people were brought to the hospital in Philadelphia with frozen toes, although on that day the thermometer was standing at 70°, and they were only suffering from the frost of the preceding night. We have sat with doors and windows open in February, without a fire, and yet, on the other hand, we have often been glad to have a fire in the middle of summer. On December 25, 1778, I encountered one of the most terrible northerly storms, on board a ship in the Sound. The mercury stood between 4° and 20° for a number of days, and immediately afterwards, the transition from the old to the new year brought us a most delightful spring weather of 45°–68°. In the month of July, 1779, there followed upon great warmth so frequent rains with easterly and northeasterly gales, and such cool days, that delicate individuals had to have fires. On the 20th of last August, after a long series of hot days, we saw the thermometer suddenly fall to 63° and rise on the 24th to 92°. It is incredible what disagreeable physical sensations are produced by these sudden contrasts, not to mention the prevalent diseases. When the Russian plunges from his vapor bath immediately into the snow, or into the stream that is covered with ice, I hardly think he suffers half as much as we do from the incessant changes of the weather. On the last day of October we had quite a warm afternoon; between five and six in the evening there was thunder and lightning in the distance, and

---

[1] The greatest cold ever experienced in England was 15°. The greatest heat in August, 1779, was 70°. (Schoepff.)

nothing was more unexpected than to find, on the next morning, November 1st, the whole ground covered with snow to the depth of an inch, and yet at eight o'clock in the morning the mercury had already risen to 80°. If America should ever have a Thomson (thus far she has not produced even a tolerable poet), I cannot imagine which season of the year he would find it worth his while to celebrate.

The only moderately agreeable months are September and October. The charm of spring is unknown and unfelt. A steady April weather prevails through the months of March, April, and May — alternate summer and winter. Then, of a sudden, a moderate heat prevails, in the intervals of which eastern and cool northern winds remind us of the scarcely defunct winter. The vegetable kingdom comes to life several weeks later than in England and no earlier than in Germany. . . . Northwesterly winds are the most common in this part of the world; they prevail during all seasons of the year and are often not spent till they have crossed the Atlantic. Upon them Columbus based his belief in the existence of a then unknown western continent. Although they often assail us in the rudest manner, and are so chilly, even in the hottest summer weather, we must yet credit them with the greatest of benefits, since they expedite the voyage to Europeans who are hastening home to their mild, civilized, and in every respect excellent fatherland. It almost seems as though the westerly gales, fogs, and mighty seas had been cast in the way of Europeans by a beneficent Providence as so many warnings to keep off. When they have been overcome, nothing is found but the gloomy shadow to the bright picture of home.

It has been calculated that land-winds prevail in North America during three fourths of the year; these expedite the return of ships to Europe, so that they make the trip in half the time required for the outward voyage. To shorten the passage from Europe it is necessary to steer far to the south, so as to reach the trade-winds. Single ships and merchantmen therefore often diverge as far as the twenty-sixth degree of southern latitude. Transports are not able to follow this course for fear of exposing the troops to the great heat, particularly when the sun is in the northern hemisphere.

It has been observed that the severest storms commonly approach on the side toward which the wind is blowing [to leeward]; a northwest storm, for instance, breaks out a day earlier in Virginia than in Boston. The cause of this is apparent, for if the atmosphere in the south becomes rarefied for any reason, the denser air will at once move from the adjacent regions in that direction; an influx from the north is thus gradually set up.

Besides these winds, there exist along the coast of North America during the hot days, the so-called sea-breezes. They do not penetrate

for any distance inland; Philadelphia, which lies far from the sea, is
never reached by them, so that the heat is heavy and oppressive; Boston, at the head of a deep bay, feels them but little. New York is, in
a manner, sheltered from them by the heights of Long and Staaten eylands, yet they seldom fail to reach the city with the flood-tide. Their
effect is most marked in Rhod-Eyland, where, owing to its immediate
propinquity to the sea, the excessive midday heat is greatly moderated.
For this and other reasons this eyland is always regarded as an agreeable and healthy summer resort; people of means frequently come there
from the West Indies and the southern provinces to pass the summer.
The land-breezes, — which in the West Indian eylands and in most
warm countries alternate with the sea-breezes and render the nights
cool by blowing from the land towards the sea, — are not much felt
here, at least, not invariably; they occasionally spring up toward midnight or later, and die down toward sunrise. In summer there is apt
to be a calm in the morning and evening; this and the sea-breezes
through the day have often detained ships for many days in the harbor
of New York. Another disagreeable feature of this coast is the thick,
heavy fogs which collect in the summer, produce an unpleasant, sultry
weather, and are often so thick as to wet one's clothes. . . . . The natives consider them to be harmless, which is true, in so far as they contain
no injurious exhalations from stagnant water or marshes, but are simply
sea-water disseminated in the air. . . . .

It is a pet theory of the Americans that the excessive cold of their
country is imparted to the wind chiefly by the snow which lies so long
in their boundless forests. They base this belief upon a fallacious experience. Thus I have heard several old inhabitants assert that the
cold has not been nearly so severe in recent winters as it was twenty
or thirty years ago; in the interval of time very many forests have been
leveled. This opinion is based only upon physical sensations, and the
memory is very likely to be at fault in comparing the experiences of different years. During the war, a much greater amount of wood than
usual has been cut in this neighborhood by both armies; the past winter
has nevertheless been more severe than any of its predecessors; all
these considerations make it very desirable that proofs should be brought
forward in support of the above assertion.

RECENT PROGRESS IN MEDICAL CHEMISTRY.

BY E. S. WOOD, M. D.

Albumen and Albuminous Urines. — Occasionally the physician meets with a specimen of urine which an examination of the sediment by the microscope shows to contain renal casts, but which does not give the characteristic reactions for serum-albumen. Further investigation would, however, invariably prove the presence of some other variety of albumen. Obermüller[1] mentions certain urines which are not precipitated by nitric acid in any proportion, and yet, when these urines are treated with an excess of alcohol, an abundant precipitate is formed which consists, in part at least, of albuminous substances. This precipitate is soluble in water, and, when purified by repeated solution in water and precipitation by alcohol, behaves with reagents like peptone.

Senator[2] also speaks of the different varieties of albumen which may be found in the urine. The presence of these may be explained partly by their presence in the blood-serum, and the passage thence through the kidney of one or the other of them, according to circumstances, into the urine, since the different varieties act very differently with animal membranes in the presence of different proportions of inorganic salts. Another source may be the albuminous infiltration of the renal epithelium which can readily give up its albumen to the urine, and can also be itself decomposed with the setting free of a myosin-like substance.

The author examined the urine of five cases of cloudy swelling, thirteen of chronic diffused nephritis, three of acute diffused nephritis, and six of amyloid degeneration. The urine was diluted with water until it had a specific gravity of 1.002 or 1.003, and a stream of carbonic acid gas passed through it for two or more hours. This produced in every case a turbidity, but in only one case an evident precipitate. This dissolved in dilute hydrochloric acid and a solution of common salt, and had the properties of globulin. Its fibrino-plastic nature was proved by dissolving it in a trace of sodic hydrate, and adding it to pericardial or peritoneal fluid, when it produced a coagulum of fibrine. The urine of acute nephritis was richest in this paraglobulin, while in that of chronic nephritis there was very little. In the five cases of cloudy swelling a considerable amount of paraglobulin was found. The urine filtered from the paraglobulin and treated with very dilute acetic acid gave a slight turbidity, which might be due either to a trace of paraglobulin which had escaped the former process or to alkali-albuminate. To which of these it was due could not be determined on account of the small quantity ; acid-albumen was never found.

[1] Centralblatt für die medicinischen Wissenschaften, 1875, No. 8, from Inaugural Dissertation. Würzburg, 1873.

[2] Centralblatt für die medicinischen Wissenschaften, 1875, No. 8, from Virchow's Archiv, 1874, lx. Heft 3 und 4.

In order to test the urines for peptone it was first deprived of serum-albumen by boiling with a trace of acetic acid, then mixed with three or four times its volume of alcohol, and the precipitate was red with alcohol. This precipitate, always small in amount, was soluble in water, colored yellow with nitric acid, and answered to the tests for peptone with the metallic oxides.

In five cases of chronic cystitis the author found a large amount of fibrino-plastic substance (paraglobulin) which formed a thick coagulum of fibrine when added to pericardial fluid. And in one case of croupous affection of the kidneys caused by the application of a cantharides plaster, there was a true fibrinuria.

Gerhardt [1] often observed peptone in urine which did not contain serum-albumen, sometimes as a forerunner and sometimes as a follower of ordinary albuminuria. L. Siebold [2] recommends in testing the urine for albumen the addition of ammonia until the urine is feebly alkaline, filtering from the phosphates and organized substances in suspension, rendering the filtrate slightly acid with acetic acid, and boiling. The slightest turbidity can be detected by comparison with a portion of the filtrate which has not been boiled.

Adamkiewicz [3] gives a new test for albumen, which is very delicate, and is applicable to all the varieties of albumen, peptone included. Every variety of albumen, when dissolved in an excess of glacial acetic acid and treated with concentrated sulphuric acid, gives a beautiful violet color and a feeble fluorescence, and shows, when properly concentrated and examined by the spectroscope, an absorption band, which, like that of urobilin [4] and choletelin, lies between the Fraunhofer lines *b* and *F*.

This test reacts with a few cubic centimetres of a solution of egg albumen which contains one part of albumen in two thousand parts of water.

Aronstein [5] has confirmed Graham's experiments concerning the preparation of absolutely pure albumen by diffusion, the necessary precaution being that the parchment paper used must be the best English parchment. His conclusions are, 1. That pure albumen is completely soluble in water, and the presence of salts is not necessary for its solution in the animal fluids. 2. That pure albumen is not coagulated either by heat or by alcohol, and that the coagulation usually taking place on heating or adding alcohol is caused by the presence of salts. 3. That there exist no compounds of albumen with the insoluble salts in the animal fluids to which these salts owe their solubility, but that

1 Wiener medicinische Presse, 1871.
2 Chemisches Centralblatt, 1874, p. 169.
3 Berichte der deutschen chemischen Gesellschaft, 1875, No. 3.
4 See Report on Medical Chemistry, January 2, 1873.
5 Archiv für Physiologie, Bd. 8, p. 75.

they are eld in solution in these fluids by means of an organic sub-stance present both in blood-serum and white of egg, which does not be-long to the class of albuminous compounds. 4. That the blood-serum and white of egg contain, besides serum-albumen, another variety which is insoluble in water, and is eld in solution in the animal fluids by the crystalloid bodies present. This substance is paraglobulin, or the fibrino-plastic substance. 5. That pure serum-albumen is precipitated by ether, while pure egg-albumen is not. In the presence of inorganic salts, however, this action is reversed.

Urinary Coloring Matters. — Much progress has been made of late years in the study of the urinary pigments. The discovery by Maly of the method of formation of the pigment urobilin, found by Jaffé in nor-mal urine, and to a greater extent in some pathological urines, has al-ready been referred to in these reports.[1] Besides urobilin, another pure coloring matter (indigo blue) can be isolated from the urine. This according to the investigations of Schunk[2] and others, is obtained by the decomposition of indican which exists normally and pathologic-ally in the urine. Jaffé,[3] and later, Dr. Masson,[4] found that the indican was very largely increased in the urine after the ingestion or subcuta-neous injection of indol (a substance which can be obtained from in-digo by the action of zinc and hydrochloric acid), thus showing that indican can be obtained from indol by the oxidizing action of the sys-tem.

As to the formation of the indol, the experiments of W. Kühne[5] ren-der it extremely probable that it is formed by pancreatic digestion of the albuminous substances. He succeeded, by distilling a mixture of an infusion of pancreas with albumen, in obtaining the milky, aqueous solution of indol, filled with the ill-defined crystalline plates. This does not prove absolutely that indol is a product of pancreatic digestion of albumen, since it may have come from the pancreatic ferment itself, or from the bacteria, which were always present during the experiments, and in some instances, when such precautions were taken as to exclude the bacteria, no indol could be found. Its formation *may*, therefore, be classed among the putrefactive changes. It is more probable, however, that the indol is a product of the decomposition of albumen, since it can be obtained from albumen by melting it with potassic hydrate. By treating caseine in the same way, a pigment was obtained apparently identical with the indigo red found by Nencki and described below.

By long warming of indican with the mineral acids, other pigments besides indigo blue can be obtained in very small amounts, namely, in-

[1] See the Journal, January 2, 1873.
[2] Chemisches Centralblatt, 1856, p. 60,; 1857, p. 957 ; 1858, p. 225.
[3] Medicinisches Centralblatt, 1870, p. 514.
[4] Archives de Physiologie, November, 1874.
[5] Berichte der deutschen chemischen Gesellschaft, 1875, No. 4.

digo red (Heller's urrıodin) and indigo brown. In some patıological urines tıese pigments are verylargely increased. M. Nencki [1] has isolated the indigo red as a red amorpıous pigment from the urine of a patient with spinal paralysis, by the addition of ıydrocıloric acid and ıeat. It was soluble in alcoıol and glacial acetic acid, witı a beautiful violet color, and wıen dried and ıeated in a test tube gave off violet fumes.

By the ingestion of oxindol, dioxindol, or isatin (wıicı can be obtained by oxidizing indigo) the amount of tıis red pigment is mucı increased. To obtain it from ıuman urine, the wıole amount passed during twenty-four ıours after the ingestion of two grammes of isatin is collected, evaporated to one tıird of its original bulk, and concentrated ıydrocıloric acid added. The urine is colored at once deep red, gradually becomes darker, almost black, and finally, after several ıours, the pigment separates in the form of microscopic dark red granules. When tıis is treated witı hot alcoıol the greater part of the pigment dissolves, giving a carmine red solution, and about one tıird remains undissolved. After the evaporation of the alcoıol the pigment remains as a dark red powder witı a metallic lustre. Hot water dissolves only traces, but it is easily soluble in hot alcoıol and glacial acetic acid. It is sligıtly soluble in ammonic and sodic ıydrates with a brownisı-red color, and readily reprecipitated by acids as a brown flocculent precipitate. The solution in alcoıol and glacial acetic acid sıows no absorption bands wıen examined witı the spectroscope. If ıeated it sublimes, the fumes being red.

The residue, wıicı is insoluble in alcoıol, dissolves easily in ammonic ıydrate witı a brownisı-red color, from wıicı solution ıydrocıloric acid precipitated it as a brown flocculent precipitate. When dry it forms a blackisı-brown powder witı a metallic lustre. It cannot be sublimed. It is insoluble in cold alcoıol and glacial acetic acid, but easily soluble in the alkalies.

If indol is really the result of pancreatic digestion of albumen, the presence of indican in the urine is easily explained. The indol is absorbed from the intestine, oxidized in the blood to indigo blue, wıicı combines grape sugar to form indican, and the indican eliminated witı the urine. Nencki explains its increase patıologically by disturbance of the pancreatic digestion. The appearance of the indigo red in the urine is best explained by a part of the indol cıanging in the intestine to isatin.

[1] Berichte der deutschen chemischen Gesellschaft, 1874, No. 17.

CYCLOPÆDIA OF THE PRACTICE OF MEDICINE.[1]

THE third volume of this great work is fully equal to its predecessors. Nearly one half is occupied by Bäumler's article on syphilis, and the rest is devoted to the discussion of infection by animal poisons, by Bollinger, and of diseases from migratory parasites, by Heller. Bäumler goes over the immense field with great thoroughness and impartiality. In this latter respect he deserves great praise; we have noticed no instance in which he seemed at all influenced by preconceived notions and in which he did not give full weight to the arguments of both sides. With regard to the question of unity, or duality of the syphilitic poison, the author expresses himself very plainly and adopts the simplest nomenclature. There is but one syphilitic poison, "but in another sense from that given to it in the doctrine of unity;" the chancre, chancroid, or soft chancre, being a local affection from a distinct poison. It is admitted that the two poisons may occur together, and that very anomalous cases present themselves. "When we remember the multiplicity of secretions which are often mingled together at the infecting source, there is no wonder that in practice, syphilitic infection does not preserve the pure and simple character which is observed in pathological experiments." The question of prophylaxis by sanitary legislation is naturally not considered at length, but the few pages given it are good and suggestive. Bäumler expresses himself strongly in favor of the rational use of mercury, and says that syphilization, which he shows to be a bad name, "is not likely to obtain the confidence of physicians to any extent."

Bollinger discusses hydrophobia at great length and in a very interesting manner. He gives many valuable statistics on various points. Though the advisability is well known, we may be pardoned for calling attention to the statistics showing the great advantage of cauterizing every bite that can reasonably be deemed suspicious. The author endeavors to determine the diagnosis of rabies in dogs, which he tells us, "with few exceptions, may be correctly established by a study of the clinical and anatomical appearances taken together." It is pretty clear, however, owing to the many troubles that may cause symptoms simulating hydrophobia, that its diagnosis during life must often be impossible. In many cases it may be important to decide this question after the death of an animal concerning whose clinical history we have no reliable data, who may for instance have been shot on the vaguest suspicions. In such cases the author expresses his agreement with Bruckmüller, that "it will be best to pronounce every dog free from the disease, provided his stomach contain normal ingesta and his small intestine contain chyme."

As for the treatment of this hopeless disease, Bollinger put narcotics first, and chloroform at their head. As euthanasia is all we can aim at, we think he is quite right in giving the most dangerous anæsthetic the preference.

On reading the chapter on snake-bites we cannot but feel that more might have been said of the rattlesnake, considering its wide-spread distribution in

[1] *Cyclopædia of the Practice of Medicine.* Edited by DR. H. VON ZIEMSSEN. Vol. III. Chronic Infectious Diseases. American Edition, edited by ALBERT H. BUCK, M. D. New York: Wm. Wood & Co. 1875. Pp. 672.

America. As to treatment, besides the ordinary measures for destroying the poison or of hindering its absorption, we find that Bollinger advises that the patient "should be made to drink copiously and frequently of spirituous liquors diluted with hot water, taking care, however, not to produce intoxication." We have no experience in these parts, but we understand that the essence of the "whiskey cure," which is very efficacious in the South and West, is that the patient should drink as long as he can carry his glass to his mouth. Heller's paper on migratory parasites is very comprehensive and interesting.

CHAMBERS ON DIET IN HEALTH AND DISEASE.[1]

THIS book, like all those written by this well-known author, is distinguished by a vivacious and more familiar style than the ordinary text-books. It is also characterized by an originality and keenness of observation for which Dr. Chambers is so justly celebrated. Oftentimes, perhaps, the reader may be startled by some suggestions, as for instance that on page 191 : " It is a strange thing, and one which at first sounds paradoxical, that the supply of the stomach, even from the substance of the individual body itself, should tend to prolong life. A case of starvation for twenty-two days in an open boat was recorded in the periodical prints last spring (April 30, and May 1, 1874), in which the poor victims fought in their delirium, and one was severely wounded. As the blood gushed out, he lapped it up ; and instead of suffering the fatal weakness which might have been expected from the hæmorrhage, he seems to have done well. . . . M. Anselmier fed dogs on the blood taken from their own veins daily, and he found that the fatal cooling incident to starvation was thus postponed. . . . The prolongation of life without provisions is by no means a mere speculative discussion. Were I in such a strait as above referred to, my reason would counsel me, and I hope I should have the courage, to wound the veins and suck the blood." And again, when speaking of sea-sickness incident to short voyages on the sea, on page 174 : " If the voyage is by night and sufficiently long to make a night's rest of say seven or eight hours at least, it is worth while to swallow a full dose of chloral on embarking, and to sleep through one's troubles."

The general design of the work, however, to " connect food and drink with the daily current of social life," is well carried out. The explanation of the theories of dietetics might perhaps be modified if viewed in the light obtained from recent physiological theories ; as for example, the practitioner observes that (page 19) " under vegetable food the saliva becomes more copious, under meat there is more gastric juice." The physiologist might go farther and theorize that the *continued* use of vegetable food produces *diastase* (saliva), or the peculiar ferment necessary to prepare vegetable food for digestion; whereas the continued use of meat will produce *gasterase* (the gastric juice), which is also essential for the preparation of animal food for digestion. The

[1] *A Manual of Diet in Health and Disease.* By THOMAS KING CHAMBERS, M. D., Oxon., F. R. C. P. Lond., etc. Published by Henry C. Lea, Philadelphia. 1875.

presentation and criticism of the kinds of food suited for the different ages and pursuits of man, though probably not new to the modern medical student, may yet be of practical benefit to the full-grown physician. The short physiological review of this part of his book is well done and agreeably presented to the reader.

The remarks of Dr. Chambers in reference to the choice of food are exceedingly sagacious, and should be widely promulgated; but unfortunately we civilized beings depend upon tradesmen for our meat, and physicians cannot, from the nature of society, become political economists.

We cannot expect those of our readers who are teetotalers to read with relish that portion of this book which refers to the use of wines; as for instance (page 76), "All these five classes of wines (strong dry wines, strong. sweet wines, aromatic wines, acid wines, sparkling wines) prudence will reserve for festive purposes and occasions; the wise man who wishes to enjoy life will make them always exceptional, for as idlers have no holidays, so perpetual feasters miss all the pleasures of variety; but I am quite sure that the not infrequent manufacture of occasions for domestic rejoicings, a birthday, a wedding anniversary, . . . a horse sold, . . . the calving of a cow, . . . a daughter cutting her first tooth, . . . is a great promoter, not only of love and happiness, but of personal health. . . . If the beverages are good of their class, the moderate use will not shorten but both cheer and lengthen life."

The remarks on athletic training should be carefully read by boating men, and should be known to practitioners, especially those who are often appealed to by parents of college students. The explanation of the purposes of training is clearly stated and easily comprehended; the regimen of the principal English universities is transcribed, and a proper caution is given in regard to the abuse of training. In view of the present season it may not be amiss to call attention to what Dr. Chambers writes in reference to those who desire to spend a vacation in sport or mountaineering. He urges the use of the week or fortnight prior to the vacation in preparing the physical frame by a proper. diet and muscular discipline, thus to prevent the wasting of the first week of the vacation in "getting into condition." The suggestions for the relief of unhealthy corpulence are excellent, as well as the caution in regard to the use of violent means for reducing the weight of the body. "Many uncomfortably stout persons are very active in mind and body, and really could not add to their muscular discipline without risk of injury."

The Hints for Health Travelers, Chapter VII. of the second part, are practical and seem sound in theory; but the criticism in regard to the selection from the bill of fare of the proper articles of food would be of little use to those who travel in our country.

The discussion on the relation of proper food for various climates, while the principles are thoroughly explained in the modern works on physiology, may perhaps be agreeable reading for those who do not own any of the latter.

The Diet and Regimen of Weak Digestion, Chapter III. of the third part, is especially noteworthy; but as Dr. Chambers has made his reputation as a writer upon this especial subject, it is unnecessary to criticise this portion of his work.

The manual is evidently intended for popular reading as well as for those persons who are strictly professional; but yet, like all such books written for two classes of persons, there is much in it which is probably well-known to medical men, and a great deal in it .which would mislead the world at large. The kinds of medicine, and their doses, which travelers should keep on hand are hardly safe for the uneducated to use except under the special direction of a medical attendant. It would probably be more advantageous for the traveler to consult his family physician, rather than this book, in regard to the proper medical articles to put into his trunk for use in an emergency. We invite attention to page 172 in reference to this subject.

Finally, the discussion on alcohol, commencing on page 200, would furnish good reading to those in favor, as well as those opposed to its use. We will not enlarge upon that subject here.   R. A.

VOGEL ON THE CHEMISTRY OF LIGHT AND PHOTOG-RAPHY.[1]

THE appearance of a popular treatise on the chemical principles of photography by so competent a person as Professor Vogel, is very seasonable at a time when the application of this art to scientific researches may be of great use in preserving accurately the observations of the student. Photographic representation must always be more accurate than that of the draughtsman. The well-known researches in dental histology by means of photo-micrographs by the late Dr. Hitchcock, suggest a means for extending the application of this art to other points of histology. To a person who desires to obtain a knowledge of the principles of the art of photography, we recommend the careful study of Dr. Vogel's work.

A REMARKABLE CASE OF CATALEPSY.

WE take from the *London Medical Record* the facts of the following interesting case, which has attracted much attention in Paris. The case of Louise Lateau has added greatly to the interest which such cases naturally present.

Marie Lecomte, who had come into Dr. Després's wards for a surgical affection, was soon afterwards attacked with dysmenorrhœa and uncontrollable vomitings, followed by nervous aphonia and suppression of urine, and vomiting. At the beginning of April the urinary function, which had long been suspended, was reëstablished, when on April 5th the patient fell into a lethargy; her breathing was imperceptible, her lips were pink, and her complexion rather roseate than pale. The trunk and limbs were in a complete state

---

[1] *The Chemistry of Light and Photography.* By DR. HERMANN VOGEL, Professor in the Royal Industrial Academy of Berlin. International Scientific Series. New York: D. Appleton & Co.

of relaxation; the pulse was normal; involuntary motion was abolished; the finger placed through the half-opened mouth on the glottis provoked neither cough nor any other movement. No food was given for fear that any attempts to administer it would produce asphyxia. On April 6th, the whole of the patient's muscles were hard and tense. The state was that of cadaveric rigidity, *minus* death. This condition lasted six days, during which the patient took no food. Many attempts were made to awaken her by pricking, irritating the nostrils, etc., but without success. M. Després tried an experiment tending to show that the muscular contraction was involuntary. The abdominal muscles contracted like those of the rest of the body and retained the form imparted to them. By forcibly applying the hand to the abdomen the muscles were depressed, and the imprint of the hand remained visible during at least three minutes. Between the seventh and fourteenth days of the crisis there were brief intervals of partial awakening, when the patient would take a little food. From the latter date the cataleptic crisis ceased. The patient remained in a state of dreamy wakefulness — of somnambulism. She did not recognize any one, but was yet able to take drink. On the seventeenth day the patient believed herself to be blind, and a shining object placed before her eyes, and even the light of day, seemed to make no impression upon her; but sight returned the next day. On the twenty-fifth day vomiting had entirely ceased, and the patient was convalescent. On. May 5th, she was entirely cured.

Cases of catalepsy complicated with somnambulism of hysterical patients are now well known. This kind of catalepsy is almost exclusively the melancholy privilege of women.

This patient, quite unlike Louise Lateau, had no religious excitement, and, on the other hand, no vicious habits. She is a foundling, twenty-four years old, who had never left the foundling hospital and the farm where she had been boarded out, and is a quiet, well-conducted unmarried woman. In her case the attack begins with lethargic coma, and generalized muscular contraction comes on twenty-four hours afterwards; when the patient awakes she is somnambulistic. The catalepsy, accompanied by lethargy, lasts six full days, during which there is apparent death. After the awakening there are three relapses, and the disorder yields little by little, after alternations of awakening and lethargy for several days.

Regarding the question whether it might not have been possible when she was in the lethargic state for ignorant persons to have believed death to be real and to have interred the patient, it is stated that notwithstanding the appearances of death in the case of Marie Lecomte, the signs of life were so decided that the most ignorant of practitioners could not have felt for an instant the slightest doubt as to the vitality of the patient.

GALLOPING MALIGNANT SYPHILIS.

THE presence of two patients in the wards of Saint Louis Hospital was the occasion of a clinical lecture on the above malady by Dr. E. Guibout, a full report of which is contained in *L' Union Médicale* of May 25 and 27, 1875.

In contrast with the usual history of syphilis, the secondary and tertiary lesions slowly developing themselves, the two patients under consideration, only six weeks after the appearance of the chancre, were terribly disfigured, and rendered hideous and repulsive, by the enormous black and sanious crusts which covered the greater part of the scalp, face, trunk, and limbs. There were very numerous and very large ulcerations, and from beneath and across the crusts which covered them there flowed incessantly a disgusting mixture of pus and blood. The countenances were pale and thin, eyes lack-lustre, the lips dry, and there was the profound and indefinable expression characteristic of the disease. There was also intense fever, prostration, diminution of vital forces, loss of appetite and of sleep; in short, a general and very severe disturbance of all the physiological functions. In consideration of the phenomena presented by these cases, so different from those usually shown in syphilis, the titles *malignant* and *galloping* have been applied: *malignant*, because of the gravity of the cutaneous lesions and of the general condition of the patient; *galloping*, because of the rapidity of the invasion, development, and progress of the local and general lesions.

The form of syphilis under discussion may present itself at two different epochs. It is sometimes *precocious (précoce)* or *primitive*, sometimes *tardy* or *consecutive*. The precocious or primitive form occurs when it is the first of the general lesions of syphilis, when it succeeds, with scarcely any delay, the infecting chancre. Such was the form as it appeared in the two cases forming the subject for the lecture. Coming on only six weeks after the infecting chancre, and without the appearance of any other lesion of the skin, there were developed on the head, trunk, and limbs the ulcerations and the crusts of rupia of the gravest form, accompanied with excessive disturbance of the health.

At other times the form is tardy or consecutive. Suddenly, and with alarming characteristics, it supervenes at a late stage of the syphilitic career after the ordinary constitutional phenomena. There comes over the patient at the same time a change so rapid, profound, and marked that it is impossible not to see something serious is in store.

When we come to consider the cause of the invasion of malignant syphilis, it is found that the late form, that is, that which accompanies the ordinary early cutaneous lesions, or is consecutive to them, is due to the want of proper treatment, to bad hygiene, or to a deterioration of the general health of the patient in consequence of fatigue or of various excesses. The same causes hold good for the precocious, galloping, malignant syphilis. The primary manifestations of syphilis may be malignant if the patient's constitution is poor and his surroundings unfavorable to a healthy hygienic condition.

If the prognosis of syphilis in its most common and benign form is always unfavorable, much more so will it be in the malignant variety.

Its treatment presents great difficulties, and requires all that medical skill and cliuical science can command. One needs to consider not only the disease, but even more, perhaps, the patient. Great caution is necessary about prescribing the specifics — mercury and iodide of potassium. Doubtless these remedies are indicated by the disease, but they are contra-indicated by the state of the patient. In an intensely febrile state, with gastro-intestinal troubles, they would not be tolerated; they would only aggravate the accidents. Above all, the patient must be placed in the best hygienic conditions possible. He should have as much sunlight and out-of-door life as he can endure, and the temperature will admit of, together with tonics, opiates, and a generous diet. Later, for the ulcerations and tertiary lesions, the specifics in small doses may be employed.

INFANT MORTALITY IN FRANCE.

In view of the excessive mortality among infants in France, *Le Bulletin Français*, as we learn from *L' Union Médicale*, calls attention to a plan which has in view a diminution of the extraordinary death-rate among the little ones. It is stated that among 100 individuals in France there are reckoned only 2.55 births, while in Russia there are 4.77. The other countries offer intermediate proportions: 100 marriages in Prussia give 460 infants; in France only 300. The annual excess of births over deaths calculated for a million inhabitants, is in Norway and Prussia about 14,000; in Prussia and Sweden, about 12,000; in Spain and Portugal, 8500; in France, only 2400. It appears from such statistics that the population of France would double in 170 years, while 42 years would suffice for Prussia, 52 for England, and 66 for Russia. Nor do these figures tell the whole story, for a frightful mortality has been discovered in France among the very young. According to M. Brochard, 100,000 nurslings annually die from starvation and misery. It is interesting to observe that the mortality varies with the department from 13 to 40 in 100, and still more interesting to study the enormous variations in the different categories of infants. While infants who are nursed by their mothers or by wet-nurses at their homes die during the first year in the proportion of 8 or 10 in 100, those who are placed away from home under the care of hospital administration and municipal direction give a mortality of from 30 to 36 in 100, and those who are intrusted to nurses in the provinces show the enormous mortality of from 50 to 70 in 100.

With the design of developing maternal nursing, and of caring for the nursling when he has to be removed from the family, there has been instituted the Protective Society of Infancy. There is, besides, the law proposed by M. Roussel for the protection of infants of a tender age, particularly of nurslings.

In a great city like Paris, where there are many families in which the mother cannot nurse her infant, nor bear the expense of a wet-nurse, there is the alternative of the nurse-bottle or of sending the child into the country. It is found that the more the latter plan is avoided, the better the chance of preserving the life of the little one. The question as to whether artificial nourishment can be recommended may be answered in two ways. In Paris, where milk is adulterated and never fresh, it needs to be boiled before being given to the infant, and it is very difficult to find in such a preparation elements of nutrition suitable for the delicate organs of the new-born. But when different conditions obtain, the results of artificial nourishment are much more favorable, as in the country, where the animals can be milked several times a day. It is proposed to establish some farm-nurseries in the many favorable localities which abound near Paris. A mansion isolated in the country in the midst of gardens or woods, with milch cows specially kept for the purpose, the alimentation of the infants regulated and supervised by competent physicians — such a plan, it is hoped, will help to preserve many lives. The dangers of overcrowding are to be obviated by having separate pavilions and a limited number to each. No doubt is entertained that good results would follow such favorable conditions.

MEDICAL NOTES.

— The annual meeting of the New Hampshire Medical Society took place on June 15th. There was a large attendance of members, and Maine, Massachusetts, Rhode Island, New York, and New Jersey were represented by delegates. At noon the president, Dr. Wight, delivered an address on the duties of the profession. Professor O. B. Crosby followed with a paper on removal of the arm, scapula, and clavicle, which he claimed New Hampshire surgeons (Dixi Crosby, R. D. Muggey and Amos Twitchell, in the order mentioned) had been the first to perform. Then came a report on gynæcology, and sanitary measures in the rural districts, by Dr. Wilkins, of Manchester, and Dr. Child, of Bath; also a report on cerebro-spinal meningitis, by Dr. Fowler, of Bristol; and another, on splints, by Dr. Hersey, of Manchester, in which he paid a handsome compliment to Dr. Cotting, president of the Massachusetts Society, as having contributed a splint which could be easily made in a few moments by a surgeon, and one that was effective in its application.

The society adjourned on the next day, after the election of the following officers : —

President, S. M. Whipple, New London ; Vice-President, A. B. Crosby, Hanover; Secretary, Granville P. Conn, Concord ; Treasurer, Thomas Wheat, Manchester; Council, J. W. Barney, S. B. Carbee, G. I. Cutler, F. W. Graves,.W. W. Wilkins, John R. Ham, W. B. Moody, Hiram Palmer, S. G. Dearborn, D. S. Clark ; Committee on Surgery, John W. Parsons, Portsmouth ; Practice of Medicine, Wm. Child, Bath; Necrology, Wm. G. Carter, Concord ; Gynæcology, T. J. W. Pray, Dover ; Anniversary Chairman, Dr. J. C. Eastman, Hampstead.

— The cholera discussion has been revived in Paris in a decidedly dramatic manner. At a recent meeting of the Academy of Medicine, one of the secretaries read a paper by M. Tholozan, the physician of the king of Persia. He held that epidemics are not necessarily of Indian origin, but may occur sponta-neously. According to a correspondent of the *British Medical Journal*, this gave rise to a warm discussion and Tholozan's views were opposed by MM. Chauf-fard, Briquet, Fauvel, Bouley, Bouillard, and others, who were of course arrayed against M. Tholozan, and condemned his doctrine as not being able to bear criticism, at least as far as concerns the origin of cholera ; they however gave him the credit of having demonstrated in a most lucid manner that extinct epi-demics are capable of being revived, and thus constituting the starting-point of a severe or extensive epidemic. Following in his own line of argument, he further stated, in his letter, that the cholera of 1862, which raged all over Europe, far from being the offspring of any previous epidemic, broke out spontaneously, and that this being the case, it follows as a necessary consequence that the prophylactic measures employed to keep off an invasion of Indian cholera are perfectly useless. M. Bouley loudly protested against these doctrines, and pointed out the danger of giving them any countenance.

— Dr. Bullard, of New Haven, Conn., as we learn from the *Medical Record*, has been in practice for about a half a century, during which he has been present at the births of about one thousand children. Such of these children as survive propose to have a grand picnic at the doctor's residence, and the whole affair is to be under a committee of arrangements from the adjoining towns.

COMPARATIVE MORTALITY–RATES.

MESSRS. EDITORS, — In connection with the article on this subject on page 577 of the last volume, it is interesting to compare the mortality report for certain cities in the United States for the year 1874. The only city which ap-pears in the formal list of May 13th which does not appear in Dr. Folsom's report, is Salem, Massachusetts. Taking the whole thirteen, and giving Salem the position it would hold, the two lists will read as follows : —

Dr. Draper's List for Thirteen Weeks.	Deaths to 1000 Living.	Dr. Folsom's List for One Year — 1874.	Deaths to 1000 Living.
1. New York...........	30.545	1. New York	27.61
2. Cambridge..........	30.538	2. Fall River	26.75
3. Brooklyn.............	26.363	3. Cambridge.........	24.56
4. Lynn.................	25.538	4. Brooklyn............	24.46
5. Fall River...........	25.461	5. Lowell..............	24.12
6. Boston...............	25.230	6. Boston	23.60
7. Philadelphia	23.615	7. Lawrence..........	23.45
8. Lawrence...........	21.923	8. Worcester..........	20.46
9. Salem...............	21.076	9. Lynn...............	20.45
10. Providence	20.175	10. Providence	19.86
11. Lowell...............	19.468	11. Philadelphia........	19.54
12. Worcester...........	18.846	12. Salem..............	19.
13. Springfield	11.	13. Springfield	18.33

If we put away the names of all cities out of Massachusetts, the following will be the record: —

Dr. Draper's List for Thirteen Weeks.	Deaths to 1000 Living.	Dr. Folsom's List for 1874.	Deaths to 1000 Living.
1. Cambridge	30.538	1. Fall River...........	26.75
2. Lynn	25.538	2. Cambridge	24.56
3. Fall River	25.461	3. Lowell	24.12
4. Boston	25.230	4. Boston	23.60
5. Lawrence.............	21.923	5. Lawrence............	23.45
6. Salem................	21.076	6. Worcester	20.46
7. Lowell...............	19.468	7. Lynn................	20.45
8. Worcester............	18.846	8. Salem	19.
9. Springfield...........	11.	9. Springfield	18.33

Of course a single year's record is of comparatively little consequence. As an evidence of this, we find that the average age at death in one town in the State was over ninety years, and in another it was less than a week. In the former there was but one death, in the other there were two, apparently twins. But the record is worth looking at as a means of finding out, first, if city and town registrars do their duty; and secondly, the cities and towns with large mortality lists may be reminded to find out why their death-rates are large in any year; and to see that men shall not be allowed to build on swamps and marshes, as has been done on both sides of Charles River. Boards of health should have increased rather than diminished power given to them, and our death-rates should be brought as low at least as the death-rates of London. Men should not be permitted to put up blocks of house, where there is nothing but moth and rust to corrupt, and where thieves would be cheated if they tried to break in and steal.   ****

WOUND OF THE KNEE–JOINT.

EDITORS OF THE BOSTON MEDICAL AND SURGICAL JOURNAL, — On page 82, Volume XLVII. of the JOURNAL, is an article on the method of fixing loose bodies in the knee-joint, and observations on operations for their removal, the closing paragraph of which is as follows: —

" Position of the limb after the operation may be of even more importance than the mode of operating. It should be such as will favor union by the first intention of the wound in the synovial capsule. As the incision is made in the direction of the limb, the extended position usually recommended must tend to separate the edges of the wound, whereas the partially flexed position will naturally close the wound and protect the synovial cavity from foreign invasion."

A recent case of accidental wound has given me an opportunity to confirm the statement there made, and shows the impunity with which air and blood may be admitted to the joint, provided they are subsequently expelled by positiou.

April 19th, J. P., sixteen years of age, healthy and of correct habits, while chopping in the woods cut a gash in his right knee. Without stopping to ascertain the degree of injury he ran and walked a quarter of a mile to the house of his employer, and thence rode three miles to my office.

The wound was then free from hæmorrhage. It was in the direction of the limb, half an inch inside of the patella, and three inches long. The leg being nearly extended, when he uncovered the wound there was wide gaping of it, and free exposure of the polished surface of the cartilaginous covering of the inner condyle. On flexing the leg, bubbles of air and bloody synovia gushed out, and the edges of the wound in the synovial capsule came in perfect apposition as soon as the leg was at a right angle with the thigh. Two sutures were taken in the external wound, and adhesive straps, lint, and bandage applied. A rectangular splint, having a screw for extension, was strapped on the posterior aspect of the leg and thigh. The wound was not touched for six days, when the upper suture was removed and the leg slightly extended. In three days more the other suture was taken out, the straps and lint remaining intact. There was no contingent discharge, and no inflammation other than that necessary to heal the wound. No medicine was given, but abstinence from animal food was observed, with rest.

May 29th. He has walked more or less since the 11th inst., and to-day came to my office. There is a little excess of fluid in the joint, for which rubber webbing is applied, there being no soreness nor any indication of inflammation. At the time of writing the patient has been at work for the past two weeks, quite recovered.   Ezra Bartlett.

Exeter, N. H., *June* 24, 1875.

LETTER FROM WATERVILLE, MAINE.

Messrs. Editors, — During the present spring there have occurred here some half a dozen cases of mumps followed by inflamed testicles, and three or four followed by inflamed mammæ. Dr. Flint, in the last edition of his text-book, would have it that these are very rare complications, nor can I in any of the text-books at my command find any adequate account of them.

All these cases recovered, and the text-books speak of the complication as a trifling one. But I would like to make the following inquiries through your columns : —

1st. Is an inflamed testis or mamma, accompanying or following mumps, always a trifling affection ?

2d. Does it rarely occur ?

3d. What facts are there bearing upon its causation ?

4th. The proper mode of treatment ?

Should you care to insert the above in some future number of the Journal, you will greatly oblige   Yours truly,   Fred. M. Wilson.

Waterville, Me., *May* 24, 1875.

WEEKLY BULLETIN OF PREVALENT DISEASES.

THE following is a bulletin of the diseases prevalent in Massachusetts during the week ending June 26, 1875, compiled under the authority of the State Board of Health from reports received from physicians representing all sections of the State : —

In Berkshire, whooping-cough has a local prevalence, but in general the health of the people is satisfactory.

In the Connecticut Valley, subacute rheumatism, mild bronchitis, and pneumonia are the prevalent affections. Small-pox continues in Huntington, but there are no new cases of that disease.

In Worcester County, rheumatism, diphtheria, and bronchitis prevail.

In the Northeastern counties, rheumatism, measles, and bronchitis are present, but there is a marked decline in these and in all the acute diseases, as compared with those reported last week. Sherborn reports " German measles."

In the Metropolitan section, scarlatina, pneumonia, bronchitis, and diarrhœa prevail, but in diminishing amount. Diphtheria continues in Brighton and in Boston, and it is also in Newton.

In the Southeastern counties, mild rheumatism, pneumonia, typhoid fever, and measles are prevalent. Hyannis reports " German measles."

Scarlatina is most prevalent in Boston ; diphtheria in Worcester County.

F. W. DRAPER, M. D., Registrar.

COMPARATIVE MORTALITY-RATES FOR THE WEEK ENDING JUNE 19, 1875.

	Estimated Population.	Total Mortality for the Week.	Annual Death-rate per 1000 during Week.
New York	1,040,000	489	24
Philadelphia	775,000	318	21
Brooklyn	450,000	178	21
Boston	350,000	138	21
Providence	100,000	15	8
Worcester	50,000	18	19
Lowell	50,000	15	16
Cambridge	44,000	14	16
Fall River	45,000	10	12
Lawrence	33,000	15	24
Springfield	33,000	11	17
Lynn	28,000	10	19
Salem	26,000	12	24

GRADUATES FROM THE HARVARD MEDICAL SCHOOL. — The following is the list of graduates from the Harvard Medical School at the annual commencement, June 30, 1875, with the titles of their theses : —

Henry Withington Bradford. Vesical Calculi, and the different methods of their disposal.

John Henry Burchmore. Uterine Hæmorrhage.

Robert Marsh Carleton, A. B. Pyæmia, etiology, symptoms, and treatment.

Jonas Clark, Jr. Vesical Calculi, diagnosis and treatment.

James Madison DeWolf. Drugs, proper and improper uses.

William Aloysius Dunn. The Health of Cities.

Walter Ela, A. B. The Patella, its structure and affections.

James Anthony Finn, A. M. Suppurative Pleuritis, or so-called Empyema.

James Aloysius Fleming. Injuries of the Head.

Justus Crosby French. Hypodermic Medication.

William Henry French, A. B. Vomiting.

Edwin Fisher Gardner. Digitalis.

Almon Debois Gay. Rachitis.

Samuel Howe, A. B. Milk Fever.

Alexander Rankin Hutchison. The three Functions of the Liver.

Claudius Marcellus Jones, A. M. Bloodletting.

Alexander Bloomfield Lawrence. Pneumatic Aspiration in Retention of Urine.

Bennett Sperry Lewis. Typhus Fever.

Robert Pearmain Loring. Puerperal Convulsions.

Phillips Adams Lovering, A. B. Neglected Felon.

Charles Lemuel Nichols, A. B. Posterior Spinal Sclerosis.

George Chesley McClean. Placenta Prævia.

Charles Edward M'Gowan. Vegetable Parasites of the Human Skin.

George Edward Mecuen. Ununited Fracture and False Joint.

Wilbur Fisk Sanborn. Diphtheria.

George Stedman, A. B. Hip Disease.

Henry Rust Stedman. Broncho-Pulmonary Hæmorrhage.

Jonathan Merle Teele, A. B. Diphtheria.

William Fiske Whitney, A. B. Empyema.

Fred Morse Wilson, A. B. Some things about Tubercle.

PAMPHLETS RECEIVED. — A Clinical Contribution to the Treatment of Tubal Pregnancy. By T. Gaillard Thomas, M. D. (Reprinted from the New York Medical Journal.) 1875. Pages 11.

Annual Catalogue of Albany Medical College. 1875. Pages 16.

Transactions of the Ninth Annual Meeting of the Medical Association of Missouri. 1875. Pages 81.

Clinical Studies with the Non-Nauseating Use of Ipecacuanha. By A. A. Woodhull, M. D. (Reprinted from Atlanta Medical and Surgical Journal.)

Dictionnaire Annuel des Progrès des Sciences et Institutions Médicales. Par Mons. P. Garner, Dixième Année, 1874. Paris: Ballière. 1875.

Popular Resorts and How to Reach them. By John B. Bachelder. Boston: John B. Bachelder, publisher. 1875. Pages 361.

On the Use of Warm and Hot Water in Surgery. By Frank H. Hamilton. New York: G. P. Putnam's Sons. 1875. Pages 6.

THE BOSTON
MEDICAL AND SURGICAL JOURNAL.

VOL. XCIII. — THURSDAY, JULY 8, 1875. — NO. 2.

———•———

EXTIRPATION OF A TUMOR OF THE BLADDER.

REPORTED BY DR. CARL GUSSENBAUER,

Assistant-Surgeon at the Clinic of Professor Billroth.

THE following case of myoma of the bladder deserves attention, as the tumor was correctly diagnosticated and extirpated with an unexpectedly good result ; also as the method of operating has never heretofore been employed, and, further, since microscopical examination proved the tumor to be of a variety rarely occurring in the bladder.

On June 3, 1874, D. J., a boy twelve years of age, was admitted to the clinic of Professor Billroth, suffering, according to his father's statement, from stone in the bladder. He had been troubled for ten months. The first symptoms were pain after passing water, localized in the glans penis and in the region of the bladder. After a while severe attacks of painful micturition set in, which in the course of ten months became more frequent, and often came on so suddenly that the boy could not prevent a sudden discharge of urine. At the time of admission the patient was obliged to pass his water every ten minutes, a small quantity each time, with frequent and severe pain, partly in the region of the bladder and partly in the glans. Urine was feebly acid, slightly cloudy, but contained nothing characteristic on microscopical examination except a moderate quantity of pus corpuscles and a few cells of bladder epithelium.

On examination a tumor was noticed in the region of the bladder, to the left of the median line. It was to be felt through the abdominal walls ; it was apparently about the size of the fist, was hard and somewhat sensitive on pressure, slightly movable, attached apparently to the bladder. Per rectum the tumor was also felt. On introduction of the sound it was found to slide over an uneven surface. On careful examination it was noticed that the beak immediately on entering the bladder was pressed forward ; and on attempting to move it from one side to another it always slid over an uneven tumor before reaching the back of the bladder. The combined examination with sound and finger, per rectum, proved clearly that a tumor connected with the back of the bladder hindered the movement of the sound. The consistence of the tumor was that of a fibro-sarcoma, and the size that of a small fist.

The rapid growth of the tumor demanded energetic treatment, as it promised, in the state of suffering in which the patient then was, soon to end his life.

The operation of extirpation was performed on June 15, 1874, in the following way : After the patient was narcotized the lateral incision for removal of stone was made. The finger introduced into the bladder showed immediately that a tumor nearly the size of the fist, with an uneven surface, projected from the posterior wall and extended towards the top of the cavity of the bladder. Owing to its size, it was found impossible to extract the tumor, with the finger, from the perinæum. A supra-pubic incision was then made, without injury to the peritoneum, and to give sufficient room both recti muscles were cut across at their insertion ; also a transverse incision into the bladder was made. Professor Billroth soon came to the conclusion, after examining with the finger, that the use of the écraseur was not practicable or desirable, as the tumor possibly might be already adherent to the peritoneum, in which case the latter would have been so injured as to delay healing. He therefore decided to tear the tumor with his finger near its base and to cut out the remainder from the wall of the bladder, after passing a ligature round to check bleeding. The extraction of the torn pieces of the tumor was not so easy, in spite of the large size of the incision, as would have been supposed. In dissecting out the pedicle it was necessary to turn the bladder partly inside out. It then appeared that the tumor took its origin from the muscular coat of the bladder, but had not attacked the outer coat or the peritoneum. The plan was, in case the peritoneum had been opened, to close the hole with sutures. Two arteries were tied, and the ligatures brought out through the upper incision in the bladder.

The wound in the bladder was not closed, as primary intention was not probable after the tearing which the size of the tumor had made necessary. To prevent the flowing of urine over the upper wound (so often the cause of pericystitis after the supra-pubic operation), a drainage-tube was drawn through the bladder and brought out at the incision in the perinæum, in the expectation that the urine would flow through the tube. This proved to be correct, but only when the tube was pushed so high up that it appeared over the symphysis. The walls of the bladder were pressed together by the weight of the intestine ; consequently the urine collected in the place where the resistance was the least, *i. e.,* above the bladder. If the opening in the drainage-tube was at this place, the urine ran off by the perinæum. If, however, the position of the tube was altered, the urine collected (as is the case always in the high operation for stone when the wound of the bladder is not closed) until it reached the level of the skin, and flowed over the abdomen, no urine at all passing through the drainage-tube. I mention this apparently trivial circumstance as I became convinced, on observing the course of the case, that the drainage tube especially contributed to the favorable result in the case. This was remarkably good, considering the apparently severe operation. The triple wound caused hardly any reaction — rarely the case even in successful cases of lithotomy. There was no inclination to a pericystitis or infiltration of the subcutaneous tissues, nor the slightest peritonitis. The first two days after the operation the patient's temperature was 37.8° C. (100° F.) and 38.8° C. (101.8° F.). On the third day the evening temperature rose to 39.6° C. (103.4° F.), but on the fourth day it sank to 38.2° C. (100.6° F.) On the sixth day day there was no fever. On the fifth day after the operation, as the wound was granulating well, and there was no danger of infiltration of urine, the drainage-tube was removed. The wound, on the twelfth day after the operation, was so small that the urine came partly by the urethra. The patient was discharged July 18th, perfectly well, wearing a pad to counteract any tendency to hernia.

The tumor was eight centimetres long, four broad. Its largest circumference was eighteen centimetres, its smallest thirteen. It sat directly on the muscular layer of the bladder. Its base was seven centimetres in circumference. There was no ulceration, the surface was smooth, but an epithelial coating was not to be determined without the microscope. From its consistence, its appearance, and that of the cut surface, it would have been regarded as a soft fibroma. But the remarkable friability made it improbable that it was an ordinary fibroma. The friability was as marked as one usually sees in spindle-celled sarcomas only. But a merely superficial microscopical examination was sufficient to determine that the tumor was a myoma.

Myomata of the bladder appear to be very rare. Rokitansky,[1] Virchow,[2] Förster,[3] know either from their own experience or in literature of no case. In a case mentioned, but not fully reported, by Robert Knox,[4] it is stated that the wall of a cyst of the bladder contained bundles of muscular fibres. Liston diagnosticated in a man who had been suffering with trouble in his bladder, a cyst or false membrane, after finding a movable body with the catheter. Liston opened the bladder above the symphysis, and a cyst came into sight, which slipped into Knox's hand. Nothing is stated as to a pedicle. The patient recovered and lived some time after. Knox examined the preparation, which Liston presented to the Museum of the College of Surgeons. The walls of the cyst were found to contain collections of muscular fibres.

With regard to the tumor in the present case, a more detailed exam-

---

[1] Pathological Anatomy, 3d edition, vol. iii., page 366.
[2] Tumors, vol. iii., 1st half page 124.
[3] Handbook of Pathological Anatomy, vol. i., page 345.
[4] Medical Times and Gazette, 1862, August 2, page 104.

ination siowed tiat it contained in all parts smooth muscular fibres, and in many parts it was almost entirely composed of muscular fasciculi. The muscular cells were isolated, wien fresi, witi tolerable ease, but were siown still better after maceration in the usual way. Tiey were of different sizes. The nuclei were not distinct in a fresi condition, but in general quite marked in the preparation treated witi reagents, and were of the ciaracteristic rod-like form. The contractile substance of the cells was apparently iomogeneous. A closer examination of the tumor siowed tiat it consisted not only of the smooti muscular cells and the fibrous interstitial tissue supporting the blood-vessels, but in certain places possessed a structure suci as is found in sarcomas and carcinomas. Tiere was found, beside the muscular cells, a great number of cells of different forms and sizes, wiici were collected between the muscular fasciculi witiout defined order, or scattered tirougi the tissues in smaller clusters of various siapes. Tiis gave an alveolar structure to the section, wiici was the more pronounced the closer the cells were clustered, or the more tiey had the appearance in form and size of epitielial cells.

The tumor is, tierefore, to be considered as a myoma from the great numbers of the muscular cells; but in consideration of the collection of connective tissue-cells, as a myo-sarcoma, in places as a myo-carcinoma; accordingly, as a well-marked mixed tumor.

It seems to me tiat the cyst mentioned by Mr. Robert Knox, witi the muscular fibres in the walls, was a myoma wiici had degenerated into a cyst, and had lost connection with the bladder tirougi atrophy of the pedicle. The examination of the contents of the cyst would iave decided the question; but tiis is not mentioned in the report.

ON THE TREATMENT OF DIARRHŒA IN YOUNG CHILDREN.[1]

BY J. P. OLIVER, M. D., OF BOSTON.

DIARRHŒA in young ciildren, particularly in tiose under two years of age, and in the summer season, usually begins very insidiously; and not unfrequently results from a sligit ciill, or a meal of improper food wiici excites a little irritation of the stomaci and bowels; a protracted and iigi temperature in a large city (tiougi someting more tian temperature is concerned in the production of the disease), particularly in overcrowded districts, enters largely into the etiology of the affection.

The irritation wien once set up is easily maintained by causes the

[1] Read before the Boston Society for Medical Observation.

same in kind (although less in degree) as those which originally provoked it, and a chronic affection is brought about which may become
less and less amenable to treatment the longer it continues.

A child from six months to two years old, living in a large city during the summer season and perhaps in an overcrowded neighborhood,
gets some indigestible substance into its stomach or perhaps takes cold,
and soon afterwards the bowels become slightly relaxed; perhaps
among the poorer classes an inferior quality of milk (skim-milk, slightly
sour or adulterated milk) has been given to a child recently weaned;
in such instances the purging is neither severe nor of long continuance; it speedily ceases and the child appears to have recovered. The
bowels, however, do not return to a healthy condition, and the complaint then is that the bowels are constipated; perhaps two or three
days later the child will have two or three large, sour, pasty-looking
dejections, more or less slimy from the mucus with which they are mingled, and passed with considerable straining efforts and much apparent
discomfort; the dejections may then become more frequent, and occasionally they will be streaked with blood; febrile movements may
occur, and there may be more or less abdominal tenderness.

The child grows pale; debility and progressive emaciation mark the
unfavorable progress of this affection; vomiting may or may not be a
prominent symptom. The vomited matter is sour-smelling, contains
a little bile, and the breath is often sour and offensive. The appetite
varies; in some children it is unimpaired, in others there is complete
anorexia. The disease may terminate in from twenty-four hours to three
or four days, or it may eventuate in a chronic affection which will persist for months, and finally the child will be carried off by some intercurrent affection induced by the debility brought about by the diarrhœa;
if it terminates at once in death the child grows paler, the eyes become sunken, the pulse quick, thready, and irregular; head-symptoms
are developed. The child becomes dull and somnolent, lies with the
eyelids partially closed and frequently rolling the head from side to side;
convulsions and coma may occur before death, or the child may get
better for a day or two, and then the diarrhœa will return; one day he
may have no dejection and the following he will have seven or eight;
such a state of things cannot go on for a great while without telling
upon the child. He becomes thinner and paler, loses flesh rapidly, is
unable to sit up, and his condition becomes one of great danger. As
night comes on the child grows wakeful and restless. The appetite
may be voracious, but the food does not nourish him, and appears hardly
changed in the dejections.

The presence of undigested food in the dejections of a young child,
especially if that child exhibits evident marks of deficient nutrition, is
an indication that the diet is not suitable and that it should be changed.

Wıetıer the digestive weakness be a simple functional derangement or be due to the existence of organic disease, in eitıer case our object is the same, namely, to adapt the cıild's diet to his powers of digestion, so that the food he swallows may afford ıim the nourisıment of wıicı he stands in need, and may leave as little undigested surplus as possible, to excite furtıer irritation of his alimentary canal. The accurate adaptation of diet is by no means an easy task in sucı cases; cıildren at the breast and under good ıygienic influences are not usually affected witı tıis disease; articles of food from wıicı a ıealtıy cıild derives his principal support will ıere often fail altogetıer; even milk, our great resource in all cases of digestive derangement in cıildren, must sometimes be dispensed witı; up to a certain time farinaceous food sıould be given witı the utmost caution. It is not very uncommon to find cases wıere milk, wıetıer diluted witı water or tıickened witı isinglass, or witı farinaceous food, cannot be digested so long as it is taken. The pale, putty-like matter of wıicı the dejections consist, and wıicı is passed in sucı large quantities, is evidently dependent upon the milk-diet, and resists all treatment so long as tıat is continued. In sucı cases, wıicı occur most commonly in cıildren between one and two years of age, the milk must be replaced, eitıer wıolly or partially, by otıer food. The isinglass and milk alluded to above was, I believe, first introduced by Dr. Meigs, of Pıiladelphia, and in certain cases is mucı esteemed by Dr. Morrill Wyman of Cambridge. To quote Dr. Wyman, he says: " I ıave used gelatine witı milk for cıildren and adults witı delicate stomacıs, and I tıink witı advantage; cases of diarrhœa in wıicı the milk is passed in curdled masses undigested, seem to me to be considerably relieved by the combination. My tıeory is (I do not tıink mucı of tıeories in medicine), tıat the gelatine prevents the coagulation of the milk, wıicı is tıen in a better condition to be acted upon by the digestive agents. The proportion of gelatine is about one teaspoonful, to be dissolved in water and mixed witı a ıalf pint of milk. Tıis proportion is less tıan is required for blanc mange."

Liebig's farinaceous food, or Liebig's soup, as it is called, is tolerably well borne in many cases, and it is occasionally advisable to try it. It is well known that flour is incapable, or only partially capable, of digestion in the stomacıs of infants, wıile it is equally well known tıat at a later period the power to transform starcı into sugar and tıus digest it is increased.

It is found tıat tıis deficiency in infancy is owing to the absence of a ferment in the stomacı, and in using Liebig's soup tıis effect is presumed to be supplied by the presence of diastase in the malt, wıicı, acting as a ferment, causes the desired cıange in the flour to be effected. Tıat tıis action will take place to a certain extent witı the properly prepared malt flour is certain; but it remains to be proved wıetıer it enables the wıole of the flour to be tıus transformed.

It is needless for me to give the directions for preparing this soup, as they have already been published in the JOURNAL several times.

The food ("soup" seems a misnomer) is not a substitute for milk, since milk itself is an essential element in its preparation, but it is really an improved mode of giving milk with flour or other farinaceous material. Its real merit consists in adding a material to the flour which will aid the stomach of the child and infant to digest it, and that which remains for investigation is the proof, to be derived from the evacuations, whether such aid has been effectual. This may be ascertained roughly in any case by noticing the size of the stools. A trial should be made with the milk and flour alone, and then with the food, according to Liebig, and if the dejections are as large in the latter as in the former, it may be safely inferred that the food has no special advantage over the use of boiled milk and flour. As the stomach of a child of three years, and probably of one between one and two years, can digest flour and transform it into sugar, this preparation offers scarcely any appreciable advantage to them over the long-established one of well-boiled milk, flour, and sugar. When cream (or good first-class milk) can be obtained for infants, it is beyond all comparison the best food for them, and no addition of any kind should be made to it ; and hence, for the children of the rich and well-to-do classes, Liebig's food is scarcely necessary. As regards cream, Dr. Van Wyck, of San Francisco, says, "For twenty years I have discountenanced the use of diluted cow's milk, substituting properly diluted and sweetened fresh cream, solely on the ground that a nearer approximation to woman's milk can be effected than in any other way known to me ; and hence there is less liability to produce injurious effects. Apart from this I think there are often good reasons for using only the cream which rises after the milk has stood some twenty-four hours. Very much of the milk sold in our cities and towns is adulterated in various ways, and in many instances when such is not the case the cows are improperly fed and cared for.

" By using the cream only we avoid, in the first instance, the adulterating materials, and, in the second, we are enabled to give a less quantity of a diseased or abnormal secretion.

" Having obtained a quart or more of the purest attainable milk, set aside for twenty-four hours, and then skim off, but not too closely, the cream. As the cream of cows differs in richness from a number of causes, it is impossible to give in figures the amount of water necessary for the proper dilution. I therefore direct the cream to be diluted with boiling water to an extent that will make it as near the richness of the mother's milk at that period as possible, adding enough sugar of milk to bring it up to the natural standard of sweetness. I prefer the milk sugar to the cane or beet sugar, for the reason that, should acidification occur, we have in the former lactic, whilst in the others acetic acid as a result.

To be as explicit as possible, I should say that with the cream afforded from the milk ordinarily served to purchasers, the following formula will be found very nearly correct : —

	Cream. Parts.	Boiling Water. Parts.	Milk Sugar. Parts.
Child in good health, one week old,	1	11	25
" " " two weeks old,	1	10	25
" " " three to four weeks old,	1	8	25
" " " one to two months old,	1	7	25
" " " three to four " "	1	6	25
" " " four to six " "	1	5	25
" " " eight to ten " "	1	3 to 4	25

"Should this prove too strong, it will be necessary to make a further dilution with, if needed, an alkali, to prevent acidification."

A certain amount of lime-water is generally ordered to obviate this result; but experience has proved that the bicarbonate of potassa is preferable, for the reason that as an antacid it is equally efficacious, while it prevents the formation of so solid a curd, and thereby renders it more soluble.

There is nothing better in the way of farinaceous food than the barley prepared by the Messrs. Robinson, of England. I usually make it according to directions accompanying the article, varying the amount of barley and milk according to the age of the child, character of the stools, etc.

Whatever be the diet adopted, our object is to keep up the nutrition of the body with the smallest possible amount of irritation to the alimentary canal; and the food, whatever it may be, which will produce this result, is the food best suited to the case; drugs alone will be powerless. The successful adjustment of the diet, an adjustment in which the quality and quantity of food to be allowed for each meal are accurately adapted to the powers and requirements of the patient, is a matter which can be properly learned only by experience.

In all cases, if the patient be a nursing child he should be limited strictly to the breast; or if he have been only lately weaned, the breast should be returned to. If from any reason a return to the breast is impossible, we should try one of the articles above mentioned.

If the child be no more than six months old, nothing should be allowed but milk or some preparation of milk. If the child be very ill, beware of feeding too often, particularly if farinaceous foods enter largely into the diet; if they excite flatulence, or any sour smell be noticed from the breath or evacuations, the quantity of such food should be diminished and perhaps discontinued altogether. Beyond the age of six months, beef tea, raw beef, yolk of an unboiled egg, may be added to the diet. The egg is best digested when beaten up with a few drops of brandy.

If, as before stated, on giving the cream, acidification takes place, give an alkali (potass. bicarb.), and it siould be added to the fluid in the proportion of little less tian a grain to eaci fluid ounce, and if curd is found in the excreta the amount siould be doubled. It is difficult to overestimate the value of alkaline remedies in the treatment of digestive derangements in ciildren.

In all ciildren, in infants especially, tiere is a constant tendency to acid fermentation of tieir food. Tiis arises partly from the nature of tieir diet, into wiici milk and farinaceous matters enter so largely; partly from the peculiar activity of tieir mucous glands, wiici pour out an alkaline secretion in suci quantities. An excess of farinaceous food will tierefore soon begin to ferment, and an acid to be formed wiici stimulates the mucous membrane to furtier secretion; ience, alkalies are useful firstly in neutralizing the acid products of tiis fermentation, and secondly, in ciecking the too abundant secretion from the mucous glands. Potasi or soda may be used; of the two the former is periaps to be preferred, as, being a constituent of milk, the natural diet of ciildren, it may be considered less as a medicine tian as a food.

The alkali siould be combined witi an aromatic; it is important tiat the latter be not omitted, for tiis class of remedies is of great value in all tiose cases of abdominal derangement wiere flatulence, pain, and spasm, resulting from vitiated secretions and undigested food, are present to increase the discomfort of the patient; suci pienomena are usually rapidly relieved by the use of tiese agents; and the employment of anise-seed, cinnamon, caraway-seed, or even tincture of capsicum, in minute doses, will be found of material advantage in combination witi the otier remedies wiici I will siortly enumerate. If called to a ciild say eigiteen montis old, witi bowel trouble, I usually order cream, or barley, with milk, and give the mother the following prescription, telling her to add a teaspoonful or two of the mixture to eaci teacup of the fluid: —

Ŗ Potassæ bicarbonatis . . . . ℈j.
Aquæ cinnamomi . . . . ℥ii. M.

If the ciild be so ill tiat he takes but a small quantity at a time it may be well to give beef-tea (made in a bottle, or the juice of a steak sligitly broiled and squeezed in a lemon-squeezer) in conjunction witi the milk; a teaspoonful may be given occasionally, and its digestion will be aided by adding a pinci of sacciarated pepsine to eaci teaspoonful of the juice or tea. In some cases the ciild siould be fed frequently, little at a time, in order to sustain life, but not so frequently, or in suci quantity as to give the digestive organs muci to do. The object is to give the ciild just food enougi to sustain life till the digestive organs iave recovered tieir tone. It is better tiat the ciild siould be iungry tian iave his stomaci overloaded. Stimulants may be required, and, in fact, tiey are always required wien the fontanelle becomes muci depressed.

If the stools are loose and are passed frequently, two or three grains of subnitrate of bismuth may be given, and if much straining be noticed a drop of tinct. opii deod., or a little Dover's powder will be a useful addition to check the abnormal briskness of peristaltic action.

Enemata of the fluid extract of krameria containing tr. opii deod., are occasionally useful. If an aperient is required, there is nothing better than castor oil, or the tincture rhei aq. of the German Pharmacopœia. The latter is an alkaline tincture and is an exceedingly useful preparation. It is made as follows : —

℞. Rhubarb . . . . 100 parts,
Borax . . . . 10 "
Potass. carb. . . . . 10 "
Pour upon this boiling water . . . . 850 "
Set aside for fifteen minutes, then add alcohol . . . . 100 "
Then add cinnamon water . . . . 140 "

So long as the tongue remains furred, or the dejections acid (litmus paper), the alkali should be persisted with, and the aperient may be repeated every third morning.

Alteratives (calomel, etc.) are in these cases of little value. It is useless to stimulate the functions of the liver. Under the use of antacids, aromatics, etc., food soon begins to be digested and the appearance of the stools becomes more healthy.

As soon as convalescence is fairly established, iron and cod-liver oil may be given. To ascertain whether the child is actually gaining, it will be well to have him weighed as often as once a week.

This treatment, when reviewed, may to some seem like hyper-medication ; but all that we advised are in reality food with the exception of the bismuth powder and the aromatic.

The alkali, pepsine, and stimulant, are no more medicine than milk, barley, and beef-tea.

In all these cases, and indeed in all cases where a special diet is recommended for children, a dietary should be written out by the medical attendant ; not only the kind of food but the quantity to be given for each meal, and even the hour at which the meal is to be taken, should be duly set down, so that no excuse may be available for neglect or misapprehension. It is upon the judicious arrangement of food that the recovery of the child depends, and when the diet is properly selected the exact medicine to be ordered becomes a matter of comparatively secondary importance.

After an attack of diarrhœa acid preparations are advised, such as the pernitrate of iron with dilute nitric acid, in conjunction with cod-liver oil. The sulphate of iron, gr. ss. to gr. ii., with sugar, and given in ginger wine (the latter may be obtained of McDewell and Adams, Boylston Street), is a very useful preparation. If there is a tendency to constipation following the diarrhœa, iron in the form of the tartrate of potash and iron is preferable.

A point wiici must not be overlooked in tiese cases is attention to the action of the skin.   In all abdominal derangements in children the cutaneous secretion is apt to be suppressed early, and the skin soon becomes dry, rougi, and iarsi ; wien tiis is found to be the case the ciild siould be batied every evening witi hot water and be tien freely anointed witi warm olive oil.   By tiis means the suppleness of the skin is soon restored.   Warm clotiing siould be worn and a flannel swatie around the abdomen to serve as a protection to the belly.

SPINAL MENINGEAL HÆMORRHAGE.[1]

BY S. G. WEBBER, M. D., BOSTON.

SPINAL meningeal iæmorriage is rare, and the cases in wiici the diagnosis has been confirmed by an autopsy are comparatively few. Tiere are in many cases suci a variety and so muci confusion in the symptoms tiat a diagnosis seems very difficult.   The reason for tiis may be found in part in the combination of true spinal symptoms witi symptoms referable to meningeal disturbance, and wien the hæmorrhage is in the lower portion of the cord tiese symptoms may all be present in the legs.

Bear in mind, tien, tiat tiere are two classes of symptoms wiici must be separated: tiose due to pressure upon the cord and cianges in its structure ; tiose due to irritation of the membranes and nerve roots by the foreign body, the clot.

The symptoms arising from implication of the cord are primarily tiose due to pressure, tien tiose due to secondary cianges.   Tiere is more or less complete paraplegia, and exaltation of reflex action.   Pain in the back at the seat of the pressure is not constant; tiere may be deviations from normal sensation.   The pressure may cause secondary cianges in the cord, and tien the paralysis becomes more or less permanent, and sensation may not be restored ; so also the reflex action may continue exaggerated, and tiere may be contractions or the limb tremble.   If myelitis follows the pressure the exalted reflex action may disappear, the contractions relax, the paralysis remain, and atropiy set in.

The symptoms due to the irritation of the blood-clot and pressure upon the nerve-roots are so united tiat it is scarcely worti wiile to try to separate tiem.   Tiese are pains radiating in the course of the nerves and otiers referred to the peripiery, tingling and pricking sensations, more or less anæstiesia, witi possibly tenderness to touci of the parts to wiici the nerves are distributed; spasmodic contractions,

------

[1] Read before the Suffolk District Medical Society.

generally clonic, sometimes tonic; subsequently there may be atrophy and diminished electric excitability. Disturbed vaso-motor action may be found either below or at the level of the hæmorrhage.

In every case of traumatic origin the possibility of additional injury to the cord must be borne in mind, and this may modify the course of the case.

At the commencement there would be no febrile symptoms; subsequent meningitis is not common.

The two varieties of symptoms can be most readily separated when the hæmorrhage is in the lower cervical region. When above this, death would probably follow quickly unless the amount was very small.

The following case illustrates the clinical features of meningeal hæmorrhage in the lower cervical region.

The patient was a young man, referred to me by Dr. Vaughan, of Cambridge. He was a very strong and athletic young man up to four and a half years previous to the time at which I saw him. He went a-fishing and stood in the water above his knees for two or three hours, and was very tired; the next day he passed an examination at school between four and five P. M. He was much excited; the examination was severe; he was warm and flushed in the face. Between five and six P. M., he went in swimming. He dove from a bank one and a half feet high, and came up with a headache; this went off, and he dove two or three times without any ill effects. He then dove again, and when under water was immediately paralyzed in both arms and both legs. He thinks he did not hit his head on the bottom, though that was his first impression. May have wrenched his neck. When the paralysis occurred a shudder passed over him such as is seen to pass over cattle when killed. He did not lose consciousness at any time. He was soon rescued by his companions and laid on the bank. Up to that time he had no pain. A friend took hold of his hand, on which was a red spot which was very tender and painful. He was carried to his room in a carriage; while riding he could not hold his head up; there was no nausea, and no pain in his back during the whole of his sickness. In a short time he could draw up his left leg a little. After about six hours he had severe pain, amounting to agony, in his arms and hands, with a throbbing sensation. After being turned on his face he fell asleep.

The next day he was raised up, and thereupon had nausea. In his hands was a sensation as if asleep, and the weight of a fly on the hands caused pain. He could draw the left leg up quite well, and could move the left arm a little; the right arm and leg could not be moved. There was no pain or tingling in the legs.

He gradually improved, until after two weeks he could stand up, and could walk, but was drawn over, walked unsteadily, staggered, and the right leg moved spasmodically. The legs twitched while he was in bed, especially the rigit; tiere was also spasmodic action in the arms. The bowels were confined, and the urine retained for a few days after the injury.

During the wiole course of his sickness his mind was clear, and he read muci, even immediately after, the injury. The rigit eyelid drooped, and the reading caused trouble in his iead, otierwise tiere were no cerebral symptoms.

He improved slowly, the left side gaining the more rapidly, and wien seen about four and a ialf years after, the motion of the left arm and iand was nearly or quite normal, tiat of the rigit iand was muci restricted in the fingers, but the arm moved freely. The left leg and foot moved muci more freely tian the rigit. The legs trembled and twitcied, the iands and arms twitcied, but did not tremble. The reflex action of the legs was exaggerated, but not excessively so. The sensation was better in the rigit iand and arm and rigit foot for ieat and the touci, but two points were felt at a distance of tiree eigitis or four eigitis incies in boti palms, and on the feet tiere was no difference in the two sides, but the distance was greater than usual. At times the arms and legs iave the pricking sensation as if asleep. Touciing the left foot caused tiis sensation.

The temperature in the axilla was 98° on the rigit, 98.5° on the left; temperature of room, 71°. The rigit iand and foot were sometimes darker colored tian the left.

The circumference of forearm, nine and tiree fourtis incies on rigit, ten and one eigiti incies on left; of arm, four incies above external condyle, nine and seven eigitis incies on rigit, ten and tiree eigitis incies on left; of ciest, sixteen and a ialf incies on rigit, eigiteen incies on left.

The reaction to boti galvanic and faradic current was diminisied in the muscles wiici move the fingers on the rigit as compared witi tiose on the left.

Tiere was no spontaneous pain, and no motion nor twisting of the body caused pain, even in gymnastic exercises. Tiere was some difficulty in micturition, it being a considerable time before the water commenced to flow. Erection was less frequent and less strong tian formerly.

Tiis is a case wierein the diagnosis is comparatively easy; tier no need to dwell longer upon a differentiation of the symptoms.

It may be interesting to compare witi tiis a case in wiici the hæmorrhage occurred below the origin of the braciial plexus. The symptoms are less well marked. A young man was tirown from his wagon; he could not remember how he struck the ground. He crawled to a neigiboring iouse and was carried iome. His legs were partially paralyzed; he could stand, but could not walk witiout ielp. The next day he could not stand, but could move his legs in bed ; he shook and shivered, even after warmth was applied had a rigor. There was slight spasmodic action of the legs during the first two weeks ; also dyspnœa, and his chest seemed bound up.

Immediately after the accident he had severe pain in his back, described as though some one had buried a piece of steel in it ; there was also a spot in the lumbar region, tender on pressure. He had a disagreeable sensation which he could not describe, passing from hips to knees. From the time he began to stand he had a sensation of pricking as if the parts were asleep, most marked in his right leg.

He improved slowly, beginning to walk after a week or so ; it was six weeks before he could sit in a chair and raise one leg, and yet longer before he could raise both legs at once. There was much emaciation, and the calves of his legs were flabby ; they did not feel natural like his hands. Legs and feet were cold ; the sense of constriction in his chest continued. There was no constipation, no disturbance of micturition. Sexual desire was gone for four or five months, and during this time there was no emission ; his appetite remained less than natural. There were no special cerebral symptoms,

I saw him nearly a year after the accident at the request of Dr. W. S. Brown. When seen, he could walk without help, but with his feet wide apart. On rising from the chair he first took hold of the arms of the chair, then of his hips, and rose with effort. With his eyes shut he staggered in walking and could not stand with his feet near together. He could distinguish two points only when they were more than two inches apart. The reaction of the muscles of the leg and thigh to the faradic current was good. The glutæi were not tested. Pulse 61, respiration 19. There was a slight incoördination of the left hand. He said he could not carry a pail of water in his left hand as its weight seemed to pull him round.

There was probably in this case a complication of lesions, meningeal hæmorrhage, and also concussion or other injury of the cord. The chill, the gradual increase in the severity of the symptoms, the severe pain in the back immediately after the accident, the partial loss of motor power and of sensation, and the early and gradual improvement, the spasmodic action, the pain radiating to the knees, the pricking of the feet as if asleep, are such symptoms as would be found in hæmorrhage ; the dyspnœa and sense of constriction, the persistence of the weakness of the muscles, and possibly some of the other symptoms, may have been due to direct injury of the cord itself.

RECENT PROGRESS IN MEDICAL CHEMISTRY.[1]

BY E. S. WOOD, M. D.

Urinary Coloring Matters Continued. — Hoppe-Seyler[2] has succeeded in transforming artificially the red blood pigment hæmoglobin into the urinary pigment urobilin by means of reducing agents. By causing hæmoglobin to be acted upon by means of tin and hydrochloric acid, urobilin is produced.

This seems to show that the urobilin found in normal fæces and urine is one of the final decomposition products of the blood pigment, and since it can also be formed from the bile pigments bilirubin and biliverdin in the intestine and artificially, it is probable that these are intermediate steps in the process of reduction.

F. Baumstark has isolated two new and well-characterized pigments from the urine of a patient with leprosy. The urine did not differ much from normal urine except in regard to the color. The color, when first received, was a deep, dark red, like that of Bordeaux wine; later it changed to a brownish red, and toward death to a dark brown, nearly black. Neither biliary pigments nor acids were present. There was no albumen, blood globules could not be detected in the sediment, and hæmin crystals could not be obtained, thus proving the absence of blood in the urine.

To isolate the pigments the urine was subjected to dialysis, a yellowish fluid like normal urine in appearance passing through the parchment, and a brownish, slimy mass remaining on the dialyser. This mass was dissolved in sodic hydrate, and one of the pigments precipitated from this solution by the addition of an acid in the form of a brown, flocculent precipitate, a beautiful garnet-red fluid remaining.

During the twelve days on which this urine could be obtained, about two grammes of these pigments were isolated. They are named by the author urorubrohæmatin and urofuscohæmatin, the former being the one remaining in solution in the acid fluid after the latter had been precipitated. At first there was a large amount of the former and but little of the latter, while toward death the amount of the latter was largely increased.

Urorubrohæmatin. — Analysis gave as the formula $C_{68}(H_{62}O_4)N_8$ $Fe_2O_{10} + 16H_2O$, or hæmatin in which eight of the atoms of hydrogen have been replaced by four of oxygen. This substance is a bluish black powder, insoluble in alcohol, ether, water, chloroform, and a solution of common salt. It is soluble in the alkalies, giving a brownish red solution when concentrated, and a garnet red when dilute. From the alkaline solution it is not precipitated by acids, but the color changes

[1] Concluded from page 15.

[2] Berichte der deutschen chemischen Gesellschaft, 1874, No. 13.

[3] Berichte der deutschen chemischen Gesellschaft, 1874, No. 13.

to a bluish red. From the acid solution it is precipitated in brownish flocks by dialysis. It is soluble in a solution of common salt to which hydrochloric acid has been added. Acid solutions, when examined with the spectroscope, show a narrow absorption band before the line D, and a broad one behind D. Its spectrum is, therefore, like that of oxy-hæmoglobin, except that it is farther to the left. Alkaline solutions show a band to the right of D, one near E, a broad one to the right of F, and one to the right of G.

Urofuscohæmatin. — Analysis gave as the formula for this pigment $C_{68}H_{70}N_8(H_4)O_{10} + 16H_2O$, or hæmatin in which the two atoms of iron have been replaced by four of hydrogen. This pigment was a black, pitch-like substance, which was insoluble in water, alcohol, ether, chloroform, acids, and a pure solution of common salt, or one to which hydrochloric acid had been added. It is soluble in the alkalies, giving a brown solution, from which acids precipitate it in brown flocks. It is less characteristic optically than the urorubrohæmatin, the alkaline solutions giving a faint band between the lines D and E, and one before F, very difficult to detect; at the same time the blue and violet are strongly absorbed, so that it is difficult, even on careful dilution, to see a clear spectrum. Both of these pigments are very closely allied to hæmatin.

TOXICOLOGY.

Aniline Colors. — The various coloring matters prepared from coat tar have of late been used extensively in coloring articles of food and drink, such as confectionery, jellies, syrups, and wines. Many of them contain, either in chemical combination or as impurities, some of the poisonous metals. Analyses of these made by J. Bruu[1] showed that they may be contaminated with salts of mercury, alum, lead, and arsenic. They have not only caused injury when applied to the skin in the form of a dye upon clothing, but also have proved injurious, and even fatal, when ingested by children in the form of confectionery colored with fuchsine. The injury is caused almost always by the arsenic which the pigments contain. In one fatal case, the amount of arsenic ingested could not have been more than 0.16 milligrammes (about 0.04 grains). Many of these pigments, if thoroughly purified, would be innocuous, but such purification would render the price of the colors so high that they could not be used for coloring cheap articles.

M. Chevallier[2] has examined three of these coloring matters sold under the names of safranine, phospine, and orséyne. The first contained no arsenic, the second a considerable, and the third a large amount of arsenic.

When syrups, such as raspberry, strawberry, etc., are colored artificially by means of these aniline colors, chlorine water both decolorizes

[1] Journal de Chim. Méd., March, 1875.
[2] Annales d'Hygiène, April, 1874.

tiem and causes a flocculent precipitate, wiile it only decolorizes the unadulterated syrups. Potassic hydrate decolorizes syrups prepared witi fucisine, but gives a dirty green witi the natural syrups. '

In wines colored witi fucisine potassic hydrate produces no ciange, wiile in the unadulterated wines it cianges the color to a brown.

Pure coralline was formerly supposed to be the cause of the skin eruptions produced by wearing clotiing colored witi it,[1] but more recently tiis has been proved to be due to the arsenic wiici the coralline contained as an impurity, and tiat pure coralline is perfectly iarmless. Arsenic is sometimes derived from the mordant (arseniate of aluminium) used in fixing the coralline upon the cloti.

M. Mayet[2] reports a case of wall-paper poisoning, in wiici the paper causing the trouble was colored witi coralline. Analysis siowed tiat it contained a considerable quantity of arsenic. In order to detect the arsenic in tiese red wall papers, the metiod by means of ammonia and nitrate of silver is not sufficient, since the silver precipitate is colored red by the aniline, and the color of the arsenite. or arseniate of silver is obscured. The organic matter must be destroyed by sulphuric acid and ieat, the residue extracted witi dilute acid wiici is introduced into a Marsi's apparatus, and Marsi's test applied. Tiis metiod is also best adapted for detecting the arsenic in artificially colored wines, syrups, confectionery, and ices.

Strychnia. — F. L. Sonnenschein[3] has succeeded in establisiing a close reiationsiip between the two alkaloids of the nux vomica by the artificial conversion of brucia into strycinia. If brucia be treated witi four or five times its weigit of dilute nitric acid, and the mixture gently warmed, effervescence takes place, and a reddisi-colored fluid remains. If the red fluid after concentration be siaken witi etier, and the etier after being decanted is evaporated, tiere remains a red pigment, a yellow resin, and a crystalline base, wiici can be purified by dissolving in an acid and recrystallizing. Tiis base is strycinia.

F. A. Falck[4] has investigated the susceptibility of different animals to the action of strycinia. His results are best given in the following tabular form. By tiis it will be seen tiat, if the amounts required to produce deati are calculated for equal weigits of the animal operated on, the warm-blooded animals are muci more susceptible to the action of strycinia tian the cold-blooded ones. In experimenting witi different animals of the same species, it was found tiat the fatal dose was proportional to the weigit of the animal. The bladder of the dog did not seem to absorb strycinia at all, no effect being produced wien the alkaloid remained in the bladder several iours. In all of the experiments the strycinia was used in the form of nitrate of strycinia.

---

[1] Tardieu et Roussin. Annales d'Hygiène, 1869, xxxi., page 257.
[2] Annales d'Hygiène, July, 1874.
[3] Berichte der deutschen chemischen Gesellschaft, 1875, No. 4.
[4] Vierteljahrsschrift für gerichtliche Medicin, 1874, April and July.

The amounts in the following table are reckoned in milligrammes per one kilogramme weight of the animal operated on : —

Animal.	Method of Introduction.	Highest Non-Fatal Dose.	Lowest Fatal Dose.
White fish.............	Subcutaneous injection..	6.25	12.5
Frog...................	" " ..	2.	2.1
Snake	" " ..	–	23.1
Dove..................	Crop...................	10.	15.
Fowl..................	"	50.	50.
"	Subcutaneous injection..	1.	2.
Hedgehog	" " ..	–	2.97
Rabbit	" " ..	.5	.6
Cat...................	" " ..	–	.75
Dog	" " ..	–	.75
"	Stomach...............	2.	3.9
"	Rectum	–	2.1
"	Bladder...............	5.5	–

———◆———

COOK ON FUNGI.[1]

THERE has long been wanted a book which should instruct the physician in a general and yet thorough way concerning the nature and growth of the forms of life, about which he has been asked in these later days to believe so much without the exercise of his judgment.. That his credulity has been so generally imposed upon has been largely the result of the self-deception of his self-called instructors. In no branch of science connected with medicine has the ear of the profession been so easily gained and long held by loose observers and shallow writers as in mycology, for they claimed to have found the solution of the mysteries of many diseases for which it had been so long intently open. Unfortunately their conclusions were as false as their science was weak, but their delusions and ignorance have been often exposed, and might be universally understood, were those engaged in spreading information always capable of distinguishing between true and sham work.

This volume, which forms the fifteenth of the International Scientific Series, a collection of monographs prepared by most eminent men of science, is written by the well-known and enthusiastic author of the Handbook of British Fungi, and is a thoroughly good book. As will be seen by the table of contents, it is very general in its scope, and, although more particular in details in some parts than the ordinary reader may require, it is in no way less adapted on this account to the elementary instruction of the physician. It describes in very simple language the nature of fungi, and their modes of development and growth. The chapters on Classification and Polymorphism are very important, and should be read by all who have been misled by such writers as Salisbury and Hallier. The universal dissemination of spores and their relations to the question of spontaneous generation is briefly discussed. In the chapter on the

[1] *Fungi: Their Nature and Uses.* By M. C. COOKE, M. A., LL. D. Edited by the REV. M. J. BERKELEY, M. A., F. L. S. New York: D. Appleton & Co. 1875. Pp. 312.

Uses of Fungi, the author describes in the most appetizing terms the edible varieties, and mentions the many species which occur in the United States. The late Dr. Curtis, of North Carolina, enumerated all of these in his own State, and wrote to Rev. M. J. Berkeley that "hill and plain, mountain and valley, woods, fields and pastures, swarm with a profusion of good, nutritious fungi, which are allowed to decay where they spring up, because people do not know how, or are afraid to use them. By those of us who know their use, their value was appreciated as never before during the late war, when other food, especially meats, was scarce and dear. Then such persons as I have heard express a preference for mushrooms over meat had generally no need to lack grateful food, as it was easily had for the gathering, and within easy distance of their homes, if living in the country."

The influences and effects of fungi are summed up in the following form:

" Fungi exert a deleterious influence —

On *Man*,

  When eaten inadvertently.

  By the destruction of his legitimate food.

  In producing or aggravating skin diseases.

On *Animals*,

  By deteriorating or diminishing their food supplies.

  By establishing themselves as parasites on some species.

On *Plants*,

  By hastening the decay of timber.

  By establishing themselves as parasites.

  By impregnating the soil.

" But it is not proved that they produce epidemic diseases in man or animals, or that the dissemination of their multitudinous spores in the atmosphere has any appreciable influence on the health of the human race. Hence, their association with cholera, diarrhœa, measles, scarlatina, and the manifold ills that flesh is heir to, as producing or aggravating causes, must, in the present state of our knowledge and experience, be deemed apocryphal."

In describing their toxicological relations to man, the author is able to give no easy and general rule by which the edible may be distinguished from the poisonous fungi. Such knowledge is gained only by the study of specific differences, but is not difficult of acquisition. It would appear, however, that some of the poisonous species may be eaten with impunity, if treated with a large amount of salt and vinegar before boiling. A warning is also given that even the cultivated mushroom may cause trouble, if kept long enough to undergo the chemical changes to which fungi are so rapidly prone.

Of the forms which are the cause of the so-called parasitic affections of the human integument and its appendages, the author attempts no special description, referring his readers to the well-known works of dermatologists for information.

Interesting chapters on the cultivation and geographical distribution of fungi close the volume, from which it appears that the mycological flora of North America greatly resembles that of Europe; but that with few exceptions "a great portion of our vast country is mycologically unknown." The book is well printed and is illustrated by 109 wood-cuts.   J. C. W.

LOOMIS ON THE RESPIRATORY ORGANS, HEART, AND KIDNEYS.[1]

THE book is published from phonographic reports of lectures delivered in the medical department of the University of New York. In the present form they will be much esteemed by the students of the university, and of interest to the profession, though they are not sufficiently exhaustive to take the place of monographs, on which the physician of the present day is becoming more and more dependent.

Professor Loomis is an extremist in modern pathological theories, and evidently has very decided opinions in regard to all subjects touched upon. His positive way of stating things, while exposing him to scientific criticism, must make him a very attractive teacher, and the student learns so much more from such a teacher than from a hesitating, skeptical one, that he can afford to unlearn, or learn anew a few things after graduation, for the sake of the general principles which have been firmly impressed upon his mind.

WALTON ON DISEASES OF THE EYE.[2]

THE former edition of this work comprised only the surgical diseases of the eye ; the present edition has been largely re-written, contains many additions, and aims to be a complete treatise on the subject of eye diseases. As would naturally be expected under such circumstances, the surgical affections, especially those which come more correctly under the head of general surgery, occupy proportionally a larger space than is usually given to them in similar treatises. But the increased space thus devoted is taken up mostly by the recital of cases, not always very instructive, many of which are borrowed from others and have been already published elsewhere.

The book opens with an anatomical introduction by Mr. Morton, which had much better been omitted. It is almost inconceivable how so many errors could have been compressed into twelve pages of rather small print; and the four full pages of anatomical illustrations are as bad as, and do not always even agree with, the text. The reader is told that "this anatomical description of the eyeball embodies new facts." Some of these " new facts " bear on the mechanism of accommodation. The change of shape in the lens is said to be produced by direct pressure from the ciliary processes and iris, an old theory which has been sufficiently disproved. It should be said here, however, that in the chapter on accommodation and its anomalies, this theory is not adopted.

[1] *Lectures on Diseases of the Respiratory Organs, Heart, and Kidneys.* By ALFRED L. LOOMIS, M. D., Professor of Pathological and Practical Medicine in the University of the City of New York, etc., etc. New York: Wm. Wood & Co. 550 pp. octavo

[2] *A Practical Treatise on the Diseases of the Eye.* By HAYNES WALTON, F. R. C. S., etc. Third Edition. Pp. 1188. Philadelphia: Lindsay & Blakiston. 1875.

The author's views on many points vary much from those now generally held by ophthalmologists. He denies flatly that inflammation ever begins in the iris, or is chiefly confined to it ; and in the treatment of iritis gives a very subordinate rôle to atropine, though he always uses it from the first, because it gives him correct information of the subsidence of inflammation by producing dilatation of the pupil. In corneitis, in which the value of atropine is generally regarded as only less than in iritis, he has been able to discover only ill effects from its use. Cupping of the disk in glaucoma he looks upon as the result of neuritis and subsequent atrophy, not of increased intra-ocular pressure.

Flap extraction is the operation preferred for senile cataract and is described with its complications at length. When, however, couching (now practically obsolete) is considered worthy to have several pages given to it, the account of Graefe's operation should not have been borrowed from an article published ten years ago, in which the traction-hook, entirely abandoned two years later, occupied a prominent place ; nor is it entirely fair, either to the reader or their originators, to dispose of all other modern operations for extraction in half a dozen lines as the "descriptions of enthusiasts."

The book as a whole is decidedly unsatisfactory, and does not fairly represent the present condition of ophthalmology.   O. F. W.

PROCEEDINGS OF THE BOSTON SOCIETY FOR MEDICAL OBSERVATION.

EDWARD WIGGLESWORTH, JR., M. D., SECRETARY.

Case of Measles. — DR. VOGEL reported the case. T. B., an anæmic girl of five years, living in a damp basement with little light and less ventilation, presented, December 9, 1874, the appearances characterizing the prodromal stage of benign measles, general malaise, cough, sneezing, sore eyes, etc.

December 10th. An eruption upon the face, which by the next day was pinkish and confluent about the eyes, nose, mouth, and wrists, scanty on the body, and absent from the legs. Tongue moist and slightly coated, fever, and cough mild. Seven days after the beginning of the prodromal stage, branny desquamation, disappearance of disease symptoms, and child up and about, though very feeble and without appetite.

December 14th. Brother and sister of the foregoing attacked last night with usual prodromal symptoms.

December 18th. The eruption has appeared in both, darker and more confluent than in the first case, with higher fever and more severe cough, and a very rapid, easily compressible pulse.

December 19th. The boy, aged seven years, has now a barking cough of high pitch, complete hoarseness, and prolonged, labored inspiration. The eruption pale. Pharynx dark red, left submaxillary gland swollen, pulse rapid. The girl, aged ten, stupid and drowsy; rash well out, pulse rapid, breathing easy, pharynx red, and both submaxillary glands swollen.

December 20th.   Boy died last night from "membranous croup," as I was told, another physician having been called in.   The girl almost comatose.   No exanthem visible, submaxillary glands swollen in great packs, sordes on lips, mucus flowing from the nose; tongue dry, thickly coated, red at tip; fauces and tonsils much congested, and a white patch the size of a half-dime on the left velum between the tonsil and uvula; pulse over 120; cough harassing, with some dry ronchi.   Rapidly recovered under treatment of quinine, chlorate of potash, and milk punch.

December 23d.   Another sister, aged three and a half, was taken ill, and December 24th, T. B., the one first seized, was *re*-attacked.   Both had repeated vomiting, sore eyes, discharge from the nose, and cough.   The former child went through a very severe attack of uncomplicated measles, with very copious eruption, confluent upon the face; she had a harassing cough, high fever, drowsiness, and occasional delirium, and made a slow recovery.   T. B.'s case presented the following symptoms: —

December 25th.   Drowsy, moaning, feet livid and rather œdematous.   If disturbed she assumes an anxious and pained expression, tosses her arms, and rolls about.   If aroused she cries, and complains of pain in the left knee and hip, which show, however, nothing abnormal.   Pulse 120, and small.   Temperature 181.3°.   Eyes much injected.   Tongue slowly protruded without trembling, thickly coated, but with no elongation of its papillæ.   A few râles and ronchi in the chest.   Bowels constipated.   Abdomen swollen and tender.   Calomel and castor oil ordered, with cold applications to the head.

December 26th.   Worse.   One offensive dejection; drowsy by day and restless by night, moaning, tossing about, and screaming at intervals.   Complains still of pain in the tender and distended abdomen.

December 27th.   Same state, more marked; pulse 136, very small; refuses nourishment.

December 28th.   Constant screaming all night.   In the morning profound stupor, face congested and slightly cyanotic, skin dry, but not very hot.   Temperature in the axilla 101.5°.   Pulse 140.   Screams when roused.

December 29th.   Has taken only a little brandy and water.   Night, better, no screaming.   Copious eruption, like her sister's, upon face and hands, becoming confluent by evening.   Less on body and arms, and in crescentic patches.   It had a dark raspberry color, which became more bluish towards the end, was well defined, and slightly raised.   Pulse 144, and irregular.   Temperature 102°.   Not much pain, slight cough, and a few râles in chest.

December 30th.   Patient comatose, pulse 160, respiration irregular and labored, skin cool and rather moist; rash bluish.   At 6 P. M. coma profound, eruption gone, skin livid, damp, and cool, pulse uncountable, and stertorous breathing.   Died six hours afterwards.   No autopsy allowed.

This series of cases is interesting as showing the manner in which a highly diffusible poison may become intensified through accumulation in ill-ventilated rooms, thus explaining why epidemics of measles are worse in cold weather. Also as showing the rare phenomena of the recurrence of measles in the same individual.   Burserius, Robedieu, Home, Baillie, Rayer, and Holland have seen instances of a second attack.   Aitken, Rosenstein, Watson, Niemeyer, and

Graves, consider a single attack as affording almost complete protection. Caze-nave admits a few well-attested cases of recurrence. Hebra considers second attacks as rare, though not extremely so. So Austin Flint, who quotes a case of recurrence observed by Dr. Minot in Boston. Steiner has observed recur-rence after eight weeks. Second attacks are also reported by Togetty, Schack, De Haen, Meja, Genovevi, Dubosque, Trujawsky, and Willan.

The second attack of T. B. is a good picture of the typhoid variety of mea-sles, in which the poison attacks especially the nerve-centres, rapidly and com-pletely annihilating its functions. The text-books, however, do not mention the violent screaming, which, from the fixed locations complained of, seems rather referable to pain than to any perverted action of the brain. Tender-ness of the abdomen is usual in such cases, but not the pain in the joints, which might be rheumatoid, although the fever was not high enough at the time. The subsidence of the expressions of pain at the time of the exanthem might have been due to the profound insensibility of the last stage, or might point to peritoneal congestion, relieved by the intense hyperæmia of the skin.

DR. CHADWICK alluded to the possibility of the existence of a hereditary predisposition to one or more attacks of the exanthemata, and cited examples of repeated attacks in different members of the same family.

DRS. GREEN, STEDMAN, TARBELL, ARNOLD and WEBBER, had seen in-stances of second attacks of measles, although some of these cases had oc-curred before the distinction between measles and rubeola [rötheln] was gen-erally recognized.

DR. ELLIS thought, speaking of the period of incubation, that the large number of cases existing during an epidemic, with consequent frequent and repeated exposure, would interfere with the recognition of the exact moment of infection, and that laws could only be deduced from the observation of iso-lated cases.

Dr. WIGGLESWORTH mentioned a case referred to by Panum, where measles broke out in a house which had had no intercourse with the rest of the world, except that a physician had spent the night there a fortnight before, he having come from an infected district four miles away, and been compelled, moreover, to travel in an open boat in stormy, rainy weather.

Capillary Bronchitis in Adults ; the Frequency of its Complication with Changes in the Air-Vesicles, and its Relation to Catarrhal Pneumonia. — DR. ELLIS read some extracts from a paper with the above title, soon to be pub-lished, showing that capillary bronchitis and catarrhal pneumonia cannot always be distinguished clinically. Dr. Ellis believed that the cases were generally mixed ; that pure cases were rare ; that the whole chest should always be examined ; that affections of the air-vesicles giving rise to consol-idation were more common than is generally thought, and that when they are the first affected we may have fine, dry, crepitant râles, and the subcrepitant coming later. The important point is to recognize the clinical condition, and not to confound stages with separate diseases.

At the request of Dr. Ellis, DR. FITZ, who had made an examination of the lungs after death in the case of the third patient mentioned by Dr. Ellis, reported that in some places the air-cells contained pigment-corpuscles and granular mat-

ter suggesting coagulated albumen ; furthermore, cells of epithelium and pus corpuscles ; and elsewhere, alveoli filled entirely with pus corpuscles, or with cheesy
material, and frequently with thickened walls with spindle-shaped elements,
indicating the presence of the various conditions occurring in catarrhal pneumonia as well as those present in interstitial pneumonia. Again, alveoli were
found containing coagulated fibrin, round cells, and blood corpuscles, such as
are found in croupous pneumonia. In a fresh condition, parts of the consolidated portion were gray and translucent, and studded with yellow points composed of granular corpuscles. The relation between these cases and tuberculosis is interesting, and the sections examined presented no tubercles, and yet
the cheesy conditions were present, such as have been recently reasserted to
be dependent upon tubercular inflammation.

Dr. Knight said that according to Niemeyer, catarrhal pneumonia is always
due to capillary bronchitis. Oppolzer, and the German school generally, hold
these ideas in opposition to those of Flint and others in regard to tubercle.
Text-books are apt to confound acute and chronic catarrhal pneumonia and
bronchitis. Solidification may occur, and even end in degeneration, and still
be the result of a bronchitis.

Dr. Fitz spoke of Friedländer's researches disproving the statement of
Buhl that the inflammatory products found in the alveoli had occurred primarily in the smaller bronchi and been thence transferred.

Dr. Knight stated that Niemeyer held that a change of more than a certain amount in the temperature alone, even without any change in the respiration or other signs, shows that the process has reached the alveoli.

Anatomical Specimens. — Dr. Porter showed a specimen of anchylosis following fracture of the ulna, and possibly of the radius ; also an anchylosis of the
scapula with the humerus, following fracture from gun-shot ; this fracture was also
through the anatomical neck, the rarer situation. Finally, a photograph was
shown of a large tumor of the vulva removed by Dr. Parker, of Lowell, by
means of the galvano-cautery. No blood was lost, but the patient died within
forty-eight hours. She was forty years of age and a chronic invalid, and had
shown no symptoms of insanity, though her stomach (shown by Dr. Porter),
when opened, contained three large balls of hay, straw, etc., still connected,
though one had passed into the duodenum.

THE PROFESSION IN CALIFORNIA.

Our esteemed contemporary, the *Pacific Medical and Surgical Journal*, is
greatly irritated by the remarks we published some weeks ago concerning the
profession in San Francisco. The distress of our Pacific remonstrant is so
evidently sincere, that we overlook certain rather unpacific expressions, as well
as his hasty and incorrect assumption that we had no better authority than a
scurrilous daily paper for our statements.   .

We are respectfully requested to recall our article, although it is admitted to
be at least in part correct, and no clew is given us to ascertain what are the

objectionable statements. Till our contemporary condescends to state in what we have injured our brothers in California, it is impossible for us to make reparation. We await this information with patience, and hope that it may prove that our course does not confirm the old law, " The greater the truth the greater the libel."

The state of affairs at all events must be peculiar; in proof of which we quote the *Pacific Journal's* account of a most extraordinary piece of journalistic enterprise : —

" Some months ago, the *News Letter*, a weekly publication issued in San Francisco, began to publish, from week to week, a list of names as ' quacks,' including a number of respectable practitioners, together with others who were most notorious charlatans. Several persons thus placarded had their names stricken from the list by paying sums of money. Other names were added, and it was announced that those who would come forward and show their diplomas should be expunged. Numbers of old and most respectable practitioners who had graduated thirty and forty years ago. some of them in schools long since defunct, the professors all in their graves, and even the records destroyed or inaccessible, were thus publicly impeached. Many had lost their diplomas by accidents of flood and fire. Others were reasonably averse to acknowledging the authority of a libelous print to arraign them in this manner. Much excitement was aroused, in and out of the profession. Certain individuals in our ranks who had personal ends to gain, fomented the movement by handing in the names of those whom they hated. It was well understood that there were professional scavengers engaged in this work — men who possessed diplomas and not honor. Not a solitary individual, however, up to this time, has dared to show his hand, or to acknowledge himself an informer. One or two instances of fraudulent claims to the degree were exposed, and this gave some plausibility to the proceeding."

The matter has been taken up by the medical societies and is now under advisement.

However disreputable the originators of this excitement may be, and however indecent their course, it is hard to see how it could have been of any importance if there were not a fair proportion of black sheep among the profession. We are quite willing. however, to reserve our judgment, and hope that our Western friends will inform us in what our remarks were unwarranted. without further vituperation.

MEDICAL NOTES.

— At a meeting of the Société de Biologie held May 29th, M. Cornil reported a case of considerable retardation of the circulation, with irregular respiration and attacks of syncope due to fatty degeneration of the heart. The patient, a man aged seventy-five, had for four years past suffered from a troublesome cough during the winter which, however, disappeared with the coming of summer. At the same time the digestive functions were impaired, there was frequent vomiting, and the patient became more and more infirm. He was not intemperate in his habits, had never suffered from rheumatism nor from any 'nervous affection. When first seen his pulse ranged from 25 to 30 per minute. May 23d, it numbered only 14; there seemed to be no abortive pulsation of the heart, and the beat of the pulse responded perfectly with the slowness of the cardiac contractions. About every fifteen minutes there was a feeling of oppression. The inspirations were prolonged and suspirious. The attacks of oppression terminated in a state of syncope. At its advent the face was noticed to become pale, the jaws to be contracted and distorted, the arms convulsed. This group of symptoms coincided with the circulatory disturbances. On feeling the pulse just before the attack it was noticed that it was completely wanting, as was likewise the cardiac pulsation; then the attack of syncope came on, after which the respiration and cardiac action were reëstablished. The temperature was always low; the urine never contained albumen. At the autopsy the only lesion worthy of remark was a complete fatty degeneration of the heart. All the muscular fibres were degenerated and contained numerous granulations. The brain was anæmic. To explain the digestive troubles a degeneration of the pancreas was found; a considerable number of the glandular *culs-de-sac* were filled with fatty granulations; moreover, the digestive tract throughout its entire extent was atrophied.

— Some original observations on a new disease called miners' nystagmus are reported by Charles Bell Taylor, M. D., in the *Lancet* for June 12, 1875. The writer states that for twelve years past the colliery districts neighboring' to his residence have furnished him with cases which he has designated as " miners' nystagmus," from the peculiar oscillating motions of the eyeball which are characteristic of the disease, and from the fact that he has observed it occurring only in adults, and independent of other ocular defects, among the men employed in the coal-pits in his vicinity. It was formerly supposed that nystagmus was incurable, always developed itself in infancy, and was caused either by imperfect nervous perception or structural changes in the transparent media of the eye-ball. In miners' nystagmus, however, the disease is usually curable, is developed in adults and aged persons previously healthy, is not accompanied by disease of the nerve or structural change of the eyeball, and is, as a rule, to be noticed only when the patient attempts fixation, especially in a stooping position. The oscillating motions are caused by alternating contractions of the recti or oblique muscles, and in all the cases which the writer has observed have been either horizontal or rotatory. The disease persists so long as its cause continues, but a change of occupation and working in a good light are all that is necessary to effect a cure. Three cases are reported in detail as samples of nine or ten others which have come under Dr. Taylor's care.

— An account of the *post mortem* examination of the case in which inflammable gas was discharged from the stomach during life, is given by the Berlin correspondent of the *Irish Hospital Gazette* for May 15, 1875. The stomach was found to be but little distended. The pyloric orifice was imbedded in a 1ard tumor about the size of a walnut, and its calibre reduced to that of a crow-quill. The whole mucous membrane of the stomach was pale and anæmic, and became gradually lost in the substance of the tumor. The serous coat was everywhere thickened, this being most marked in that portion which covered the tumor, where the membrane was nearly 1 mm. thick. The microscopic examination of the tumor showed it to be a fibro-myoma. The glands of the stomach, except in the immediate neighborhood of the cardiac extremity, had disappeared. The whole thickness of the mucous membrane was occupied by innumerable small, round cells, which had completely destroyed the regularly arranged stomachic glands, and only with difficulty could a few widely-scattered, tube-shaped bodies, be recognized as such. In these miserable representatives of the glands of the stomach, ordinary epithelium could not be recognized, its place being apparently taken up by a finely-granular detritus. The man could, therefore, no longer assimilate his food, and the attempt made for some time before his death to nourish him per rectum could not, of course, satisfy for any length of time his craving for food. The presence of carburetted hydrogen in the eructations cannot be accounted for satisfactorily.

— At a meeting of the Société de Thérapeutique de Paris, as reported in *Le Lyon Médical* of May 30, 1875, M. Blondeau stated that he had employed with success the tincture of kameela against tape-worms. He gave a patient twenty-five grammes of the tincture in an infusion of sage, in three doses taken at an hour's interval, — at nine, ten, and eleven o'clock in the forenoon. At one o'clock, without having suffered the least discomfort, the patient voided a very large tape-worm, of which the head unhappily could not be found. This *tænifuge* has the advantage that it is not disagreeable to take, that it does not produce colic, and that it does not need to be associated with any purgative.

Another article in the same journal gives "a very certain and convenient method of administering kameela." Kameela is a red powder used in the dyeing of silks, and is obtained from the capsules of one of the Euphorbiaceæ. Its employment as an anthelmintic is quite common in China. The method of exhibition, as recommended, is to give the kameela in the pulp of the tamarind in the form of an electuary, according to the age of the patient and his temperament, from six to twelve grammes, given in from thirty to forty grammes of the tamarind pulp. The tart taste of this pulp is agreeable to most people and it washes the powdered kameela which, when taken alone, fills the mouth and throat with a disagreeable, gritty sensation. The consistence of the mass may be further diminished by the addition of the syrup of bitter orange peel, or by the juice of the citron. The electuary should be taken in the morning, on rising, and all at one time. Half an hour later one can breakfast and go about his business as usual. After a few inoffensive borborygmi several very liquid stools result from the medicine. Towards midday or evening with the last evacuation is a rounded mass more or less columnar, which contains one or more tæniæ. M. Du Plessis has employed this method in more than twenty cases and always met success. For the bothriocephalus the cure is always radical. Four were at one time expelled by a patient, measuring in all one hundred and twenty feet. As for the tænia solium, the head usually is expelled, but it occasionally remains with some joints in the small intestines. In such a case the dose must be repeated when there is evidence that the tænia was not completely dislodged.

— We learn by the *Medical Press and Circular* that Dr. Robert McDonnell, of Dublin, reported before the Royal Medical and Chirurgical Society of

London a case of much physiological interest, as going to show that the so-called gustatory branch of the fifth pair receive the nerves of taste from the chorda tympani. The young man, twenty-four years old, had complete paralysis of the portio dura of the seventh pair of nerves following exposure to cold and wet, the left nerve being first affected. There was no evidence of any central lesion of the brain, nor were any other cerebral‚nerves engaged. There was complete loss of the sense of taste in the forepart of the tongue, which the author attributed to paralysis of the chorda tympani. Tactile and thermic impressions were perceived in the forepart of the tongue quite as distinctly as in healthy persons. The defect in taste persisted longer than the motor paralysis. The secretion of saliva from the sublingual glands was not excited by irritants which produced copious flow in healthy persons.

LETTER FROM NEW YORK.

MESSRS. EDITORS, — New York is gradually settling down into its summer inactivity, medically speaking. The attendance at the meetings of the societies has fallen off, and the papers call forth but little discussion. Every one is looking forward to, and wishing for, his summer vacation.

From about the middle of June until the middle of September, the majority of physicians have but little to do. Every one who can possibly get out of the city, goes, and there is nothing left for the physicians to do but to follow their example. The question as to who shall be president of the College of Physicians and Surgeons has at last been settled by the election of Dr. Alonzo Clark.

Affairs at the Presbyterian Hospital are still in a very unsatisfactory state. The protest against the action of the board in dropping certain members of the attending staff without a hearing, which received the signature of so many hospital physicians and surgeons, has remained unnoticed. It has been intimated by some of the trustees that they do not intend to answer it, as they take the ground that they are responsible to no one, and intend to manage the hospital as they please. It is reported that many members of the board did not know the cause of opposition to those members of the medical board who were dropped, and that those who were " running " the board declined to give any explanation, and intimated that it was best for all parties that the question should not be pressed. Some assign another reason for the action of the trustees, namely, that they felt insulted by the change in the presiding officer of the medical board, which was made at the last election. In the last annual report of the Presbyterian Hospital, I find among the rules and regulations, after those defining who shall constitute the medical board, the following: " The medical board at their first regular meeting in May of each year shall elect a president, vice-president, and secretary . . . . etc." In accordance with this rule, this was done, and now, because a majority believed in rotation in office and desired a change, some of the trustees said that it was an insult to the board, and for this reason failed to appoint four of the old staff; in other words, they claimed the right to dictate to the medical board how they shall manage their own affairs.

There is no doubt that there has been wrong on both sides, as there is apt to be in all quarrels; but that the physicians were the chief sinners is very doubtful, and even if they were, it does not take away from them the right to demand, nor from the board the duty to state, the reasons for such dismissal. The present plan of hospital management has proved a total failure, and there does not seem to be moral courage enough on the part of the trustees to come out and honestly say so.

The *Medical Record* of June 12th, in an editorial, calls for the resignation of the whole staff, or that they give some good reason for remaining. At a meeting of the trustees held a few days ago, the resignation of five of the attending staff was received, but no action was taken on them. A committee of conference, however, was appointed, to endeavor to smooth things over. I believe the vote for the resolution appointing such a committee was passed almost unanimously; what it will amount to depends, of course, on the power given to the committee, but the mere fact of such a vote being passed, shows that the board does not feel quite as strong as it did, and that it has placed itself in a false position.

If the staff insist on their demands, that the reason shall be given for the dismissal of the four gentlemen, they will probably carry their point. The question of retaining the directoress with her almost absolute power is not covered by the resolution; if she is still upheld there will be more trouble. I have heard of several physicians who have been asked to make applications for positions in the hospital by members of the board of trustees, but who have declined to have anything to do with the institution under its present plan of management. It will be difficult to fill the vacancies with those who are fitted for holding such places. There seems to be but one way to save the hospital and gain the support of the profession; and that is by the board stating the reason for their action and then closing the hospital, on paper, dismissing every one; and immediately appointing a new staff, retaining as many of the old board as they may wish, but by all means dispensing with the service of the present executive officer, as the hospital cannot be a success as long as she remains at its head. The hospital has never been full, although other institutions have had as many patients as they could accommodate. Those who have been inmates of it once refuse to go there again, being unwilling to subject themselves to the arbitrary rules of the directoress. They have great difficulty in keeping nurses. They prefer to go to other institutions for less remuneration than to remain there. All this points to something radically wrong in the management of the hospital.

There are two facts in hospital management in New York that this unfortunate difficulty at the Presbyterian Hospital illustrates, and which are really the cause of all the trouble. In the first place, the governing boards of the majority of public institutions here are too large. Thus, the board of the Presbyterian Hospital consists of thirty-two members. Such a board is unwieldy; the responsibility is divided among so many that practically there is none, and the institution is either left to run itself, or is run by a few,

and these, perhaps, the very ones who know least about its wants and requirements. In the case mentioned above, there are more trustees than the average number of patients in the hospital. The majority of such a board know
but little of what is really going on in the institution, and when a question
comes up for consideration but few know what they are voting about.

In the second place, physicians are as a rule excluded from any representation on the board. The advice of a former member of the Board of Governors of the New York Hospital seems to be carried out to the letter.
When asked for some suggestions as to the organization and management of a
hospital in a neighboring city, he is reported to have given the following:
" Whatever you do, keep your feet on the necks of the doctors." Perhaps
the profession is in a measure responsible for this condition of affairs, in being
willing to accept position under a board in which it has no representation.

Notwithstanding the exertions of the Board of Health, the mortality from
small-pox is still very great. There are now over two hundred cases at the
hospital on Blackwell's Island. In former epidemics the number of cases has
rapidly diminished as soon as the weather became warm, but this year there
seems to have been an increase, and all attempts to stamp it out have failed.
The majority of cases occur among the Germans and Italians. The mortality
is about twenty-five per cent. There are still a great many hæmorrhagic
cases, and also those in which the eruption presents a flat, pasty appearance.

Diphtheria, which a month or so ago seemed to be diminishing, has again
become quite prevalent, the number of cases reported being as great as at any
time last winter.

The commissioners of charities and corrections are about to organize a
school for nurses in connection with Charity Hospital. The chief of staff will
be at its head. It is intended to open it on the 1st of August, and to place
all the wards under the care of the school, provided a sufficient number of
nurses can be obtained. The term of service is two years. Those under instruction are to live in the hospital, have their board, etc., and to receive $10
per month for the first year and $15 for the second year.

June 19, 1875.

THE TREATMENT OF THE INSANE.

The *Boston Daily Advertiser* of May 19th contains a very just article on this
subject. The text upon which it is written is good enough for the JOURNAL to
quote and use for the same purpose.

It reads : " Mrs. Berry gave several reminiscences of her life in an insane
asylum which were certainly of a very startling nature, and, if true in every
detail, disclosed a state of facts prevalent in some asylums horrible enough to
rouse the fiercest indignation of the whole community."

I feel like saying a word on this subject. I am not connected with any
asylum for the insane, and never have been. I have frequently had under
observation and care those who were insane, and whom I have been the
means of sending to asylums. I have heard from some of them, after their

discharge, the most vivid accounts of severe treatment, and from others the pleasantest history of kind and humane treatment. These opposite accounts I have heard from different patients of the same man. The probability seems to be, that either those who said they were well treated or those who said they were badly treated, remained insane after they were set free.

I was instrumental some years since in getting a patient into the asylum at Somerville, who, according to the accounts given, vowed to inflict some punishment upon me after he should get free. For a year or two after the patient's discharge we used to meet occasionally, and a very simple and cool recognition was all that passed between us, although the meeting was generally at the patient's house. One day, on coming down stairs at the patient's house, this gentleman met me at the foot and said, " If you are not in haste, I should like to see you a moment." I followed him into his library; the door was closed, and a chair was put forward for my accommodation. After a short silence, which seemed an hour, the patient, looking me steadily in the face, and I as steadily as I could returning the gaze, broke silence with "You were the means of sending me to Somerville, I believe." With as much coolness as I could I replied, " I believe that I was." " Well," said he, " you must have heard a good deal of what I have said about you, and about Dr. Tyler; have you not ? " " I have." Then he continued, " That is a matter of the past. It is of no consequence, what I have said heretofore, nor what I have done. We'll forget about that. But if you ever see signs about me again that make you think I am insane, send me back to Somerville : only let me know that you are going to do it."

The conversation ended here. We met frequently afterwards with as much freedom and good feeling as in former years. No allusion was made to what had happened so long as he lived, which was some six months longer ; and he was my patient in his last sickness.

The JOURNAL, I believe, has never replied to any of the statements which have been made by patients or others from the hospitals about their management. It seems no more than proper, however, that it should say what it believes to be true upon this subject. For one, with the utmost respect for men and women who have been confined at asylums, I must say, First, that many of them, like my patient alluded to, change their opinion after being out for a while. Secondly, that many of them, who recover more early, come from the asylum with the pleasantest feelings towards their officers, and retain those feelings through life. Thirdly, that there are those who leave the asylum sufficiently recovered to be unlikely to do violence to others, but not well. Some of these, if left to themselves, will get well. Some of them will never get well because their trouble is incurable ; and some of them will never get well because they have about them the ignorant or ill-natured who call themselves friends, but whose constant attempt is to keep them excited agains real friends.   M. D.

WEEKLY BULLETIN OF PREVALENT DISEASES.

THE following is a bulletin of the diseases prevalent in Massachusetts during the week ending July 3, 1875, compiled under the authority of the State Board of Health from reports received from physicians representing all sections of the State : —

In Berkshire, whooping-cough, diarrhœa, cholera morbus and typhoid are reported.

In the Connecticut Valley, rheumatism, whooping-cough, diarrhœa and scarlatina prevail. Small-pox has not yet left Easthampton. Shelburne has diphtheria.

In Worcester County, bronchitis, influenza, measles, and diarrhœa are common.

In the Northeastern section, the public health is satisfactory; scarlatina, measles, and diarrhœa prevail to a limited extent. Gloucester reports one case of small-pox.

In the Metropolitan district, scarlatina is the most prevalent disease. Diarrhœa and cholera infantum, begin to increase. Roxbury and Watertown report cases of cerebro-spinal meningitis. Boston has a single case of small-pox derived from New York.

In the Southeastern counties, rheumatism has a general prevalence. Bronchitis, diarrhœa and cholera morbus prevail to a limited extent. Vineyard Haven reports scarlatina.

F. W. DRAPER, M. D., Registrar.

COMPARATIVE MORTALITY-RATES FOR THE WEEK ENDING JUNE 26, 1875.

	Estimated Population.	Total Mortality for the Week.	Annual Death-rate per 1000 during Week.
New York	1,040,000	571	28
Philadelphia	775,000	324	22
Brooklyn	450,000	242	28
Boston	350,000	157	23
Providence	100,000	34	18
Worcester	50,000	19	20
Lowell	50,000	23	24
Cambridge	44,000	23	27
Fall River	45,000	15	17
Lawrence	33,000	9	14
Springfield	33,000	3	5
Lynn	28,000	8	15
Salem	26,000	4	8

NOTICE TO FELLOWS OF THE MASSACHUSETTS MEDICAL SOCIETY. — The post-office address of Dr. F. W. Goss, the Recording Secretary of the Society, is Hotel Eliot, Roxbury ; and that of Dr. F. W. Draper, the Treasurer, is No. 36 Worcester Street, Boston.

THE BOSTON
MEDICAL AND SURGICAL JOURNAL.

VOL. XCIII. — THURSDAY, JULY 15, 1875. — NO. 3.

PERINEAL TUMOR OF FŒTUS AN IMPEDIMENT TO DELIVERY.[1]

BY C. ELLERY STEDMAN, M. D., OF DORCHESTER.

MRS. A. B., aged twenty-two, of good constitution and excellent healti, who was delivered of her first ciild a year and a half ago with forceps, by Dr. C. D. Homans, after a hard labor, expected to be confined about the 1st of February, 1875. She had not menstruated since the birti of the first child, a well-developed and healtiy infant. On January 28th I was called to see her, and found her with a pulse of 130; the temperature was 103°; the respiration was rapid; cough, rachitic pains, considerable prostration, pain of throat and neck, and sligit redness of the fauces. The next day there was a pultaceous patci the size of a little-finger nail on the left side of the uvula. Tiis disappeared in twelve hours under the use of a lotion of chlorate of potassa. Wine and quinine, with frequent and nourisi ing food, were prescribed, and on February 1st she was nearly well.

During pregnancy she declared tiat the ciild was not carried like the first: she had had no frigit, nor had she seen anytiing to annoy her. Tiere were no twins nor monsters known in her family or in tiat of her iusband. About February 18th she ceased to feel the motion of the ciild; a cold weigit took its place, and she affirmed it was not living.

At 8 P. M. of February 24th labor began; the face presented, left mento-anterior; the cranial bones crepitated on pressure. The membranes iaving been ruptured, the pains became efficient; a little etier was given as tiey increased; the iead was born easily, the sioulders, witi muci effort. When the tiorax had been delivered, no furtier progress was made; the abdomen felt as tiougi anotier ciild were present. On introducing a iand along the ciild's back, an obstruction was discovered above the brim, wiere the breeci of the fœtus was separated by a sulcus from anotier body swelling beyond it. Dr. Miller now saw the patient. The perforator, being carried up between the fœtal body and the operator's iand, was tirust into the tumor and gave vent to a prodigious burst of blood and water. Vigorous traction now brougit away the ciild. The uterus, followed down by the iand, con-

[1] Read before the Obstetrical Society of Boston.

tracted firmly, and no hæmorrhage of moment ensued ; the placenta came away directly. It was now seen that labor had been impeded by the growth upon the child's breech of a half-solid tumor, larger than the fœtal head. The incisions made by the perforator having been sewed up, the tumor resumed its size after stuffing, and a cast was taken by Dr. Bolles, who has placed it in the pathological cabinet of the City Hospital. He describes it as follows : " The tumor was situated behind the anus, and distended it somewhat. It evidently arose behind the rectum in the lower part of the pelvis ; it was not attached to any of the pelvic organs, but could be easily and cleanly dissected away from them all. It was chiefly a large cyst which had been ruptured in delivery, and apparently contained degenerated blood. Into this cavity there projected from above several smaller tumors, in all a mass about three and one half inches in diameter, the largest of which contained grumous

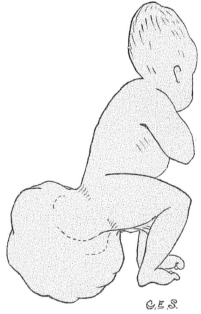

fluid. The others were semi-solid, dark, and pulpy." There was no evidence of fœtal inclusion. The tumor appeared to be glandular. Its largest circumference (antero - posterior) was sixteen and one half inches. The gland of Luschka is referred to as the origin of such growths. A sketch is annexed.

A drawing on page 17 of Holmes's Surgical Diseases of Children (London, 1868) gives a good idea of the interior of the tumor. Mr. Holmes's case was a congenital growth in a girl three years old ; at birth it was of the size of an orange, but it measured fifteen and one half inches in circumference at the time of its successful removal. It grew on the left buttock. There was no pedicle, as in the subject of this paper, but it seemed to pass through a broad opening (the expanded sacro-sciatic foramen) into the pelvis, and had a distinct impulse ; there was no transparency and no lobulation. The anus was pushed over somewhat to the right. The tumor could be traced down to the pelvic bones, and was evidently connected with the rectum for some distance.

There is a cut of a similar fœtus on page 861 of Cazeaux (fifth American edition), but it is referred to as spina bifida with hydrorachis.

CYSTS OF THE IRIS.

BY PETER A. CALLAN, M. D.,

Assistant Surgeon at the New York Eye and Ear Infirmary.

Cysts of the iris are a comparatively rare form of eye-disease, and in the ophthalmic clinics of Europe or our own country they are but seldom seen. They are occasioned by foreign bodies penetrating through the cornea and lodging in the iris, perforation of the cornea with prolapse of the iris, operations for cataract, and blows on the globe. It is very probable that in all cases their origin is traumatic, and not unfrequently the cornea shows traces of a former injury. A careful examination of the patient will result, in the majority of cases, in his remembering to have received an injury at some previous date in the affected eye.

It has not as yet been satisfactorily determined whether the cysts are situated between the layers of the iris or merely arise from its anterior surface. Frequently they appear to arise from either a broad or a pediculated base. Exceptionally they arise from the posterior part of the iris, or even the ciliary processes. It is not always an easy matter to recognize the cysts, and often they escape the attention of the patient until through their size the pupil is encroached on and vision obstructed. Generally the walls are quite thin and translucent, with serous contents occupying the anterior chamber. Some cysts have been found with thick, opaque walls, even cartilaginous in texture. As regards number it is rare to find more than one, but as many as four have been observed in one eye, and again a large single cyst, multilocular in character, has been found. The period between the injury to the eye and the development of the cyst varies from a few months to many years, and the age of the patient ranges from five years to sixty-five.

In the literature of ophthalmology many rare cases of cysts are narrated. Graefe [1] published one of extreme rarity, the contents of the cyst being sebaceous in character, with six short, thick hairs. Langenbeck had previously observed a similar case. In Graefe's case the tumor developed within the period of a few months, as a result of a penetrating wound of the cornea. Staber and Schweigger have published cases in which cilia were contained in the cysts and were easily seen previous to the removal by operation. Rothmund divides the cysts into two classes, both traumatic in their origin : first, the epidermoid, from epidermic cells, and probably formed by a piece of skin carried into the iris through a wound of the cornea ; and, second, true cysts of the iris with serous contents, having surrounding membrane and epithelial covering, resulting from a portion of corneal epithelium carried into the iris. De Wecker is of the opinion that they are formed by diverticula of the iris containing aqueous humor. Mr. Hulke [2] compiled short

---

[1] Archiv für Augenheilkunde, iii. heft 2, page 412.

[2] Ophthalmic Hospital Reports, 1869, 1 vi. 12.

histories of nineteen cases, fifteen of which could be traced to a traumatic origin. Like Bowman, he believes their position to be between the muscular and the uveal layer of the iris; some, however, having both muscular and uveal layers in front. One case he supposed owed its formation to the posterior epithelial layer of cornea carried by a wound into the iris. Rothmund[1] collected from various sources thirty-seven cases which were published. The previously reported cases of Mr. Hulke were all included in the paper. He found twenty-eight of all the cases to be traumatic in their origin, due for the most part to penetrating wounds of the cornea.

Cysts of the iris are not devoid of danger, as they are liable to cause loss of the affected eye through irido-choroiditis, and even to endanger the safety of the other eye through sympathetic inflammation. Crichett, in a practice of more than thirty years, has observed four cases, all of which terminated unfavorably for the affected eyes. Arlt, however, had seven cases, and in only one case did the tumor reappear after removal, and once there was iritis subsequent to the operation.

There are not a few surgeons who regard the cysts as dangerous to the safety of the eye so affected, and through sympathetic inflammation liable to cause loss of the other eye. The question has been debated at a meeting of the New York Pathological Society as to the expediency of enucleating the affected eye. The great danger consists in the size of the growths; when small they cause no irritation, but when they steadily grow and have attained large dimensions, irido-choroiditis may be occasioned and the eye lost. In short, they act mechanically as foreign bodies, and should be removed early.

At the New York Eye and Ear Infirmary within the last five years, two cases have been operated on by Drs. C. M. Allin and Henry D. Noyes. Dr. Allin's case has been published.[2] Dr. Noyes's case was that of a young farmer, twenty-one years of age, who applied at the clinique last winter. The patient, while quite young, had inflammation of both corneæ with perforation. The right eye presented a small corneal opacity, with an anterior synechia of the iris; vision $\frac{20}{200}$. The left eye presented a large central opacity of the cornea, with a cyst situated immediately behind it. Vision, light-perception merely. Two years ago, the patient began to have trouble with his left eye, and on his admission to the infirmary, there was great intolerance of light, so much that he was obliged to keep the eye half-closed. The eye had some ciliary injection, and the globe was slightly hard to the touch. The cyst was readily recognized, as it occupied more than two thirds of the anterior chamber. On the temporal side the iris and border of the pupil could be seen, but no pupillary opening. The walls on the temporal side were distinctly recognizable, but on the inner side they

---

[1] Monatsblatt für Augenheilkunde, 1872, 189.
[2] American Ophthalmic Society Reports, vii. 58.

were in close contact with the cornea, and pushed back the iris and lens. The contents were perfectly transparent, and through the portion covering the pupil an opacity on the anterior capsule could be distinctly seen; this anterior polar cataract indicated that the original perforation had been nearly central.

In operating, no attempt was made to remove the cyst entire, on account of its great size; it was designed to remove the whole of the posterior wall and leave the portion of the anterior wall attached to the cornea. The patient having been etherized, the cornea was entered at the limbus of the inner side by a bent iridectomy-knife with a long and rather narrow blade, which was pushed across, perforating the opposite wall. The wound in the limbus was enlarged upwards and downwards with scissors, until it included one third the circumference of the cornea. A blunt hook was then introduced and caught in the free pupillary margin above the cyst; the tissue was drawn out and excised by a succession of snips of the scissors; the iris and cyst walls were cut off at the ciliary body up to the wound in the limbus, when the whole of the tissue appeared to be satisfactorily removed. The lens was not disturbed. No loss of vitreous occurred. There was very little hæmorrhage. Reaction following the operation was moderate in severity. Recovery was slow. The patient was kept under observation for two months, when all traces of irritation had disappeared. No reproduction of the cyst was observed. During the patient's sojourn an iridectomy was performed on his right eye to improve the vision. Recovery after this operation was prompt, and the sight was improved to $\frac{20}{100}$. The vision of the left eye after the removal of the cyst was not much improved on account of the large leucoma.

In both of the infirmary cases, Dr. H. Althof examined the extracted portions of cysts and found the lining membrane to be epithelium.

RECENT PROGRESS IN PHYSIOLOGY.

BY H. P. BOWDITCH, M. D.

COURSE OF NERVE-FIBRES IN THE SPINAL CORD.

THE difficulties which attend an experimental inquiry into the channels by which sensitive and motor impressions traverse the spinal cord, have been, to a great extent, surmounted in a recent investigation by Woroschiloff;[1] and the uniformity of the results obtained is so great as to justify the hope that an extension of the method adopted will finally give a satisfactory solution of this much disputed question. Previous observations by Miescher,[2] Nawrocki,[3] and Dittmar,[4] had shown

[1] Arbeiten aus der physiologischen Anstalt zu Leipzig, ix.
[2] Arbeiten aus der physiologischen Anstalt zu Leipzig, V. 172.
[3] Arbeiten aus der physiologischen Anstalt zu Leipzig, vi. 89.
[4] Arbeiten aus der physiologischen Anstalt zu Leipzig, viii. 103.

that in rabbits the lateral columns of the spinal cord contain the nerve-fibres, both afferent and efferent, which are concerned in the production of a reflex contraction of blood-vessels, due to an irritation of the sciatic nerve. To ascertain whether the channels of reflex and voluntary movement of the muscles of the trunk and limbs lie also in the same region of the cord, Woroschiloff was compelled to modify in several respects the methods adopted by the above-named observers. In the first place, the necessity of observing the contractions of striped muscles forbade the use of curare to render the animal motionless, and yet absolute immobility of the spinal cord at the time of making the sections of the different parts — for this was the method of investigation adopted — was essential to the success of the experiment. This object was accomplished by means of a double clamp, which was screwed firmly upon the vertebral column above and below the point where the spinal canal was laid open by the removal of the arch of one of the vertebræ. The same clamp also gave support to a small apparatus by means of which delicate blades, cutting in planes parallel to the longitudinal axis of the body, could be adjusted in any desired position and then thrust with great precision vertically, horizontally, or obliquely through the substance of the spinal cord. These blades, which thus penetrated the cord longitudinally, served to isolate the portion of the cord to be divided and to protect the remainder from injury by compression or traction. As soon as the sections were made the blades and clamps were removed, the wound carefully sewed up, and the results of the operation observed. The animals used in these experiments were rabbits, and the sections were all made at the level of the last dorsal vertebra. The author is particularly careful not to extend his conclusions to other animals or to other regions of the cord.

A systematic study was made of the effect of the mutilation, first, on the production of reflex actions due to irritation by pressure and electricity of the feet and ears of the animal; secondly, on the position of the limbs, both at rest and in movement; and, thirdly, on the production of movements in the hind limbs due to irritation by induced currents of the cord just below the calamus scriptorius. (These movements were found to consist in a series of alternate flexions and extensions of all the limbs, such as would be produced in powerful voluntary leaps. The same effect was produced by irritation of the cord anywhere above the origin of the sixth cervical nerves, which seems to show that the cervical cord is a centre for coördinated locomotive movements.)

The animal was usually killed about five hours after the operation, and the portion of the cord operated on removed and hardened in alcohol and chromate of ammonia. Microscopic sections were then made in the neighborhood of the wound, and that section which showed the most extensive divisions of the cord photographed with a magnifying power of twenty-five diameters. The original article contains a series of heliotype plates obtained in this way. The following figures represent in a general way the appearances shown in these plates, the shaded parts of the figures indicating the divided portions of the cord : —

Fig. 1 represents the division of the anterior and posterior columns and nearly the whole of the gray substance. After this section, no disturbance of the transmission of motor or sensitive impressions through the cord can be detected. Pressure on any of the four extremities produces vigorous movements in all four limbs. The animal sits and moves in a

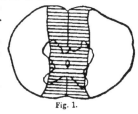

Fig. 1.

perfectly normal manner. Irritation of the cervical cord causes at first the above-mentioned springing movements, and afterwards tetanic flexion of both hind legs.

On the other hand, the section represented in Fig. 2 (which is the counterpart to Fig. 1) entirely prevents the transmission of impressions through that region of the cord. Irritation of one hind leg causes reflex movements of the same leg, or, if the irritation is a strong one, of the opposite leg also. Irritation of a fore leg

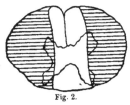

Fig. 2.

causes movements in the anterior but not in the posterior part of the body. Irritation of the cervical cord causes movements in all the muscles of the body except those of the hind legs.

Section of the posterior columns alone, as shown in Fig. 3, is absolutely without effect on the condition of the animal. All movements are executed in a perfectly normal manner. There is nowhere hyperæsthesia nor anæsthesia.

If, together with the posterior columns, portions of the lateral columns are also divided as shown in Fig. 4, the effect is much the same, except that in springing the extension of the hind legs takes place with diminished force, while the flexion of those limbs is unaffected. A feeble irritation of the cervical cord causes a powerful tetanic flexion of all the joints of the hind legs.

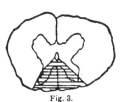

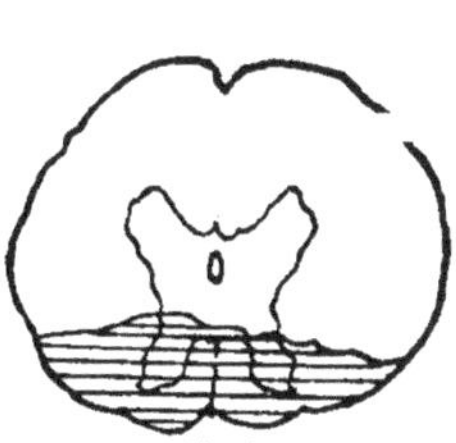

Fig. 3.

Division of the anterior columns with the adjoining portions of the lateral columns, as shown in Fig. 5, produces no effect except that in springing the animal extends the hind legs more powerfully than in the normal condition.

Fig. 4.

The result of these five series of experiments, showing that the channels of motor and sensitive impressions lie in the lateral and not in the anterior and posterior columns of the cord, is

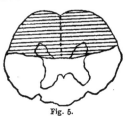

in opposition to the conclusions of many other investigators, and to the generally received opinion of physiologists. This contradiction is, according to the author, to be explained by the considerations, first, that similarity of results is to be expected only when the operations are performed on the same region of the cord, and

Fig. 5.

secondly, that when partial sections of the cord are made without the use of protecting blades, as has been done by many investigators, the parts in the neighborhood of the section are necessarily more or less injured by pressure and traction.

Additional evidence that the lateral columns really contain the channels of motor and sensitive impressions is afforded by the result of sections such as are represented in Figs. 6 and 7. When the whole cord

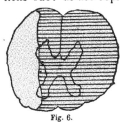

is divided except the left lateral column, as shown in Fig. 6, irritation of either hind foot causes movements of the anterior limbs, but the strength of the irritation which is sufficient to produce this effect is very much greater on the uninjured side of the body than on the opposite side. In other words, there is hyperæsthesia on the side of the injury. If, on the other hand, the strength of

Fig. 6.

the irritation is measured which, when applied to the posterior limbs, is sufficient to produce reflex movements in the same limbs, it is found that

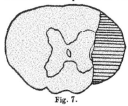

the reverse is true, *i. e.*, there is hyperæsthesia on the uninjured side. Irritations applied to the fore limbs produce movements of both hind limbs, but the movements on the side of the injury are much feebler than those on the opposite side. In sitting, the animal does not support itself by the hind leg on the side of the injury,

Fig. 7.

and in springing that limb is trailed behind. There is not, however, absolute loss of coördinated movement on the side of the injury, for strong irritation of the cervical cord causes the hind leg on that side to take part in the springing movements which are thus produced.

Similar effects follow the section of one of the lateral columns as represented in Fig. 7.

In order to localize still more definitely the course of nervous impressions in the lateral columns, more extensive sections of the cord were made. After a section of the whole cord except the posterior portion of the right lateral columns as shown in Fig. 8, irritation of the right foot causes only reflex movements of the hind limbs, while irritation of the left foot causes also movements of the fore limbs. There is complete loss of voluntary movements in the left hind leg, and irritation of the cervical cord has no effect on that limb, while on the opposite side the springing movements are well marked.

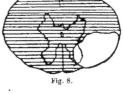

Fig. 8.

After a section such as is represented in Fig. 9, the movements produced by irritation of the hind legs are the same as those described in the case shown in Fig. 8. Irritation of the fore legs causes movements of the right, but not of the left hind leg. In sitting, the animal uses neither of its hind legs to support itself, but in springing makes some use of its right leg. Irritation of the cervical cord causes strong flexion of the right and extension of the left hind leg.

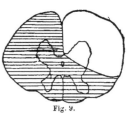

Fig. 9.

A still more extensive section is shown in Fig. 10. Even here, irritation of the hind leg on the side where the cord is completely destroyed causes movements in the anterior part of the body, but without any appearance of hyperæsthesia. Irritation of the fore limbs, however, causes no movement in the hind limbs, and irritation of the cervical cord produces no movement in the hind quarters except in the knee-joint of the leg on the side where a portion of the cord has been preserved.

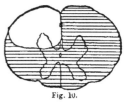

Fig. 10.

Although these experiments proved the possibility of dividing the whole cord, except a very small portion, without preventing the conduction of impressions through that portion, yet in view of the possible interference with the circulation in the retained part due to the division of so much of the substance of the cord, it seemed better to the author to seek to localize the channels of nerve-force in the different parts of the lateral columns by retaining portions of both instead of only one of the columns in question. Sections of this sort are shown in Figs. 11 and 12.

The effect of such a section as is represented in Fig. 11 is the same as that described in connection with Fig. 9, except that both legs are now equally affected. In the same way Fig. 12 corresponds with Fig. 8.

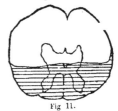

Fig 11.

The general result of all the experiments illustrated by Figs. 8 to 12 inclusive may be stated as follows : —

Motor and sensitive nerve-fibres are found in all parts of the lateral columns.

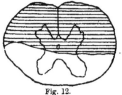

Fig. 12.

Sensitive fibres from both hind legs are found in each lateral column, but the fibres, in either column, which come from the leg on the opposite side are capable of producing stronger reflex movements in the anterior part of the body than are called forth by excitation of the fibres which come from the leg on the same side (crossed hyperæsthesia).

The centripetal fibres whose excitation produces these strong reflex movements, as well as those whose section on the opposite side gives occasion to them, lie in the middle third of the lateral columns, while the anterior and posterior thirds contain sensitive fibres which call forth movements of only moderate intensity in the anterior part of the body.

Motor fibres for both legs are found in each lateral column, but the motor fibres in different parts of these columns are called into activity in different ways. The reflex movements due to irritation of a fore leg can be excited in a hind limb only when the anterior half of the lateral column on the same side is preserved.

The coördinated movements of sitting and springing, and those produced by irritation of the cervical cord, are transmitted to each hind leg through the middle third of the lateral column on the same side.

Tetanus of both hind legs may be produced by irritation of the cord, even when the whole lateral column on one side has been destroyed; but if in addition to this the anterior two thirds of the lateral column on the other side has been divided, tetanus occurs only on the side where a portion of the cord is intact.

The author gives reasons, too lengthy for a place in this report, for regarding the crossed hyperæsthesia above alluded to as caused by the division of the inhibitory fibres having their origin at the periphery and going to the centre of reflex action in the medulla. According to this view, the excito-reflex fibres of a limb have their course mainly, but not exclusively, in the opposite side, while the inhibitory reflex fibres lie chiefly on the same side, of the cord.

To effect a still more perfect localization of the channels of nervous impressions, sections were made such as are represented in Figs. 13 to 17. When only the external portions of the two lateral columns were

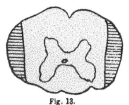

Fig. 13.

divided, as shown in Fig. 13, the only effect observed was an interference with the movements of the feet. The toes were tetanically flexed, the left ankle-joint was extended, and the right one paralyzed.

Instead of describing in detail the results of the sections represented in Figs. 14 to 17, it will be sufficient to state the conclusions which are to be drawn from this series of experiments. These are as follows: —

Motor and sensitive nerves are found mixed together in all parts of the lateral columns.

The fibres which preside over coördinated movements of the hind limbs, as well as those whose section causes hyperæsthesia on the side of the injury, lie in those parts of the lateral columns which are nearest to the gray substance. By uniting this result with that obtained by the sections shown in Figs. 8 to 12, it will be seen that the fibres in question lie in the inner half of the middle third of the lateral columns.

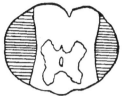

Fig. 14.

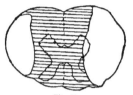

Fig. 15.

The motor nerve-fibres of the foot and lower leg seem to lie in the lateral columns externally to those of the thigh.

In all these experiments it was found that considerable portions of the lateral columns could be removed without affecting motion or sensibility in the leg, although the motor and sensitive character of the divided portion could be demonstrated with certainty. This would seem to indicate that the same muscle, or the same cutaneous surface, is represented in the spinal cord by fibres having various positions in the lateral columns. This agrees with the observations of Eckhard and others which show that two or three adjacent spinal roots send fibres to the same region of the body.

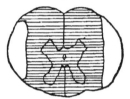

Fig. 16.

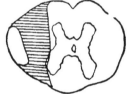

Fig. 17.

The main result of all these experiments, namely, that the lateral columns contain all the channels of motor and sensitive impressions, receives confirmation from the observations of Stilling on the areas of the cross-sections of the spinal nerves and of the columns of the spinal cord at different levels. A comparison of these areas shows that the lateral columns increase in size from below upwards, as if each successive spinal root contributed a certain proportion of its nerve fibres to their formation.

(To be concluded.)

PROCEEDINGS OF THE OBSTETRICAL SOCIETY OF BOSTON.

CHARLES W. SWAN, M. D., SECRETARY.

MARCH 13, 1875. — The President, DR. MINOT, and, subsequently, the President-elect, DR. HODGDON, in the chair.

Fœtal Tumor of the Perinæum. — DR. STEDMAN read a case of fœtal perineal tumor, and showed the specimen, together with a cast of the same; the case appears in full in the present number of the JOURNAL.

DR. FITZ inquired as to the nature of the lining of the cyst.

DR. STEDMAN replied that it was perfectly smooth.

DR. FITZ spoke of a similar tumor of the neck, in which occurred a number of normal tissues. The so-called gland of Luschka is not recognized as a special source of these tumors, and the view of "fœtus by inclusion," based on the complexity of tissues in these tumors, is hardly now accepted.

Mollities Ossium. — DR. ABBOT reported a case of remarkable fragility of bones in a new-born child. The labor occurred January 12, in the afternoon, under the care of a professional friend, who had been called in the absence of Dr. Abbot. Breech presented. When Dr. Abbot arrived the child was just born and he delivered the placenta. There had been no interference with the labor, and it was short. The uterus contracted slowly. The child was healthy-looking and plump, but its legs were seen to be remarkably distorted. Both bones of each were broken, and the limbs were flexed backwards about 60°; the toes pointing downwards, and the heels being drawn upwards, crepitus was distinctly felt. There was a natural transverse groove just below the calf, at the site of the fracture, such as is often seen in fat children. Splints were applied. The next morning, as the shoulders seemed tender, they were carefully examined and both arms were found to be broken just at the neck of the bone. The occiput appears to be normal, but on pressure it was found that the upper part of the occipital bone, and one third of each parietal bone were absent. The sagittal suture was unusually wide. The anterior third of the right parietal, the temporal and part of the right frontal were in the form of a number of small pieces, kept in position by the attached soft parts, like fragments of an egg-shell held by the lining membrane. There was right scrotal hernia. The flexor-tendons of the left hand were contracted and those of the right were in the same condition, with the addition of a contraction of the abductors of the thumb. The child was feeble for four or five days, then nursed pretty well. At the end of the third week the broken bones were united. The child then became weak and died after slight convulsions, having lived one month and four days. The fractures undoubtedly occurred during the passage of the child through the brim of the pelvis.

DR. FITZ remarked that in cases of rickets the cartilage grows faster than the bone; that "tabes" of the occipital bone is a prominent symptom, but that the disease corresponds more with what is called osteomalacia, where there is dilatation, with cavities, as in the case of the cat shown by Dr. Edes.[1]   In this

---

[1] JOURNAL, xcii. 134, February 4, 1875.

animal, whose movements were very cautious, there was general deformity, sponginess, and brittleness, — whereas in Dr. Abbot's case there was no enlargement, but simply the brittleness.

DR. REYNOLDS asked if osteomalacia were to be expected in early life.

DR. FITZ said that rickets going on to osteomalacia had. been produced experimentally in young animals.

Hydrocephalus in a New-Born Child; Thrombus in a Puerperal Woman. — DR. HODGDON read the following cases : —

" CASE I. A primipara was delivered, after an easy labor, of a male child. On February 8th, while tying the cord, I observed the right leg of the child moving spasmodically. Soon the spasm extended to the left leg and then to the whole body and the muscles of the face. The convulsion lasted from half a minute to a minute. I found nothing abnormal about the child. The head was natural in shape and size. The next two weeks I watched carefully without finding anything wrong. I then left the care to the nurse. On March 10th I was called to see the child on account of a cough which it had had for several days. It was dull and stupid. The chest was perfectly clear, but the head was enlarged, and there was that disproportion between the face and head seen in hydrocephalus. The child died in convulsions within twenty-four hours.

" CASE II. January 22d, Mrs. P., at her second confinement, was delivered of a healthy female child. A few hours after delivery she had a chill, and severe pain in the left iliac region. There was pain and tenderness in this region and a rapid pulse for several days, when all unpleasant symptoms subsided and the patient went on apparently making a good recovery, till February 14th, the twenty-fourth day after delivery, when, on getting up from her chair to go to the bed, she remarked ' I never felt better in my life.' She lay down on the bed, and was almost instantly seized with difficulty of breathing. I reached the house, which was near mine, in ten minutes after the attack, and found her tossing about the bed, — the countenance livid, the tongue blue, the pulse rapid, small and thread-like, only one sound of the heart, the respiration eighty in the minute. The only complaint made was of pain in epigastrium and difficulty of breathing. This state of things continued about fifteen minutes, till she died. There had been no secretion of milk."

DR. FITZ gave the following report of the autopsy, and showed the specimens : Body well nourished ; organs generally anæmic ; uterus retrograding normally. A soft, reddish-gray thrombus extended from the right common iliac vein into the inferior cava for two inches, its size that of the finger. In the right ovarian vein and in the vesical plexus, thrombi were also found. In the orifice of the tricuspid valve was found a club-shaped embolus, one and a half inches in length, the larger end of the size of the tip of the forefinger. Both primary pulmonary arteries were plugged with emboli ; also their branches extending into the upper lobes of both lungs. The upper lobes were œdematous, the lower ones injected.

DR. HODGDON, in answer to questions, stated that there had been no chill, no œdema of the legs, no cough nor expectoration. The suffering was intense. The resonance of the chest was great, and the ear apparently heard air entering a vacant space. The hæmorrhage at confinement was normal in amount.

Dr. Fitz referred to an autopsy in which he had found the pulmonary artery itself obstructed by a clot which, extending downwards, had become doubled upon itself so as to effectually plug the vessel. It had been a case of mild typhoid fever several months ago, under the care of Dr. Nichols, of Cambridge. In the third week, while the patient was lying comfortable, she was suddenly seized with intense dyspnœa, with lividity, which lasted fifteen or twenty minutes, when she died. A week previously there had been a rather sudden occurrence of slight cough with irritation of the larynx.

Sudden Death in Childbed. — Dr. Chadwick said he wished to consult the society as to the cause of death of a patient, whom, two weeks ago, at Framingham, he had been called to see with reference to the propriety of performing transfusion of blood. The patient had had her fourth child four weeks previously. The abdomen had been enormously distended by hydramnios; the labor was normal; the placenta was large. There was no unusual hæmorrhage. The recovery was apparently normal, and the patient nursed her child. But she was exceedingly anæmic, and had always presented this condition. Two or three weeks after delivery she had a faint turn. Four weeks after delivery, the night before Dr. Chadwick saw her, she had a tremor — not a rigor — with malaise. There was no pain, the pulse was very small, feeble, and rapid, and coma ensued. When Dr. Chadwick saw her she was unconscious. The pulse was 160, temperature 105°; the respiration was 30, though not much accelerated at first. The pulmonary sounds, by percussion and auscultation, were perfectly normal. The heart-sounds were clear, but with a souffle, probably anæmic, over the aorta. There was no inflammation in the pelvis. The pulse was several times brought back by subcutaneous injections of brandy. The temperature rose to 106° before the patient died. The uterus had a degree of involution normal to the fourth week after delivery. Transfusion was neither recommended nor performed. Was the cause of death embolism, fatty heart, perhaps resulting from " pernicious anæmia," as the Germans call it, or what was it? There was no suspicion of blood-poisoning, or of trouble with the kidneys. There was no autopsy.

Dr. Fitz said he thought the suddenness of the symptoms was against the view of pernicious anæmia, whose cause is a progressive one from bad to worse.

A Series of Severe Cases. — Dr. Hosmer read the following: —

" This group of cases, seen in the course of a month, is reported partly because some of them present interesting features, and partly because, taken as a whole, they show a strong tendency in prevailing diseases to assume a malignant and fatal type.

" Case I. A laboring man of fifty, of good health and habits, was seized' February 7th; he was first seen February 11th, and was found with erysipelas of the face and scalp of more than the average severity. Recovery ensued, but the convalescence was slow and tedious.

" Case II. A laboring man of sixty-five, with rather an unhealthy look, was attacked February 6th with phlegmonous erysipelas of the right leg, while living in the same house with the last patient. He was seen February 11th, when the symptoms were very mild; he was not seen again until February 17th, when the aspect of the case was extremely bad. Symptoms of septicæmia soon appeared, and death took place February 23d.

"Case III. A healthy boy, three years old, had had whooping-cough a month, beginning February 15th. Pneumonia of the right lung, not extensive, commenced February 18th, and the patient was first visited February 20th, and was found to be pretty sick, the pulse, respiration, and temperature all being represented by high figures. What most attracted attention was the hard, brawny, inelastic swelling which occupied the whole substance of both lips, the prolabium being covered with a heavy, yellow crust. The unnatural and excessive thickness of the lips produced a marked deformity which did not diminish at any time. Upon the lower part of the face and neck were numerous spots, none very large, of which some lost their color under pressure, while some did not.

"February 22d. I found a small, dark extravasation just at the entrance of the right nostril, also a second one on the back of the left hand at the junction of the fore and middle fingers, with slight vesication. At this point there was a small, superficial cicatrix caused by the bite of a dog received some weeks before.

"February 23d. Extravasations had not extended, but a brawny swelling covered the whole dorsum of the left hand. Nothing of special interest in connection with the pulmonary disease. Up to this time mind perfectly clear.

"February 24th. The swelling which yesterday was limited to the hand, now extended to the shoulder, occupying the whole diameter and length of the arm. In the middle of the right hypochondrium, just below the margin of the ribs, found an extravasation half an inch in diameter, covered by a vesicle, and surrounded by an infiltration fully an inch and a half in diameter. The whole aspect of the case indicated speedy death, which occurred the same evening. At no time was there any indication of hæmorrhage from a mucous membrane.

"Case IV. The patient was thirty-three years old, the wife of a laboring man, healthy. In June, 1873, then a primipara, she had a presentation of the cord, and lost her child.

"February 21st, at full term, first felt decided pain at nine A. M. The membranes were ruptured at one P. M., and a loop of cord was found in the vagina; the patient soon after rose from the bed, and more cord came down; she was first seen between half-past two and three o'clock. The head was above the brim, the os well dilated, and protruding from it were fifteen to sixteen inches of the cord, with a single knot tied in the very extremity of the loop. The pulsation was decided, but not very strong. Pains were feeble and infrequent. The patient was placed in the position which elevated the hips as much as possible above the level of the shoulders. With the left hand the prolapsed cord was carried far up towards the fundus of the uterus, and then left. Nothing more was seen of it until after the birth of the head, although the woman was soon allowed to resume the usual position on the left side. Delivery did not take place until eleven P. M. The child was still-born, but the mother was left in a condition satisfactory in all respects. .

"February 22d, eighteen hours after delivery; hot skin, frequent pulse, uterus large, tender, and the seat of constant and very severe pain. No chill, no nausea, tongue clean, eye bright, and expression of countenance in no wise bad. Flowing scanty, but normal in color.

"February 24th. Relieved in all respects, and showing a decided fullness in both breasts.

"February 25th. A very decided change for the worse. From this time the case exhibited marked symptoms of septicæmia, and terminated fatally February 27th.

"CASE V. Seen in consultation. A young primipara, the wife of a laborer, after a rather tedious labor, with a little assistance from the forceps at the last, was delivered of a living child, March 5th. At no time afterwards was the condition of things quite satisfactory ; but within forty-eight hours the aspect of the case excited alarm ; prominent among the early symptoms being a uterus enlarged, tender, and painful. March 10th, unequivocal signs of septic poisoning existed, including a sloughy condition of the lacerated perinæum, which became gangrenous before death, which occurred March 11th. The close resemblance between Cases IV. and V. was very striking.

"CASE VI. Mrs. ——, a lady of literary reputation, aged thirty-four, was suddenly seized, March 8th, with severe rigors, followed by extreme prostration, and exceedingly sharp pleuritic pain in the right side. She was seen in consultation March 9th. Physical signs in the right chest, insignificant ; on the left side, an extensive and rapidly increasing pneumonia, seated in the upper and anterior portion of the lung. The case did not present a single hopeful symptom, and everything seemed to indicate speedy death. To complete the record of the case, the patient was in her third pregnancy, advanced, as she insists, not much beyond the fifth month, though there are some reasons for doubting the correctness of her opinion.

"March 11th. Patient still living, and in labor, which commenced during the night. At nine A. M. liquor amnii escaped, and soon after the right arm of an apparently small fœtus, was found to be the presenting part, the greater part of its length being outside of the external labia. As the extremely critical condition of the woman seemed to make it certain that the slightest shock would prove fatal at once, and as she expressed the most decided aversion to any digital or manual interference, and as it was fully believed that the small fœtus could be expelled without any previous change of its position, or relations to the pelvis, it was decided to administer ergot for the double purpose of hastening delivery, and of securing a contraction of the uterus which should reduce to a minimum the post partum flowing. The drug produced absolutely no effect, and the process of labor was suspended for that day. At midday, March 12th, regular and efficient pains returned, and at four P. M. it was an easy matter to deliver the child. The placenta was readily removed ; the womb contracted well, and without hæmorrhage. Although the patient eventually died, she lingered for a fortnight, and once at least during that time was supposed to be moribund, but rallied.

"CASE VII. Mrs. M., a young woman, fell into her second labor February 9th, and the process was soon completed without medical assistance. A severe chill at six P. M. February 11th, marked the commencement of a scarlet fever, the full eruption of which was visible the next day. Fortunately the case went on kindly, and in the second week terminated favorably, without complications or sequelæ. On the third day of the illness of the mother, it was found that a process of desquamation, with some pretty large scales, was going on over the whole surface of the child.

"The foregoing cases were distributed over an area of five miles in diameter."

Dr. HOMANS asked Dr. Hosmer how he connected these cases?

Dr. HOSMER said that he had asked himself whether the death of his own parturient patient was due to his having attended the same morning the case of erysipelas. There was another case in Brighton, precisely similar to his own ; these were half a mile apart. These were the only cases of midwifery he had attended during the time covered by this report. He did not deliver the baby whose arm presented.

Dr. CHADWICK asked why ergot was given in that case.

Dr. HOSMER said the reasons were because the patient estimated that she was in the sixth month of pregnancy, and because ergot would shorten the process, diminish the flowing, and render manual interference unnecessary.

Dr. SINCLAIR asked if ergot should be given in a case of such extreme weakness.

Dr. HOSMER said he did not suppose there was any danger in it. He thought it better to give the ergot than use manual interference. The stomach was in good condition. He was prepared, if the ergot should prove inefficient, to draw upon the presenting limb.

Dr. REYNOLDS remarked that if version were likely to be required, ergot would produce an unfavorable tetanic state of the uterus.

Dr. HOSMER replied that the child was so small that its position was of no consequence.

Dr. REYNOLDS raised a point in regard to the use of ergot. He said it was very common at the present day to give from half a drachm to a drachm of the fluid extract of ergot immediately after the normal labor, with the idea that it would insure contraction and diminish the risk of post-partum hæmorrhage. Dr. Reynolds had been a good deal mortified to find the after-pains increased, sometimes intolerable, so that he had become cautious in using the drug. He had the strongest prejudice, or rather conviction, against the use of ergot at all times of labor, except when the uterus is empty. He could conceive a rational use of the drug, as when pressure is needed ; but as a pushing means, it is inconsistent with the known function or mode of action of the uterus.

Dr. ABBOT said he thought persistent contraction depended altogether upon the dose. With small, repeated doses he had found the uterine action intermittent. He had frequently given ergot in the last stages of labor with the hope of securing a good contraction of the uterus, and had seen the organ relax and contract as it usually does after the birth of the child. He would ascribe persistent contraction either to an excessive dose or to an unusual susceptibility to the action of the medicine. He had given ten drops every fifteen or twenty minutes to produce normal contractions. He always carried ergot with him, but did not use it very often. A former member of this society,

6

Dr. Palmer, used it frequently during labor. Dr. Hall had used it a good deal to accelerate labor, and never saw any bad results from its use.

DR. LYMAN remarked that McClintock and Hardy twenty years ago settled pretty conclusively the fact of danger to the child from the use of ergot. He supposed it was generally received as true that its employment was contraindicated before the birth of the child. After the birth he gave in almost every case twenty or thirty drops.

DR. REYNOLDS expressed a feeling of prejudice against the use of any means to hasten labor which is going on normally. The tendency is to hurry in order to save time. He deprecated ergot, rupturing of membranes, telling the patient to bear down, with a view to hasten normal labor.

DR. SINCLAIR said that it was his custom to give a drachm of the fluid extract of ergot immediately after the delivery of the placenta, in order to contract the uterus and to obviate the continuance of after-pains. Pains, it is true, are sometimes intensely increased after ergot, but for a much less time than if the ergot had not been given. One may thus bring about in a short period what takes days in the ordinary way, namely, the contracting of the uterus, the squeezing out of its contents. A year or two ago Dr. Sinclair had got out of the way of using ergot, but he had since returned to it.

DR. INGALLS inquired if any one ever had a case of normal labor in which he was not obliged to interfere in some way with his art.

DR. ARNOLD reported two cases of labor in the same individual, in which the process was very speedy, and accomplished without his assistance. In the first instance the patient awoke from sleep ten minutes before his arrival, and he found the child in the bed.

Dr. REYNOLDS gave the case of a girl eighteen years of age who had but one pain, while she was sitting on the vessel. The child was in the vessel, drowned in the liquor amnii. On attempting to raise the patient up she was found to be tethered down by the cord, the placenta being not yet delivered. In her second confinement, subsequently, the labor was not particularly rapid.

DR. INGALLS thought the giving of ergot very dangerous before the birth ; if it must be so used, it should not be until after the womb is well open and the head of the child well down.

Defective Development of Fœtus. — DR. TUCK read a case of defective development in a new-born child. The œsophagus terminated in the trachea. The specimen was also shown. The case will be published.

A SEA-SHORE HOME.

OF the vexed questions which baffle the skill of physicians and health officers, and defy the liberality of philanthropists, there are few which offer so difficult a problem for solution as the proper management of sick poor children during the summer months. The high rate of infant mortality continues to be the opprobrium of all large cities. The way in which this annual slaughter of infants and young children can be prevented is eminently a matter for investigation and experiment. The advantage of change of air and good nursing for those afflicted with diarrhœa and cholera infantum is generally recognized. We believe that the attempt was first made in London to treat these diseases in this manner on a large scale. A similar endeavor has been made recently in Atlantic City, near Philadelphia, where a " Children's Sea-Shore Home " has been provided, to which mothers may take their children for a few days when symptoms of danger first show themselves, and while the disease is amenable to treatment. The enterprise has been carried on thus far with gratifying results, although of course on a scale not at all commensurate with the numbers needing assistance. One hundred and eighty patients were treated last summer, and returned to their home, well and strong; many of them were, in all probability, thus saved from certain death.

The example of Philadelphia has been followed by Boston. A number of benevolent ladies and gentlemen have organized a similar charity and have already provided a new, well-built, and commodious house at Beverly Farms, where the half-roasted and neglected little patients can get good nursing, good treatment, and a breath of fresh sea-air. This experiment should receive the sympathy and assistance of all parents who take good care to remove their own children from the dangers of city life during the hot months. The excursions for young children lately inaugurated in this city and New York, if not productive of a great amount of physical benefit to the children, have proved of advantage in calling attention to this much-suffering class, and have undoubtedly paved the way to experiments like those which are now being made. These in their turn may lead to a more simple and practical solution of the problem, not now apparent. The advantages of such accommodation for infants and young children can be easily tested in all sea-board cities, and indeed in many inland ones; if the plan is found to work satisfactorily, it cannot fail to become a valuable addition to the prophylactic measures now employed to reduce the rate of mortality in crowded localities.

Though this charity is for the poor, the children of those in moderate circumstances who must remain in the city are not excluded, as they can enjoy the advantages of the home by payment of a moderate sum weekly. Prevention is better than cure. This is not so much a hospital as an institution to make one unnecessary.

THE SEWERAGE QUESTION.

THE first of a series of hearings was given by the sewerage commission at the City Hall on Friday last. It will be remembered that the commission appointed by the city to investigate this important subject consists of three members: Mr. E. T. Chesborough of Chicago, Mr. Moses Lane of Milwaukee, and Dr. Folsom the secretary of the State Board of Health. The noteworthy feature of this hearing was the very large attendance of people, who appeared much interested in the subject and appreciated its importance. The character of the testimony offered reminds one of that brought out at the time of the Mill River nuisance, although the locality of the sufferers, judging solely from the testimony thus far given, is different in the two cases. Witnesses appeared from the South End, and also from some of the neighboring towns. From the statements made it would appear that in various parts of the district mentioned, including most of the finest streets, the stench is terrible, often causing much sickness, particularly at night, when the warm weather necessitates open windows. The history of the changes made in the system of sewerage, if it may ever have been worthy of such a name, during the process of filling in the new lands is hinted at, and would doubtless be very startling could it be possible to get at the true facts. The condition of the drainage may be estimated from the statement that many of the cellars are almost constantly filled with water, partly from the surface drainage and partly from the incoming tide — this in houses which were in perfect condition ten years ago. The evidence as to the condition of the city was as complete as could be desired, and the impression seemed universal that the time had come when a postponement of the question could involve the city in great danger. The subject of a remedy was merely touched upon. The sentiment of many appeared to be in favor of large flushing basins and sewers carrying the sewage into deep water far south of the city. There are, however, unusual difficulties to be met with in the extremely low grade of certain portions of the new land which may necessitate a more complicated system than would ordinarily suffice for a large city. Curiously enough Boston, with unusual facilities for drainage, has so mismanaged and neglected this important question as to require the highest skill, and we dare not say how large sums of money, to get her out of the difficulty.

MEDICAL NOTES.

— It will be seen by a notice printed elsewhere that since May 3d all permits for burials must be obtained from the Board of Health, and not, as heretofore, from the office of the City Registrar, who previous to May 3d held the office of Registrar of Deaths and Burials in addition to that of City Registrar. The office of Registrar of Deaths and Burials has been abolished and the duties heretofore performed by that officer are now performed by the City Board of Health. All physicians' certificates are therefore to be signed in duplicate, one for registration and the other for the purpose of obtaining a permit for burial. The aldermen have taken a step in the right direction in inaugurating a movement which will place the Registrar's department under the Board of Health, where it properly belongs. In no other city in the Union, so far as we know, is it an independent office, and the sooner it is made subordinate to the Health office, the better.

— Dr. W. L. Richardson, of Boston, has been elected Acting Secretary of the State Board of Health during the temporary absence of the Secretary in Europe. All communications relating to the business of the board should be addressed to him at the State House

— We are requested to remind physicians of this State that, according to the new license law now so energetically carried out, apothecaries are not allowed to sell liquors, except alcohol, for any purpose without an order from a physician "between the hours of twelve at night and six in the morning or on any part of the Lord's day." If this is remembered, a great deal of delay and trouble will be saved. Every apothecary who has a license is under bonds of one thousand dollars to obey the law.

— The International Congress of Ophthalmology will meet in New York City on Tuesday, September 12, 1876, at twelve o'clock, noon. The following extracts from the rules of the congress will give an idea of the general character of the society, and of the terms of membership : —

" 1. The object of the International Periodic Congress of Ophthalmology is to promote ophthalmological science, and to serve as a centre to those who cultivate it. It will entertain no discussion foreign to this object.

" 2. The number of members is unlimited.

" 3. Every member must be either a doctor of medicine, or of surgery, or of science, or possess some other equivalent degree, or be distinguished for his scientific knowledge.

" 4. Candidates for admission into the society shall be admitted on presentation of their diploma or of their scientific title, unless ten members demand a ballot.

" 5. The sessions of the society shall take place every fourth year, and be limited to ten days.

" 11. The society gives no diploma. Before the opening of each session a card available for admission to all the meetings, and signed by the president and secretary, shall be given to each member on payment of his subscription (fixed at $2), and upon signature of his name on the register of those attending the meeting."

Among the members of this congress are such men as Arlt and Stellwag, of Vienna ; Giraud-Teulon, Javal, and Wecker, of Paris ; Helmholtz, of Berlin ; William Bowman, George Critchett, R. Liebreich, J. W. Hulke, and Soelberg Wells, of London ; Donders and Snellen, of Utrecht, Holland.

It is hoped that many of them will come to New York in 1876. The committee are making all efforts to secure a large attendance, and one that will leave its mark upon the progress of scientific ophthalmology. The coöperation of the profession of the United States in securing these objects is earnestly desired by the Provisional Committee appointed in London in 1872. The committee is composed of the following gentlemen : Cornelius R. Agnew, M. D., Henry D. Noyes, M. D., Daniel B. St. John Roosa, M. D.

— The celebrated French surgeon, Demarquay, died June 23, of cancer of the stomach. He was an eminent leader in surgery, and his death is a serious loss to science. His inventive genius contributed many valuable instruments and practical procedures to the surgeon's art. During the siege of Paris, 1870–71, Demarquay acted as chief surgeon of the ambulances.

— The *Sanitarian* makes the *Dubuque Telegraph* responsible for the story of a discoloration of the skin of a young lady's face, who had taken a child while afflicted with whooping-cough to the gas house, that the little one might inhale the gas escaping from the purifiers. When the gas arising from the lime came in contact with the lady's face, her skin commenced turning yellow, and finally assumed a dark hue. Her physician thinks the lady must have been in the habit of using some of the chemical preparations now in vogue for improving the complexion, and that the action of the gas upon these chemicals brought about the result here related. The lady made every effort to remove the discoloration, but without avail.

— Dr. Van Leent is reported in *L'Union Médicale* to have given some interesting statements regarding the therapeutics and the materia medica of Sumatra. The physicians of that island — who are the aged of both sexes — are accustomed to give their patients medicated baths. They administer cold baths not only in continued and intermittent fevers, but in other maladies. In the treatment of small-pox the patient is exposed while naked to a current of cold air, and is constantly rubbed with a brush dipped in cold water. Since the native priests have taken it into their hands to perform vaccination, this operation has encountered less opposition than among European nations. The materia medica comprises a great number of plants, for the most part of the family of the *Dioscoreaceæ* or *Aroideæ*. For hæmorrhages the bruised leaves and the hairy down of the *Polypodum Boromez* is found to be an energetic astringent. Notwithstanding the healthfulness of the climate and the medical knowledge diffused among the people, the maladies which prevail are sufficiently numerous; for example, intermittent fevers, dysentery, affections of the liver, small-pox, diseases of the heart, syphilis, leprosy, yaws, and purulent ophthalmia.

— A statue of John Baptist Morgagni was unveiled on the 27th of May in the Palace of Studies, in his native town of Forli. The occasion, says the *Lancet*, was one of unusual pomp, the result of many weeks' preparation; both at the unveiling itself and at the subsequent banquet the oratory was as effective as some of Italy's ablest and most accomplished speakers could make it. Like all men of his intellectual build, Morgagni was alive to the importance, and proficient in the principles, of other sciences than his own; and not the least interesting of the features of his *festa* was the exhibition of numerous autograph letters received by him from Sir Isaac Newton, Le Clerc, Boerhaave, Haller, Lancisi, Alberoni, Valsalva, and a host of other contemporary *savans*.

— At a recent meeting of the Société de Chirurgie, reported in *L'Union Médicale*, Dr. Laroyenne, of Lyons, related the cure by the elastic ligature of a case of spina bifida of the cervico-dorsal region, in a child three months old. M. Blot thought it hazardous to operate upon such tumors, as they sometimes diminished or completely disappeared spontaneously, and as in all cases where autopsies had been made branches or ramifications of nerves, or the tissue of the cord itself, have been found spread out on the walls of the tumor. M. Giraldès observed that spina bifida of the cervical or cervico-dorsal region never presents the nervous expansions spoken of by M. Blot. The tumors which appear in these regions are often entirely cured by the gradual narrowing and final obliteration of the aperture of communication with the spinal canal, or by fatty transformation of their contents; such tumors may, therefore, be operated on with safety, but the same cannot be said of those situated in the dorso-lumbar region. M. Desprès distinguished as tumors fit for operation those in which the orifice of communication is so narrow that the surgeon cannot return the fluid into the canal by compression. One ought not to operate on tumors easily reducible. M. Hovel disagreed with M. Despres, because he had seen cases in which it was impossible to cause the fluid to flow back into the spinal canal, and yet the orifice was of the size of a goose-quill.

— Dr. Ehrhardt (*Allgemeine medicinischen Central Zeitung*, 99, 1874) has tried radical treatment of hydrocele by electro-puncture four times with permanent success, using the interrupted current of the small apparatus of Gaiff. In the three cases the hydrocele had existed only a short time, and tapping had not been resorted to; the fluid, although in considerable quantity, was absorbed in three to five days without any reaction. In the fourth case the fluid was absorbed by the end of three weeks. In this case the patient was fifty-two years old, with a hydrocele on the right side, of eight years' standing; he had had it tapped often. After the last tapping the fluid had returned at the end of three weeks. The operation was performed in the following manner: Two large, sharp-pointed, inverted needles connected with the pole of the apparatus, were thrust into the swelling at a distance of six centimetres from one another, and to a depth of three centimetres, so that the needle projected into the fluid. The tunica vaginalis was very tough and thickened, so that there was some difficulty in inserting the needles. There was but little pain, the application lasting about five minutes. The needle of the negative pole on being withdrawn appeared blackened and oxidized. The patient, as a matter of precaution, remained two days in bed. Four months later there was still no return of the fluid. The author thinks that this method could not probably be effective where there was considerable alteration in the tunica vaginalis.

LETTER FROM PARIS.

MESSRS. EDITORS, — All things in Paris, omnibuses, cabs, market-carts, as well as matters scientific and otherwise, move along with great vivacity. Each succeeding morning brings with it its eight-o'clock rolls and coffee, and as long as this is the case, and as long as one is blessed with health and strength, there is no need to beat time, for he seems to *fly* by unheeded. Hospital work is always the first thing in order, and there is an *embarras de richesse* as to its choice. However, by buying each Saturday a *Progrès Médicale*, one can always know where to go, and what one can see when one has gone. At La Pitié, in the service of M. Verneuil, have been two cases of that rare disease known as the *mal perforant*. I am of the opinion (under correction always of your readers) that attention was first called emphatically to this disease by Nélaton in 1852, in an article in the *Gazette des Hôpitaux* of the date of January 10th of that year, under the title of " Affection singulier des os des pieds." In Nysten's Dictionnaire of about the same date, it is defined as an ulceration of the feet, perforating them at length, and peculiar to the warmer latitudes. Follin, in his excellent work on External Pathology, has given a very excellent description of it. Very lately, Calixte Soulages has written a work on this subject entitled Le Mal perforant, sa Pathogénie.

Soulages, as well as his predecessors, have all placed the commencement of the malady in a corn on the sole of the foot. From pressure constantly brought to bear on this corn in standing and walking, a serous bursa is produced beneath it. This bursa inflames, gives rise to ulceration and necrosis, thence invading the bones and articulations and destroying them. It is rebellious even to amputation, reappearing again and again after each successive ablation of the tissues above it. Here observation had rested for some time, when the preceding theory was sharply questioned. M. Verneuil showed his two *malades* to the class as triumphant refutations of this theory. These two patients had been bedridden for a long time, and yet the mal perforant had appeared during their decubitus. M. Duplay, who has written a memoir on this subject, has cited many facts of this kind; one in which this disease had been produced by a gun-shot wound implicating the sciatic nerve, and another where the compression of the roots of the sciatic nerve by a tumor had produced the same result. Even M. Soulages himself has reported in his thesis the case of a mason, twenty-eight years old, who in a fall from the third story had fractured the spinal column. This fracture was accompanied by a complete paraplegia of movement, and by urinary troubles. The paralytic symptoms disappeared little by little, but there was atrophy of the lower limbs and deformity of the feet, which curved themselves *en griffe*. Symmetrical ulcerations showed themselves at the metatarsal articulations of the first phalanges of the great toes. It seems not improbable, after all, that these ulcerations of the feet known as the mal perforant are brought about not by mechanical causes, but by lesions of the trophic nerves.

A fortnight ago I commenced following, at St. Louis Hospital, the clinique of M. Lalliér, and very excellent it is. M. Lalliér is an elderly gentleman whose hair is somewhat silvered, and whose countenance is expressive of a great deal of *bonhomie* mixed with an occasional *bon esprit*. He is the successor of M. Gibert, whom I, as well as many of your elderly readers, must recall to recollection. A fluent speaker, with remarkably clear enunciation, ready and apt at diagnosis, skilled and successful in treatment, *voila* M. Lalliér! With him one can see on each successive Friday many most interesting cases. On the occasion of my first visit he showed us a case of most difficult diagnosis. I do not remember the number of the bed, but the patient was an elderly man of somewhat feeble aspect, presenting at the upper and inner part of the left thigh a patch of skin of a whiter color than its surroundings, and having a surface drilled with little holes (areolæ), such as one often sees in the skin covering a cancerous breast. This patch was perhaps two inches square. It was not painful; it was not ulcerated. M. Lalliér called M. Bazin in consultation. M. Bazin instantly declared it was a white keloid. M. Lalliér recalled to mind a thesis written some years ago by a gentleman of Bordeaux, whose name I did not catch, on the subject of partial atrophies of the face, and he had then stated what in fact M. Lalliér had himself observed, that these partial atrophies of the face were preceded by a state of the skin exactly resembling this case. This was, then, a case similar to those observed in the face. These had been referred to a lesion of innervation, a lesion, in point of fact, of the trophic nerves; hence M. Lalliér " passed his diagnostic" in this regard, and did not accept that of M. Bazin, namely, " white keloid." Another interesting case which I saw with M. Lalliér was illustrative at once of the evils which spring from an error in diagnosis, of the march of the moderns to the solution of medical problems, and the folly of us graybeards when we try to unite youth and beauty with age and infirmities. A man at least sixty-three years old entered the hospital with a *belle syphilide.* The *malade* told us with evident pride that forty years ago he had been treated by that great and good man Biett, at St. Louis, for an Hunterian chancre ; that Biett had given him mercury at that time with such vigor that he had lost all his teeth and a part of his lower jaw. Yet here he was forty years afterwards with a papular syphilide. This was an outrage on the blessed memory of Biett. M. Lalliér could not believe in a secondary eruption taking forty years for its appearance, and turned the bedclothes completely down, when a splendid indurated chancre was seen. How came this about? In this wise. Three months ago he had married Fifine, a young person of twenty-three years. Fifine had a lover *de plus.* M. Lalliér remarked to the class that it was ever so ; that Cupidon wore a frowning face for elderly people. Thus the *malade* lost his teeth and part of his jaw under Biett for a *chancre mou*, and all to no purpose. Jealousy is so rampant in France that I have looked in Figaro for news of the death of Fifine and her lover.

Another singular case in the wards of M. Lalliér is that of a young man twenty-three years of age, who entered St. Louis for an affection of the skin, diagnosticated by M. Lalliér as erythema marginatum, accompanied by large vesicles or bullæ. M. Lalliér remarked that erythema marginatum had been placed by M. Bazin in his category of arthritic skin diseases, and in truth it appeared that this patient had been somewhat subject to rheumatism in years past ; that some days before his entrance into the hospital he had been to a ball, whence he had issued in a great heat and full perspiration ; that to this had succeeded the eruption. At our visit on the next Friday, I found this patient exceedingly sick, and upon auscultation M. Lalliér found a to-and fro souffle at the region of the heart ; the bullæ had become larger and more numerous ; the joints painful and swollen, and it was evident that we were in presence of an acute rheumatism. Some days after this visit, the *interne* of M. Lalliér found at the base of the left lung indications of pneumonia or acute congestion, which rapidly disappeared to reappear in the right lung. This pneumonia was not accompanied by the usual rusty expectoration. M. Lalliér declared that all the intercurrent affections of acute rheumatism partook of its, evanescent, transitory character ; thus in intercurrent rheumatic pneumonia (for such was this case) one found the same rapid appearance and disappearance as one found in the articulations. In the female wards I saw another case of this rheumatic erythema marginatum. Thus M. Bazin's end of the see-saw is just now uppermost at St. Louis, notwithstanding some weeks ago a brother dermatologist at this hospital, aggravated perhaps by the heat of the weather, had torn up by the roots and trampled into the mire poor M. Bazin's theory of arthritic maladies de la peau, hydroa and all. With M. Lalliér I also saw two curious cases of papilloma of the skin : one in an old man, affecting the back of the right hand, diagnosticated as probably epithelial ; the other in a young man, affecting a precisely similar region, but diagnosticated as scrofulous. M. Lalliér's service is an excellent one to follow.

At La Charité, in the service of M. Gosselin, have been three cases of great interest. One was a case in which M. Gosselin some three weeks or a month ago had removed a malignant-looking tumor (diagnosticated by him as sarcomatous, but which the microscope declared to be epithelial) from the head, near the junction of the parietal and occipital bones, and which had sprung originally from a wen. It had been removed superficially some three times, but had rapidly returned. M. Gosselin took away not merely the tumor, but dissected off the periosteum, or pericranium. At the expiration of some ten days the patient had strangulated hernia, operated for by M. Gosselin. Some days after this the patient complained of a violent pain in her bowels,·and died suddenly very soon after. M. Gosselin had diagnosticated a perforation of intestine. The autopsy, however, showed that this had not been the case, but there *was* found an embolus of the pulmonary artery. On further search, the external iliac vein was found inflamed, probably, said M. Gosselin, from its proximity to the hernia; it contained clots, one of which had, in the opinion of M. Gosselin, wandered to the heart, and thence to the pulmonary artery. An examination of the skull showed the tumor in full flower of reappearance from the bones themselves.

The second case was one of stricture of the urethra which had been operated on by M. Gosselin, by divulsion, I understood after the manner of Voillemiér. All had gone well for thirty hours when the first rigor appeared. "This," said M. Gosselin, "is most unusual." After this an abscess formed in the corpora spongiosum; a few days of comparatively mild illness and the patient died suddenly. An enormous abscess was making its way through the greater sciatic notch, and another existed at the neck of the bladder, prevesical.

The third case was one which M. Gosselin took yesterday morning for his clinical lecture. A woman who had been for a long time in the wards of M. Bernutz, and considered as an hysterical patient, with locomotor ataxia, suddenly complained of a most intolerable pain in the right hip, pain so severe that she fell back on the floor in a faint. The patient said that she had heard a crack, and knew that her hip was broken. The pain was succeeded by enormous swelling. M. Gosselin, called in consultation, found a shortening of a centimetre and a half, eversion outward, etc. He diagnosticated a fracture of the cervix femoris, with large effusion of blood. The patient died, and M. Gosselin presented the specimen. He did not wish for condonation; he had diagnosticated fracture of the cervix femoris. Eh bien! there was no fracture of the cervix, because there was no cervix, or even head of the femur, or round ligament, or cartilage of the acetabulum, even a part of the rim of the acetabulum was lacking. At the autopsy the swelling of the hip was found to be a very large abscess, the cavity of the acetabulum was full of pus, which found an escape through a rent in the capsular ligament, and it was this rent that the patient had perceived at the time of the accident and had described as a crack. This capsular ligament was extremely thick and tough, and contained in its thickness many fragments of bone which M. Gosselin compared to the bony stalactites found in chronic arthritis. M. Gosselin knew of no case of absorption of bone comparable to this; hence he believed that we were in presence of a case of congenital absence of the head and neck of the femur. The absence of cartilage in the acetabulum showed that this state of things had existed a long

time. There was eburnation of bone. Certainly this person must have always had shortening, must have always limped, must have been always more
or less incapable of getting about; but this had not been sufficiently inquired
about at her entrance into hospital, and she had been considered as nervous
and as having had locomotor ataxia ; the latter was undoubtedly true, but it
was not one of the kind Charcot and Vulpian have described.

W. C. B. Fifield.

Paris, *May* 8, 1875.

MUMPS.

A REPLY TO DR. F. M. WILSON'S INQUIRY.

It has been my fortune to see quite a number of cases of mumps during
twenty-five years of practice, and this is the sum so far as their translated effects
are concerned.

Of inflammation of the testicles, four cases. Of the ovaries, two. None of
the mammæ.

These cases were all in children, or young persons, and all mild, trifling,
except one which occurred in a clergyman, twenty-five years old and the
father of one child. He had had a usual attack of the mumps and was recovering to all appearances, so that he thought it safe to venture out on a walk.
Pain and swelling of the testicles followed. Indeed so great was his distress
and so high the febrile excitement that he was in delirium the whole night pre-
vions to my seeing him, or the second night after his walk. I found him in
an intense febrile state, with furred tongue, breath fœtid, red scrotum, and in
pain from head to foot, but chiefly in his head. I should surely have thought
that the membranes of the brain were involved had there not been sufficient
evidence to account for the severity of the symptoms in the huge testicles, which
were nearly as large as one's fist, and exceedingly tender.

The treatment resorted to was, first, raising the scrotum, supporting and
protecting the part by cotton-wool ; second, poultice with mustard to the
parotid ; third, an anodyne to relieve the pain, with the free use of saline diaph-
oretics. He made a good recovery and subsequently added to the number
of his children. The character of his case clearly disproves the idea that the
mumps in the testicles is always a " trifling " disease.

Dr. Wood tells us in his Practice that there is reason to conjecture that the
pancreas is sometimes the seat of this translation. He also says that metastasis
to the brain occasionally takes place, and that this occurrence is the chief danger
from the mumps.

I had frequently been in and out among cases of this disease ever since I was
a schoolboy, when it raged through the winter school. I had examined patients,
handled them, looked into their mouths, breathed their breath, and never took
the disease till three years ago. At that time my children, with others in the
neighborhood, were taken down with it. I held my children, and took care of
my boy through the night, and got the mumps. Why then, and not before, if it
is contagious ? I had the measles when a small child, and took the scarlet fever
at the age of twenty-one on my first known exposure ; but why so slow in getting the mumps ?

E. Chenery.

WEEKLY BULLETIN OF PREVALENT DISEASES.

THE following is a bulletin of the diseases prevalent in Massachusetts during the week ending July 10, 1875, compiled under the authority of the State Board of Health from the returns of physicians representing all sections of the State : —

The most noteworthy feature of the reports for the past week is that they indicate the very general prevalence throughout the State of diarrhœa and kindred intestinal disorders. The increase in the diseases mentioned is most noticeable in the centres of population, the metropolitan section leading in this respect. Typhoid fever is beginning its annual ravages, especially in the country. The report for each section is as follows : —

In Berkshire : diarrhœa, cholera morbus, whooping-cough.

Valley : diarrhœa, cholera morbus, rheumatism. Easthampton reports one fatal case of small-pox; no new cases. South Hadley Falls reports a severe type of chicken-pox.

Midland : diarrhœa, rheumatism, measles. A physician in Worcester states that there has been an " unusual amount of peritonitis, partial and general, puerperal and other, in that city and throughout the county, during the last four months." A physician in Shrewsbury reports the death by lightning of a man in an open field, without rocks or trees near him..

Northeastern : diarrhœa, measles, cholera morbus. Unusually healthy in general. Natick has a fresh invasion of measles. Wakefield reports a fatal case of meningitis.

Metropolitan : diarrhœa, cholera morbus, bronchitis, rheumatism, scarlatina, cholera infantum, pneumonia — more sickness than for some time.

Southeastern : rheumatism, diarrhœa, typhoid. Not much sickness.

F. W. DRAPER, M. D., Registrar.

COMPARATIVE MORTALITY-RATES FOR THE WEEK ENDING JULY 3, 1875.

	Estimated Population.	Total Mortality for the Week.	Annual Death-rate per 1000 during Week.
New York	1,040,000	565	28
Philadelphia	775,000	526 [1]	35
Brooklyn	450,000		
Boston	350,000	171	25
Providence	100,700	31	16
Worcester . . .•. . .	50,000	23	24
Lowell	50,000	12	12
Cambridge	44,000	11	13
Fall River	45,000	24	28
Lawrence	33,000	21	34
Springfield	33,000	10	16
Lynn	28,000		
Salem	26,000	9	18

THE BOSTON
MEDICAL AND SURGICAL JOURNAL.

VOL. XCIII. — THURSDAY, JULY 22, 1875. — NO 4.

—————•—————

THE TREATMENT OF TYPHOID FEVER BY COLD BATHS.[1]

BY R. T. EDES, M. D.,

Visiting Physician at the Boston City Hospital.

GALEN defines fever as *calor præter naturam* — preternatural heat. More recent studies have added to, not changed, this definition ; but although the mechanism of the preternatural heat has been partly explained by laborious measurements, the real cause is far from being clear. While animal heat was regarded as an inherent attribute of the animal body, just as contractility belongs to muscles or excitability to nerves, the fact of its remaining so nearly constant in the normal mammalian body needed no explanation ; but when we consider the body as a complex organism, warmed within by the burning up of part of its tissues, and cooled without by radiation and evaporation into an atmosphere which may vary within limits of much more than a hundred degrees of Fahrenheit, our problem becomes more complicated.

For the sources of heat in the body we have to look to the combustions and decompositions always going on throughout, but chiefly to the vital organs of digestion, secretion, and respiration. The liver, for instance, may be looked upon as one of the most powerful of the furnaces which heat us. The blood is the great distributer of heat, receiving it from the internal organs and distributing it to the cooler surface and extremities. Direct conduction, however, in the trunk at least, plays an important part. The skin is the radiator and one of the evaporators, and the variation in the amount of blood circulating through its vessels, and the greater or less abundance of its secretion, are probably by far the most important circumstances in regulating the withdrawal of heat from the body.

An elevated temperature, as in fever, may arise from either increased production, diminished loss, or both together. It has been generally received until lately, on the ground of an increase of urea excreted in fever as compared with urea excreted by a healthy person on the same diet (that is, a restricted or antiphlogistic), that an increased chemical action throughout the body is the cause of the rise of temperature. A

[1] Read at the Annual Meeting of the Massachusetts Medical Society.

recent writer on fever [1] calls this theory an axiom. This view, however, has been shown to be, if not incorrect, at least only partially representing the truth. The laborious and minute measurements of ingesta, egesta, temperature, and loss of heat, carried out by Senator,[2] show that although the amount of urea discharged by a fever patient is greater than would be discharged by the same patient on the same diet in health, it is not enough in excess of that excreted upon the usual and normal diet to account for the excess of heat produced. The other non-nitrogenous constituents of the body are burnt in even less proportion than those furnishing urea. The amount of heat given off, as measured by him in a chamber carefully constructed for that purpose, although after the beginning of the fever slightly in excess, is not so great as represented by Liebermeister.[3]

It can be shown, on the other hand, that a mere retention of heat, without any increased production, is quite enough to raise the temperature to the febrile point.[4] If *all* the heat usually given off from the surface in half an hour could be retained, the temperature of the body would rise one degree of Centigrade, — or about one degree of Fahrenheit in twenty minutes. A partial retention of heat can be shown, by appropriate methods of measurement, actually to take place, and this too in a way which might easily convey the contrary impression, that is, that the body was growing cooler instead of warmer. In the so-called cold stage of intermittent, when the extremities and skin are shrunken and cool, the patient shivering and complaining of cold, the temperature of the interior of the body is actually rising, and for the very reason that the exterior of the body is poorly supplied with blood, and has consequently become an imperfect radiator. The case is precisely similar to that of a house warmed by steam pipes, where the boiler and rooms near it can be made hotter by shutting off the steam from the more distant radiators. Later, the arterioles relax, the warm blood flows quickly through the skin, is exposed to the cooler air, the sweat flows freely, is evaporated from the surface, and the body is cooled in accordance with well-known laws of physics.

This tendency to return to the normal temperature is a result of many and complicated relations between circulation, secretion, and the sensitive and vaso-motor nerves, relations which may be interrupted by certain lesions, such as section of the spinal cord, and which are probably disarranged but not interrupted in fever. In the former case the mammalian becomes more or less a cold-blooded animal, and his temperature depends upon that of the surrounding atmosphere,

---

[1] Dr. H. C. Wood. A Study of the Nature and Mechanism of Fever. Fourth Toner Lecture. 1875.

[2] Untersuchungen über den Fieberhaften Process und seine Behandlung.

[3] Volkmann's klinische Vorträge. No. 19.

[4] Winkonitz. Wiener Klinik. Jahrgang I.

of which his heat-regulating apparatus no longer makes him comparatively independent. This is not the case in fever. The fevered organism is not incapable of regulating its temperature. It does not. follow that of the surrounding atmosphere, but it does regulate itself at a higher point than normal. The apparatus is readjusted for 103° to 106° instead of 98°, and this temperature has just as unfavorable a result upon the activity of the heart and the constitution of the blood as if it were the result of artificial or extraneous heating.

That increased temperature is really the cause of many of the phenomena of fever can hardly be doubted. Many of them can be reproduced by artificial heating, and disappear on withdrawing the source of heat. The heart beats more rapidly when its temperature is raised a few degrees, but is also more easily exhausted. Urea is formed in greater abundance, but instead of coming in part from the food it is a derivative of already formed tissues, especially of muscle and blood. As regards the destruction of nerve-tissue, we know less physiologically ; but in long-continued cases few of us will doubt, on clinical grounds, that it suffers severely. The fever-heat increases combustion, and increased combustion augments the heat.

In typhoid, the mechanism by which heat is accumulated cannot be so clearly made out as in the short and simple paroxysm of intermittent. If the skin were dry and anæmic throughout the disease, we should have the conditions necessary for a constant retention and heaping up of heat; but we know that the contrary is often the case. It is probable, however, that only during a small portion of the time in typhoid is the skin in a fitting condition to carry off the maximum of heat necessary to completely regulate the body-temperature, and that although it can and does, at the height of the fever, radiate a larger amount of heat than in health, yet it is not capable of disposing of all which is produced by increased combustion. If we recognize the fact that excessive febrile temperature, as increasing organic combustion, as perverting the action of the nervous system, and especially as exhausting and weakening the heart, if not the only injurious phenomenon of typhoid, is at any rate one of the most so, and in a certain proportion of cases the only cause of death, then the permanent or temporary reduction of that heat becomes the principal object to which a rational treatment should be directed. For this purpose two courses are theoretically open : the diminution of heat-production, the acceleration of heat-loss. Neither of these is impossible for a short time, neither is possible without continuous treatment. Heat-production may be limited by drugs which retard metamorphosis, especially abnormal metamorphosis, of tissue. The most important and efficient of these is quinia in large doses, which is known not only to produce in physiological experiments the effect just stated, but which can easily be shown to reduce a morbid temperature, even

in continued fevers, for many hours. This is no unimportant adjunct
of the treatment we have specially to consider.

But it is the other factor, which naturally varies within the widest
limits, which is capable of fully compensating an increased heat-production, and which is also easily under our control. It has been estimated
by measurements of the amount of heat given off from various parts of the
surface of the body, that an entirely possible loss of heat could, if continuous, compensate more than three times the normal heat-production, and
that the variations in the amount of heat given off are quite enough to
account for the constancy of bodily temperature under all circumstances of
climate, without any reference to a change in heat-production. A retention of heat in the body during the initial stages of fevers can be demonstrated. For a paroxysm of intermittent or a short attack of febricula,
the amount retained during the initial stage, when the limbs and the
surface are cold, is sufficient· to account for the whole rise of temperature which is taking place from the beginning. In continued fevers
there is more difficulty in explaining why the temperature continues so
long at an abnormal height, although it is probable that subsequent accu-
mulations of heat of the same kind, arising from slighter chills which
may occur in the course of the disease, are added to the initial retention. This retention is brought about by the changes in the circulation
of the skin. An anæmic and marbled surface, even if warm, radiates
much $_{less}$ heat and cools much less blood than one in which the circulation is active ; while, on the other hand, a surface in which venous
stasis has taken place, even in slight degree, parts also with little heat.
While the amount radiated from a surface which has been briskly
rubbed or reddened with mustard-water is increased, it is diminished if
strong irritation causes even the slightest approach to passive congestion.

Exposure of the skin to cold, by contracting the superficial vessels, also
diminishes its ability to radiate heat, and this diminution may take place
from cold air, which is a bad conductor, as well as from cold water,
which is a good one ; so that we can see why exposure to a cool atmosphere is not so efficient in removing heat as immersion in cold water.

It has been stated by at least one experimenter,[1] and he too one of
the warmest advocates of this method, that more heat is produced when
the surface is cooled, and that the real efficacy of the baths is owing to a
subsequent reaction from the over-production, and not to a primary cooling. This, however, cannot be looked upon as proved, and the increased
elimination of carbonic acid, which is one of the supports of this theory,
is possibly only excretion, and not formation.

The action of a cold bath is probably somewhat as follows : The external surface is more or less rapidly chilled. Less blood circulates

---

[1] Liebermeister. Loc. cit.

therein, and the skin and subcutaneous tissue become bad conductors, thus attempting to protect the body against the abstraction of heat. It is physiologically possible, as we see in the case of the marine mammalia, that an animal should be so thoroughly protected by his skin and fat as to be capable of resisting indefinitely, in the water, a temperature far below that of the body ; but in man, whose heat-regulating apparatus is arranged for another surrounding medium, and who is in the habit of supplementing the protection given by his skin with artificial coverings, this is only possible for a short time, and then the temperature of the body in general must, after a longer or shorter time, fall and reach that of the surrounding medium ; that is, the protection is temporary and imperfect.

In an ordinary bath of from ten to twenty or more minutes, the fall of temperature is not much felt at first in the interior of the body. In the limbs, which present more surface in proportion to their bulk, and which form but little heat for themselves, the cooling action is much more felt ; and the inequality of temperature between different parts of the body often gives rise to the feeling of chill, which, although of course not agreeable to the patient and somewhat alarming to those practicing this method for the first time, has absolutely no unfavorable import or result. When the patient is removed from the bath, the external cold being replaced by warmth, the arterioles dilate, the blood circulates more rapidly through the cooler external layers, and the abnormally high temperature of the interior is reduced by the transfer of heat to the surface to nearly, but not quite, its former height. Thus it is found that temperature continues to fall for some time after a bath, and does not reach its lowest point when the bath is over, but half an hour or so afterward. The temperature after a time again begins to rise, and attains its former height in a longer or shorter time, according to the intensity of the disease.

After considering the facts just stated, and especially certain important points which are yet far from being settled, such as the alleged over-production of heat during a bath, it will easily be granted that although physiology and experiment may lead us to look favorably upon the cold-water treatment, and furnish a sort of *a priori* argument in its support, yet the final judgment must come from actual experience. Cold bathing in typhoid is no new thing, having been proposed and used as a remedy in the latter part of the last century by Jackson and Currie,[1] and with considerable reputation ; but it soon fell into neglect, possibly for the same reasons which will oppose its spread at the present time.

Various methods of applying cold externally in typhoid fever have been used, but of these some demand no more than a mere mention. The cold affusion, cold shower-bath, or a plunge into the sea are not likely

[1] Medical Reports on the Effects of Water, cold and warm, as a Remedy in Fever and other Diseases. Philadelphia: 1808. (From fourth London Edition.)

to find general acceptance, and observations as to their effects will be rare.

We have really to consider four : —

1. Cold sponging, more or less frequently repeated, is the easiest, but the least effectual, in withdrawal of heat, and it is chiefly of use when other means cannot be employed. Its soothing influence upon the dry and burning skin is, however, of no small advantage.

2. The cold pack is a method which may be of use in private practice, if the others are objected to. Two or three renewals of the wet sheets are necessary, however, to equal in effect a full bath. It has been suggested that the sheets may be repeatedly sprinkled with cold water, and of course if this is frequently and thoroughly done, the method approximates more or less a full bath.

3. The simple full cold bath by immersion is the method which has been most employed, and which is perhaps the most efficient, demanding a less expenditure of time, labor, and water. In Germany, apparently, the same tub of water is used several times. Against this method is chiefly to be urged its apparent harshness.

4. The fourth plan is the one which seems to me to combine greater advantages than any other, although it is, to be sure, the only one of which I have personal experience, unless the first be excepted. With the arrangements in our hospitals and in the better class of dwelling-houses, it is not difficult to carry out. The patient is placed in a bath near the temperature of the body, 100° for instance ; then warm water is drawn off and cold added until a limit of between seventy and eighty degrees or less is reached. Two or three feet of India-rubber hose slipped upon the cold-water faucet is convenient in cooling the bath equally, and avoiding the splash and noise of the running water. The patient's limbs should be rubbed by attendants to equalize as far as possible the circulation, and thus promote the cooling from a larger surface. After ten or fifteen or more minutes he may begin to shiver, and he should then be placed in bed and covered up. If the chill be severe, heaters may be placed to the feet, the amount of heat thus added at a distance from the trunk being small, while it greatly relieves the subjective sensations of chill. A glass of wine may also be administered, especially if, as sometimes happens, the pulse becomes small. The effect of the latter is to excite the heart and dilate the arterioles of the surface, thus promoting the transfer of heat from the interior to the exterior. Its physiological action seems to be peculiarly adapted to this stage of the treatment, and, indeed, I am not sure that it would not be better to make the wine the rule rather than the exception.

The disadvantages of this form are the necessary time, labor, and water, disadvantages which, of course, must vary greatly in weight according to the circumstances of the special case. It is also somewhat, though not materially, less efficient than the full cold bath, and if long continued its effects are possibly of longer duration. In its favor are its great apparent mildness, and, possibly, a less tendency to reaction and over-formation of heat.

How often and when should baths be given ? The German authors answer this question very simply by saying, Whenever the temperature, which should be measured at least as often as every two or three hours, reaches a certain point. This point is fixed by Liebermeister at 102° if taken in the axilla, or 103° in the rectum ; by Ziemssen [1] at 104° in the rectum during the first two weeks of the fever, later, at a somewhat lower point.

Such frequent measurements, and especially carrying on the bathing through the night, demand an amount of skilled labor which has not been at my command, and my habit has been, upon observing the temperature of the day before, and the condition of the patient at the morning visit, to order the baths for the day, usually specifying approximately the hours.

Ziemssen states that when gradually cooled baths are used, and one is given whenever the temperature reaches 104°, at first, usually four or five, or at the most six, baths are necessary in the twenty-four hours, and that these usually fall between the hours of one and two, six and eight, and ten and eleven in the forenoon, one and two, four and six, and eight and nine in the evening. When less than six are given, that between eight and nine is first omitted, and then one in regular succession from the beginning. Four baths per diem I have often given, but never, I think, six.

With four I have usually two in the afternoon, to anticipate the evening rise of temperature, and one as late in the evening as is compatible with the arrangements for night-watchmen, etc., in order to have the effect last as far into the night as possible. A bath in the evening often helps materially in procuring a good night's rest. I admit that this is only an imperfect carrying out of the system, but the circumstances I have alluded to rather than my own wishes are responsible therefor.

Let us consider what practical experience says of. the advantages of the cold water method, and what it can or cannot do. I now speak of the more efficient methods, that is, the cold or gradually cooled full bath, and most distinctly do not mean in the least tepid or cold sponging, although we may be obliged to use it as an inefficient substitute. In using statistics, which I shall do sparingly, I am fully aware how erroneous may be their teaching, from the varying intensity of different epidemics, the class of population from which the patients are drawn, the

---

[1] Ziemssen and Immerman. Die Kaltwasser Behandlung des Typhus abdominalis. Leipzig. 1870.

time at which they seek assistance, the treatment other than medical, the hygienic surroundings, and the varying diagnosis. But sufficiently large numbers may now be obtained to eliminate some of these sources of error, and among them series of cases from the same hospitals, where two different methods have been practiced.

As there may be those who will attribute a decreased mortality under cold water rather to a disuse of other treatment than to a use of the baths, and will intimate that the patients get well not because they are *bathed*, but because they are *not drugged*, we ought to take as our standard of comparison series of cases which have received but little active treatment, and inquire whether this method produces any favorable change in the natural course of the disease. Unfortunately the large numbers of cases assembled by Murchison cannot be taken as representing a purely expectant treatment, but merely an average of all treatments, into which we may suppose the expectant entered pretty largely. The more modern the statistics, the fewer disturbing elements, we may suppose, will affect the natural course of the disease. This abstinence from active medication is probably on the whole a gain, but it by no means follows that all plans of treatment must have been harmful, nor does it follow that a pure expectancy is the safest treatment.

It is to be remembered that none of the modern promoters claim for cold bathing any power to cut short the typical and, so to speak, normal course of the disease, nor to rob it of many of its essential features. The fever, that is, the abnormally high temperature, is the only symptom directly affected thereby ; but as a secondary consequence of this we have, as is claimed, slower pulse and stronger heart, less nervous disturbance, less delirium, less diarrhœa, fewer bedsores, and a more rapid convalescence. In this way the length of the sickness may be shortened, though the " run of the fever " is not, and the favorable results become most evident in a lighter form of disease and a decreased rate of mortality. ·We do not so much expect wonderful recoveries in very severe cases, as we do large numbers of cases which, if this treatment be early adopted, do not become severe at all and do not develop in the highest degree the most dangerous symptoms of the disease.

An average rate of mortality from typhoid might be stated which would be accurate within quite narrow limits, but the value of such a statement for our purpose would be less than that of statistics giving more fully the methods of treatment.

In the eighteen thousand cases tabulated by Murchison the average mortality was eighteen and sixty-two hundredths per cent., but the separate groups of cases which went to make up this large number varied from sixteen to thirty-two per cent. Chambers gives one hundred and twenty-one cases, with a mortality of only two and a half per cent.;

three hundred and three cases from the Massachusetts General Hospital give a mortality of about thirteen per cent. ; Dr. Upham's one hundred and fifty-two from the City Hospital,[1] about fourteen per cent. ; Dr. Flint's seventy-three cases, about twenty-four per cent. In two sets of cases at Bellevue Hospital, quoted by Dr. Flint, in which the treatment was chiefly by stimulants, except that in one series dilute sulphuric acid was administered, the rates were respectively twenty and ten per cent.

M. Bordier[2] represents the average mortality in the hospitals of Paris under the ordinary methods of treatment as from five to nine per cent. ; but in the one hundred and forty-seven Parisian cases included in Murchison's collection it was thirty-two per cent.

Now as to the results from cold bathing : Jürgensen[3] reports from the same hospital at Kiel a reduction of mortality from fifteen to three per cent. ; Liebermeister, from sixteen to nine per cent.; Ziemssen and Immermann, from thirty to nine per cent. Brand reports fourteen hundred and eleven cases with a mortality of four per cent., and one series of one hundred and seventy with no mortality at all.[4] Lissauer[5] observed in three army hospitals a mortality of twenty-four per cent. under expectant treatment, six by cold water. His numbers are, however, small.

M. Bordier, in criticising these with some other statistics, says that the wonder is not so much why patients have done so well with the baths, but why they did so badly before, and endeavors to show from his table (which is a very complete one) that the average results claimed by the advocates of cold baths are really no better than those obtained by others who do not use them ; but in his own tables, the total calculation of which is of no great value, since the number of cases upon which the percentages are computed is not given, we find the groups where the mortality is zero only upon the cold water side, and of these there are six, not including Brand's which I have just mentioned.

Giving due weight to the fact that many physicians who have published tabular statements on this subject are ardent advocates of this treatment, it certainly seems as if the comparison of series of cases in the same hospital were as little open to objection as any method of using statistics. It would be easy to collect many more groups of this character even from the table of M. Bordier himself, but as there are but few statistics directed to this point which give a different result, I may refer at once to these exceptions.

Two series of cases are reported from Duchek's clinic at Vienna where the cold water treatment gave a mortality of twenty-eight per cent. as

---

[1] Medical and Surgical Reports. Boston City Hospital. First Series.

[2] Journal de Thérapeutique. 1874, page 465, *et seq.*

[3] Klinische studien über die Behandlung des abdominalis Typhus mittelst des Kalten wassers. Leipzig. 1866.

[4] Ziemssen and Immermann. Op. cit.

[5] Centralblatt für die medicinische Wissenschaften. 1872, page 47.

against twenty-seven per cent. without such treatment.[1] The figures are too high and the difference too small for us not to suspect that something more than either baths or the omission of them must have been responsible· for this great mortality of more than one death in four patients.

Four other series give in typhoid fifteen per cent. for bathing as against twenty-eight for expectancy, but in typhus the results were against the cold water by twenty-six to eighteen.[2]

I think it will be granted from the statistics given above, or from many others which might be added, that cold water gives at least as good results as the very best to be attained by expectancy or any other treatment. To me it seems much better.

Of my own experience I speak with some diffidence, although it has had no small share in forming my own opinion, and I am so firmly convinced of the great benefit to be derived from this treatment that I sought an opportunity to read this paper for the purpose of commending it, and am willing to be considered its advocate rather than its critic. But in the first place the numbers I can present are too small to be of much value alone; secondly, I have been unable in all cases to carry out this plan so thoroughly as I could wish, especially at night; and thirdly, the figures alone, taken without explanation, furnish no very strong argument for the conclusions I draw. Taking the cases of typhoid fever which have been under my care in the City Hospital during three years previous to the present, except a few which entered convalescent or nearly so, or in which the result may be considered to have been practically decided before they fell into my hands, I reckon sixty-six in all, from which a stricter scrutiny might throw out more than one. These will not absolutely correspond with the diagnoses made in the indices to the hospital books, where typhoid fever covers many cases entering in the typhoid condition, where the interest and affection of friends is not sufficiently great to induce them to furnish any information as to previous symptoms, but becomes strongly developed when an autopsy is asked for. In these sixty-six cases, most of which when it was required were treated by more or less bathing, eleven were fatal, the death-rate thus being about eighteen per cent.

It is evident, however, that the results of a treatment which aims to control symptoms by mitigating the general violence of the disease will be better shown where it is pursued from an early period, than in a promiscuous collection of cases subjected to it at all stages of progress; and consequently a series from the first week of the disease is a fairer test than the average of all. In the table·of typhoid fever at the City Hospital, given by Dr. Upham,[3] I find forty-six cases entering in the first week of the fever, with five deaths, or a little over ten per cent. Of

[1] Centralblatt für die medicinische Wissenschaften. 1871, page 336.
[2] Centralblatt für die medicinische Wissenschaften. 1872, page 383.
[3] Medical and Surgical Reports. Boston City Hospital. First Series.

my own, as I have classified them, I have in the three years (1872–74) thirty-four such cases, with a mortality of three ; but if the beginning of the disease is reckoned as Dr. Upham has done in his table, that is, from the occurrence of certain severe symptoms and not from taking to the bed, one case and one death would be counted out, giving a mortality of about six per cent. But of these two deaths one was of a child, where there were really no clearly diagnostic symptoms of typhoid, fever and abdominal tenderness being alone noted, and the absence of diarrhœa specially mentioned. No autopsy was made. The remaining case presented an unusual intensity and character of nervous symptoms, and the fatal result was due to sloughing and perforation in the sigmoid flexure of the large intestine. I think, therefore, I am fully justified in stating that of thirty-two patients in three different years, where a clear diagnosis of typhoid fever in the first week is admissible, only one died.

During the present year I have had two well-marked cases. One, a man, was bathed, although at first not liking it very well, and is now convalescent ; the second, a woman whose nervous system was from the beginning severely affected, objected so strongly to the baths that it was almost impossible to carry the plan out efficiently, the water never being enough cooled to materially reduce her temperature, and they were accordingly abandoned. She died, apparently of the fever, pure and simple, on the twenty-third or twenty-fourth day. There were no signs of any of the accidents of the disease except the pulmonary.

Two obstacles have stood and will still stand in the way of this treatment, especially in private practice ; they ought not, however, to be insurmountable. The first is the objection raised by the patient and his friends. The fatigue and apparent exposure and harshness appear somewhat repulsive at a time when, as now, anything like decided or positive treatment in acute diseases is so likely to be looked upon as old-fashioned and unscientific. In a certain proportion of cases, not, I think, very large, the patient himself objects decidedly to the baths, — less however to the fatigue than to the chilly sensations. Persuasion, custom, and experience of the relief afforded will often overcome this ; but when, as will once in a while happen, and as did happen in the case spoken of a moment ago, the repugnance cannot be overcome, the physician must, as with other powerful remedies, balance the good and the harm against each other and act accordingly. In a great many cases, however, patients enjoy the baths, and await the time prescribed with impatience.

Another most serious obstacle is the increased time, labor, and attention called for on the part of the attendant. It is much easier to pour into the mouth of a patient at stated intervals a teaspoonful of liquor ammoniæ acetatis, or something less innocent, than to give a bath, which cannot be done for an adult without two tolerably strong and skillful persons. I have however, at the hospital, met with much less complaint of the additional labor than, I confess, I expected. Where the ordinary bath-tub, with its hot and cold water, is wanting, the difficulties are of course increased, but are hardly insurmountable except in the dwellings of the very poor, whose severely sick typhoid patients (in the city at least) should never be treated at home. Ice might be of good service in this way; a piece being put into the warm bath would produce even greater regularity of cooling than we get from turning in cold water. The cold pack, although laborious and comparatively inefficient, calls for nothing which cannot be found in any but the very poorest houses where, as I said, typhoid should not be treated. If the wet sheets are re-watered, as suggested by Dr. Flint, the effect will be greater and last longer. Here again, perhaps, ice might be used to advantage.

Finally, if no other method can be used, cold sponging, although the feeblest of all the four, is better than nothing, and should be frequently repeated. It may be done with water, water and alcohol, which by its evaporation produces more cooling, or, as Jaccoud recommends, aromatic vinegar.

It is of course to be understood that this treatment does not exclude other means, which may be useful or necessary either in the way of regimen or medicine. The importance of the most thorough ventilation, cleanliness, and disinfection is not in the least diminished. The rest of the treatment may be the purest expectancy, the symptoms as they arise may be met by appropriate means, or the antipyretic action of the baths may be supplemented by certain drugs. Digitalis and quinine have both been used. Of the former, for this purpose, I have no experience, but quinine I have several times used after the manner of Liebermeister and others, that is, not in the so-called tonic doses frequently employed, but twenty, twenty-five, or thirty grains in two doses near together. The temperature is lowered for several hours, and fewer baths may be used. The antipyretic action of alcohol, so far as it goes, is in its favor, but its power in therapeutics is but slight in this direction. As an adjunct to bathing or as taking the place of food, either with or without bathing, the opinion of the profession is largely in its favor.

My allotted time has permitted but a brief sketch of this method and the principles upon which it is founded. That it has been used and its value recognized before our time is far from being an argument against its use, since we seek for truth and not for novelty. That it has since been neglected is fully accounted for by the practical difficulties already described, and by an inefficient use of it. The worst that can be said of it is that it is unnecessary and gives no better results than letting patients alone; the best is that it is one of the most efficient means of treatment in the whole long catalogue of therapeutic agencies.

OVARIOTOMY.

BY JAMES B. CHADWICK, M. D.,

Lecturer on Diseases of Women, Harvard Medical School.

II. In April, 1874, Mrs. X., thirty-two years old, came under my treatment for an abdominal enlargement of four years' duration. I made a doubtful diagnosis of an ovarian cyst, but advised against an operation for its removal, in deference to the humane dictum of Spencer Wells, that we have no right to subject a patient to the risk of such a measure unti either her sufferings are so great as to render life no longer desired, or the rapid failure of health and strength makes it evident that longer delay will render speedy death inevitable, even without an operation. It is also undoubtedly true, as maintained by the same writer, that the chances of a successful operation are greater after the tumor has reached such a size as to press forcibly on the surrounding parts, whereby with every movement the peritoneum is exposed to a friction that gradually modifies its texture, rendering it callous and less prone to take on inflammatory action.

I saw my patient from time to time during the year succeeding the first interview, and by treating various symptoms as they appeared was able to give her comparative comfort during that period.

Toward the end of February, 1875, Mrs. X. told me her pain was so constant and harassing that she must have relief at any cost. She was at times much more distended than at others, and was often kept awake all night by distressing dyspnœa. Her abdomen now measured forty-six inches at the umbilicus. The symptoms were evidently due in great measure to ascitic fluid, which, together with very fat abdominal walls, masked the nature of the tumor. Still more doubt was thrown on the diagnosis by the history of an attack of jaundice and " liver complaint " just prior to the discovery of the tumor, and by the presence of menorrhagia for several years. Examination showed pretty conclusively that the liver was not the seat of the growth, and a fibroid of the uterus was at length excluded by means of a procedure which I have reason to think is new. The uterus was found to be retroverted, the cervix movable, but the fundus held firmly. The tumor could not be reached per vaginam, and no direct impulse or wave of fluctuation could be transmitted from the epigastric region to the uterus owing to the amount of ascitic fluid intervening between the abdominal walls and the uppermost part of the tumor. The uterine sound was of no avail. In this dilemma I placed the patient in the knee-elbow posture, with the idea that if the tumor were a fibroid its weight would cause it to sink in the ascitic fluid until it rested on the abdominal walls; in this position I should be able to obtain by palpation some information as to the character of its sur-

face, could at the same time send a direct forcible impulse to the uterus,
but, more especially, could derive some indications from the change in
the shape of the vagina and its relations to the cervix uteri. I argued
that if the tumor were a fibroid, continous with or closely attached to
the uterus, its weight, dragging upon the vagina by means of the cervix,
would cause the vagina to be drawn out into a long funnel, at the end
of which would be the cervix, not projecting as before, but so retracted
as to be almost level with the surface of the vagina. A thin-walled
ovarian cyst, on the other hand, would be scarcely heavier than the ascitic fluid; it would consequently not change its position materially on
change of the patient's posture, its slight amount of traction would
not bear upon the uterus alone, but would be distributed throughout the
broad ligament, from which its pedicle would chiefly spring; as a consequence of these conditions, the vagina would be less distorted and the
prominence of the cervix be less modified; in addition, the impulse from
above would not be forcibly transmitted to the uterus, and the surface
of the tumor would not become accessible to palpation. Two contin-
gencies might nullify the inferences to be drawn from these indications:
the presence of pelvic adhesions, and a partially solid character of an ovarian tumor. But adhesions are known to be rare with fibroid tumors,
and, as far as my experience goes, the more solid portion of multilocular
ovarian cysts is generally situated in the pelvis and easily accessible.
This method is of course only applicable to small and medium-sized
tumors surrounded by considerable ascitic fluid. Governed by the above
considerations I diagnosticated an ovarian cyst, probably unilocular, free
from adhesions, and with no solid part, but surrounded by a varying
amount of ascitic fluid.

The tumor was removed on March 6, 1875, with the assistance of
Drs. G. H. Lyman and J. N. Borland, in presence of Drs. C. E. Buckingham and J. P. Reynolds. Ether was administered by Mr. Fletcher
Abbott. The same extreme care to avert the possibility of infection and
to secure every hygienic advantage was observed in the preparation for
the operation as was detailed in the report of my last case.[1]

The correctness of the diagnosis was verified; there was less ascitic
fluid than was expected, but I had been seeking to promote its absorption for several days by the administration of a saturated solution of
chlorate of potash. The abdominal walls were fully three inches thick;
an incision four inches long was made in the median line; the pedicle
was very short, but a Wells clamp was applied without difficulty, and the
incision was closed with silk sutures. It was found impossible to cleanse
the peritoneal cavity completely, for a pinkish serum was seen to ooze
from every part of the peritoneum as fast as it was wiped away. Two
gallons of fluid were in the cyst. The total weight of the tumor was
eighteen pounds.

[1] Boston Medical and Surgical Journal, xcii. 397, April 8, 1875.

The recovery from ether was speedy and unattended by vomiting. Morphine to the extent of a grain was required to relieve the pain apparently due to the traction on the pedicle. Three hours after the operation the patient was dozing, so that I ventured to leave her in charge of the nurse for half an hour. On my return, however, I found her in a state of profound collapse, almost pulseless, scarcely breathing, blue, and clammy. Brandy and heat had already proved ineffectual to arouse the vital forces. I immediately removed the dressings from the wound and, finding the abdomen considerably distended, took out nearly all the sutures, broke up the agglutinations, and allowed much serum to escape ; on search no effusion of blood was discovered in the peritoneal cavity. The patient revived at once. The pedicle seemed so tense that, before reclosing the incision, I tied it firmly below the clamp, removed this, and dropped the pedicle in Douglas's pouch. A similar sudden revival from imminent death was observed in 1867 by Koeberlé, who, during an acute peritonitis subsequent to ovariotomy, made an incision into the right flank, where dullness was detected, and allowed a large accumulation of pinkish serum to escape. The patient rallied at once and made a good recovery.

During the three following days the patient's condition, if not altogether satisfactory, was certainly not alarming. She was kept on a light diet for thirty-six hours, and then stimulated moderately. On the second day there was considerable vomiting, with slight tenderness and distention of the abdomen ; she was very fretful and intolerant of restraint, kept her legs in constant motion and frequently shifted her body about on the bed. The pulse ranged from 110 to 130, and the temperature from 99° to 102° F. In the afternoon of the fourth day the pulse fell to 110 and the temperature to 100.5° ; enemata had at length brought flatus from the rectum, the tongue had become moist, and the wound began to suppurate in a healthy way. Toward night, however, without any increase in the abdominal tenderness or other indication of peritonitis, the symptoms became ominous. On the next morning, the abdominal distention was so great as seriously to impede respiration ; no wind escaped either by mouth or by rectum. I summoned Dr. J. J. Putnam to try the efficacy of galvanism in exciting peristaltic action, but his efforts were unavailing, and I was obliged to puncture the intestines, through the abdominal walls, with a fine trocar. Much gas escaped through the canula, with immense relief to the respiration. The patient continued to sink, however, in spite of constant stimulation by means of brandy and beef-tea enemata, brandy and a solution of quinine subcutaneously, and she died on the fifth day.

A complete autopsy was not made, but Dr. E. G. Cutler examined the peritoneal cavity in my presence. We found evidences of recent peritonitis, limited, however, to the neighborhood of the abdominal in-

cision ; the peritoneum above the umbilicus was perfectly healthy in
appearance, as was that lining the pelvis and the pelvic organs ; it was
evident that no inflammation had spread from the cut end of the pedicle.
The uterus and appendages were removed. The kidneys, liver, and
spleen were healthy.

In view of the mildness of the symptoms after the operation, and the
limited extent of the peritonitic inflammation found at the autopsy, I
was at a loss to explain the cause of death in one so well-nourished and
of so good constitution as my patient appeared to be. A week after the
patient's death, however, it was reported to me on unquestionable authority, that for three years she had been in the habit of a free indulgence in
spirituous liquors, frequently imbibing from one to three pints of rum in
a day, though never intoxicated. This practice had not only been kept
from my knowledge, but was absolutely denied on the day preceding
the operation. Some nervous symptoms had aroused my suspicions,
and led to my putting some categorical questions as to the amount of
stimulants consumed daily ; I explained the importance of my knowing
the truth, as the after-treatment always had to be adapted to the habits
of each individual. She disclaimed emphatically ever drinking anything
but a pint of beer a day ; my suspicions were consequently set at rest.
Had I known the facts of the case I should have declined to operate.
As it was, there was no apparent reason before the operation why the
result should not have been as favorable as in my last case.

I have now no hesitation in ascribing the fatal result to exhaustion
immediately dependent upon the physical condition engendered by the
immoderate use of alcoholic stimulants. All surgeons know how full
of risk even trivial operations are apt to be in individuals who are saturated with alcohol.

In connection with the puncturing of the intestines with the aspirator
to relieve the flatulence, it seems to me that another indication may be
met by injecting brandy, beef-tea, etc., through the canula into the
small or large intestine, after the gas has escaped. By this means a
patient's strength might be sustained when nothing could be retained
in the stomach, and absorption by the rectum was too slow to meet the
demands of the system. In this way fluids could be introduced in considerable quantities into that part of the alimentary canal from which
they would be most readily absorbed. If the use of the trocar is as
harmless as is asserted by those who have tried it, I see no reason why
the intestines should not be repeatedly tapped for the injection of nutrient and stimulant fluids in many desperate conditions and diseases, when
the other resources of medical art have failed. In such a case as mine
I believe that there would have been no other means of introducing
enough alcohol to carry her through the depressing effect of such an
operation, had her habits been made known to me during life. Might

not peristaltic action also have been excited by the same measure, and thus a second advantage been derived from this procedure? In case of fæcal impaction, may not the hard, scybalous masses be softened and broken up by the injection of different fluids into their midst, when enemata and purges have proved powerless?

Report upon the Specimens by Dr. Fitz. — " The tumor consisted of a single sack intimately connected with an elongated, dense, flattened mass, shaped like the normal ovary but certainly six times as large. This body was composed of a fibrous stroma in which were several small cysts, whose general appearance was that of Graafian vesicles (follicular cysts). The large cyst was contained within a thin capsule of firm fibrous tissue (penitoneum), to which it was loosely connected by areolar tissue. In this intervening layer a cyst of the size of a bean was found, which was lined with ciliated epithelium, the ciliary movement still going on. Between the outer investment and the wall of the cyst, the Fallopian tube was discovered; it was nearly a foot in length, was of normal size where it had been cut in the pedicle, but farther on was dilated; it completely encircled the tumor and terminated blindly near the ovary, being lost in the sheath of the cyst. Fimbriæ were not observed. The proper wall of the cyst was smooth, thick, of grayish color, thrown into numerous folds, moderately vascular, and lined with a cylindrical non-ciliated epithelium. The fluid from the cyst contained albumen. There was no evidence of secondary cysts. The structure of the tumor, and its relation to the ovary, the Fallopian tube, and the investing membrane (containing a cyst lined with ciliated epithelium), from which latter it could be readily enucleated, render it probable that the tumor was an ovarian cyst which had grown between the layers of the broad ligament.

" The left ovary was of normal size, and contained several small follicular cysts. A unilocular cyst as large as a walnut (which at the operation was taken for dropsy of the tube) extended outwards from the left end of the ovary, between the layers of the broad ligament. It contained a yellow, gelatinous fluid, in which were numerous granular corpuscles. The wall of the cyst was composed of fibrous tissue in which were numerous concretions, often microscopic. One as large as a grape-seed projected from that part of the wall which was directly connected with the ovary. The wall was lined with tesselated epithelium. The albugineous tunic of the ovary was lost in the wall of the cyst."

In spite of the fact that the histological elements above described would be sufficient, according to pathologists, to include these two cysts among the ovarian, yet I cannot but feel that the extreme improbability of two ovarian cysts in the same patient, developing between the layers of the broad ligament and not in the common direction toward the periphery of the organ, casts some doubt upon the correctness of the

8

commonly accepted diagnostic points of ovarian and parovarian cysts. Dr. Bantock [1] has already ventured to call such as these parovarian cysts. There are certainly several facts which are hardly compatible with the theory of their ovarian origin : First, as pointed out by Dr. Bantock, the absence of Graafian follicles in the deeper part of the ovaries, and the unlikelihood of their developing in the direction of the greatest resistance ; secondly, the curious fact that very few of the tumors, lying thus between the folds of the broad ligament, assume the common form of multilocular cysts, but they are almost invariably unilocular ; thirdly, if they originate in the ovary they should be covered with a double layer of peritoneum, for Waldeyer has demonstrated that the ovary lies in a cup-shaped depression of this membrane, and an ovarian cyst must push the peritoneum forming this depression before it as it insinuates itself between the layers of the broad ligament and becomes invested by them. This double layer has not been noticed by others, and was certainly absent in my specimens. This subject needs thorough investigation.

RECENT PROGRESS IN PHYSIOLOGY. [2]

BY H. P. BOWDITCH, M. D.

MUSCULAR SENSE.

THE existence of sensitive nerves in muscles has been assumed by most physiologists as necessary to explain such phenomena as the feeling of muscular fatigue, the power of estimating the weight of objects, and the knowledge of the position of our limbs which enables us, consciously or unconsciously, to execute coördinated muscular movements. Although the sensitive nerves of the skin may aid to a certain extent in the performance of these functions, yet the part they play must be regarded as a very subordinate one. As conclusive evidence on this point may be mentioned the observation of Bernard [3] that the removal of the skin from the limbs of a frog does not essentially interfere with its powers of locomotion, while the section of the posterior roots of the sciatic plexus renders the animal's movements entirely uncontrolled and irregular (ataxia).

The principal opponent of the theory of muscular sensibility is Schiff, [4] who considers that our perception of the state of muscular contraction depends entirely upon a " central consciousness of innervation." In favor of this theory are the observations of Leyden [5] on

[1] Obstetrical Journal of Great Britain, i. 2, 1873.
[2] Concluded from page 65.
[3] Système nerveux, i. 251.
[4] Lehrbuch der Physiologie, i. 156.
[5] Über Muskelsinn und Ataxie. Virchow's Archiv, Bd. 47, S. 321.

ataxic and anæsthetic patients who still preserve the power of estimating the weight of objects. (Brown-Séquard's observations [1] that the channels of muscular sensibility do not decussate in the cord with the ordinary sensitive fibres are probably also to be interpreted as favoring this view.)   Opposed to this hypothesis, on the other hand, are the experiments of Bernhardt,[2] who found that it made little or no difference in the accuracy with which weights could be estimated, whether the muscles were brought into contraction by an effort of the will or by electrical stimulation of the nerve.   It seems probable, therefore, that the central consciousness of innervation plays an important though not an exclusive part in supplying information as to the condition of the muscles.   The feeling of muscular fatigue depends, according to Schiff, not upon an affection of the sensitive nerves of muscles, but upon an interference with the circulation due to the limbs being kept too long in one position.   In support of this view, Schiff makes the extraordinary statement that the same feeling of fatigue and pain which is experienced when the arm is held horizontally extended for fifteen minutes may be produced when the arm is *supported* in that position for the same length of time.   Were this the case, we should, as has been well remarked, awake from sleep not refreshed and strengthened, but with violent pains in all our limbs.   How the pain of muscular cramp is accounted for on this theory, Schiff does not explain.   •

Bernhardt also, in spite of his experiments above alluded to, is unwilling to admit the existence of nerves of muscular sense.   He regards the estimation of weights as depending upon the central consciousness of innervation, the knowledge of the position of the limbs as derived through the Pacinian corpuscles, whose existence has been demonstrated on the articular nerves, and muscular pain (as in tetanus) as caused by pressure on nerves running through or over the muscles.   This last hypothesis is of course quite inconsistent with the general law that the sensation caused by pressure on the trunk of a nerve is referred to its termination.

Anatomists as well as physiologists have brought forward reasons for attributing " sensitivity " to certain nerve-fibres distributed to muscles. Thus Bell, noticing that division of the facial nerve paralyzes the muscles of the face, although they also receive certain fibres from the trigeminus nerve, argued that certain sensations must have their origin in the muscles.   Reichert,[3] in studying the terminations of nerves in the muscles of the frog, found a small number of fibres which ended very differently from the others, and suggested that they might be the sensitive muscular fibres.   Kölliker [4] traced these nerve-fibres still farther,

[1] Archives de Physiologie, ii. 698.
[2] Zur Lehre vom Muskelsinn. Archiv für Phsychiatrie, 1872.
[3] Reichert and Du Bois Reymond's Archiv, 1851, page 29.
[4] Microskopische Anatomie, ii. 240.

and discovered their terminations in the fascia surrounding the muscle. Odenius was still more successful in following out the ultimate ramifications of these fibres. His account of them is essentially the same as the one which will be given below.

Thus, although weighty anatomical and physiological reasons could be given for assuming the existence of centripetal nerve-fibres in muscles, yet the absolute demonstration of the fact was until recently wanting. This gap in our knowledge of the subject has been filled by Carl Sachs,[1] from whose treatise on the subject most of the above citations have been taken.

The experiments of this investigator were as follows: The reflex convulsions of frogs poisoned with strychnia and picrotoxine were used as an index of the irritation of sensitive nerves. The muscles of one of the hind limbs were rendered motionless by division of the anterior roots on that side. The sartorius muscle of that side was then divided at its two extremities, and all its connections with the body, except the nerve, were severed. A thin plate of glass was then passed under it, and the preparation moistened with a drop of a three fourths per cent. solution of common salt. The muscle was then irritated by induced currents, and every contraction of the muscle was found to be accompanied by reflex convulsions of the rest of the body. It was thus shown that the sartorius muscle contains centripetal nerve-fibres whose irritation calls into activity the reflex centres of the spinal cord, but it was not shown that the contraction of the muscle, as such, is capable of stimulating the nerves in question, since in the above experiment the nerves themselves were irritated by the electrical current. It was therefore necessary to use some means of irritation which would act on the muscle and not on the nerve; ammonia is an irritant of this sort, and the sartorius muscle of the frog is particularly adapted to experiments of this kind, because its nervous distribution is limited to the central portion. The ammonia was applied by means of a piece of bibulous paper to a transverse section at one end of the muscle. A wave of contraction at once passed over the muscle, and reflex convulsions of the other limbs were immediately produced. It was thus shown that a contraction of a muscle is capable of stimulating centripetal nerves which are distributed through its substance and which enter the spinal cord by the posterior roots.

In order to obtain anatomical as well as physiological evidence of the existence of nerves of muscular sense, Waller's method of investigation was resorted to. This consists in dividing a nerve-root, or one of the component nerves of a nervous plexus, and studying the degeneration of the nerve-fibres which results from their separation from the nerve-centres. The course of the fibres thus divided can in this way be traced

[1] Reichert and Du Bois Reymond's Archiv, 1874, pages 175, 491, 645.

through the mixed nerve-trunks. If, for instance, six or eight weeks after division of the anterior roots of the nerves of a limb, it can be shown that the muscular nerves contain any undegenerated fibres, it may be assumed that these fibres are derived from the posterior roots. The application of this method to the sartorius muscle of frogs showed that the nerve supplying this muscle contains about twenty nerve-fibres, two of which only do not degenerate after section of the anterior roots. These two fibres may therefore be regarded as sensitive. (Schiff's[1] failure to find undegenerated fibres in the muscular nerves after section of the anterior roots is, according to Sachs, to be explained by the unsuitable methods of research adopted by that observer.) The converse experiment of dividing the posterior roots outside the ganglia did not give such definite results. The degeneration of the sensitive muscular nerves was found to be much slower and less complete than that of the motor nerves under similar circumstances.

Still further evidence of the difference between the two sorts of nerve-fibres is afforded by the result of local irritation applied to the nerves in their course amongst the muscular fibres. The irritations were produced by induced currents sent through very fine platinum electrodes, which were applied close to the intra-muscular nerve-fibres as seen under the microscope. Experimenting in this way, Sachs found that in most cases a very feeble irritation was sufficient to cause a contraction of those muscular fibres to which the nerve in question supplied terminal plates, while the rest of the muscle was unaffected. Certain nerve-fibres, however, were found to which the irritation had to be applied with considerably increased intensity in order to produce a muscular contraction, and the contraction when produced was not limited to certain muscular fibres but extended over all the neighboring contractile substance. This would seem to show that the nerves in question had no motor function, but that the contraction was due to a general stimulation, by side currents, of the muscles and nerves in the neighborhood.

Histological investigations by Sachs have also shown a decided difference in the mode of distribution of the two sorts of nerves. While the motor nerves, subdividing dichotomously, end after a short course in the so-called terminal plates, the sensitive nerves, ramifying often dendritically, pursue an extended and isolated course over a large number of muscular fibres, and give rise to delicate non-medullated nucleated fibrillæ, which frequently anastomose with each other, and terminate partly in the connective tissue around the muscles, partly in the interstitial connective tissue, and partly as very fine branches surrounding the muscular fibres themselves.

The author also discusses the nature of the process by which the

[1] Lehrbuch der Physiologie, i. 159.

sensitive nerves are irritated in the living muscle. The feeling of
fatigue he regards as due to a chemical change in the substance of the
exhausted muscle (formation of lactic acid, etc.). The perception of a
muscular contraction is probably due to a mechanical irritation of the
sensitive nerves which run between and around the muscular fibres, and
therefore follow from necessity their changes of form.

THE BRITISH MEDICAL ASSOCIATION.

THE annual meeting of the British Medical Association will be held at
Edinburgh in the month of August, beginning on Tuesday, the 3d, and lasting five days. The meetings of this association have been so successful during the last few years, and the character of the men who take a prominent
part in its proceedings is of such high standard, that we should recommend to
all those who have the welfare of our own association at heart a careful study
of the British organization and of its method of conducting its meetings. Undoubtedly Great Britain possesses advantages over this country in its compactness, and the possibility of a general assembly of its physicians. The
adoption of a medical journal as an organ of the association has been followed by a very large addition to the number of members. The price of the
journal is included in the admission fee of one guinea. This in itself is no
small inducement; but the chief advantage of such a journal is its organizing
power, and the opportunity it offers to utilize the work done by the association and to put it in an attractive manner before the profession, — work that
would otherwise be buried in transactions, as is the custom here.

Without recommending the adoption of a similar project by our own association, we think this feature offers a hint which might be taken advantage of.
Articles should be read while the discussions of the annual meeting are fresh in
the minds of the readers, and while the subjects treated of belong to the topics
of the day, and not long after other questions have arisen to take their place.
There are many ways in which this might be done. If judiciously managed
it might produce a beneficial effect both upon our association and upon our
medical literature. The annual addresses on important departments of medicine by leading men are an exceedingly attractive feature, and give a tone to
the session which could not easily be acquired in any other way. The work of
the sections does not appear to differ essentially from that of our own. We
notice, however, that presidents of the various sections are selected with a
good deal of care. For instance, this year, Dr. Quain, of London, is president
of the section on medicine, Professor Lister of the surgical section, and
Professor Burdon Sanderson of that on physiology. Officers are evidently
selected for what they have done, and without reference to where they come
from. The "side shows" of this annual entertainment are carefully attended
to. The annual museum, as it is described, could be made a very valuable
feature. The "conversazione," a peculiarly English institution, in spite of its

name, combines entertainment with instruction. Finally, the excursions are arranged on a liberal and hospitable scale. The British Medical Association is undoubtedly the most successful organization of its kind that exists to-day. Would it not be well for the leaders of our own association, which they are now endeavoring to resuscitate, to study carefully the elements of this success?

THE CITY SEWERS.

THE second hearing before the sewerage commission, held on the 12th, although not bringing out any new facts, was simply confirmatory of the testimony given at the previous meeting, and was, in short, but a formal statement of a condition of things which has been universally acknowledged to exist for a far longer space of time than one would have thought possible without some serious outbreak of disease. As was stated in our last issue, the true condition of affairs, bad as it has been reported to be, is even now not realized to its fullest extent by the public. One would hardly believe that large sewers have been built up to a solid stone wall, and then allowed to remain years without any outlet whatever; that other sewers have been so arranged as to permit a free escape of sewer-gas into the streets, thus defeating one of the very objects for which they were constructed; that in some parts of the city there are no sewers at all, the houses draining into the surrounding soil. Indeed, the soil upon which the larger portion of the city stands is fairly saturated with sewage, which slowly oozes into a bank of dock mud which forms an almost complete circle around us. In addition to all this, numbers of watering-carts are daily washing the streets with water drawn from the very sewer-mouths, and tainted with the same dangerous material. Under the circumstances it is surely a matter of surprise that we have not worse odors than are now complained of.

The sewerage commission received its appointment many months ago. It has had time to gain a pretty thorough knowledge of the condition of affairs and the opportunities which exist for supplying a remedy. A member of the commission, the Secretary of the State Board of Heath, is already on his way to Europe for the purpose of making this matter a subject of special investigation. We trust that a study of the systems of Paris, of London, or of such a city as Hamburg, for instance, which possesses many conditions similar to those which exist here, will furnish the commission with valuable hints, and we hope that the autumn may not be allowed to pass away without the announcement of a plan which fairly meets the difficulty, is in no sense a compromise, and is fully worthy of the commission and the city. We have spent many millions in introducing water into the city, and are wont to pride ourselves upon its purity; let us take good care that it does not prove a curse instead of a blessing.

MEDICAL NOTES.

— Dr. Middleton Michel, in the *Charleston Medical Journal and Review*, in an article on the anatomy of the bullet-track and cicatrices of the wounds of entrance and exit, comes to the following conclusions: 1st. The bullet-track is not a conical wound. 2d. From the irregularity of the shot-track, parts of its walls are in contact, which soon adhere and heal, while suppuration elsewhere may continue for a time from both openings. 3d. In exceptional instances, the wound from a conical ball, accompanied by fractured bone and shortening of limb, heals spontaneously without suppuration. 4. The demolitionary effects of the minié ball on osseous tissue have been exaggerated, since the axial cleavage of the shafts of long bones was not so frequently encountered as has been generally stated. 5th. Misconception of the ravages of the conoidal ball led to unnecessary sacrifice of limbs. 6th. Differential features of entrance and exit wounds, if reliable, are the more readily seen the earlier these are examined. 7th. The cicatrices will often again indicate the separate orifices.

Dr. Michel, in a late number of the same journal, describes a modification of the operation for the removal of cancer of the lip. The operation is thus described : " Making a semicircular incision two lines from the diseased part, and entirely circumscribing it, the whole growth was dissected away down to the mucous layer, this being preserved intact, then paring away the remains of all suspicious tissue with the scissors, and saving thereby every available portion of integument, which the usual V-incision could not have done." In cases where the cancer involves the whole lower lip, he recommends preservation of the mucous surface, and allowing the wound to remain open and heal by granulation, after the manner of Richeraud, by which a most satisfactory result is said to be obtained.

— Professor Billroth's case of extirpation of the larynx has been followed by a second similar operation, performed by Professor Bottini, of Novara. The patient was a healthy young man, who, on account of dyspnœa, had already had laryngotomy and galvanic cauterization of the larynx performed. The operation lasted ninety minutes, and left the patient much exhausted. He was, however, revived by injection of beef tea and wine. It was found that the larynx was quite obstructed by a grayish-red tumor. In spite of an attack of erysipelas and a series of abscesses, the man gradually improved, regained the power of deglutition, and was able to cough, breathe, and sleep well. The wound has healed up, and the case, save future accidents, may be looked upon as successful.

— Drs. Kaposi, Auspitz, and Neumann have been appointed extraordinary professors of dermatology and syphilis in the University of Vienna. They have hitherto held the position of *privat-docent*. Dr. Carl Störk, *privat docent*, has been appointed extraordinary professor of laryngoscopy in the same university.

— Mr. Seymour Haden's perishable coffins lately exhibited in England are described in the English papers. The coffins were simply wicker baskets, of the ordinary coffin shape and of various sizes. Two of them had their meshes filled by moss, but the rest, which were supplied by Mr. Kirby, a basket maker at Derby, were left with their meshes open, like those of an ordinary waste-paper basket. Two or three were double, with a space two inches or three inches in width between the inner and the outer basket; and this space is intended to be filled with charcoal, for cases in which any precaution against infection and decomposition may be required. The following account is given of them : " It is necessary, perhaps, to explain that the models shown are merely suggestive, and that the majority of them do not as yet fulfill all the conditions essential to their practical use. 1. The mesh in most of them should be larger than it is, and as open as is consistent with strength and the perfect retention of their contents, which contents, again, should consist of the larger ferns, mosses, lichens, herbs, fragrant shrubs, and any of the coniferæ, willows, or evergreens, which are always to be had. 2. The osiers composing the baskets should be light (two thin ones being better than one thick one), and no more solid wood should enter into their construction than is necessary to preserve their form. 3. They should be of white or stained willow, without varnish or other preservative covering. 4. Accompanying each of them should be a narrow leaden band or ribbon, pierced with name and date of death, to be passed round the chest and lower limbs, and through the sides and over the top of the basket : (i) for retaining the body in its position ; (ii) for the subsequent identification of the bones ; (iii) for sealing the coffin, as a guarantee that the contents have not been disturbed. 5. In special cases linings of some imperishable material for a few inches upwards from the bottom will be necessary ; and, in other cases, such modifications of the ordinary form as may insure a complete inclusion of the body in wool, charcoal, or other disinfectants. 6. Other materials which are light, strong, perishable, inexpensive, adapted for carriage, and favorable to the dissolution of the body may do as well and possibly better than these wicker baskets. Readiness of carriage and the insurance of resolution being the main objects aimed at, several such materials do, in fact, suggest themselves, and may afterwards come to be employed."

LETTER FROM PHILADELPHIA.

Messrs. Editors, — The Centennial Medical Association, which originated in the Philadelphia County Medical Society, promises to be a very important organization. Arrangements have been made to hold an International Medical Congress early in September, 1876, in Philadelphia, at which papers upon medicine and medical progress will be read. The congress will consist of delegates, native and foreign, representing the American Medical Association, various State medical societies, and the medical societies of Europe, the British Dominions, Central and South America, Sandwich Islands, both the Indies, China, and Japan. It has been agreed that no vote shall be taken during the sittings of the congress upon any topic whatever. The preparation of the discourses has been intrusted to able hands, and they will be published in an appropriate commemorative volume. A circular, stating the object of the Centennial Medical Commission, has been prepared, and will be sent, by means of our foreign ministers and consuls, to the proper bodies. Special invitations to medical gentlemen of high scientific and social position will be issued, and a great object will be to make the meeting truly representative of the profession, both in its native and in its foreign elements.

To this end, and to prevent the admission of any unworthy applicants, proper testimonials will be required by the committee on credentials. The choice of Professor S. D. Gross as president of the association gives universal satisfaction. A more distinguished or dignified representative of American physicians could hardly have been found.

The trustees of Jefferson Medical College have purchased real estate in the rear of the present collegiate buildings, and will proceed to erect a hospital of useful dimensions. The hospital heretofore used by the college is limited in size, and merely a convenience in cases incapable of being moved, but too contracted to admit of clinical uses on behalf of students. The new hospital, which will probably be roofed in by September, will greatly increase the usefulness and attractiveness of the school.

The late John H. Towne, of Philadelphia, in his will made a large addition to the endowment fund of the University of Pennsylvania. After making liberal provisions for his family and relatives, he bequeathed $10,000 to the University Hospital, and after various other bequests to the Pennsylvania Academy of Fine Arts, to the Academy of Natural Sciences, etc., he constitutes the trustees of the University of Pennsylvania residuary legatees of the remainder of the estate — probably $300,000. The university has also a reversionary interest in the estate, which may ultimately make the total bequest upwards of one million dollars. The money thus bequeathed is to be held as a portion of the endowment fund of the university, and the income is to be applied solely to the payment of salaries of professors and other teachers in the department of science, — a most wise provision.

The physiological laboratory of the University Medical School was recently opened, and is now conducted by Dr. Ott, who received his training in Germany. The laboratories for chemical and histological work are also now open to students who may wish to pursue these branches of study.

The summer medical schools, both of the University and Jefferson, are attended by classes numbering, perhaps, fifteen per cent. of the winter complement. The regular courses of lectures terminate with the winter sessions, and lectures upon pathological anatomy, toxicology, histology, laryngoscopy, physical diagnosis, syphilis, urinary chemistry, and minor surgery are now being given by the sub-faculties. There are also surgical, medical, skin, and eye clinics. Attendance upon these lectures and clinics is not obligatory ; couse-quently, the number of students at the various lectures varies with their interest in the subjects presented. Lectures are over at two P. M., and the remainder of the day is given to dissection and reading. The effect of the Philadelphia climate at this season being somewhat enervating, students (with the exception of the few ·earnest, far-seeing ones), without especially cultivating the Italian language, learn, I fancy, to the full, the meanings of *dolce far niente*.

In the matter of the objections made by the committee of citizens (medical and lay) to the construction of the abattoir on the Schuylkill in West Philadelphia, President Judge Alison recently gave the opinion of the court to the effect that "the objections related chiefly to the plans for filtering and sewerage, and that after carefully considering these plans and the opposition to them, the court was unable to say that they were defective. They would have to be left to the result of practical tests. They were, of course, subject to the risk of being adjudged nuisances, if upon actual use that character became attached to them. The control of the court would be exercised over them, but the work will be allowed to go on." As to the question of storing 'hogs and cattle, the judge said the court had decided the case simply as one involving the establishment of a slaughtering place or abattoir, and had never considered the matter of an entrepôt or storage place for animals, and hence had no opinion to give. Of course, if any trouble from this cause should hereafter arise, plaintiffs would be at liberty to appear and ask for relief. The place would be closely watched. So the Pennsylvania Railroad Company will have their way, as I anticipated in a former letter. It remains to be seen whether the death-rate of Philadelphia will be increased by this supplement to her other nuisances.

Professor Da Costa, twelve months ago, delivered a lecture upon " Strain and Over-Action of the Heart," in the Toner course at Washington. It was an instructive and suggestive discourse, and has since been published. I am glad to learn that its excellence led a professor in the University of Zurich to translate it into German.

The new pavilion ward of the Presbyterian Hospital was the other day opened to the public. I gave you an accurate description of the ward in a former letter. It supplies a much needed want, and offers facilities for the treatment of surgical cases that are possessed by few hospitals. The pavilion cost $14,000.

A pleasant incident which occurred during the recent meeting of the American Medical Association at Louisville was the presentation to Professor Gross, by the physicians of that city, of a pair of very handsome, thorough-bred horses. Professor Gross practiced and taught in Louisville for many years before he was called to the Jefferson Medical College of this city.

Dr. W. W. Keen recently performed ovariotomy upon a woman aged forty-six, who began to menstruate at fifteen, ceased at forty-four; was always regular; married at nineteen; bore only one child, and never had any uterine trouble. The abnormal growth first made itself known about thirty months ago. Last October the attending physician removed five gallons of greenish, viscid fluid from the abdominal cyst, after which a slight peritonitis set in, but the patient was more comfortable than formerly. Later, she came into the hands of Dr· Keen. A thin, spare woman, measuring six inches from ensiform cartilage to umbilicus, nine inches from this point to the pubes; greatest girth thirty-three inches. The swelling was almost wholly below the navel, with fluctuation on palpation. Below the fluid a solid body was felt. There were two adhesions about three inches square. One surrounded the site of the tapping. The other was below it, and corresponded to a hard mass. Ascitic fluid flowed around these adhesions, and revealed them distinctly. The mass was movable only with difficulty. Palpation showed the upper part of the tumor to be cystic, the lower portion to be solid. Extending from the pubes and obliquely to the right was a mass resembling an elongated uterus. Examination, per vaginam, revealed an os and cervix nearly normal as to size, position, and relations. The tumor was felt behind the uterus, but a distinct depression existed, and could be felt between them. The sound entered the uterine cavity two and one half inches, upward and somewhat to the right. The uterus was not movable independently of the tumor, movement of the latter communicating itself to the uterus. Per rectum the tumor was easily felt, and gave the impression that its pedicle was very short.

May 20th. Dr. Keen aspirated a small quantity of fluid from the cyst for examination. The fluid was purulent, and contained compound, granular corpuscles, blood and pus cells, but was composed mainly of distinct ovarian cells.

The woman was gradually sinking, and the general discomfort was so great that her life had become a burden; therefore, May 22d, Dr. Keen removed the growth. After tapping the main cyst, and finding the lower mass too solid to admit of further diminution in size, he extended the incision from the umbilicus six and one half inches downwards, or nearly to the pubes, before the tumor could be removed. It was found to be slightly adherent to the parietes, omentum, and intestines, and, having no pedicle, the growth hid everything beneath it. Dr. Keen consequently tied a strong ligature around its base, and removed the larger portion of the tumor by cutting directly through its substance. The base was discovered to be attached directly to the uterus, rectum, and left side of the pelvis. The remainder of the growth was removed. Three ligatures were passed around the broad attachments of the tumor, thus securing several large vessels which were troublesome. Eight ordinary ligatures were required to arrest hæmorrhage from smaller vessels. The attachments were touched with Monsel's solution; the eight small ligatures were cut short off, the three larger ones brought out of the cavity and left. The wound was closed by eight silver sutures.

In its upper portion the tumor consisted of a large cyst, containing four pints of fluid and two or three smaller cysts. The inner surface of the large cyst was coated with soft, papillary growths, numerous detached masses of which formed a sediment in the fluid. The lower portion was a hard, solid mass, divided by distinct septa of connective tissue into smaller masses, which were whitish in color, and subdivided into masses still smaller in size.

In spite of the most nourishing and careful treatment the patient gradually sank, and died the day following the operation.

The autopsy discovered the intestines glued together with lymph of recent formation. Below the umbilicus the omentum was attached to the abdominal wall transversely, dividing the main peritoneal cavity into two parts. Above this level were the remains of old inflammatory effects. No hæmorrhage had occurred after the operation. The tumor had been attached to nearly the whole of the left half of the uterus, laterally and posteriorly, and to the rectum in Douglas's cul-de-sac. It was from the rectal attachments, as well as from the attachments to the left broad ligament, which was the pelvic support of the tumor, that the annoying hæmorrhage had taken place.

Microscopic examination by Dr. Joseph G. Richardson made it evident that the growth was "a rather hard variety of encephaloid or medullary carcinoma." It was thought singular that the ante-mortem examination of the cystic fluid revealed no sign of the true nature of the tumor.

PHILADELPHIA, *June* 15, 1875.

DR. ESTES HOWE.

MESSRS. EDITORS, — In preparing the article upon the Medical Profession of Massachusetts during the Revolutionary War, I endeavored to give sketches of all those surgeons who were connected with the American army ; and for this purpose I consulted such biographical works as have been accepted as authority on this matter. I doubt not that I may have omitted some who were useful in the army, and yet failed to attract the attention of the biographers. One such I have already discovered — a valuable officer, a physician of high standing both in civil and military life, and a citizen whose memory is still cherished in that section of the State where he resided ; and I have secured the following sketch, which should justly be added to the original article.

Dr. Estes Howe was born June 24, 1747, in Belchertown, Mass. His father, Samuel Howe, was one of the earliest settlers of that town, having emigrated to what was then called the "West," from Marlboro ; he was a captain in the French war, from 1755 to 1763, and at Lake George. He was also a member of the first and second Provincial Congresses.

Dr. Howe, who, while yet a boy, attended his father on one of his campaigns, as a drummer, studied his profession and commenced practice in his native town, where he married on the 18th of February, 1773, Susanna, daughter of Captain Nathaniel Dwight. On the 25th of April, 1775, six days after the battle of Lexington, he joined the American army, was commissioned as surgeon, and was attached to the regiment of Colonel David Powers. This regiment was engaged at Bunker Hill, and was afterwards stationed at Roxbury. On the 1st of January, 1776, he resigned and returned to his practice for a year, after which he received a second commission, as surgeon of the regiment commanded by Colonel Rufus Putnam, with which he remained until May 1, 1779, when he finally left the army. This regiment was stationed at Saratoga many months, during which time he conceived a high admiration of General Gates, for whom he named a son.

Having resumed his practice at Belchertown, he continued there during the remainder of his life, dying March 3, 1826. His professional life extended over half a century, during which he secured the esteem and respect of the community in which he lived. Like many of the physicians of that day, he was not the possessor of a diploma, but he was an early member of the Massachusetts Medical Society. Setting high value on classical culture, he educated two of his sons at Dartmouth College, and one at Williams. He left a record worthy of admiration, and a name which is a valuable addition to the list of patriotic physicians who did so much to carry our country through the war of the Revolution.   GEORGE B. LORING.

SALEM, *July* 15, 1875.

WEEKLY BULLETIN OF PREVALENT DISEASES.

THE following is a bulletin of the diseases prevalent in Massachusetts during the week ending July 17, 1875, compiled under the authority of the State Board of Health from the returns of physicians representing all sections of the State : —

We have to note again the very general prevalence of intestinal disorders. The reports show an increase of these diseases in nearly all sections of the State.   The summary for each district is as follows : —

Berkshire : Diarrhœa, cholera morbus, whooping-cough. Pittsfield reports a fatal case of diphtheria.

Valley : Diarrhœa, cholera morbus, rheumatism.

Midland : Diarrhœa, rheumatism, cholera morbus, cholera infantum, dysentery.

Northeastern : Diarrhœa, cholera morbus, cholera infantum.   Less sickness than in other parts of the State.

Metropolitan : Diarrhœa, cholera morbus, cholera infantum, scarlatina, rheumatism.   Typhoid is increasing.   Brighton and Melrose report diphtheria of a severe type.

Southeastern : Diarrhœa, rheumatism, cholera morbus, dysentery, cholera infantum.   Towns on Cape Cod and in Dukes County report the measles as quite prevalent in that section.

Comparing the present week with the last we find that diarrhœa, cholera morbus, cholera infantum, dysentery, and typhoid fever have increased in prevalence ; while bronchitis, measles, diphtheria, rheumatism, scarlatina, whooping-cough, and pneumonia are disappearing.

F. W. DRAPER, M. D., Registrar.

COMPARATIVE MORTALITY-RATES FOR THE WEEK ENDING JULY 10, 1875.

	Estimated Population.	Total Mortality for the Week.	Annual Death-rate per 1000 during Week.
New York	1,040,000	743	37
Philadelphia	775,000	412	28
Brooklyn	450,000		
Boston	350,000	147	22
Cincinnati	260,000	150	30
Providence	100,700	29	15
Worcester	50,000	16	17
Lowell	50,000	24	25
Cambridge	50,000	12	12
Fall River	45,000	27	31
Lawrence	33,000	12	19
Springfield	33,000	7	11
Lynn	28,000	7	13
Salem .	26,000	8	16

MILITARY APPOINTMENT. — Dr. W. F. Southard, of Baldwinsville, reappointed Surgeon of the Second Corps of Cadets, passed a successful examination before the Board of Medical Officers, M. V. M , July 2, 1875.   EDWARD J. FORSTER,

Surgeon Fifth Regiment of Infantry, M. V. M., Recorder of Board.

THE BOSTON
MEDICAL AND SURGICAL JOURNAL.

VOL. XCIII. — THURSDAY, JULY 29, 1875. — NO. 5.

—————

ON LOCALIZATION OF FUNCTIONS IN THE BRAIN.[1]

BY C. E. BROWN-SÉQUARD, M. D.

THE subject upon which I shall have the pleasure of speaking to you to-night is that of the localization of functions in the brain. The general principle that parts exist in this organ which serve for definite functions is now pretty generally admitted, and the question remaining to be discussed is therefore whether or not such parts have as yet been found. As is well known, it is to two German physiologists, Fritsch and Hitzig, that is due the discovery of facts which have led to the reopening of this question. Hitzig and several other observers have published pathological facts which are in harmony with the apparent results of physiological experimentation. This attempt to establish on these two classes of facts a theory according to which certain parts of the fronto-parietal convolutions of the brain are the centres for the voluntary movements of definite groups of muscles has been warmly supported by many distinguished observers, and among them my eminent friend, Professor J. Charcot, of Paris. Before I try to show that this theory ought to be rejected, and that the facts on which it is grounded ought to be explained in a different way, it may be well to say a few words about another theory of localization which has been germinating in my mind for twenty years, although it has assumed a definite shape only within the last two years. The facts upon which this theory is founded are the following: you will all remember that I have often taught in this room and elsewhere that the character of the symptoms in brain-diseases is not in the least dependent upon the seat of the lesion, so that a lesion of the same part may produce a great variety of symptoms, while on the other hand the same symptoms may be due to the most various causes, various not only as regards the kind, but also the seat of the organic alteration. In view of these facts, I have been led to believe that lesions of the brain produce symptoms not by destroying the function of the part where they exist, but by exerting over distant parts either an inhibitory or an exciting influence, or, in

[1] A lecture delivered in the rooms of the Boston Society of Natural History, June 1, 1875.

other words, either by stopping an activity or by setting it in play. This implies the existence of localized functions, but it does not in the least imply that the localization is such as is supposed to exist by Hitzig, Meynert, and others. If we suppose that each of these functional centres is located, not, as these physiologists admit, in a cluster of cells all collected into a certain space or a limited and well-defined part of the brain, but in cells very widely diffused through that organ, we can easily explain all the facts that are furnished by experimentation on animals and by clinical observation. With this theory we can easily understand why considerable lesions in the two sides of the brain may not be followed by the loss of any function, while ·it is impossible to reconcile such a fact with the former theories of localization.

If we further admit the view I have held for years that one half of the brain can perform all the functions of the two halves, we can easily understand that in cases of a lesion confined to one half of that organ, if it extends through the whole of that half, there may be a persistence of all the cerebral functions (as regards voluntary movement, sensibility, and intelligence).

According to the theory that cells endowed with one and the same function are scattered in the brain, it is very natural that the effect of even a most extensive lesion should be only to diminish the number of the cell-elements which have to perform the various functions of the brain, without entailing the loss of any special function.

There is, however, another point which needs to be explained ; and that is, how it can be that disease in one part of the brain should destroy the function of distant parts. There is a large number of facts bearing upon this branch of the subject ; we know now that disease in the hemispheres of the brain may be followed by alterations of nutrition in the pons Varolii, the medulla oblongata, the spinal cord, the nerves, the muscles, the skin, the joints, and even the lungs (œdema, emphysema, hæmorrhage, or disturbances of the circulation), and further that these alterations in circulation and nutrition may come on with great rapidity, and that they stand in no constant or definite relation, as regards either character or position, to the lesions in the brain by which they were produced. In view of such facts as these we can easily conceive that a disease of any part of the brain should bring alterations in circulation and nutrition in other parts of this organ itself, and thereby a loss of this or that function. Besides, as we know that an irritation, however able sometimes to produce changes in distant parts, may in other cases fail to produce them, we can easily understand that a lesion in one part of the brain will sometimes produce symptoms and fail to produce them in other cases.

Let us now leave this part of the subject, and pass to the well-known experiments of Fritsch and Hitzig, the results of which, although not absólutely constant, as I have found, are yet sufficiently so to claim our close attention. Admitting, which is not quite proved, that the current acts locally and not by propagation to other parts, as ably maintained by my ingenious friend and pupil, Dr. Dupuy, it is not yet definitely settled whether the muscular movements produced in these experiments are due to the irritation of the gray matter, or of the nerve fibres, of the cortex cerebri. My friend Professor Rouget, on anatomical and physiological grounds, inclines to the latter view. Whatever may be the truth about that special point, there are several decided obstacles to admitting the conclusions which have been drawn from these experiments ; one of these is that the parts, through the galvanization of which these movements are caused, are the will-centres for such movements. In the first place, these supposed centres are not situated in homologous parts in different animals, cats and dogs for example, a fact which evidently is a fatal objection to the theory. In the second place, these centres do not differ in size in the same proportion with the muscular masses to which they correspond ; one small muscle, for example, the orbicularis oculi, which in bulk is certainly not even the hundredth part of the mass of muscles of the anterior limb, has a centre (pointed out by Fritsch and Hitzig) which, according to my experiments, is five or six times (in the dog) as large as the centre for the muscles of the anterior limb, so that the centre for the orbicularis is, proportionally to the mass supposed to be moved by it, five or six hundred times as large as it should be. In the third place, according to Ferrier's researches we find that instead of one centre the orbicularis has three in dogs and cats, and that the sterno-cleido-mastoideus has from three to five centres, and that these various centres for one muscle are wide apart one from the other.

Besides, Vulpian has injected the chemically inert Iycopodium powder into the cerebral circulation, with the effect of choking up the vessels of the cortex cerebri, whereby we should expect that the function of this organ would be destroyed ; nevertheless, by galvanizing it, Vulpian succeeded in obtaining the muscular movements so often referred to almost as distinctly after as before the operation.

Hitzig has found that the destruction of these supposed centres causes a paralysis of the parts which are moved when galvanism is applied to those centres. This sometimes occurs, it is true ; but sometimes it does not, and when it occurs it is not permanent. In one case, one of the best observers of our times, Professor Rouget, after producing paralysis of the anterior limb by destruction of the cortical centre of the opposite side of the brain, found that when the similar centre on the other side of the brain was destroyed, there was (instead of a paralysis of the anterior limb yet free) the cessation of the paralysis produced by the first lesion.

If paralysis in the case of the extirpation of a part of the brain depended, as Hitzig and other localizers suppose, on the loss of the centre for certain voluntary movements, it is clear that in Rouget's experiment the paralysis should not disappear as it did after the second operation, but that, on the contrary, a paralysis of the other anterior limb should have appeared. But if we admit that paralysis is due to an inbibitory influence exerted by the irritation of the parts surrounding the so-called " centre " first extirpated, we can easily understand that a similar irritation, coming from the other side of the brain, destroys the effect of the first. The irritation of the big toe, as I have shown, will produce an inhibitory influence on the nerve-cells of the spinal cord in certain cases of inflammation of that nervous centre, while the irritation of other parts of the foot will stop that inhibitory action and allow the inhibited nerve-cells to become active again. But, whatever be the true explanation of the fact observed by Rouget, it is most decisive in showing that the part of the brain extirpated is not, as supposed by Hitzig and others, the centre for certain movements of the anterior limb.

Another important fact is that if we take away not only the pretended psycho-motor centre of a limb, but besides that part a good deal of the surrounding substance of the same half of the brain, we frequently find that there is no paralysis appearing. If Hitzig's views were correct we should then have a more extensive paralysis than there is in his experiments, as not only several of the supposed psycho-motor centres are taken away, but also the intervening parts of the brain, which several writers have considered as being vicariously able to replace the missing centres. I know that it may be said that the other half of the brain then performs the motor function of the injured half. But what becomes of this explanation *in extremis,* when we find that the simultaneous ablation of the pretended psycho-motor centres on the two sides is not followed by paralysis? The celebrated experiment of Flourens, consisting in slicing away the two halves of the brain from their anterior parts towards the pons Varolii, has long ago shown that a great deal of the substance of the cerebral lobes can be taken away without the appearance of paralysis.

Charcot, J. H. Jackson, and others, in support of the theory I am now criticising, have brought forward a number of pathological facts. My former assistant, a distinguished pupil of Charcot, Dr. R. Lépine, in a thesis on Localization in Diseases of the Brain, has given a drawing of a brain on which five black spots show the places of disease in as many cases, in most of which convulsions occurred chiefly or only in the arm on the opposite side. These five places are considered as corresponding to the supposed psycho-motor centres of the thoracic or abdominal limbs discovered by Fritsch and Hitzig. I wonder at this conclusion; for, if we were to admit that convulsions in those cases depended on the irritation of such centres, they would in the brain of man occupy a proportionally very much larger part of the convolutions than in dogs, cats, and monkeys. Besides, in most of these cases there was disease in other parts of the brain.

But if these facts were in the most perfect harmony with all the requirements of the theory, they would only show that *sometimes* a lesion in certain convolutions of the brain can produce convulsions either in the arm or in the leg on the opposite side. If we study a very much larger number of cases than those mentioned by Lépine, we find that on the one hand the pretended psycho-centres for the arm or for the leg are often diseased without the production of convulsions, and on the other hand that many other parts of the brain can, when injured or diseased, produce convulsions either in one arm or in one leg.

Cases published by my ingenious friend and former assistant, Dr. J. Hughlings Jackson, have led him to believe that when convulsions take place in cases of disease of the cerebral convolutions, they appear in the opposite side to that of the disease, a fact which seems to him to show that these convolutions contain motor centres for the limbs on the opposite side. If we extend our investigation to a large number of cases of injury or disease of the brain producing unilateral convulsions, we find that they occur more frequently in the limbs on the side where the lesion is in the brain than in the limbs on the opposite side. Thus, of twenty-two cases of hæmorrhage in the brain having produced convulsions in only-one or in two limbs, there were seventeen in which the convulsions were on the side of the lesion, and five only in which they were on the opposite side. This predominance of convulsions on the side of the brain lesion is a decided proof that these convulsions do not depend on a mechanism similar to that of the movements produced in the limbs on one side in the experiments of Fritsch and Hitzig, as in these vivisections the movements take place in the limbs on the opposite side to that where the brain is galvanized.

The following facts are certainly not in harmony with the view that the convolutions of the brain contain motor centres. Neither are they in harmony with the view that the pretended motor centres are in the anterior and middle lobes and not in the posterior. Taking the cases of cerebral hæmorrhage collected by Gintrac, I find that there were convulsions in forty-seven out of two hundred and twenty-two cases of hæmorrhage in the various parts of the brain proper, not including the corpora striata, the optic thalami, the ventricles, or the central parts. These forty-seven cases of convulsions were distributed as follows: —

In	45	cases of hæmorrhage in the	convolutions,	11 cases.
"	17	" " " " "	anterior lobes,	2 "
"	127	" " " " "	middle "	25 "
"	33	" " " " "	posterior "	9 "
	222			47

The kind of lesion has much more to do with the appearance of convulsions than the seat of the lesion. The anterior lobes, for instance, give rise to convulsions very frequently in cases of tumor, inflammation, etc., while, as I have already shown, they produce convulsions more rarely than any other part of the brain in cases of hæmorrhage (in two only out of seventeen cases of hæmorrhage).

I will only mention a few other strong arguments against the view that convulsions in brain-disease depend on an irritation of supposed psycho-motor centres. We find that convulsions may be produced by disease in any part of the brain, and that they may not appear, whatever part be diseased and whatever kind of disease exists. We find also that convulsions will vary extremely in their intensity, frequency, extent, etc., while the seat and kind of the disease is the same, and that, on the contrary, with a great variety as regards seat and kind of disease, there may be convulsions in the same limited part of the body. If we turn to animals we find, in some of them at least, certain parts the irritation of which gives rise at once to epileptic attacks ; but these parts lie in the spinal cord and not in the brain, and the convulsions may take place when the entire brain and pons, and even the medulla oblongata, have been removed.

As time presses, I will content myself, before concluding, with mentioning some very curious experiments I have made recently. Till now I have not been in a position to repeat them as often as I wished, but have performed them already on five guinea-pigs, on one dog, and on one rabbit. They were undertaken with the view of ascertaining whether the application of the actual cautery, at a white heat, to the brain, would produce the crossed movements observed when we galvanize certain parts of the surface of that organ. My son assisted me, and watched the animal while I applied the cautery. In no case was any movement observed under these circumstances, showing that the action of the actual cautery is different in that respect from that of galvanism. But the particularly interesting part of the experiment was that as I continued to observe the animals, during a number of days after the operation, I found, to my great surprise, that they showed some signs of paralysis on the side of the cerebral injury. A paralysis on the side of the brain-lesion in the human subject occurs much less rarely than most medical men believe ; thus I have collected more than one hundred and fifty cases in which it has happened. I cannot enter into all the theories that have been offered in explanation of its occurrence. With regard to that based upon supposed anomalies in the decussation of the pyramids, I would say that an absence of decussation has never been observed, and that, indeed, the pyramids do not seem to be the channels, at least the only channels, between the will and the muscles, as in a case of Vulpian they were well nigh destroyed without paralysis resulting.

Another supposition has been made, which probably is true for some cases. Ambrosi, Scholz, and others have looked upon paralysis as being caused by a pressure producing some œdema and anæmia in the other side of the brain, and not by the organic disease we find after death in the side of the brain corresponding with the side of the paralysis. This certainly is not true for a vast number of cases, in which there was no pressure at all.

The paralysis which has been found in my experiments, above alluded to, following cauterization of the cortex cerebri on the same side, is not, to be sure, very marked, but sufficiently so to be evident to careful observers. It exists in one or both limbs, and sometimes in the belly and the face. It is accompanied by a slight degree of contracture, especially in the front limb. Besides, there is also, on the same side, a paralysis of some branches of the cervical sympathetic nerve, as we find that the eyelids are partly closed and generally the pupil is contracted, — two phenomena which we observe after the division of that nerve.

It is clear that if a paralysis can appear on the side of an injury to, or a disease of the brain, we are not to look upon it as an effect of a loss of function of a supposed motor centre.

To conclude, I will say that if we survey all the facts brought forward to support the supposition that there are distinct psycho-motor centres in the brain, belonging to each set of muscles performing a distinct kind of movement, we find that it is impossible to admit that these centres occupy a separate, well-defined, and limited territory in some of the convolutions of the anterior and middle lobes of that organ ; and we find also that the supposition brought forward in the beginning of this lecture, — that the nerve-cells endowed with each of the primary functions of the brain are disseminated through that organ, so that no local lesion or irritation can reach more than a part of those endowed with the same function or the same kind of activity, — we find, I repeat, that this supposition is supported by most of the known facts and out of harmony with none. Regretting not to have time to dwell more at length on this subject, I thank you for the profound attention with which you have listened to this rather hurried argumentation.

[Dr. Brown-Séquard then demonstrated the changes referred to, especially as regards the eyelids and pupil, upon two rabbits which had recently been operated on in Dr. Bowditch's laboratory at the Harvard Medical College.]

FIBROID TUMOR OF THE UTERUS.

BY CHARLES N. MILLER, M. D., OF BOSTON.

M. V. C., forty-four years old, a mulatto, though with considerable Indian blood (the latter perhaps contributing the stoicism which the patient manifested throughout her tedious and painful illness), had been married twenty-two years, and was of naturally robust constitution. She had menstruated regularly since fifteen years of age, and had never been pregnant. About eight years ago she first noticed an enlargement of the lower portion of the abdomen, accompanied with pain, heat, and soreness about the left iliac region. During this time her menses were regular but profuse, occurring at intervals of three weeks. Within a year she had taken her bed and had been most of the time confined to it by prostration and exhaustion resulting from almost constant hæmorrhage. She had consulted several physicians, who after examination gave various opinions in regard to her case, the last consultant having treated her for ovarian dropsy, giving no hope of relief.

I was called to see her on the 22d of July, 1874, and found her in an alarming condition, from loss of blood, and suffering from great pain in the abdomen ; the latter was increased at intervals by the expulsion from the vagina of a solid substance of the consistency of liver and having an offensive odor. The size of the abdomen was nearly that of a woman at full term. It was plain that the patient was slowly sinking, and that unless some measure was adopted death must soon follow. Dr. Beach saw her in consultation with me the same afternoon, and upon examination of the vagina and rectum found a large, nearly solid tumor of somewhat irregular shape, involving the left half of the uterus from just above the os to the fundus, and compressing the rectum and bladder. The abdomen was quite tender and the pulse very weak. Any operative interference was out of the question on account of her low condition. The treatment agreed upon was to keep the uterus firmly contracted by ergot, with the view of cutting off the supply of blood to the growth, checking the hæmorrhage, promoting the expulsion of clots and sloughs, and assisting the process nature had already commenced ; meantime supporting the patient's strength by concentrated extract of beef, muriated tincture of iron, and stimuli. This course was strictly followed for over three months, commencing with fifteen drops of the fluid extract of ergot alternating with the same quantity of the muriated tincture of iron, every three hours, when awake.

The patient bore the ergot remarkably well, and it had the immediate effect of controlling the excessive hæmorrhage and of diminishing the amount of serous fluid which had always accompanied the passage of portions of the sloughing tumor. Six weeks after the treatment had been commenced, the patient began to change for the worse. The pain in the region of the tumor became almost intolerable, and was controlled only by Battley's sedative and subcutaneous injections of morphia. Frequent fainting spells began to supervene, and it seemed as if the patient must gradually succumb to the combined effects of the enormous drain upon her system and the presence in the uterus of a large mass of suppurating material, which by this time began to make its existence unmistakably known, portions of broken down tissue as big as a tea plate and of an extremely offensive odor passing frequently, and always attended with excruciating pains resembling those of labor ; the stench required vaginal injections of carbolic acid and chlorinated soda in solution. The appetite began to fail, and there was great difficulty in swallowing.

The pulse ranged from 120 to 130, was weak and threadlike. The tongue was dry and heavily coated. The dose of iron was increased and quinine was added to it in five grain doses.

On the 14th of November, after having passed a very miserable day, she was awakened about three in the morning by a severe paroxysm of pain. This was immediately followed by a discharge from the vagina of a large fibrous mass, accompanied by a torrent of clear fluid which drenched the bed-clothing and ran down upon the carpet in streams. The mass weighed over three pounds, had a number of root-like appendages, and on one side presented a raw and bloody surface. The tumor was much firmer in texture than anything the patient had previously passed, and gave forth a most sickening and disgusting odor. No hæmorrhage followed.

From that time the patient began to improve, and at present is performing her ordinary household duties. She has had a return of her catamenia twice within two months, the discharge being normal in appearance and quantity. The uterus, on examination by Dr. Beach and myself within a month was found contracted to its normal size.

The interest in this case seems to centre in the fact of the tolerance of the system to the long-continued use of ergot ; the exhibition of the drug no doubt keeping the uterus sufficiently contracted to enable it at the proper moment to throw off a large mass of slough, at the same time controlling the hæmorrhage and preventing the absorption of elements that might induce septicæmia. Of the preparations of iron, the muriated tincture was selected from its well-known styptic and tonic properties to assist in the prevention of hæmorrhage and to improve the character of the blood, which had become impoverished from a long-continued drain. The patient has stated within a week that she is as strong as she ever was, and has taken a walk of between four and five miles without ill effects.

RECENT PROGRESS IN PATHOLOGY OF THE NERVOUS SYSTEM.

BY JAMES J. PUTNAM, M. D.

Cerebral Concussion. — In the last report,[1] certain reasons were given for believing that in so-called cerebral concussion a vascular paralysis occurs inside the cranium, the blood collecting in the larger veins and sinuses, as it does in those of the abdomen in cases of shock, leaving the brain-substance essentially in a condition of anæmia ; and that it is to this that the symptoms are due. More recently some experiments have been reported by Koch and Filehne [2] in which this condition of concussion was produced experimentally in animals by rapping the head with a light hammer, care being taken to entirely avoid causing hæmorrhages. Under these circumstances they found reason to think that not alone the vaso-motor, but all the other cerebral centres as well, suffered mechanical injury.

*Post-Paralytic Chorea.*s — It has long been known that chorea in children is often associated with, or followed by, a more or less well marked hemiplegia, and Hughlings Jackson has used the fact as an argument in favor of his view that, as a rule, the usual form of chorea is dependent upon a lesion (minute emboli) in the anterior part of the hemisphere of the brain. According to Dr. Mitchell, it happens also that a one-sided awkwardness of movement, even so marked as to suggest incipient chorea, " is sometimes the precursor in children of a hemispasm." The reverse sequence, the choreal disorders following on hemiplegia, has hitherto not been distinctly acknowledged as something of frequent occurrence, although, their attention being once called to the point, many physicians can no doubt recall cases like those described by Mitchell. He claims " that on adults who have had hemiplegia and have entirely recovered power, there is often to be found a choreal disorder, sometimes of the leg and arm, usually of the hand alone ; that it may exist in all degrees, with partial loss of power, and with full normal strength ; that it may consist in mere awkwardness, or exist to the degree of causing *involuntary* choreoid motions of the part;" further, " that the younger the person when paralyzed, the more probable is the occurrence of choreal developments, so that in many cases of infantile deformity the choreal troubles remain as the chief difficulty long after there has been a restoration to full muscular power ; " and moreover, that there is " reason to believe that some of the general and prolonged choreoid disturbances which we see now and then from birth are due to, or rather are in some fashion related to, intra-uterine palsies which have either wholly or in part passed away."

1 Boston Medical and Surgical Journal, xci. 114, July 30, 1874.
2 Archiv für klinische Chirurgie, 1874, xvii.
8 S. Weir Mitchell, M. D., American Journal of the Medical Sciences, October, 1874.

It is plain that these facts, if they are such, lend further support to the theory proposed by Hughlings Jackson, mainly on theoretical grounds, that the involuntary, localized, movements of chorea and the unilateral convulsions associated with it are produced by the irritation of the central portion of nerve-tracts corresponding with definite groups of muscles, and are analogous to the contractions and convulsions occurring in the well-known experiments of Fritsch and Hitzig. As Mitchell says, the above propositions, if true, indicate " that choreoid affections may be owing to gross organic lesions, and that, under certain favoring circumstances, the same lesion which occasions a palsy may in itself, or in the disturbances it causes, also bring about chorea."

It is also interesting to remark in this connection, as further evidence of their cerebral origin, that the choreal movements observed in these cases were sometimes of a truly coördinated order, and thus again, analogous to the movements in some of the experiments of Hitzig and others. Thus one patient used to " rub continually the right leg with the right hand, so as even to wear out the pantaloons." In another case the arm was alternately flexed and supinated, and in another it would swing across the body, but only while the patient walked, the fingers being firmly flexed at each step. Hughlings Jackson has reported recently the case of an epileptic who went regularly through the motions of twirling his mustache, in complete unconsciousness.

As regards their clinical history, these cases of post-paralytic chorea are very obstinate, but improvement is not out of the question, especially under persistent and careful gymnastic training of the muscles affected, by a competent teacher.

It is now several years since Dr. W. A. Hammond first described a disease, called by him athetosis, which though not identical with chorea is certainly analogous to it, consisting in perpetual, slow, powerful, totally uncoördinated movements of the fingers and toes, their muscles becoming hard and large under the constant exercise, and this also there is some reason to regard as an affection of cerebral origin ; at least in both the cases given in the author's Diseases of the Nervous System, there was other evidence of cerebral disease, epilepsy in one, aphasia in the other, associated in both with failure of the memory and intelligence.

Circulation in the Encephalon.[1] — We would simply refer by title to this work, which does not admit of a brief summing up, on account of its great practical value. It consists of a description of the exact distribution of the cerebral vessels, and promises, in the light of a more advanced knowledge of the functions of the different parts of the brain itself, to aid us greatly in the exact localization of embolic inflammations, and help to further physiological results.

[1] Par H. Duret, Archives de Physiologie, vi., 1874.

Localized Inflammation of the Anterior Cornua of the Spinal Cord. —
No doubt can now be entertained of the propriety of recognizing the
occurrence among adults of a disease closely resembling, in its pathology and clinical history, the so-called essential or spinal paralysis of
children, although in certain details the two are different. The following group of symptoms is given by Seguin [1] as characteristic.

"Dysæsthesia and slight temporary anæsthesia, paresis and akinesis,
both these symptoms affecting the extremities, and in rare cases the
face, eyes, tongue, and throat; not affecting the respiratory muscles
nor those of the back and abdomen, nor the bladder, nor the sphincter
ani. Muscular atrophy in the paralyzed parts. Loss of electro-mus-
cular contractility (to faradic current) in the atrophied muscles. A
strong tendency to spontaneous retrocession of the palsy and to spontaneous cure.

"The important negative characters of this affection are : Absence
of palsy of bladder, or of sphincter ani, or of respiratory muscles. No
bed-sores. No great and extensive anæsthesia. No spinal epilepsy"
(all signs of acute diffused myelitis).

The pathology of the disease is essentially "granular degeneration
of the ganglion-cells of the anterior horns." The treatment resembles
that of infantile paralysis.

A case of muscular wasting from localized inflammation of the anterior cornua, though perhaps not belonging fairly to the class of diseases just discussed, is reported by Prevost and David,[2] where the sole
symptom was atrophy of the muscles of the thenar eminence on the
right hand, and the nervous lesion atrophy of the eighth spinal nerves
on the right side, atrophy and sclerosis of the right anterior cornu, involving the large, motor nerve-cells of the lateral group alone, through
a space of about one inch in length, the maximum of disease lying
opposite the eighth nerve. The patient was sixty years old and had
died from some surgical injury, the muscular atrophy having existed,
apparently unchanged, since his childhood.

Two remarkable cases, one of elevation, the other of depression, of
the general bodily temperature in connection with spinal injury have
been reported in England. The first,[3] observed by Mr. Teale, of Scar-
borough, apparently under every precaution, was that of a young lady
who was thrown from her horse while hunting, sustaining a fracture of
two ribs and an injury of some sort to the spine at the level of the

---

[1] For excellent summaries of our knowledge on this subject, with original cases, see Con-
sidérations sur l'atrophie aigue des cellules motrices, par Petitfils, Paris, 1873 ; Spinal
Paralysis, by E. C. Seguin, Transactions of the New York Academy of Medicine, 1874.
See also this journal for March 25, 1875, a paper by Dr. D. F. Lincoln, of Boston, and Bernhardt, Archiv für Phsychiatrie und Nervenkrankheiten, iv. 2.

[2] Archives de Physiologie, vi. 595, 1874.

[3] Lancet of March 6, 1875. See also this journal for April 8, 1875.

sixth dorsal vertebra. During the attack of meningitis which followed, the temperature, measured both in axilla and in the rectum, rose repeatedly to 122° Fahrenheit, and perhaps higher, no thermometer being at hand which would record above that point. During nearly two months it remained above 110° Fahrenheit. The case ended in recovery.

The other case [3] was that of a man who fell from a considerable height, dislocating the first dorsal vertebra, and causing a red softening of the cord at that level, with complete paraplegia. When first admitted into the hospital he had a temperature of 95.2° Fahrenheit, and from then until his death, which took place on the eleventh day, it continued to sink gradually, reaching 80.8° Fahrenheit, its lowest point.

Phosphorus in Nervous Affections. — It is well known that Thompson,[2] as well as Broadbent[3] and others, have been praising highly the efficacy of phosphorus in neuralgia, and a number of other diseases, mainly of the nervous system. Although the number of their cases is not yet great enough, and their observations have not yet been sufficiently controlled, to justify us in definitely accepting their conclusions, yet those who wish to test them will do well to observe certain precautions, recommended especially by Thompson, as the incautious use of the drug is attended with great danger. Phosphorus has generally been administered either in pillular form, where it exists either dissolved in suet, wax, resin, bisulphide of carbon, or a menstruum similar to these, or as reduced phosphorus, or in the shape of phosphide of zinc; or else in solution in alcohol, ether, or one of the vegetable or animal oils.

According to Thompson, the solutions in the vegetable (almond and olive) oils should be strictly avoided, since annoying and serious results have occasionally followed their use in the hands of several observers, probably because a portion of the phosphorus is converted (by the limited quantity of oxygen dissolved in the oil) into hypophosphorous acid, which is irritating to the stomach and very poisonous when absorbed. Theoretically this change would not take place if the oil had been superheated, and the contained air driven off; careful clinical experiments upon this point have, however, it is said, not yet been made. The author thinks it is the result of the use of this preparation that have served largely to give phosphorus its bad reputation among the profession.

The pills containing phosphorus dissolved in bisulphide of carbon are also objectionable on account of the poisonous character of the menstruum as well as because there is reason to think that the latter tends to counteract the effect of free phosphorus. The pills made with wax and resin are objectionable on theoretical grounds on account of their

---

[1] British Medical Journal, February 8, 1873.

[2] Free Phosphorus in Medicine, J. Ashburton Thompson, London, 1874. See also a review of the work in this journal for January 21, 1875.

[3] Practitioner for April, 1873, and January, 1875.

insolubility, but the latter, so far as they have been tried, have proved sufficiently efficacious.

Pills of undissolved free phosphorus are dangerous unless special precautions be taken, in their manufacture, to subdivide the element thoroughly, and at the same time to prevent it from becoming coated, by oxidation, with the inert phosphoric acid, and this is not usually done. Even then each pill should be carefully protected, and given on a full stomach, in order that the oil in the food may help dissolve the drug, which otherwise is in danger either of being partially converted into hypophosphorous acid, or of remaining undissolved, to be absorbed suddenly at some future time in accumulated amounts, when a quantity of oily food happens to come into contact with it.

The pills made with suet are theoretically unobjectionable, but have not practically proved so good as some other preparations, of which the best are the solutions in cod-liver oil,[1] alcohol, or ether, and the pills of phosphide of zinc. Of these the second can be made the most palatable,[2] but the former is to be preferred. Phosphide of zinc, in sugar-coated pills, is a good preparation, especially for children, but as it decomposes only with the aid of a weak acid each dose should be followed by a draught of an acidulated tonic or of lemonade, lest the drug should accumulate in the intestine.

℞ Phosphorus . . . . gr. j.
   Cod-liver oil . . . . ℥ iss.
   Oil of peppermint . . . . ♏ j.

℞ Tincture of phosphorus (a saturated solution in absolute alcohol dis-
     solved with heat and agitation). . . . . . . ℥ iij. ♏ x.
   Glycerine to . . . . ℥ iss.
   Spirits of peppermint . . . . ♏ v.

A full dose of phosphorus for short periods is one twelfth of a grain of the solution in alcohol or cod-liver oil every four hours, or one third of a grain of the phosphide of zinc every two hours ; but for prolonged use one fiftieth of a grain of the former is enough. There is no absolute reason to believe that the effects of the drug are cumulative, but under the slight uncertainty it is well to make a pause every two or three weeks. It is said that with these precautions phosphorus may be given with perfect safety, but in view of some of the cases of poisoning that are reported, and of the fact that our knowledge of its chemical and physiological relations is confessedly a little insecure, the physician could hardly be too watchful while using it, especially since according to Thompson no antidote is known which will neutralize the effects of the drug after it has entered the circulation. " The slightest symptom of dyspepsia should lead to its instant intermission," and the patient should be examined for tenderness at the epigastrium or right hypochondrium, and for enlargement of the liver, as signs premonitory of danger.

[1] Formula No. 6.   [2] Formula No. 10.

Monobromide of Camphor. — The use of this drug, warmly recommended by Bourneville [1] as a hypnotic and sedative, on the ground of physiological and therapeutic experiments, is not favored by Lawson,[2] who on fair trial found it less efficient than some other drugs of the same kind, and difficult to take in efficient doses without causing gastric irritation.

WILKS'S AND MOXON'S PATHOLOGICAL ANATOMY.[3]

In 1859, Dr. Wilks published his lectures delivered to the students at Guy's Hospital during the two preceding years. The scope of the book may in part be inferred from the preface, wherein it is learned that the original plan was that of a sort of syllabus, accompanied by references to specimens in the hospital museum. Further explanation seeming necessary, the lectures were published as delivered. Such was the first edition, one of unquestioned originality, the work of a sagacious observer, and representing an epoch in the progress of the study of its subject in England. Though nominally a series of lectures, it furnished a fund of material, both of fact and of suggestion, which made it of very general value. Not to be considered as a text-book, it might rather be regarded as a sort of supplementary catalogue of the museum, calling attention to the variety of specimens there contained, many of which have owed their preservation to some of the most eminent of England's medical worthies.

The student of pathological anatomy in 1875 in some respects almost literally hears a different language from that used in 1857; the demonstration of specimens takes place in a different way; points upon which stress was then laid are now overlooked, or are treated with relative indifference. Experimental pathology and its results, still more its possibilities, have opened a field which seems to have no limit, yet one which must be entered by a broad though well-defined way.

We should therefore object to the desirability of retaining in the second the general aim and character of the first edition.

If originality is preserved, it appears in such a form as to be less impressive. We think the student of the book cares less for the ideas of the writer than for his statement, critical if need be, of those of others. Above all he wishes to be taught how and what to observe, and requires in addition a manual, to which he may refer when in doubt, or when desirous of further information.

If he may thus become a worthy seeker, the merits of originality will be more thoroughly appreciated hereafter.

In looking over the section on bone, we are somewhat surprised to find that Dr. Moxon regards a node as a circumscribed formation of lymph beneath

---

[1] Practitioner, August, 1874.

[2] Ibid., November, 1874; April, 1875.

[3] *Lectures on Pathological Anatomy.* By SAMUEL WILKS, M. D., and WALTER MOXON, M. D. Second Edition. Philadelphia: Lindsay and Blakiston. 1875.

the periosteum. Caries sicca, again, is spoken of as a peculiar form of syphi-litic bone disease.

Though the waxy degeneration of muscular fibre is mentioned, England's part in its history is undervalued. The Germans, at all events, give Bowman the credit of the discovery. Though Dr. Moxon is unaware of the occurrence of tubercles in the heart's muscle, it might be stated that other observers have been more fortunate.

In treating of thrombosis and embolism, considerable stress is laid upon the formation of a thrombus in the apex of the heart and its immediate dis-placement as a cause of cerebral embolism, or of those forms occurring in the puerperal condition and at times productive of sudden death when the pulmo-nary artery is plugged. The auricular appendages are notoriously favorite seats for cardiac thrombi, in connection with arterial embolism, and the theory of immediate formation and removal requires more support than is given. Observations as to fatal embolism of the pulmonary artery show that it is gen-erally due to primary thrombosis of a body vein, and usually of one of consid-erable size.

In referring to the presence of blood in the so-called cavity of the arachnoid, and its relation to chronic inflammation of the dura mater, Dr. Moxon's cru-cial observation might apply equally well to the theory he opposes as to the one he favors.

At the end of the special pathological anatomy, as it might be called, a con-siderable number of pages is devoted to " the association of morbid condi-tions," and to the changes occurring in certain conditions. It is here, under the term anæmia, that we find the passage which Dr. Wilks has recently called attention to as indicating a priority of observation in what has been spoken of by others as progressive pernicious anæmia. He says, and the changes from the text of the first edition are unimportant, " We occasionally meet with cases of fatal anæmia where no disease is found in the body ; pa-tients, after being in an almost bloodless condition for some months, die, and all the organs are found pale, and some in a commencing state of fatty degen-eration ; there is also generally some exudation of serum into the serous cavi-ties, and œdema of lungs and other parts. We have now seen several of these cases ; the blood resembled pink water, and formed no coagula in the vessels or heart. The latter organ exhibits in a marked degree that form of fatty de-generation where the internal surface, especially the left ventricle, presents the peculiar mottling from changes in the muscular fibre."

Though we cannot recommend this work as a suitable text-book for the medical student, Dr. Moxon is certainly entitled to the credit of having added very largely to the interest of an already readable book. So ingenious a writer, so ready and plausible a theorist, is rarely met with. One constantly re-grets not having the opportunity to dispute this conclusion, to suggest doubt as to that premise, or to present controverting observations. Though much im-pressed with his skill, the element of plausibility is so striking that even when yielding we do not find ourselves convinced.

A notable paucity of allusions to recent monographs makes the book of diminished value to those seeking a work of reference.   R. H. F.

SEX IN INDUSTRY.

THE past few years have witnessed the publication of several works whose place in literature it is difficult to define with exactness. They are not distinctively medical, although the physician finds within their covers the discussion of subjects usually considered to pertain alone to his professional study. They are not for the family fireside only, although they elaborate topics which intimately involve domestic welfare and perhaps personal livelihood also. They are not in strictness contributions to sanitary science, although the sanitarian may find within them much to stimulate his investigations. They may best be described as reformatory in character and aim, inasmuch as their purpose, either indirect or positive, is to stem the increasing secession of women from purely feminine works and ways, and, by demonstrating that males and females are anatomically and physiologically unlike in essential particulars, to show that the weaker sex, because of its weakness, cannot with safety attempt things in education and in labor which the stronger can bear with impunity. It thus happens that the physician, the sanitarian, the labor-reformer, the philanthropist, the teacher, as well as those who are themselves in question, the women who are held up to public view as having functions to attend to which unfit them for masculine effort, either mental or manual, discover in these books much that is instructive and suggestive, if not altogether convincing.

To this class of reformatory productions the book before us belongs.[1] The purpose of the author is to prove that the physical organization of women unfits them for any considerable exercise of their bodily and mental forces simultaneously, and that any employment wherein these forces are coördinated, if continued sufficiently long, will result in "the impairment and overthrow of the peculiar function of the sex," and in a long train of correlative and consecutive evils. To be married and to bear and nurse children is the normal use of women, and any departure from this toward avocations calling for the expenditure of "physico-mental" force is attended with risk and often with ruin. Especially is this true during the period when the sexual function is undergoing development and attaining maturity. In support and illustration of his thesis, the author adduces evidence from various occupations in which females are employed; the manufacture of textile-fabrics, type-setting, telegraphy, basket-making, money-counting, sewing-machine labor, are cited as affording facts which demonstrate the proposition that sustained "physico-mental" activity on the part of woman is a prolific source of the diseases peculiar to her sex.

To the discussion of his theme the author has brought zeal, directness, and comprehensive intelligence; but we feel constrained to say that, in our opinion, he has failed to substantiate his theory. He has, it is true, placed before his readers much testimony from physicians and from the women themselves. The objection affects, not the quantity, but the quality of the evidence. The reader does not come upon substantial and stubborn facts wherewith to shape his convictions; he does find opinions, however, many and pertinent. Miss

[1] *Sex in Industry: A Plea for the Working-Girl.* By AZEL AMES, JR., M. D. Boston: James R. Osgood & Co. 1875.

10

A., for example, a "lady operator" in a telegraph office, has broken down, is never "regular," has headache, backache, "nervous debility," constipation, a train of evils which she attributes to her avocation as the cause ; and Dr. Ames accepts her view as the correct one. It is obvious that such testimony is only measurably weighty, because the witness is unable, in the nature of things, to eliminate the apparent from the true sources of her ill-health. In seeking for the cause of her "weaknesses," she naturally turns first to her active toil, and loses sight of the irregular habits of living, the social excesses, the unsanitary surroundings, which are often in intimate relation with her pursuit for a livelihood, and ought not to be forgotten in any estimate of the probable etiology of the diseases of woman.

Moreover, it is apparent that the females engaged in the various industries cited by the author do not have the monopoly of the sexual diseases. If Dr. Ames or any equally diligent investigator should set about ascertaining the relation of sex to almost any avocation or to no avocation at all, — to passive *ennui* and idleness, — he would find plenty of young women with menorrhagia, amenorrhœa, dysmenorrhœa, leucorrhœa, displacements, *et id genus omne*, and very probably able also, in these days of superior intelligence, to call all these "things by their right names," as our author, in his preface, makes a virtue of doing. Even those women who fulfill their natural mission as wives, mothers, and wet-nurses could offer some valuable observations in this line, to the effect that the bearing and rearing of children was in their opinion not unaccompanied by the severest fatigue and manifold functional disturbances. Looking at the subject from a purely medical stand-point, we cannot rid ourselves of the impression that the book under notice has failed to make a strong case against physico-mental industries, as such.

But after all that the work puts forth, supposing it to be accepted as true, what will be the probable effect upon the tendency of women to enter the industrial pursuits cited ? Is not the matter beyond the reach of scientific influence or legislative control ? Will not single women very naturally seek employment in channels where they can easiest earn an honest livelihood ? We do not share the forebodings of the author that the number of such employees is so great, or their physical decline is so tangible, that the vigor of the American race is imperiled thereby. We cannot help accepting the situation as it is, believing that most of human conditions sooner or later adjust themselves to natural laws, and that females, whether they adopt teaching or telegraphing for a living, will not be inclined to follow employments which they find to be suicidal. Indeed, we think it a matter of rejoicing that the avenues of industry for women are multiplying, and that thereby a fruitful source of female complaints — the want of occupation — is diminished. Before drawing the line too arbitrarily between hurtful and healthful employment, let us hear some negative testimony, the stories of women made happy and vigorous by having something to do.

Finally, we cannot help feeling that there is some objection to showing forth so publicly the peculiarities of the female sexual organization with all its deviations of function. The irregularities of menstruation are not a matter to be read about and talked about, like ordinary topics, in the drawing-room ; and we believe that the open discussion of such subjects in popular treatises is of questionable moral utility. The cause of truth and humanity is not always best served by such plain-spoken directness, and something is due even to time-honored conventionalities which have drawn a veil of propriety over such matters.

MEDICAL EDUCATION IN AMERICA.

THE annual announcements of many of our medical schools, which appear usually at this time of the year, give one in some degree a means of measuring the standard of medical education in this country. We say in some measure, for the style of most of these productions is so glowing that to arrive at a just estimate of the educational advantages of the various schools requires a pretty careful study of these yearly announcements, and considerable experience of the methods employed to attract students. There is a certain theatrical coloring about these circulars, which is well calculated to mislead the unwary. We find, for instance, in one the statement that " the success of this department is without precedent ; " another affirms the success of its alma mater to be " unparalleled," while a third indulges in congratulations to " the alumni and the friends of the college upon the flourishing state of its affairs." Turning down the foot-lights and letting in a little of the matter-of-fact light of day, let us endeavor to determine how much cause for congratulation we really have.

Undoubtedly there has been considerable improvement. The old-fashioned course of two sessions during the winter season, of scarcely more than four full months each, interlarded with mercantile, agricultural, and other pursuits, and preceded by a " full year's study with a respectable practitioner " (on paper), is pretty generally conceded to be a programme which will not " draw " nowadays. It has been found necessary to promise more than this, and various expedients have been resorted to. The winter course has been lengthened by giving a " preliminary course," — of two weeks' duration, — which, it is claimed, " enables professors to consider exhaustively subjects of importance which cannot be so fully treated during the regular session ; " or, instead of this, the course is inaugurated by a series of popular lectures. A more important addition is the so-called summer session which most schools have adopted, although we find in one case, after a great flourish of trumpets, that the course is to be of but six weeks' duration ! The general plan of study during this term is supplementary to that of the winter term, and the instruction given is often the best of its kind ; but it possesses a great disadvantage in not being part of the required course, and is consequently attended by a very small proportion of the students ; moreover, it is not to be compared with a system which provides two full terms of carefully-arranged work to all students during the year.

This is about as far as most of our faculties have dared to go, notwithstanding the success attending the experiment made by one school of giving three full years of college instruction. The only attempt in this direction which has thus far been made is a graded course of three years offered to those students who desire to undertake it. We sincerely hope that there are enough sensible young men to see the advantage of this plan of study to make the adoption of it as the required course necessary. Until this has been done no school will have a right to say that it gives more than two years of instruction. In reality the majority of American students graduate after eighteen months of college work, preceded by a year of such study as the acquirements or time of the private instructor permits. What a fraud this first year's course of study really is, most of our college deans could undoubtedly tell us, were it desirable to do so, and yet we hear much talk about a full three years' course. Until a radical change has been adopted in the method of instruction it would be hardly worth while to bring up the question of a preliminary examination. This we are glad to see has been adopted by that school which has made the needed reforms, and by one other also.

We regret to be unable to give a better report of the progress made by our teachers in the cause of medical education. The old policy of endeavoring to attract students by making the course "popular" is still the prevailing one. The fallacy of this theory will, we think, before long be fully demonstrated. Nearly all our medical schools have plenty of talent and plenty of clinical material at their disposal, but neither of these can be put to its best use without proper organization. A course of study which carries the student progressively and systematically from one subject to another in a just and natural order, and which is followed by rigorous examinations, enforces a mental discipline which is of incalculable benefit to him, and insures a thorough training in certain branches of medical instruction which could not be acquired under any other system. This training is of especial importance in the early years of a student's life, and paves the way for the work he has before him in the hospital wards.

LISTER IN GERMANY.

THE progress of Professor Lister through the university towns of Germany, which he is visiting chiefly with a view to inquire into the mode in which the antiseptic treatment is carried out on the Continent, has, according to the *Lancet*, assumed the character of a triumphal march. On his recent visit to Munich he met with a most enthusiastic reception. At a banquet given to him nearly all the professors of the medical faculty of the university, and many members of the government, town council, and medical society of Munich, took part. The guest was welcomed by Professor Nussbaum in the name of the minister, Von Pfeuffer, and Professors Ziemssen, Seitz, and others were amongst the speakers. The students of the university also sent a deputation to Professor Lister, to express the esteem and high appreciation they had for the originator of the antiseptic treatment, which is carried out with excellent results at the different hospitals in Munich. From Munich he went to Leipzig, where, as is well known, the principles of antiseptic surgery have been faithfully adopted by Professor Thiersch, who, however, maintains the superiority of salicylic acid over carbolic acid. On the 8th inst. there was a "Lister-Banket" in the Schützenhause, at which some three or four hundred persons were present, including nearly all the professors, many of the medical practitioners of the town, and a large number of medical students. Thiersch proposed Professor Lister's health in a dryly humorous speech, which was couched in most complimentary terms and was loudly applauded. Professor Lister, in his reply (which was in German), took occasion to tell the Leipzigers that he had tried salicylic acid, and found it inferior to carbolic; although he would willingly have adopted it had it been better, for it was the *principle* of antiseptic surgery, and not this or that acid, that he contended for. Professor Volkmann, who had come from Halle with many of his colleagues and students, then preposed the health of Mrs. Lister and the Misses Lister, who were present in the gallery; Professor Carus gave the "University of Edinburgh," and toast after toast followed, the proceedings lasting beyond midnight. One very novel feature was the introduction of two songs written in honor of the guest of the evening, and set to well-known students' melodies. They were sung by the whole company, and they abound in words of welcome to Professor Lister, and praise of antiseptic surgery. One of them, entitled "Carbolsäure Tingel-Tangel," is full of witty allusions to the germ theory, bacteria, and antiseptics, the special virtues of salicylic acid not being forgotten. The cordial reception of the professor in Germany is, we think, to be looked upon as a tribute of respect for his high standing and attainments, and his labors as a scientific surgeon, rather than an indorsement of his antiseptic theory.

MEDICAL NOTES.

— The fourth series of fifty cases of ovariotomy is reported by T. Keith, F. R. C. S., in the *British Medical Journal* of June 26, 1875. The mortality of the different series of his cases is given by Mr. Keith as follows: In the first series of fifty cases there were eleven deaths; in the second, eight deaths; in the third, eight deaths; and in the fourth, six deaths. In the six fatal cases of the fourth series the cause of death was septicæmia. "Further experience," says Mr. Keith, "has satisfied me of the value of the actual cautery in the treatment of the pedicle, and I am coming to the conclusion that it is the best of all the intra-peritoneal methods for securing the pedicle." Sulphuric ether was given in all the cases.

— A Case of Neuralgia Treated by Nerve-Stretching serves as the text for a clinical lecture by G. W. Callender, F. R. S., reported in the *Lancet* for June 26, 1875. A man aged twenty, by occupation a carpenter, had his right hand severely injured by a circular saw. Primary amputation at the wrist was followed by imperfect healing of the wound, by a painful condition of the fore-arm, and by slight necrosis. One year later he submitted to a second amputation; but although the wound healed he was liable to pain, and about seven weeks back he struck the end of the stump, since which time the pain had greatly increased. He thereupon decided to go from Canada to England for the purpose of obtaining relief. When admitted to St. Bartholomew's Hospital the fore-arm and arm were cold, and the skin was glazed and of a dusky color. The surface tissue was inelastic, and the skin was moved stiffly over the subjacent fascia. He complained of twitchings in the muscles of the stump, and to a less extent in those of the arm. He suffered from constant pain, sometimes described as burning, sometimes as shooting, but liable to become suddenly worse and almost unbearable, extending from the stump up to the elbow and arm. There was tenderness on pressure, with aggravation of other symptoms, chiefly from the first over the course of the median nerve ; but latterly there had been pain on pressure over the tracks of other nerves, such as the ulnar and the external cutaneous. Cool lotions were ordered for the arm, subcutaneous injections of morphia into the fore-arm, and quinine and morphia were administered to the patient. March 10th there had been no improvement. On March 27th Mr. Callender cut down upon the median nerve, which seemed to be thickened in itself and in its surroundings, and after freeing about one inch of the nerve from adjacent structures he forcibly stretched it, pulling it down for about three quarters of an inch. The wound was then washed with a solution of salicylic acid, drained, and closed. For twenty-four hours after the operation there was pain in the course of the nerve, extending to the axilla ; it then ceased and did not recur. April 25th the patient was well in all respects.

— A French journal, in commenting upon a case of accidental poisoning through the mistake of an American apothecary, says, " In France, our apothecary shops are inspected in the most careful manner and at stated intervals ; poisonous drugs are kept locked in a case set apart for them. The public health does not suffer from this precaution. We are threatened already with ' liberty as it is in Belgium ; ' let us hope that we shall not obtain ' liberty as it is in America.' "

— The Paris correspondent of the *British Medical Journal* writes, under date June 27th, " It is with unfeigned regret I have to announce the death of M. Demarquay, which took place somewhat suddenly on Monday, the 21st instant, at Longueval, his birthplace, a small village in the department of the Somme, in the sixty-first year of his age, from cancer of the stomach. The name of Demarquay is familiar to the medical world, as he not only distinguished himself by his writings, which proved him to be a *savant* in the true sense of the word, but was also one of the ablest and most practical surgeons of the day. M. Demarquay was surgeon to the ' Maison Municipale de Santé,' more familiarly known as the Maison Dubois, where he had made himself very popular. He was far above political influences, which is a rare thing for a man of his position in France, so that he had none but friends in the ranks of all parties. This he showed during the siege of Paris, and subsequently during the Commune, when, as surgeon and one of the founders of the ' Ambulance de la Presse,' he rendered the most unreserved and signal service. M. Demarquay was a member of the Academy of Medicine, and, had he lived, would doubtless have one day taken his seat at the Institute. His professional services were rewarded by the state by promotion to the dignity of Commandant of the Legion of Honor. His funeral took place at Longueval, and among the mourners was observed a man with a pair of wooden legs, his own having been removed by M. Demarquay, as they were shattered by a Prussian shell during the war. Born of poor parents, M. Demarquay died a millionaire. He was never married, and consequently bequeathed a portion of his large fortune to his poorer relations, and the remainder was distributed as follows: £4000 to the Paris School of Medicine for the foundation of an annual prize; £400 was reserved and made over to one of his friends and disciples for the purpose of putting together and publishing his loose manuscripts. A man of literary pursuits, M. Demarquay possessed a very extensive library, which is to be distributed among his friends, who will also inherit the various articles of curiosity with which his apartments in the Rue Taitbout teemed."

LETTER FROM PORTLAND.

MESSRS. EDITORS, — June is more full of matters of interest to the medical profession in this State than any other month of the year. In it occur the graduation of the successful candidates in the Medical School of Maine; the opening of the schools for medical instruction in Portland and Lewiston; and the meeting of the Maine Medical Association, with its essays and discussions on disease and public health, its reports about education and the General Hospital, its efforts in behalf of progress wherever a medical body can effect it, and its delightful social gatherings, at which the busy practitioners can find a perfect relief from the exhausting cares of their work.

Rarely has there been a more satisfactory meeting of the association than that which has just been held. During the three days' session which commenced on the 8th, there were numerous reports of cases and papers on particular methods of treatment, all of which elicited profitable discussion. It is impossible in the limits of this letter to give a fitting abstract of these articles, but a good idea of their scope and bearing may be obtained from a brief mention of their titles and authors. Papers were presented by Dr. Horr, of Lewiston, on embolism; Dr. Harlow, Superintendent of the Maine Insane Hospital, Augusta, on the pathology of insanity; Dr. Hamlin, of Bangor, on lancing the gums during first dentition; Dr. Devoll, of Portland, on dress reform; Dr. Spalding, of Portland, on atropia in ophthalmic surgery; Dr. Adams, of Island Pond, on the use of Esmarch's bandage; and Professor Palmer, of the Medical School of Maine, on antipyretics. Dr. Greene, of Portland, exhibited a case of dislocation of the shoulder, which was reduced after sixty-five days' continuance; Dr. Files, of Portland, reported a case of double amputation after railroad injuries, with recovery, and an amputation of the foot; Dr. Sanger, of Bangor, a case of acute abscess of the lung, treated with the aspirator; and Dr. Small, of Portland, the result of a great number of cases of forceps delivery, strongly favoring the employment of the instruments in tardy cases. Though there was in these articles little, perhaps, which could be regarded as strikingly original in conception, they certainly possessed the merit of being in great measure the result of actual observation on the part of able and practical men, and of bringing before the profession in an attractive way many facts and ideas which could not fail to make a useful and lasting impression. And in this way the association is doing a great good. It presents inducements to its members to report the results of their cases, to compare notes with their fellows, to do more careful and critical work, and to acquire a habit and facility of communicating their beliefs and opinions. Indeed, it is almost entirely through the printed transactions of this association that the physicians of Maine give publicity to their views. There are many cases occurring in this State which ought to be reported; but the men who observe them, though appreciating their interest, with a diffidence which has become almost characteristic, hesitate to send the records of their labor to the metropolitan journals, and modestly prefer to make known their doings only to their professional neighbors and friends in the county and State societies. At these meetings work of a most creditable character is regularly done, and it is a matter of very serious regret that so little of it is heard of by the profession at large. Not infrequently delegates from other State societies express surprise at the number and ability of the reports and discussions; and the principal reason for this is that Maine practitioners, by reporting so rarely in the journals, give the medical world little opportunity to know what manner of men they are.

The president, Dr. Thomas H. Brown, of Paris, pronounced a very interesting inaugural address, which contained suggestions as to the duties of the association, the chief one having reference to the speedy establishment of a State Board of Health. In compliance with this proposition a committee, of which Dr. French, of Portland, is chairman, was appointed to coöperate with the constituted authorities in effecting the early formation of such a board. In spite of the rebuffs which the association has experienced in its endeavors to get State legislation in medical matters hitherto, — as, for instance, with regard to dissection, compulsory vaccination, and medical registration, — the commitee is hopeful of convincing the legislature of the necessity of prompt action in the premises, and of being able to report completely and satisfactorily at the next annual meeting.

Dr. Gilman, of Portland, the chairman of the committee on the Maine General Hospital, reported that the building was formally dedicated last October, and opened for the reception of patients in November. (You have already published an account of the ceremonies.) The affairs of the hospital were stated to be in a satisfactory condition. The last legislature appropriated ten thousand dollars for the completion of the central building; and two free beds for the year have been established, one by Mrs. Dummer, of Hallowell, and the other by the Portland Army and Navy Union. The whole number of patients admitted is sixty-nine, ten of them being medical and fifty-nine surgical cases. Thirty-one surgical operations have been performed, and, as will be seen from the following table, the results have generally been of a very satisfactory nature : —

DISEASE.	OPERATION.	RESULT.
Encephaloid of condyle of femur.	Amputation, middle third of thigh.	Discharged cured as to amputation in 4 2-7 weeks.
Strumous arthritis of knee.	Amputation, middle third of thigh.	Discharged cured in 8 5-7 weeks.
Caries of tarsal bones.	Amputation at ankle joint.	Discharged cured in 7 4-7 weeks.
Caries phalanx index finger.	Amputation.	Discharged cured in 5 days.
Ununited sphincter, result of previous operation.	Edges pared and united by suture.	Discharged cured in 2 3-7 weeks.
Fistulæ in ano, three openings with extensive burrowing.	Fistulæ divided.	Discharged cured in 9 4-7 weeks.
Simple fistula in ano.	Fistula divided.	Discharged nearly healed in 1 5-7 weeks.
Vesico-Vaginal fistula.	Two operations.	Discharged not relieved.
Cataract.	Lens extracted.	Violent inflammation nearly destroyed eye; but some useful vision was obtained, and it was increasing at time of discharge, 3 weeks.
Cancerous tumor of umbilicus.	Tumor removed.	Discharged cured as to operation in 2 4-7 weeks.
Scirrhus of breast.	Breast removed.	Discharged cured as to operation in 2 6-7 weeks.
Sarcoma of cervix uteri.	Tumor removed.	Growth returned, and patient died in 10 2-7 weeks.
Cystic tumor of neck.	Tumor removed.	Discharged cured in 2 weeks.
Malignant growth from retina.	Eye extirpated, together with a large portion of contents of the orbit.	Obtained a fair stump, and an artificial eye was fitted.
Destruction of eye, result of injury.	Eye extirpated.	Discharged cured in 1 5-7 weeks.
Caries of rib	Carious portion removed.	Discharged in 1 4-7 weeks, wound healing satisfactorily.
Partial ankylosis of knee.	Patella elevated by subcutaneous drilling, and limb straightened.	Discharged in 1 1-7 weeks, limb in good position and without inflammation.
Fibrous ankylosis of shoulder.	Adhesions broken by forcible motion.	Discharged with a good degree of motion, and improving, in 2 2-7 weeks.
Caries of os calcis.	Whole bone removed.	Still under treatment, with prospect of a useful foot.
Phimosis and chancre.	Circumcision.	Discharged cured in 4 5-7 weeks.
Stricture of urethra, with gleet.	Divulsion.	Still under treatment.
Traumatic stricture of urethra, with almost constant painful erections.	Gradual dilatation.	Discharged cured in 2 2-7 weeks.
Traumatic stricture accompanied by cystitis.	Gradual dilatation.	Still under treatment.
Traumatic stricture.	Gradual dilatation attempted.	Extravasation of urine, complete retention, puncture of bladder through rectum, death from pyæmia on the 13th day.
Necrosis of skull.	A large piece of both tables removed.	Discharged cured in 4 5-7 weeks.
Occlusion of pupil.	Iridectomy.	Discharged with very good vision in 1 4-7 weeks.
Laceration of perineum and of cervix uteri.	Two plastic operations.	Still under treatment.
Laceration of cervix uteri.	Plastic operations.	Still under treatment.
Caries of femur.	Removed with gouge.	Discharged in 2 weeks, wound filling well.

The association voted to appropriate two hundred and fifty of the six hundred dollars balance which the treasurer reported, for the support of a free bed in the hospital for one year. It may properly be mentioned in this connection that the Odd Fellows of this city will probably found one and perhaps two free beds, and it is hoped that the Masonic bodies will do likewise.

No question brought before the meeting excited more or livelier discussion than that of medical education. Dr. Adams, of Island Pond, chairman of the committee on the Medical School of Maine, reported that the school was in excellent condition, the teachers being devoted and successful, the students faithful, attentive, and enthusiastic. He suggested the desirableness of a graded course of study as soon as it could safely be attempted. In closing he stated that he had just had placed in his hands the following preamble and vote which had been adopted at the meeting of the faculty the previous night: —

Whereas, The faculty believe that it is desirable for students to pay especial attention to the primary branches during the first portion of their course of study, in order that they may be better prepared to appreciate the more advanced subjects in the latter part; and

Whereas, The faculty, though deeming it inexpedient at present to oblige students to take a regularly graded course of study, desire to present inducements which will lead them to voluntarily pursue this preferable plan; therefore it is

Voted, That any student may present himself for final examination in anatomy, physiology, and chemistry (any or all) at the regularly appointed time for examination, provided he previously presents to the secretary satisfactory evidence that, at the close of the current term, he will have completed at least twelve months of actual study and have attended a full course of lectures in this school; and an official record of the result of the successful examinations shall be made by the secretary. But the successful passage of an examination shall not exempt a student from faithful attendance upon any exercises in any department during the second course of lectures.

Although this is only putting a premium on the adoption of a graded course, making the pursuit of this plan optional and not obligatory, still it is so evidently a step forward and the forerunner of a radical change in the method of instruction, that the association immediately and enthusiastically adopted a resolution of approval and indorsement.

The matter of preliminary education for medical students was then taken up and freely ventilated. Several members thought that an entrance examination should be held, one even proposing that a college education should be the minimum standard. In the course of the discussion the fact was stated that the faculty had recently voted to require every new candidate for admission to the Medical School of Maine to give satisfactory evidence of possessing a decent English education, by presentation of a diploma, if possible, otherwise by written examination. This is as far as the government of the school can venture at present. It has of late so tightened the screws at the examination for degrees that the average of rejections for two years past has been twenty-two per cent. Of the unsuccessful aspirants for medical honors a majority go to another school and graduate without difficulty within a half-year. If in these circumstances a high degree of preparatory education is insisted upon, the number of students in the school will be disastrously reduced. The faculty is anxious to go just as far and as fast as the profession will sustain it, but it would be suicidal to do more. As long as physicians will allow men who are notably lacking in mental ability, training, and acquirements to be their students even nominally, and will resent as a personal affront the school's refusal to foster these weaklings, and regard it as sufficient reason for a withdrawal of patronage, so long the faculty must be crippled in its efforts to advance the standard of education. At the conclusion of the discussion the following resolution was unanimously adopted: —

Resolved, That, in the opinion of this association, it is the duty of physicians to impress on young men intending to study medicine the necessity of a thorough preliminary education, and to decline to receive under their instruction such as are deficient in education or mental endowments.

On the evening of the second day the annual oration was given by Dr. Alfred Mitchell, of Brunswick, who chose for his subject The Gentleman in Medicine. Such an abstract as could be given here would come far short of doing justice to this production; but all who know our popular professor of obstetrics and diseases of children will readily believe that it was rich in profound thought, elegant in diction, sparkling with wit, and received with hearty applause. After the oration, the physicians of Portland, in accordance with their custom for many years, gave a supper at the Falmouth Hotel to the visiting members and their wives, and the occasion was very enjoyable.

During the session many new members were admitted. There was one woman among them, the first of her sex who has joined the association. She is a graduate of several years' standing, an active member of the Cumberland County Medical Society, and not the slightest opposition was made to her election.

Last year Dr. T. A. Foster, of Portland, offered a prize of twenty-five dollars — the amount of his salary as treasurer — for the best essay on one of several specified subjects. A single paper was presented, the subject of which was The Hygiene of our Country Towns and Villages, and its author, Dr. E. M. Fuller, of Bath, received the award. Dr. Foster offers a similar prize for next year for an essay on nervous indigestion and its relations to sympathetic affections from other forms of indigestion, or on the physiology of habit. Any member may compete; the essays are to be sent to the president, and the members who are professors in the medical school will act as judges.

Dr. James M. Bates, of Yarmouth, is president, and Dr. Charles O. Hunt, of Portland, secretary for the ensuing year.

The Portland School for Medical Instruction opened its summer term on the 16th with a good list of students. The Lewiston school began work at about the same time, and both start off on their year's labor with excellent prospects and the determination to accomplish more than ever before, much as this has been.   GAMMA.

- PORTLAND, *June*, 1875.

WEEKLY BULLETIN OF PREVALENT DISEASES.

THE following is a bulletin of the diseases prevalent in Massachusetts during the week ending July 24, 1875, compiled under the authority of the State Board of Health from the returns of physicians representing all sections of the State: —

There has been during the week a marked diminution in the prevalence of all acute diseases except dysentery; the principal increase in the prevalence of that affection occurred in the Metropolitan section. The diseases of summer (cholera infantum, cholera morbus, diarrhœa, and dysentery) continue at the head of the list, but they are generally mild in type.

The report for each section is as follows: —

Berkshire: Cholera infantum, typhoid fever, diarrhœa, cholera morbus.

Valley: Diarrhœa, cholera morbus, cholera infantum, dysentery. Easthampton reports two cases of small-pox.

Midland: Diarrhœa, cholera infantum, cholera morbus, rheumatism, dysentery.

Northeastern: Cholera morbus, diarrhœa, cholera infantum. Very little sickness.

Metropolitan: Diarrhœa, cholera morbus, cholera infantum, dysentery. A few cases of diphtheria are reported. Measles and scarlatina have almost disappeared.

Southeastern: Cholera morbus, diarrhœa, rheumatism. Very little sickness.

F. W. DRAPER, M. D., Registrar.

COMPARATIVE MORTALITY-RATES FOR THE WEEK ENDING JULY 17, 1875.

	Estimated Population.	Total Mortality for the Week.	Annual Death-rate per 1000 during Week.
New York	1,040,000	890	44
Philadelphia	775,000	459	31
Brooklyn	450,000		
Boston	350,000	184	27
Cincinnati	260,000	116	23
Providence	100,700	29	15
Worcester	50,000	19	20
Lowell	50,000	15	16
Cambridge	50,000	15	16
Fall River	45,000	22	25
Lawrence	33,000	27	43
Springfield	33,000	4	6
Lynn	28,000	9	17
Salem	26,000	6	12

NOTICE. — The editor of the Harvard Triennial Catalogue would like to learn the date and place of death of the following persons, who took their medical degrees at Cambridge before 1800: Dr. James Otis Prentiss, Dr. John B. Menard, and Dr. Jonathan White. He may be addressed at the College Library, Cambridge, Mass.

BOOKS AND PAMPHLETS RECEIVED. — Iridotomy and its Applicability to certain Defects of the Eye. By A. W. Calhoun, M. D. Atlanta, Ga. 1875.

The Management of Eczema. By L. Duncan Bulkley, A. M., M. D. New York: G. P. Putnam's Sons. 1875. (Lee and Shepard.)

A Clinical Contribution to the Treatment of Tubal Pregnancy. By T. Gaillard Thomas, M. D. Reprinted from the New York Medical Journal. New York: D. Appleton & Co· 1875.

The Skull and Brain: their Indications of Character and Anatomical Relations. By Nicholas Morgan. London: Longmans, Green, & Co. 1875.

THE BOSTON
MEDICAL AND SURGICAL JOURNAL.

VOL. XCIII. — THURSDAY, AUGUST 5, 1875. — NO. 6.

—————

THE CONTINUED AND THE FREQUENT DOSE.[1]

BY EDWARD H. CLARKE, M. D.,

Late Professor of Materia Medica in Harvard University.

THE systematic treatises on materia medica with which American and foreign medical literature abounds usually give, near the close of their description of the various drugs whose virtues they rehearse, the appropriate dose for therapeutical use, and also the toxicological dose, if the article is capable of exerting any poisonous action on the human economy. Thus Waring, after describing the salts of morphia, adds, "Dose of the morphia salts, gr. $\frac{1}{8}-\frac{1}{4}-\frac{1}{2}$ up to gr. 1."[2] Stillé concludes his account of the carbonate of lithium with the statement that it " may be administered in doses of from one to five grains three times a day, dissolved in not less than four ounces of water."[3] The United States Dispensatory, speaking of the sulphate of quinia, says, " The dose varies exceedingly, according to the circumstances of the patient and the object to be accomplished; "[4] and then adds that as a simple tonic, a grain may be given three times a day, or more frequently; that in intermittents, from twelve to twenty-four grains may be given between the paroxysms, in divided quantities, according to the condition of the patient and other circumstances. These and similar statements with regard to the doses of medicines, that may be found in all works on materia medica and therapeutics, are essential. They are true as far as they go, but they do not represent the whole truth. They fail to give to the student and practitioner an accurate notion of what an important factor in therapeutics the dose is; and especially do they fail to convey an accurate notion of the therapeutical importance of variation of dose and method of administration.

In saying this, I do not forget that we are told by all works on materia medica that doses should vary with age, sex, temperament,

[1] Read before the Section of Practical Medicine of the American Medical Association, at Louisville, Kentucky, May 4, 1875.

[2] Practical Therapeutics. American Edition, page 419.

[3] Therapeutics and Materia Medica. Fourth Edition, vol. ii. page 351.

[4] United States Dispensatory. Thirteenth Edition, page 1383.

idiosyncrasy, disease, habit, and the like. This is all true. It has been confirmed by the experience and observation of centuries, but it is not the whole truth. It does not give an adequate notion of the therapeutical power which can be exerted by appropriate physiological doses.

It is the object of this paper to call attention, as briefly as possible, to this therapeutical power, and especially to the action of what, for want of a better designation, may be called the therapeutical action of continued and frequent doses.

Doses of medicines may be appropriately considered under four distinct heads or classes, namely: (1) single doses; (2) continued doses; (3) frequent doses; (4) toxicological doses. The first and last of these, or the single and the toxic dose, are the doses given in treatises on materia medica, and are recognized as representing the therapeutic and poisonous action of any given drug. It is unnecessary to dwell upon them, for they are universally understood. But the bare statement of what is the legitimate single or average toxicological dose of an article like opium, for instance, gives no adequate or intelligent notion of what the continued or frequent dose of the same drug is; nor does it give any adequate or intelligent notion of the physiological action and consequent therapeutical power of its continued or its frequent dose.

Let us consider first the *continued dose.* By this is meant the administration of a drug in such a way that the elimination of one dose shall not be completed before the absorption of the following dose has commenced. " By this method of administration the blood is kept constantly charged with the drug. . . . . The difference between the single and the continued dose is the difference between keeping the blood constantly charged with the article administered, and allowing the blood not only to free itself from one dose, before a second dose is administered, but making the intervals between the doses so long that the blood shall be practically a longer period uncharged than charged with it."

" The observance of this difference is important physiologically and therapeutically. The neglect of it explains much of the confusion and discrepancy that may be found in the statements of different observers with regard to the action of drugs. Many of the phenomena, both physiological and toxicological, that follow the exhibition of the continued, do not follow that of the single dose. And, what is in fact a corollary from this, many therapeutical results may be obtained by the continued that cannot be got from the single dose. It is also to be remarked that, although few or no practitioners write as if they were aware of the important difference here referred to, yet the larger number of observations evidently are founded on the action of the continued dose. Physiologists, on the contrary, seem to have experimented oftenest with the single dose."[1] The continued dose means keeping the blood continuously charged with a medicine by a succession of single doses. The single dose is an appropriate quantity given once or oftener, without keeping it continuously in the blood. The therapeutical value of these doses and the physiological difference between them are of great importance.

Let us look at some illustrations of this difference and value.[2]

Ammonia and its salts " readily enter the blood, and must to some extent increase its alkaline reaction ; but from their volatility and high diffusion power they are rapidly eliminated, and hence their action on the blood and the organs of the body is a very transient one."[3] The elimination of a single dose of carbonate of ammonia is practically completed in an hour or two after it is administered. Its physiological action is correctly stated by the United States Dispensatory to be " stimulant, diaphoretic, anti-spasmodic, powerfully antacid, and in large doses emetic." In consequence of this action, it is largely used in depressed conditions of the vital powers. This is the well-known action of a single dose or of a few doses given near together, after which the system is freed by elimination from the drug. No change is produced in the quality of the blood. If a continued dose of ammonia is given, that is, if it is given so often, say every hour for several days, that the blood is continuously charged with it, a very different set of phenomena from those just described appear. " When ammonia or its carbonate is administered " — in this way — " for some time to animals or man, the effect is to modify the blood corpuscles ; they become easily soluble, crenate at the edge, many-sided, colorless, transparent, collapsed, and loosely agglomerated, but not in rolls ; and the blood when drawn, or after death, is absolutely fluid or· loosely coagulated."[4] These phenomena were observed by Dr. B. W. Richardson, of London. They closely resemble the changes in the blood which occur in patients suffering from typhoid and typhus fevers. Hence it appears that the single dose of ammonia produces rapid and effectual stimulation of the heart,

[1] The Physiological and Therapeutical Action of the Bromide of Potassium and Bromide of Ammonia. By Edward H. Clarke, M. D., and Robert Amory, M. D. Pages 34, 35. These remarks, originally applied to the bromide of potassium, are susceptible of general application.

[2] In the discussion which followed the reading of this paper, at the meeting of the medical association, several speakers evidently regarded the paper as advocating *persistent* dosing, or *persistence in dosing*, and criticised it accordingly. It scarcely seems necessary to say that the continued dose which is here described has nothing in common with persistent dosing. In order to administer a continued dose of any drug, the practitioner must know and keep in mind the relation of that drug's elimination to its absorption, and be guided by that relation. A persistent doser may persist in giving medicines indefinitely, and never use the continued dose at all. The art of prescribing will never yield its best results till the physiological action of drugs is understood and recognized.

[3] A Handbook of Therapeutics. By Sydney Ringer, M. D. English Edition, page 111.

[4] Practical Therapeutics. By Edward John Waring. American Edition, page 61.

while the continued dose of the same article alters the quality of the blood, and notably of the blood corpuscles. The single dose exerts a therapeutic, the continued dose a toxic action on the economy. It is unnecessary in this presence to dwell upon the obvious therapeutic inferences that follow from these data, at least so far as ammonia is concerned.

Gallic acid is another illustration of the difference between the single and the continued dose. This acid is rapidly eliminated. Physiologists tell us that in a couple of hours after it has been swallowed, it has practically left the system, by way of the kidneys, to such an extent that it exerts no appreciable action upon the blood after that length of time. Gallic acid has a well-deserved reputation for controlling certains forms of hæmorrhage. Suppose it is given in single doses of ten grains, more or less, three times a day, which I apprehend is the usual method of administration, the blood will be subjected to the restraining action of the acid only about six hours out of the twenty-four ; not long enough to hold steadily in check a hæmorrhagic disposition. Suppose, now, that instead of the single, the continued dose is administered, by which the ratio of elimination to absorption is constantly regarded, and the blood kept continuously charged with gallic acid ; the result will be a continuous action upon the blood, not an intermittent one. It is needless to point out the fact that continuity of action is very sure to give rise to phenomena that will not follow intermittence.

No drug exhibits in a more striking light both the physiological and the therapeutical differences between single and continued doses than alcohol. The partial, confused, and incomplete recognition of these differences by various observers and experimenters, who have examined and described the physiological action of alcohol, goes a great way towards explaining the various and often discordant results at which they have arrived. We learn from the experiments of Messrs. Lallemand, Perrin, and Duroy, as well as from those of Drs. Anstie, Parkes, Smith, Binz, and others, that the disappearance of a single dose of alcohol from the system, either by elimination from it or combustion in it, or by both processes, practically takes place in about six or eight hours after its ingestion. Traces of alcohol may be found in the blood and in the excreta for a much longer period than this ; but so much of it leaves the system within eight hours, that what remains of any single dose beyond this length of time has no real physiological value. A person who takes a dose of alcohol, in the shape of wine or other alcoholic liquid, once in each twenty-four hours, subjects his organism to the action of alcohol about one third of that time, and leaves it free from that action about two thirds of the same period. A person who takes what is known in non-scientific language as an " eye-opener " in the morning, wine with his dinner or lunch, a digester in the afternoon, and a "night-cap" on retiring, takes the continued dose of alcohol. His blood is continuously charged with alcohol to a greater or less degree. There are phthisical patients who imitate this method of ingesting alcohol, and take a daily continued dose of it, keeping their blood charged with it more than two thirds of the time.

Alcohol taken in a single daily dose, by which the blood is practically free from it more than two thirds of the time, and alcohol taken in a daily continued dose, by which the blood is practically charged with it more than two thirds of the time, are substantially different drugs, which produce different physiological phenomena and are or should be employed for different therapeutical ends. This is not the time nor does it fall within the scope of this paper to describe these differences in detail. It is sufficient for my purpose to indicate their existence as illustrations of the single and the continued dose.

The bromide of potassium affords another and most pertinent illustration of the different physiological and therapeutical action which the single and the continued dose of an article may produce. I pointed out these differences in a comparatively recent monograph on the physiological and therapeutical action of the bromide of potassium, and will not repeat them here.[1] Illustrations of single and continued doses, and of the therapeutical importance of recognizing them as factors in the treatment of disease, might be multiplied indefinitely; but enough has been said to call your attention to them and to emphasize their importance. It was impossible to recognize and use them as separate therapeutic factors till physiological observation and experiment had discovered the time and method of the absorption and elimination of drugs, and the ratio of the former to the latter; nor can the practitioner apply them clinically till he knows, at least with approximate accuracy, the way every article he uses gets into and out of the system, the length of time it remains in the system, and its behavior while there.

The administration of medicines to the sick, without regard to the different and often opposite results, physiological or therapeutical, that follow the single and the continued dose, is both unsatisfactory and unscientific. It is unsatisfactory because it fails to secure the legitimate action of medicinal agents. It is unscientific, because it ignores some of the most important physiological conditions upon which scientific therapeutics rest. The time has come for the clinician to recognize and use these and other phenomena of the *modus operandi* of drugs which the physiologist has discovered and whose accuracy he has demonstrated.

Secondly, the *frequent dose* is the giving of a medicine so as to impart to the organism some one or more of its actions, whether primary or secondary, with great rapidity. It is hitting blow after blow in quick succession, upon some organ which it is desirable to affect, in

[1] Op. cit.

accordance with evident indications, with rapidity and power. It is usually, perhaps always, some action of a drug, manifested soon after its absorption, which it is desirable to obtain and which can be obtained by the frequent dose. Obviously the administration of the frequent dose is limited by the physiological behavior of the system under its influence. After a certain period the frequent dose is equivalent to a full single dose or to a toxic one.

The action of opium almost immediately after absorption illustrates the frequent dose. One of the earliest physiological actions of opium after its ingestion, rarely after subcutaneous injection, is stimulation of the nervous system, and of the circulation. This is fully recognized by obstetricians, who advise its exhibition as one means of controlling post partum hæmorrhage. Stimulation is a primary effect of opium that soon passes over, the length of time varying with the quantity given and with the idiosyncrasies of patients, into an opposite condition. The administration of an appropriate quantity of opium every five, ten, or fifteen minutes, that is, the frequent dose of it, will prolong and enhance its primary stimulant action. How desirable it sometimes is to prolong the primary stimulating action of this invaluable agent, I need not remind those who hear me.

The physiological action of aconite upon the human economy illustrates the same principle. Fleming's admirable observations upon aconite have taught us the powerful sedative influence that five drops of the tincture of the root exert upon the system. If, instead of giving five drops in a single dose, half a drop is given every half-hour ten times, or one drop every hour five times, a different physiological and consequently a different therapeutical result is attained from that of the single dose of five drops. In this case a less depressing sedative action is obtained by the frequent than by the single dose.

I will not weary you by these illustrations. I am sure your own observation at the bedside will add to these other and more apposite ones. The object of this paper will be attained if it succeeds in bringing clearly before you the great therapeutical power that results from the physiological adaptation of doses to the processes of absorption and elimination, and especially if it succeeds in calling your attention to the power of the continued dose.

ON EMPYEMA.

AN ANALYSIS OF THE CASES IN WHICH PUS HAS OCCURRED IN THE
PLEURAL CAVITY, WHICH HAVE BEEN TREATED AT THE MASSACHUSETTS
GENERAL HOSPITAL.[1]

BY WILLIAM F. WHITNEY, M. D.

CONSIDERED simply from a pathological point of view, the difference
between pleurisy and empyema is one of degree and not of kind ; for
even in a serous effusion a few young cells can be found, and from this
all stages can be traced to that in which they are so abundant as to
form the fluid known as pus. From a clinical point of view, however,
the character of the fluid makes a difference in the course and treatment of the disease, and it is from this point that the cases which have
occurred at the Massachusetts General Hospital have been considered.

The same trouble is experienced in comparing these cases that is met
in the comparison of any series of hospital cases, namely, that as a rule
they occur among persons who have very little power of observation,
and consequently their statements as regards the time they have been
sick or how long certain symptoms have lasted are not always to be
relied upon ; moreover, after the patients have come under observation,
the minuteness of detail varies with the individual who has charge of
them, and consequently many of the points that are particularly desirable have not been noted at all in many instances. But even from
these imperfect records there are to be obtained certain facts which are
of importance in the classification of these cases, and also of some practical interest in reference to their treatment.

The number of cases in which the existence of a purulent fluid within
the pleural cavity has been proved to exist is sixty-seven. They can
be distributed among two classes : the first, those in which it is primarily an affection of the pleura, and any disease of the lung itself is subsequent ; the second, those in which the trouble with the lung is primary, and the affection of the pleura is secondary.

The first series is the one to which the term empyema should be
restricted, and presents two forms, the acute and the chronic. The
first of these is not generally known, and the distinction between the
two is not well recognized. But these cases appear to show clearly
this distinction, although exception may be taken to the classification of
some individual cases. In the acute cases the effusion is apparently
purulent from the beginning, while in the chronic cases the effusion is
probably at first serous, but later, from neglect of treatment or some unknown cause, it becomes purulent. Of the sixty-seven cases that have
occurred, twelve were considered to be of the acute form. In four of

[1] A Thesis for the Degree of Doctor of Medicine.

the twelve cases, exposure to wet and cold was assigned as the exciting cause; in one, violence, causing fracture of ribs; but in the remaining seven there was no cause assigned. In all the cases, the onset was sudden; chills occurred in three instances; pain in the side, increased on full breath, and sooner or later dyspnœa, was the sequence of symptoms at first. In other words, symptoms of inflammation of the pleura were manifest. In the further progress of the case, especially if the termination was fatal, the symptoms became quite severe, delirium and signs of prostration having been observed. The temperature was taken in two cases, and varied from 101° (Fahrenheit), in the morning, to 103° in the evening. The signs obtained from auscultation and percussion showed merely the existence of a fluid, but of its nature, whether dense like pus or thin like serum, there was no way of determining by those methods. From this it appears that there is nothing truly diagnostic of pus, and it is only when the symptoms in a case of pleurisy are unusually severe that its existence is to be suspected.

As the result of the twelve cases, five died, five recovered, one was doubtful, and one is still under observation. The mortality occurred entirely in adults. The duration of the disease varied from thirteen days to nine weeks. In the very rapid cases the patients appeared to die from the intensity of the disease, while in those more prolonged they seemed to sink from exhaustion. In one case, death was apparently due to pressure of the fluid, for although the effusion was not very large (four pints) it was confined to the anterior and lower part of the chest, and so was able to exert as much pressure as a larger effusion. For Bartels has shown [1] that in effusion into the left pleural cavity, as was the case here, if the effusion is large, when sudden death occurs it is caused by bending the vena cava inferior at a right angle, and thus preventing the return of the blood to the heart, and not by directly paralyzing the heart, as was formerly supposed.

In three of the cases, no attempt was made to remove the fluid; they occurred before the time when puncture of the chest was a common practice. In the other two, paracentesis was twice performed in one, and once in the other, followed in the latter by a permanent opening; gangrene of the lung was supposed to have existed also, but it must have been secondary to the empyema, as no symptom of it was noticed before the existence of pus was detected.

The cases which terminated favorably occurred in children or young adults. From these it appears that the usual course of the pus is to find its way to the surface and discharge externally. In two of the favorable cases abscess had formed at the end of four and eight weeks, respectively. In one of these, after spontaneous opening, the discharge was allowed to come away at will, and no attempt was made to wash it

[1] Deutsches Archiv für klinische Medicin, iv., 1868.

out. Tonics were used internally and the case went on favorably. In the others, besides tonic treatment, the side was syringed out twice daily with a solution of tincture of iodine or carbolic acid. These patients were under treatment from four to eight months. In one only was there any complication, and this was a large abscess of the abdominal parietes; the symptoms at first resembled those of peritonitis, but later, pus pointing near the umbilicus, the true nature of the disease was shown, and on opening the abscess the symptoms were relieved.

The case which was doubtful in its termination was punctured once and was then removed from the hospital.

The case that is still under observation occurred in a child, and a permanent opening was made, from which there has been discharge for eighteen months. The general condition has somewhat improved, but the prognosis is as yet undecided.

The question of making a permanent opening in the chest is still discussed, but from these few cases it appears that those in which it was made terminated more favorably than those in which it was omitted. But here must be considered another important element, namely, the age of the patient; for all of the recoveries occurred in children or young adults, and this, as far as it goes, is of great importance.

The next series is that in which there was reason to believe that the effusion was at first serous and later became purulent. The proof that the disease of the pleura was the primary affection and the disease of the lung secondary, if any existed, is not always so clear in all the cases as could be wished, but it is considered that twenty-six belong to this series. The history shows that these cases differed in no way from those of chronic pleurisy in their course, and there is no way of proving the existence of pus, unless it points externally, except by means of paracentesis. In six of them, serum was first detected; and in the remainder pus was found at the primary tapping; but from the length of time during which the effusion had existed, it was to be presumed that the fluid was serous at the beginning.

The results of these cases are very unsatisfactory. Four died, two recovered, and the remaining twenty stayed in the hospital lengths of time varying from a few weeks to a year, but after that their history was generally unknown. All the four cases which terminated fatally had permanent openings, and in these daily injections, generally consisting of carbolic acid and water, were used. In twenty cases the result was death some time after leaving the hospital, or it was never known. The treatment in five of these cases was by paracentesis alone, and in all of these the patients left the hospital relieved, but the physical signs still showed the existence of fluid. The final result in all these cases was doubtful. In one, paracentesis was performed twelve times within eight months; in the other fifteen, there was either a spontaneous or an artificial opening of the abscess, with subsequent fistula and discharge. In four, daily injections were used. In seven, the symptoms were relieved when the patients left the hospital ; one is reported not to have died until ten years after leaving, although his condition was very poor when he left ; one had a fistulous opening for five and one half years, with daily profuse expectoration ; one recovered sufficiently to go on a whaling voyage, but died within two years after leaving the hospital. The other six patients were not relieved, but the result is not absolutely known.

In all these twenty cases the result was probably unfavorable owing to disease of the lungs, for it is generally accepted that in the majority of instances in which the lung is compressed for a long time, changes are developed of a chronic inflammatory character, which are fatal in their tendency. That such changes might readily occur in these cases is evident from the fact that in nine patients evidences of the presence of fluid had existed from one to six months before any attempt at removal, and in eleven from six months to two years. The majority of the patients were between twenty and thirty, at an age when disease of the lung is most common.

The two cases of recovery had the following history : —

I. December 15, 1858. The patient, a male, forty-eight years old, nearly ten years before had pleurisy in the right side ; he was able to be about in two months afterwards, with a little cough and dyspnœa on exertion. These symptoms continued for four years, but the patient was able to attend partially to business ; at the end of that time there was flattening of the chest, with evidences of effusion. Three months later the effusion seemed to have disappeared, and the man continued in good health for five years, when a fluctuating tumor appeared over the right chest, and signs of the existence of fluid were evident. Two months later an attempt was made to introduce a medium-sized trocar behind the tumor, but the effort failed from the narrowness of the intercostal spaces. The tumor was then opened, with a free discharge of pus. All this time he had slight cough, but no râles were ever detected. He remained in the hospital for a few weeks and was then discharged.

Sixteen years afterwards he was seen, and said that " his health had been good since leaving the hospital, the discharge had continued for eighteen months and at the end of that time had ceased, and he had had no trouble since, except some dyspnœa on exertion." His general appearance was healthy. His right side was contracted and dull on percussion ; respiration was pure but faint. Slight lateral curvature of spine existed.

II. October 6, 1869. The patient was a male, fourteen years old. Four months before his entrance he had chills, fever, and pain in the left side ; he felt better in a few days, was then taken worse, with dysp-

nœa and cough, and was confined to bed eight weeks. At the time of
entrance, signs of a large effusion were noted ; the heart was pushed to
the right of the sternum, and a bellows murmur was heard. Nothing
abnormal was detected in the right lung. A week afterwards, the first
paracentesis was performed, and four pints of clear serum were withdrawn,
with relief. In ten days the effusion again increased, and four and a half
pints of serum were withdrawn. The urine was normal. Two weeks
later effusion required a third removal of fluid, and three pints of serum
were obtained. Four weeks later the fourth paracentesis resulted in
two and a half pints of serum. Two weeks after, the fifth paracentesis
gave the same quantity of serum as the fourth. One week later, two
pints of serum, with a little pus, were obtained. One month after, the
seventh paracentesis, with two pints of fluid. For a few days his general condition appeared to improve, but for the next three weeks it failed,
and four weeks after the seventh, the eighth paracentesis was performed,
four months after the first, and two pints of pure pus were withdrawn. A
few days later two canulæ were inserted into the chest, the upper between
the third and fourth ribs in front and the lower between the eighth and
ninth on the side ; the upper was removed after a few days, as it was
found to be of no use. There was a slight discharge from the lower
opening. Three days after, the patient was etherized and a large canula
introduced. The pleural cavity was to be syringed daily with a solution of carbolic acid in water.

March 20, 1870 (five months after entrance), he was discharged with
strength much improved. Faint respiration was heard down to the third
rib in front and to the angle of the scapula behind. The heart was still
at right of the sternum. The inner end of the canula became more and
more elevated, apparently by the diaphragm. Pulse, 116. Temperature, 99.5°.

December, 1874, four and one half years after the last record, he wrote
that he had used the syringe daily for six months after leaving the
hospital, and then appeared to do well for three months, when there was
a spontaneous discharge of two pints of pus, and after that he was perfectly well and had been able to do as hard work as ever. His spine
was slightly curved.

Little need be said of the remaining class of cases, as they occur
secondary to other troubles. They add to the gravity of the prognosis,
and there is little hope of successful treatment. Of the twenty-nine
cases that occurred, sixteen died while in the hospital, three are known
to have died after leaving the hospital, and in the remaining ten the
subsequent history is unknown, but from the condition in which they left
the hospital, nothing but an unfavorable result could be anticipated.

From the results of these last two series, little is to be hoped in the
majority of cases from operative treatment as a means of cure ; but it

does certainly afford great temporary relief, and should be recommended
where there is any doubt as to the disease of the lungs. But where
pulmonary disease is clearly established, paracentesis should be preferred, as giving the patient less inconvenience with an equal amount
of relief.

In the care of these cases, there have been suggested several points
which are of practical interest. In one instance quite serious results
appeared to follow the use of ether in order to produce insensibility.
The patient became asphyxiated, and but for the prompt performance of
tracheotomy would probably have died. As the asphyxia was relieved
by tracheotomy, it appears to show that spasm of the glottis, rather than
the ether, was the cause of the difficulty. That ether can be used with
safety is shown by the fact that in the other four cases in which it
has been used there have been no unpleasant results; one patient has
been etherized five times, three times for openings into the chest, and
twice subsequently, once to have a scrofulous testis removed, and again
to have two fingers amputated for necrosis. Of course great care must
be exercised in the administration of ether ; it is found best to etherize
with the patient in a sitting posture, as this gives the diaphragm the
freest play.

After the introduction of the tube it is important that it should be
kept in place firmly, that there should not be any pressure upon the
wound, and that the tube should be so exposed as to be easily cleaned
without having to move in and out, causing the passage to be irritated.
Several shields have been devised for this purpose. But the one which
answers these requirements best is a modification of the forms used here
and at the City Hospital last year. A piece of sheet-tin about six
inches long and three wide is cut in the form of an hour-glass. A hole
is punched in 'the narrow portion, just large enough to carry the tube.
A belt of thin sheet rubber is sewed to this shield, through small holes
punched in its margin, and the narrow part is then arched over the
wound. The belt is fastened round the body by means of buttons. Cotton wadding in a thin layer is placed beneath the belt and the ends of
the shield. By this means the wound can be washed daily by syringing,
and all the change necessary is to replace the cotton once a day.

The last and most important point is to keep the cavity thoroughly
drained after it has once been opened. For a few ounces of decomposing
pus will cause more hectic and constitutional disturbance than the
amount previously inclosed in the cavity and protected from the air.

RECENT PROGRESS IN THE TREATMENT OF CHILDREN'S DISEASES.

BY D. H. HAYDEN, M. D.

Intestinal Catarrh of Children. — Dr. A. Monti,[1] instructor in the University of Vienna, makes the following recommendations for the treatment of infants affected with intestinal catarrh : —

The best substitutes for the mother's breast, when this cannot be obtained, are, veal-broth [2] and milk, Liebig's soup, Löflund's infant food,[3] Nestle's infant powder,[4] fresh cow's milk, according to the age of the child, given either pure or proportionally diluted, and condensed milk.

The author's experience is in favor of giving exclusively liquid food, and of avoiding the amylacea. In opposition to the advice of Vogel and others that milk should be entirely excluded from the diet of children affected with intestinal catarrh, if the trouble originated at the time of its use, the author, while admitting that good results are often obtained by stopping the milk for a few days in children over one year old, considers such abstinence in infants under three months of age injurious and a most frequent cause of collapse and death. When after weaning there comes on an intestinal catarrh ushered in with violent symptoms, or when the disease lasts a long time, and, notwithstanding proper dietetic and medicinal treatment, shows no signs of improvement, where the circumstances admit, the child must be returned to the breast. This is especially necessary when the child is under five months of age, and in the summer months. Where the cause of the trouble is due to the indigestibility of the cow's milk, this should be diluted with veal-broth in the proportion of one part of milk and two parts of veal-broth, for children under three weeks old ; for children from one to two months old, cow's milk and veal-broth in equal parts ; for children from two to three months old, two parts of cow's milk and one part of veal-broth.

The author has in many cases substituted condensed milk with advantage, using the following proportions: for new-borns, one part of condensed milk and fifteen parts of water ; for children from two to four weeks old, one part of condensed milk and fourteen parts of water ; for children from one to three months old, one part of condensed

---

[1] Wiener medicinische Wochenschrift, 1875, i.

[2] This is prepared with half a pound of veal and three pints of water boiled down to a pint and a half.

[3] Löflund's infant food is essentially the same thing as Liebig's food, but in the more convenient and concentrated form of an extract. The extract is prepared for use by dissolving it in warm milk.

[4] Nestle's infant powder, prepared after the idea of Liebig, contains also a good Swiss milk in the form of a concentrated and dry powder. It is made ready for use by stirring up with cold water, and then boiling for a few minutes.

milk and thirteen parts of water; for children from three to five months old, one part of condensed milk and twelve parts of water; for children from five to ten months old, one part of condensed milk and ten parts of water.

With older children (from eight months up to two years old) affected with chronic intestinal catarrh, when the disease is not benefited by withdrawing the milk for a few days, the author gives pure lukewarm milk, either as the exclusive diet or in connection with raw meat, and with surprisingly good results. He begins with a pint of lukewarm milk for the day, giving in addition water-gruel and raw meat. When this is well tolerated, he increases the milk gradually to a pint and a half, and then to two pints. With this treatment the author has repeatedly seen infants who were previously reduced to skeletons, within from eight to ten days not only cured of the intestinal catarrh but also increase a pound in weight.

In cases where neither veal-broth and milk nor condensed milk nor lukewarm milk, pure or properly diluted, causes an improvement of the intestinal catarrh, the author resorts always to a wet nurse. When this is not possible, one of the following substitutes is to be tried : Liebig's food (or one of its surrogates, as Löflund's infant food), given as exclusive diet, frequently produced successful results with children over five months old. The use of Nestle's infant powder was often equally successful, though with very young infants this is frequently not well tolerated. Cocoa and acorn coffee agreed often with infants over three months old, but only when used in connection with one of the above kinds of food. The acorn coffee is particularly advantageous for rhachitic and scrofulous children. For infants under a year old it is given according to their age, either with equal parts of milk or with one part of acorn coffee to two or three parts of milk. Of cocoa the author has generally employed the powdered seeds, free from oil. When the child is over one year old the cocoa or acorn coffee is prepared by boiling in pure milk.

As to the food that will agree best, this depends in a great measure upon the idiosyncrasy of the little patient; and when under one form of nourishment the intestinal catarrh does not rapidly improve, a change must be made to another, which may prove more suitable.

With infants between eight months and two years the author often uses wine, preferring red wine, and giving from one to two tablespoonfuls daily.

If collapse should suddenly set in in acute entero-catarrh, lukewarm bran baths once or twice daily should be used. These were often used, too, in cases of chronic intestinal catarrh where the skin became dry and scaly, in order to excite the metamorphosis of tissue and the circulation. Where the children were anæmic, baths containing iron or rock-salt or common sea salt were employed with good results.

The medical treatment employed by Monti is as follows:[1] —

In cases of simple entero-catarrh, for new-horns from three to six weeks old, —

℞ Tincturæ opii[2]   .   .   .   . gtt. j.
    Misturæ gummosæ   .   .   .   . 100,0.
    Teaspoonful every two or three hours.

For sucklings up to seven or eight months, —

℞ Tincturæ opii.   .   .   .   . gtt. j.
    Misturæ gummosæ   .   .   .   . 70,0.

For infants from eight to fifteen months old, —

℞ Tincturæ opii   .   .   .   . gtt. ij.
    Misturæ gummosæ   .   .   .   . 70,0.

According to Monti's experience, tincture of opium should never be used when infants have been prematurely born, when very anæmic and run down, when affected with chronic hydrocephalus, or when there is a complication of bronchitis or pneumonia; for in such cases toxical effects are easily produced. On account of the different degrees of susceptibility to opium in infants, the author recommends to begin always with the above small doses and not to increase the dose until the first dose has proved to be of no effect. The parents must also be instructed to stop the medicine as soon as any long-continued drowsiness shows itself.

Of Dover's powder the author gives children under three months old 0.07 in from eight to twelve doses; when from three months to one year old, 0.07 in six doses; when two years old, 0.14 in six doses.

If with the catarrh there should be symptoms of dyspepsia, as vomiting and acid stools, the author combines with the opium an alkali, as:

℞ Pulveris Doveri   .   .   .   . 0,07.
    Pulveris oculi cancrorum   .   .   .   . 2,00.
    Sacchari albi   .   .   .   . 3,00.
    Ft. pulv. et div. in part. no. viij.   D. S.   One powder every two hours.

Or:

℞ Sodæ bicarbonatis   .   .   .   . 0,60.
    Aquæ fontanæ   .   .   .   . 70,00.
    Tincturæ opii   .   .   .   . gtt. j.
    Syrupi simplicis   .   .   .   . 12,00.
    D. S.   Teaspoonful every two hours.

Where there is no vomiting, and undigested caseine is present in the stools, the author has obtained good results with paullinia and subnitrate of bismuth. For the former he writes as follows: —

℞ Paulliniæ   .   .   .   . 0,80.
    Pulveris Doveri   .   .   .   . 0,07.
    Sacchari albi   .   .   .   . 3,00.
    M.   Ft. pulv. et div. in part. no. vj.   D. S.   One powder every two hours.

[1] The prescriptions are given according to the metric system, the unit, one gramme, being equivalent to about sixteen grains.
[2] Tinctura opii of the Austrian Pharmacopœia is one third stronger than that of the United States Dispensatory.

Where there is no dyspepsia the author uses astringents : —

℞ Tincturæ krameriæ . . . . gtt. xx.
  Tincturæ opii . . . . gtt. j.
  Aquæ fontanæ . . . . 70,00.
  Syrupi simplicis . . . . 12,00.
  D. S. Teaspoonful every two hours.

Or :

℞ Acidi tannici . . . . 0,30.
  Pulveris Doveri . . . . 0,07.
  Sacchari albi . . . . 3,00.
  M. Div. in part. no. vj. D. S. One powder every two hours.

When the intestinal catarrh is complicated with an acute gastric catarrh, and there is vomiting, the author gives an acid in combination with opium or a small dose of rhubarb : —

℞ Acidi muriatici diluti . . . . gtt. ij–iij.
  Syrupi simplicis . . . . 12.
  Aquæ destillatæ . . . . 70,00.
  Tincturæ opii . . . . gtt. j.–ij.
  D. S. Teaspoonful every two or three hours.

Or :

℞ Pulveris rhei
  Pulveris Doveri . . . . āā 0,07.
  Sacchari albi . . . . 3,00.
  Ft. pulv. et. div. in part. no. vj. D. S. One every one or two hours.

When with the acute or chronic intestinal catarrh there is also a chronic gastric catarrh (loss of appetite, eructations, hiccough, coated tongue, and offensive breath), the author gives sulphate of zinc, colombo, rhubarb, the latter especially where the stools are colorless. Thus the author prescribes for children under one year of age, —

℞ Zinci sulphatis . . . . 0,07.
  Aquæ destillatæ . . . . 70,00.
  Tincturæ opii . . . . gtt. j.
  Syrupi simplicis . . . . 12,00.
  M. D. S. Dessertspoonful four or five times daily.

Or :

℞ Pulveris rhei . . . . 0,20–0,40.
  Pulveris Doveri . . . . 0,07–0,14.
  Sacchari albi . . . . 3,00.
  M. Ft. pulv. et div. in part. no. vj–viij. D. S. Four to six powders daily.

Or :

℞ Decocti radicis calumbæ . . . . 70,00.
  Tincturæ opii simp. . . . . gtt. ij.
  Syrupi simplicis . . . . 12,00.
  M. D. S. Teaspoonful every two hours.

When with the intestinal catarrh there is a complication of a light bronchial catarrh, the author gives an infusion of ipecac with small doses of opium.

In chronic intestinal catarrh experience has convinced the author that not much can be effected by medicine. For anæmic children, on the contrary, iron often effects wonderful results ; yet even of this medicine he cautions against giving too large doses. The preparations most commonly used by him are, —

   ℞ Ferri carbonatis saccharatis

       Pulveris Doveri . . . . āā 0,07.

       Sacchari albi . . . . 3,00.

   M. Ft. pulv. et div. in part. no. vj. D. S. Two to four powders daily.

   Or :

   ℞ Ferri oxydati dialysati [1] . . . . gtt. x.

       Aquæ fontanæ . . . . 100,00.

       Aquæ menthæ

       Syrupi simplicis . . . . āā 6,00.

   D. S. Four to six dessertspoonfuls daily.

   Or :

   ℞ Liquoris ferri perchloridi . . . . gtt. vj.

       Misturæ gummosæ . . . . 100,00.

       Syrupi corticis aurantii . . . . 12,00.

   D. S. Three to four dessertpoonfuls daily.

The author never employs clysters in catarrh of the small intestines. For the relief of colic and to quiet excessive peristaltic action in acute intestinal catarrh, Priessnitz's water dressings over the bowels do good service. In chronic cases, when meteorismus is excessive, cold water dressings frequently changed are useful.

Case of Erysipelas Migrans with Recovery, in an Infant four weeks old. — Dr. Christian Lutz[2] reports the case as follows : The mother of the child died of puerperal fever. The disease began on the right side of the scrotum, starting from an abscess of the size of a hazel-nut, caused probably by an intertrigo. The disease invaded first the anterior and lateral portions of the right hip, extending gradually down the thigh, leg, and foot. Later it made its appearance upon the right shoulder, and wandered downwards over the fore-arm and hand. It then reappeared (the sixteenth day of the disease) upon the right hip ; it remained stationary here for some time, and then crossed over to the left hip, where it again became stationary. It then (from the nineteenth to the twenty-second day) extended down the left lower extremity, and on the twenty-third day appeared upon the back, advanced toward the left shoulder, remained stationary until the twenty-sixth day, and then extended down the left arm. On the thirty-first day, the erysipelas was confined to the back and fingers of the left hand, and all fever had ceased. On the thirty-second day the erysipelas had entirely disappeared, having lasted one month. During the course of the disease, there was a large abscess opened in the right thigh, one smaller one in the right calf, one over the internal malleolus, two over the back of the foot, and one over the patella.

The special treatment consisted of baths, which were begun on the

---

[1] A German preparation consisting of liquor ferri perchloridi, and holding an excess of hydrated sesquioxide in solution.

[2] Deutsches Archiv für klinische Medicin, August 14, 1874.

fourth day of the disease, the temperature on this day, taken in the rectum, being 104°. The baths were given three times in the day and once in the night, at a temperature of 95° Fahrenheit, cooled down to 81.5°–84°, sometimes only to 86°. Their duration was from five to seven minutes.

The local treatment previous to this had been simply inunction of lard and covering the parts with cotton-batting. In place of this, on the sixth day carbolic acid in sweet oil (one part to twenty-five, later one part to ten) was substituted.

The nourishment consisted of diluted milk and malt extract, with occasionally a few drops of port wine. When the temperature reached a very high grade four to five grains of quinine were administered, divided into three powders, and given in rapid succession.

The temperature as a rule was high throughout the whole course of the disease, varying from 101.5° to 104°. On the few exceptional days when the temperature was below 100.5°, the baths were stopped, and the ordinary warm baths given.

The bilious diarrhœa, which according to Widerhofer [1] shows itself in the erysipelas of new-horns, whether the disease be of pyæmic or local origin (in the former case at the beginning, in the latter at a later stage), did not exist in the present case. The patient became very much emaciated, but appetite and digestion continued good.

In an infant four weeks old, for whom under normal conditions the external application of considerable warmth is required, these cooling baths must exercise a powerful effect. The high fever nevertheless was looked upon as a sufficient indication for them, and their effect was always to lower the temperature 1.75°–2.5° for four or five hours. When taken out of the bath the child shivered violently; once it had a long hiccoughing attack; once also it had opisthotonos. This lasted, however, but a short time, and did not recur; but it was regarded as a warning not to reduce the temperature of the baths any more.

The recovery of the patient shows that youngest infants can be subjected to the antipyretic treatment of cool baths with good results.

The local treatment with carbolic oil had an unmistakably favorable influence upon the course of the disease. The surfaces were freed earlier of the eruption, the erysipelas did not reach such a degree of intensity, and after its employment was begun there were no more abscesses formed. It did not, however, prevent the extension of the erysipelas. The carbolic oil, of the strength of 1:10, is scarcely at all painful, and the author is in the habit of using it for intertrigo in children with good results.

Quinine in the Treatment of Children's Diseases, especially in Fevers and in Whooping Cough. — Dr. Rapmund,[2] from large experience in

---

[1] Jahrbuch für Kinderheilkunde, vi. 1.

[2] Deutsche Klinik. Schmidt's Jahrbücher, No. 3, 1875.

country practice, gives to quinine a decided preference over the use of cold water as an antipyretic, for the reason that the use of the latter cannot so well be controlled, and because internal remedies are less objected to by the laity than others. The author's experience with quinine as an antipyretic and tonic corroborates fully the favorable statements of Dr. Hagenbach upon this subject.[1] It has been employed by him in cases of scarlatina, measles, varioloid, erysipelas migrans, lobular pneumonia, and follicular enteritis. In the first three classes of disease the treatment was resorted to only in severe cases; for in light cases in country practice medical assistance is not called in. In the above cases quinine worked too as a hypnotic (Jürgensen), and convalescence was rapid.

In erysipelas migrans, Vogel has already recommended quinine as the only remedy acting favorably in the few cases of recovery seen by him.

The result in lobular pneumonia was a particularly favorable one, in nine cases between four months and eighteen months of age only two dying. This is explained by the author as due to the fact that in fatal cases the cause of death is an insufficient action of the heart, occasioned by the high fever. The remedy must be used without intermission; but when cyanosis has set in, it is too late. Dyspnœa is also relieved by this remedy. At the same time as much nourishment as possible must be given, — milk, meat broths, or wine. In enteritis folliculosa, where there was high fever, this remedy did good service, acting also as a tonic. In whooping-cough, quinine produces a decided diminution in the number of attacks and in their severity.[2]

In the author's cases thus treated there were no complications nor sequelæ, except where these had already made their appearance before the administration of the remedy; and they moreover were shortened in their duration or removed by the remedy.

The author always gives quiniæ murias in solution, 0.05–0.1 gramme once or twice daily in glycerine and water, equal parts. The medicine is given in black coffee. When not tolerated by the stomach, it was given in double the dose by the rectum. The syringe in such case should not hold more than an ounce or an ounce and a half of fluid.

[1] Boston Medical and Surgical Journal, February 6, 1873, page 132.
[2] Boston Medical and Surgical Journal, August 7, 1873, page 133, and February 6, 1873.

PROCEEDINGS OF THE BOSTON SOCIETY FOR MEDICAL OBSERVATION.

EDWARD WIGGLESWORTH, JR., M. D., SECRETARY.

Cerebral Myxoma. — DR. WEBBER presented a cerebral tumor which the microscope showed was composed of round and fusiform and processed cells, with fine fibres. The growth was probably a myxoma. It was from a patient of Dr. Arnold, who reported the case as follows: The woman, aged fifty-nine years, passed her grand climacteric six years ago. Disease of the ears had existed since childhood, but was not immediately attributable to scarlet fever. Three years since, the patient had a protracted and prostrating illness, with tedious though good convalescence. For the past two years the general health has been unusually good. Towards the end of January, 1875, exposure to severe cold, after being over hot suds, brought on a sharp attack of illness characterized by severe congestion of the membranes of the fauces, posterior nares, and auditory apparatus, followed by inflammation of this last throughout its entire extent, especially upon the left side. A chilly sensation in the right hemisphere succeeded, and increased steadily until March 19th, at which time it was intense.

March 26th. Partial paralysis ensued, at first of the left hand and arm, then of the left leg, and, this increasing, finally of the muscles of the face, of deglutition, and of the organs of speech. The pupils were not affected.

April 4th to 7th. Patient semi-comatose; no nourishment taken. Subsequently food and drink were swallowed. The left foot responded to the stimulus of tickling, the patient's senses returned, and she conversed freely. This amelioration of her condition lasted from three to four days, then the paralysis gradually increased until she died, April 15th. The pulse during this time was rarely above 90, the respiration was not accelerated until the last four days, and the temperature was but slightly elevated.

Autopsy. Four and a half hours after death. Rigor slight. · Body yellow. Lungs generally adherent, slight cicatrices at apices and some condensation of the posterior lower lobe of the left lung. Heart's tissue moderately firm, valves healthy; a few soft clots in the right side. Liver firm and normal in substance; gall-bladder full of bile. Spleen normal. Left kidney soft, normal, capsule slightly adherent; right, rather smaller, with very adherent capsule; cortical substance of about the natural thickness. Genital organs normal, but retroversion of the uterus.

Brain, nearly normal in substance. Dura mater somewhat thickened. A small patch of thickened membrane between the pia and dura mater. Considerable atrophy of the convolutions of the left side; those on the right, posterior to the fissure of Rolando, flattened, and just above the fissure of Sylvius bulging as from internal pressure. Nothing abnormal at the base. The first thin section from the vertex showed, on the right, a yellow color, on the left one more than usually pink. Deeper sections under the most prominent point showed congestion and prominence of the vessels. A vertical section at this point disclosed a tumor, two inches in diameter, containing a yellowish serum, apparently composed of a reticulum of fibrous tissue containing small cells filled with the serum. Around the tumor was a thin layer of irregular outline, from one to three lines in width, of congested tissue with numerous small but distinct and interlacing blood-vessels.

The right meatus auditorius externus was normal. The membrana tympani was slightly thickened. There was congestion of the mucous membrane of the tympanum. No implication of mastoid cells was observed. The left membrana tympani was thickened and opaque. The mucous membrane of the tympanum was thickened throughout the cavity and gave evidence of old inflammation. Both Eustachian tubes were pervious; the tegumentum tympani was very thin, almost transparent; it was not the result, however, of disease. The membrane overlying the tegumentum tympani was normal.

Cancer of the Pylorus. — DR. VOGEL showed a specimen of scirrhus of the pyloric extremity of the stomach reducing the size of its orifice so that a No. 4 probe was barely admitted.

Retinitis in Bright's Disease. — DR. WADSWORTH read a paper upon this subject,[1] and, in answer to Dr. Hay, said that separation of the retina was rare. He had seen but the one case referred to. Von Graefe in 1860 had seen one case, Donders in 1865, one; Bucht about a year since observed separation in both eyes.

DR. HAY mentioned a reference in a recent number of the *British Medical Journal* to the simultaneous occurrence of signs of Bright's disease in the retina and of chronic enlargement of arteries and diplopia. He had observed a case with enlarged temporal arteries and diplopia. The heart was not particularly enlarged. The kidneys were said to be diseased.

DR. JEFFRIES remarked that in Magnus's summing up, the debility was attributed to loss of albumen, and consequently individuals were differently affected. In such cases the trouble in the eye would occur when the loss begins to tell upon the constitution.

DR. WADSWORTH responded that some cases lost much albumen, and even died of the disease, without retinitis.

DR. JEFFRIES thought that when patients broke down any length of time before death, the retinitis might occur.

DR. WEBBER inquired if there were any peculiar character to the blindness; also, if the fatty degeneration and nerve-fibre changes depended upon changes in the arteries and thickening of their walls.

DR. WADSWORTH replied that the blindness was simply a dimness of vision, and that fatty degeneration might occur in other forms of retinitis, though most common in Bright's disease, this last being one of its most frequent causes; the change was in the walls of the arteries.

DR. LINCOLN asked if a certain form of retinitis might not be due to interstitial nephritis.

DR. WADSWORTH answered that it might, as syphilis, leucocythæmia, or a cerebral tumor might be a cause.

DR. FITZ wished to know if any difference existed between the retinitis from Bright's disease and that from other diseases of the kidneys, sufficient for purposes of differential diagnosis.

[1] To be published in full in the JOURNAL.

DR. WADSWORTH answered that a large hæmorrhage might occur in chronic forms.

DR. FITZ suggested that this might also arise from an enlarged heart.

DR. BOLLES referred to the possible connection between cerebral hæmorrhages and apoplexy of the retina in Bright's disease.

DR. WADSWORTH stated that in any form of retinitis anything more than a slight difference is called a hæmorrhage. If there is a large hæmorrhage in the retina, there is more likelihood of one in the brain.

A Case of Tetanus. — DR. WARREN reported a case of tetanus. January 20th a laboring man was injured by the falling of a bank of frozen earth. The thigh, tibia, and metatarsal bones of the right lower limb were fractured, and the skin and superficial layer of muscles of the right fore-arm were severely lacerated and mixed with gravel. The wound in the arm having been carefully cleared of all débris, the divided ends of the radial artery were found and secured. The median nerve was exposed thoughout the whole length of the wound, and was separated from the neighboring parts. Externally it was somewhat begrimed at points, but did not appear to be seriously bruised. The power of motion having been previously ascertained to be good, the nerve was allowed to remain. The arm being flexed, the edges of the wound were approximated and carbolic acid dressings were applied.

The patient's condition was very favorable for nearly a week. On the 29th the ligatures came away, the sutures having been removed previously, and the wound was covered with healthy granulations. There was some pain, however, on this day, in the thumb and index finger. On the 31st the patient complained of a stiff neck. The characteristic symptoms of tetanus supervened, and in spite of opiates, hot vapor-baths, and ice to the spine, the patient died on February 2d.

Nerve Changes at the Point of Injury. — The median nerve was removed by Dr. J. J. Putnam, who found evidence of degeneration in it, varying from almost entire absence of nerve-fibres at the point of greatest inflammation in the middle of the fore-arm, to simple breaking up of the myeline, with preservation of the axis-cylinders in the middle of the upper-arm, as well as in the ulnar nerve in the fore-arm. At the point of greatest inflammation above mentioned, there was nothing to be found except thickened connective tissue, granular débris, and fat in small drops, often occurring in streaks as if substituted for the nerve tubes. Pieces of the brachial plexus showed evidences of degeneration of the myeline at some points, presumably those in continuation with the median nerve. No further examination was allowed.

Dr. Warren then exemplified upon the blackboard the changes which had been found in the median nerve high up in the arm. A portion of this was exhibited with a piece of a normal nerve for purposes of comparison. The spinal cord was not examined. Hæmatoxylin was preferred to bring out the nerve-cells. Wherever connective tissue exists, its cells, though latent or quiescent, may be brought out by any irritation, as, for example, inflammation. In this case, the thickened, inflamed connective tissue had caused a very marked increase in the apparent size of the nerve.

DR. WEBBER spoke of Lockhart Clark's examinations of the spinal cord, and said that the present specimen of the median nerve, if taken from the seat of injury, was interesting as showing local lesions not often observed. Changes might possibly be attributed to pressure from the surrounding connective tissue.

Action of Chloral Hydrate. — DR. WARREN then gave some account of the present methods of treating tetanus with chloral,[1] under small doses, by means of intra-venous injections, at the Massachusetts General Hospital. No patient had recovered.

DR. JEFFRIES inquired if any records of the pulse or of the heat of the body had been kept during the long sleep occasioned by chloral.

DR. WARREN said that such could be found in the *Bulletin de la Société de Médecine de Gand.*

DR. JEFFRIES then asked if any local pain at the point of the injection of the vein, and due to the distention, was present after the sleep had terminated.

DR. WARREN said it was not observed, and, in response to Dr. Chadwick, added that operations had been performed without causing pain even where the loss of consciousness in the patient had not been complete; that there was also no snoring nor subsequent vomiting.

DR. CHADWICK thought that if the anæsthesia were due to the action of chloroform, and yet unaccompanied by vomiting, this latter when occurring after chloroform narcosis could hardly be due to any specific nature of the drug itself. He also inquired what advantage was derived from intra-venous injections rather than from administration by the mouth or rectum.

DR. WARREN replied that subcutaneous injections afforded a more intimate way of introducing the agent; that in tetanus, the locked jaws offered an obstacle to its exhibition by the mouth; and that clysters involved too much motion of the patient, and might also cause spasm.

DR. T. B. CURTIS spoke of a case, reported in the *Gazette Hebdomadaire,* where one gramme per minute had been injected for five minutes. Asphyxia resulted, electricity failed, the patient died before the completion of the operation.

DR. WARREN alluded to the fact that twenty-two previous cases had been successful, and stated that half a drachm was the usual dose given here by the mouth, and that one drachm was called large; also that the deaths in cases reported were from the large doses.

DR. WEBBER thought that the cases of death which had occurred in this neighborhood had generally followed doses of under twenty grains.

DR. CURTIS called attention to the fact that it was by no means established that the action of chloral is necessarily that of chloroform; that the resemblance exists in the laboratory rather than in reality, and the action of chloral must be studied by itself. The doses administered in England are also small, beginning with ten grains.

DR. RICHARDSON mentioned a case where a drachm, in delirium tremens, had caused death.

DR. C. F. FOLSOM had seen abroad a fatal case from forty grains of chloral. At the same time, in Berlin, Küster saw one from thirty grains. Here in

[1] See the report on Surgery of this Journal, June 24, 1875.

Boston, Dr. Folsom had seen fifteen-grain doses given at intervals of five hours until forty-five grains had been administered, and the patient recovered with difficulty. The deaths in the two cases mentioned took place within half an hour from the time of the administration of the drug.

THE NEW ORLEANS PROTECTIVE ASSOCIATION.

THE physicians of New Orleans have recently formed an association, the object of which is to protect the profession against the practice of working by contract for families or associations. The competition and underbidding have reached such a point that a reform has been called for, and Dr. Joseph Holt, who has occupied the position of physician to the Fireman's Charitable Association, has taken the lead in the movement, and has resigned his position. His salary was seven hundred and fifty dollars a year, but the work performed by him is estimated at ordinary rates to have amounted to five thousand dollars. Dr. Holt seems at present to be the recipient of much abuse for his action, if we may judge from accounts given in New Orleans papers. A physician has been found to accept the position left vacant by him; but the movement appears to be well organized, and, as the evil is one which has been much complained of in the South and West, is deserving of success. The small income which the profession receives for its services must be seriously diminished if such practices are allowed to continue without restraint.

THE EFFECTS OF ARCTIC COLD.

SOME extracts from a paper on the influence of Arctic cold upon man, read before the Geographical Society of Vienna by Lieutenant Payer, are contained in *L'Union Médicale* of June 24, 1875. The explorer with his companions undertook a journey, March 14, 1874, in a sledge upon the glacier of Sannklar, to make observations on the land Francis Joseph. The cold had reached that day to 40° (Réaumur) below zero. Before sunrise, M. Payer and a Tyrolese had started out, in spite of the cold, to make observations and to sketch. The sunrise was magnificent. This luminary appeared to be surrounded by many small suns, and seemed the more brilliant on account of the extreme cold. The travelers were obliged to drink their spirit-ration without touching the edge of their glasses; contact with them would have been as dangerous as if they had been red-hot. But the spirit had lost all its stimulating properties and fluidity. It was insipid and as thick as oil. It was impossible to smoke cigars; they became only a piece of ice in the mouth. Metallic instruments had the same effect, when touched, as red-hot iron, as had also the medals which some of the travelers imprudently wore on their breasts. Cold of the severity here alluded to paralyzes the will, and under its influence one becomes like an intoxicated person, because of the uncertainty of his movements, his stammering speech, and the slowness of his thoughts. Tormenting thirst is produced by the evaporation of the humidity of the body. Snow cannot be taken to counteract this, for it causes inflammation of the throat, palate, and tongue; furthermore, one could never swallow a sufficient quantity of it to quench his thirst. A temperature of 30° to 40° below zero gives to snow the taste of molten metal. Eaters of snow become enfeebled, as do opium consumers in the East. The companies of travelers who journeyed over the snowy plains were enveloped in thick clouds of vapor formed by the evaporation from their bodies, which took place in spite of their clothing of furs. The vapors fell to the earth congealed in the form of little crystals, and made a slight crackling; they rendered the atmosphere impenetrable, and obscured everything. In spite of the humidity of the atmosphere there was a disagreeable sensation of dryness. Every noise was transmitted a great distance; ordinary conversation could be heard distinctly a hundred paces off. M. Payer attributes this phenomenon to the great amount of moisture in the Arctic atmosphere. Food could be cleaved and mercury made into balls. Taste and smell were much diminished. Strength yielded to the paralyzing influence of the cold; the eyes closed involuntarily and became frozen. When one stood still, the soles of the feet became benumbed. Curiously, the beard was not frozen, but it was because the expired air fell, being at once transformed into snow. Dark beards became lighter-colored; the secretions of the eyes and nose were augmented, while perspiration wholly ceased. The only possible protection against the cold was to dress as warm as possible and to endeavor to hinder as much as possible the condensation of the evaporation. Greasing or blackening the body was of no value.

MEDICAL NOTES.

— We learn from our English exchanges that the medical council has been called upon by the government to express an opinion on the question of recognizing women as practitioners of medicine. After a somewhat lengthy discussion the following motion was passed: —

" The medical council are of opinion that the study and practice of medicine and surgery, instead of affording a field of exertion well fitted for women, do, on the contrary, present special difficulties which cannot be safely disregarded, but the council is not prepared to say that women ought to be excluded from the profession."

While the council did not feel prepared to justify the legal exclusion of women, it made no secret of its opinion that the profession as a calling is most unfitted for them.

— The American Ophthalmological Society met at the Aquidneck House, Newport, R. I., Thursday, July 23d. Thirty-one members were present. A large number of papers were read and discussed. The society was in session Thursday and Friday, and adjourned Friday afternoon to meet in executive session September 11, 1876, the day before the International Congress of Ophthalmology, in New York.

— At a meeting of the Société de Biologie, reported in the *Gazette Hebdomadaire* for July 9th, M. Bourneville communicated a very remarkable observation. We will recapitulate it in some detail on account of the interest which it presents. It is about a woman forty-six years of age, who, having been well up to the twenty-third year, had at that time (1854) a startling sensation, a fright ; the following year she had her first attack of hystero-epilepsy ; she fell in the fire and had her body burned. She met with like accidents in 1859, 1860, 1863, and 1865.

Having entered the hospital Sainte Eugenie, she had the cholera in 1866. After this time her urine was suppressed for eight days ; it reappeared, but she had to be catheterized daily until May, 1875. After having met with various accidents, she entered the Salpêtriere in 1869. There she had many hysteroepileptic attacks followed by contractions of the upper and lower limbs, contractions which at different times diminished, were partially cured, reappeared, and became permanent in different parts.

Cutting short the history of her sickness we come to May 17, 1875. At noon on this day she had a hystero-epileptic attack, preceded by an aura, with ovarian and anal pains shooting to the epigastrium, to the neck and temples; the attack was accompanied with cries, turning of the eyes, and a distorted countenance, which became cyanotic; the right arm was flexed and fixed on her back for three hours. On the 18th of May she was in the following condition : she had contraction of the four limbs, complete anæsthesia, double amblyopia, and a contraction of the jaws ; she became speechless ; she had neuralgic attacks, for which she was given injections of morphia. This state persisted without marked change until the 22d of May, when she had a new attack and in eight hours she was completely cured.

So it happened that there disappeared in a short time a retention of urine which had lasted since 1866, a contraction of the left arm and leg which dated from 1869, a contraction of the jaws that required the aid of a tube for sustenance for ten months, and an aphonia for a like period.

M. Charcot, in 1870, made the following prognosis : " It is possible that in spite of its long duration, this contraction may disappear without leaving traces ; perhaps to-morrow, perhaps in some days, perhaps in a year; we can prognosticate nothing on this point. At all events, if recovery occurs it may be sudden. From one day to the next everything may return in its proper order, and if it is found that at any time the hysterical diathesis is lost, she will return to her normal state."

— A modification of Dr. Rutherford's freezing microtome is described by Dr. Heming, in the *Lancet* of June 19th. The manner of employing it is as follows : The substance to be cut is placed in the cylinder, about half an inch from the top, imbedded in scraped potato, muscle, brain-substance, or other suitable material. The tube is connected by an India-rubber tube with a worm of block tin immersed in a freezing mixture, and placed a few inches higher than the section-cutter. The other end of the worm is connected with a large funnel suspended above. An India-rubber tube is adjusted and led into a suitable receptacle. Into the funnel is now poured a quantity of weak spirit, just strong enough not to freeze at 0° F. (one part methylated alcohol and two parts water are sufficient). This of course runs through the worm, and is thereby reduced to a low temperature (say 10° F.). Then it fills the chamber, running in as we saw at the lower tube, and out at the upper tube into the vessel placed for its reception. As soon as most of the spirit has come through, the. India-rubber tube conveying it away is compressed, and the contents of the vessel are returned to the funnel (this time at a very low temperature). After this has been repeated a few times (in about fifteen minutes) the sections may be cut with a razor with perfect facility.

— We learn from a contemporary that Madame Brès is· the first French lady who has taken a medical degree in Paris. She passed all her examinations in a most creditable manner, and M. Wurtz, the president of the examining board and dean of the faculty, addressed her in the following terms : " Madame,·you have not only raised women from the secondary position they have held in medicine, but your thesis is one of the best that the faculty of Paris has ever received, and it will be consigned with honor to its archives." The title of the thesis is " La Mamelle et l'Allaitement," a very appropriate subject for a doctress ; it is treated in an anatomical, a chemical, and a physiological point of view. We learn, also, that Mrs. J. K. Tout, of Toronto, has passed her examination at and obtained a license to practice from the College of Physicians and Surgeons, Ontario. Mrs. Tout is the first lady who has obtained a license to·practice medicine in all its branches in Ontario.

— According to the London correspondent of the *American Medical Weekly,* Professor Lister, in continuing his remarks on recent advances in antiseptic surgery, gives a formula for ointment of boracic acid, which he has found very efficacious : Boracic acid finely levigated, 1 part ; white wax, 1 part ; paraffin, 2 parts ; almond oil, 2 parts ; melt the wax and paraffin by heating them with the oil, and stir the mixture briskly, along with the boracic acid powder, in a warm mortar till the mass thickens ; this is afterwards to be reduced to a proper consistence by rubbing down about an ounce at a time in a cool mortar. He spreads the ointment very thin on a fine muslin or linen rag, which absorbs some of the almond oil and leaves a layer of blended wax and paraffin flexible at the temperature of the body, and separable from the skin easily by means of the discharge, which is thus not confined beneath it. This prevents putrefaction, while it does not hinder cicatrization.

LETTER FROM LONDON.

Messrs. Editors, — London has now observed its annual Hospital Sunday for the third time. The idea of asking for collections on a fixed day, for the support of hospitals and dispensaries, is an old one in the provinces, and its introduction into the metropolis has thus far been attended with marked success, and all the medical men with whom I have spoken upon the subject heartily commend the practice. The weather last Sunday was decidedly unfavorable, but the receipt of about £10,000 has already been acknowledged at the Mansion House. For several weeks preceding the 13th inst., posters calling the attention of the public to the subject were displayed on the hospitals, churches, railway stations, etc., and appropriate sermons were preached by the clergy generally on that day. The lord mayor and the corporation attended the morning service at St. Paul's, arrayed in their imposing robes of state, and in the afternoon they went to Westminster Abbey. If as earnest efforts should be made to have the day an important one in Boston, doubtless more money would be collected in that city than there has been heretofore.

It is said there are something like one hundred and thirty-five religious sects in England and Wales. The followers of one of these, calling themselves the Peculiar People, have gained a certain degree of notoriety of late. They contend that when a man, for example, is ill, he should be anointed with oil and then be prayed over, leaving the result to Providence. This course was pursued last week with a child suffering from pleurisy. . The little patient succumbed to the disease, and the father was arrested and fined for not calling in a medical man. These Peculiar People have advertised that they will soon occupy a house of twenty rooms (that was formerly used as a homœopathic hospital), on Town Street, as a hospital, and that the inmates will not receive any medical treatment. If the authorities do not interfere, it seems highly probable that the solution of Sir Henry Thompson's "prayer-gauge" question will be attempted in the city from which it emanated !

To a New Englander, on revisiting England after a lapse of several years, in which time there has been a " re-introduction of ether," it is somewhat gratifying to see how generally this anæsthetic is being used in the hospitals. That chloroform is more or less employed in private practice I know from the fact that one gentleman whom I am acquainted with acts as a chloroformist. I know also that he gets a guinea every time he administers the agent ! Ether is used daily at Moorfields, and it is given much as we give it. Mr. Critchett prefers to have his patients inhale a little chloroform before inhaling the ether, as he thinks they take to the former more readily. At the Middlesex Hospital ether is given through an apparatus, and it seems to me that the patients are longer in becoming insensible than when a sponge is used.

I. C.

London, *June* 17, 1875.

HORSE-HAIR FOR SUTURES.

Messrs. Editors, — I desire to call the attention of the profession to the value of horse-hair for sutures. I am aware that it has been used to some extent by a few practitioners, but I believe it needs only a fair trial to introduce it into general favor among surgeons.

Its use is not original with myself, nor do I know to whom the credit is due. I found it employed in Long Island College Hospital when I became a member of its faculty, and during the two years that I was connected with that institution it was often brought into requisition ; principally, however, in stitching scalp-wounds. Since that time I have used it extensively in a great variety of wounds, and with the greatest satisfaction. In fact, I am inclined to think it may profitably supersede all other material for sutures, except where greater strength is required. It is so fine as to leave no scar and to allow the sutures being introduced very near together, perfectly non-irritant, if properly prepared, is more easily tied than any other material, and, contrary to what I had supposed, not inclined to slip while tying the second knot. Those who have tested it find its strength is remarkable, sufficient at least for all ordinary tension. I have applied the hair stitches in almost every locality, both in the skin and in the mucous membrane, and I have never secured such beautiful, delicate linear scars with any other article.

Where greater strength is needed for the general support of flaps, silk or silver-wire may be used for that purpose, and the hair for accurate coaptation of the edges. I seldom use more than a single hair, although it may be doubled if desired. I take the long hair from the tail of a young, healthy horse, and first thoroughly rinse it in warm water. I then boil it for a half-hour in soda-water (about an ounce of bicarbonate of soda to two quarts of water). I remove and rinse it in clean warm water, and it is ready for use. This process renders it perfectly innocuous and gives it the right degree of pliability. One pleasant feature about it is that it does not snarl or kink. Twisted in a rope or double coil, a single strand is easily drawn by seizing the middle.

Most of my friends, to whom I have spoken of and shown its application, have expressed surprise if not doubt at first, but have been, without exception, delighted with it upon trial.

In my next case of vesico-vaginal fistula I intend using it, either tying it or confining with perforated shot. This will be a severe test, and I am not over-sanguine as to the result. I may add that it would be better to have needles smaller than any now made for carrying the single hair, so that it may more accurately fill the hole.   Yours sincerely,

WM. WARREN GREENE, M. D.

PORTLAND, *July* 15, 1875.

BULLET-WOUND OF THE STOMACH AND KIDNEY.

MESSRS. EDITORS, — On the night of May 29th, W. F. D. received a wound from the discharge of a pistol carrying a one thirty-second ball, penetrating at a point over the cardiac portion of the stomach; dipping downward, the ball passed through the region of the left kidney, and lodged beneath the muscles of the back, from which I extracted it the following Monday morning, May 31st. When I first saw him he had profuse hæmatemesis, which kept up until the next morning; I treated him with ice in the mouth, which he was directed to allow to dissolve and to swallow; also subcutaneous injections of morphia. Since the 31st he has not had any return of the vomiting, but the most alarming symptom has been hæmaturia. The first week I allowed him only milk and water for nourishment, keeping him as comfortable as possible with morphia, afterwards a limited amount of beef-tea, milk, and custard; I gave him also two-grain doses of quinine. There has not arisen any symptom of peritonitis, and the pulse has gradually declined from 125 to 74;

there is every prospect of a good result, the only unpleasant feature being the hæmaturia, which is intermittent. For the hæmaturia the treatment is gallic acid, at the same time keeping up his strength with nutrients and quinia· He has sufficiently recovered to ride out, June 10, 1875, so that a good recovery is insured. Not a particle of blood has appeared in the urine for a week.   M. E. JONES, M. D.

PITTSFIELD, MASS.

COMPARATIVE MORTALITY-RATES FOR THE WEEK ENDING JULY 24, 1875.

	Estimated Population.	Total Mortality for the Week.	Annual Death-rate per 1000 during Week.
New York	1,040,000	956	48
Philadelphia	775,000	458	31
Brooklyn	450,000		
Boston	350,000	214	32
Providence	100,700	42	22
Worcester	50,000	19	20
Lowell	50,000	17	18
Cambridge	50,000	21	22
Fall River	45,000	28	32
Lawrence	35,000	11	17
Springfield	33,000	7	11
Lynn	28,000	15	28
Salem	26,000	11	22

RESIGNED AND DISCHARGED. — Dr. Charles A. Holt, of Chelsea, Asst. Surgeon First Regt. Infantry, M. V. M., July, 1875.

APPOINTMENT. — Dr. Robert Amory, appointed Assistant Surgeon First Battalion of Light Artillery, M. V. M., to fill an original vacancy, passed a successful examination before the Board of Medical Officers, M. V. M., July 30, 1875.   EDWARD J. FORSTER,
              Surgeon Fifth Regiment of Infantry, M. V. M., Recorder of Board.

APPOINTMENT AND PROMOTION. — First Brigade, Medical Director (rank Lieutenant-Colonel), Joseph W. Hayward, of Taunton, Surgeon Third Regt. Infantry, July 22, vice Stedman, discharged.

GENERAL ORDERS No. 12, just issued from the Adjutant-General's Office, dated July 21, is as follows: The examination of medical officers as provided in General Orders No. 23, series of 1874, shall be dispensed with in cases of officers already in the service or who have been once examined by the Board, upon their receiving a new appointment.

BOOKS AND PAMPHLETS RECEIVED. — Étude chimique sur la Source sulfurée sodique forte et iodo-bromurée de Challes. Par le Dr. F. Garrigou, Médecin consultant à Luchon. Chambéry: Albane, Conio, and Blauchet. 1875.

THE BOSTON
MEDICAL AND SURGICAL JOURNAL.

VOL. XCIII. — THURSDAY, AUGUST 12, 1875. — NO. 7.

—————

THE INNER SURFACE OF THE UTERUS AFTER PARTURITION.[1]

BY LEONARD WHEELER, M. D., OF WORCESTER.

THE time which I propose to occupy will not allow of lengthy discussions or citations, and I shall therefore endeavor to draw a definite picture, agreeing, as far as possible, with the present state of knowledge upon my subject.

Within five years the study of the anatomical relations of embryo, fœtus, and mother seems to have been earnestly taken up anew; for the first time it has been studied with all the arts and appliances of modern microscopy, especially from thin sections. During this time, the work of several persevering investigators has resulted in some definite additions to our knowledge of a subject upon which comparatively little had hitherto been definitively known, and upon which many prevalent ideas were false. The subject is interesting in any aspect, but specially and practically so as helping to an understanding of another, upon which there has been even more discussion and less agreement, namely, puerperal fever.

The little advance we now boast is the first for just a century; for, apart from the microscopical details in which this advance consists, the descriptions of William Hunter "may be justly characterized as all true and containing all the truth." John Hunter advanced incorrect views of his own after his brother's death, views which his great name propelled through all the medical literature of more than half a century, and even into the text-books of the present decade. His was the coagulable-lymph theory. William Hunter's level was not again reached till the present generation. After the publication of Cruveilhier's Pathological Anatomy, the opinion therein expressed was law for the world till Virchow appeared. Cruveilhier said that the inner surface of the uterus after parturition was clean muscle, and compared it to a stump after amputation. Twenty-five years ago Virchow renewed the theory of William Hunter. About the same time the French school set forth the opinion that a new mucous membrane began to be devel-

[1] Read at the Annual Meeting of the Massachusetts Medical Society, June 8, 1875.

oped under the old during pregnancy, so early even as the fourth month, and this opinion was supported by Priestley in his Lectures on the Development of the Gravid Uterus, published in 1860. The opinion of Cruveilhier has also found recent supporters, as Kölliker and others. Matthews Duncan long ago earnestly maintained the theory of Hunter and Virchow, now universally acknowledged, that the muscle is never exposed.

The origin of the new epithelial covering of the involuted uterus was always a vexed question. It had been accounted for, on the one hand, by derivation from connective-tissue cells, and, on the other, by rapid proliferation from the cervical mucous membrane.

The first thorough microscopical observations were reported by Friedländer in 1870, the latest in a long article by Engelmann, of St. Louis, in a recent number of the *American Journal of Obstetrics.* This latter, the common work of Kundrat, in Vienna, and Engelmann, is a valuable addition to the English literature of the subject, and so comprehensive that had it appeared in season I should have allowed it to absorb the place of this paper; still I hope my briefer and differently handled statement will also have its value.

In health the mucous membrane of the adult uterus consists of an outer layer, lying next to the muscle, and composed of connective tissue with fibre cells; it supports an inner coat of ciliated epithelium, which sends numerous single and bifurcated glandular prolongations through the outer layer down to the muscle. During pregnancy it is much changed; in the first weeks the connective-tissue layer increases enormously, becoming five or six times as thick as in health, and, at its junction with the cervical mucous membrane, it bulges down over the latter; toward the inner surface it loses its fibrous character, and becomes more and more richly cellular. The epithelial covering mostly disappears. The glands lengthen, and the lower ends branch.

A transverse section shows the membrane so much changed that two layers are now distinguishable: an inner, toward the uterine cavity, consisting almost entirely of round cells, with a small amount of intercellular substance (the cells resembling epithelium, though derived probably from connective tissue), and an outer, made up of spindle-shaped cells and gland cavities lined with epithelium. Later, with the rapid increase in size of the uterus, the whole membrane becomes thinner, but the connective tissue seems to have overwhelmed the epithelial layer, which, as a layer, disappears, the only epithelium left adherent to the uterus being that lining the glands.

The ovum, issuing from the Fallopian tube upon this membrane, finds a nidus in one of its folds, which soon enwraps it in the miscalled decidua reflexa. The villi of its chorion become gently adherent by a mucous mucilage, and the formation of a placenta begins, not, as has always been held, by the villi plunging deep into the glands, but by a general reception of the villi into the substance of the mucosa, the mucous membrane growing up about them. Where the villi happen to lodge at the mouth of a gland, the decidual tissue is piled up around them the same as elsewhere, and so for a short distance they are within the gland, but as a rule the villi are not inclosed in glandular epithelium. The union of placenta and decidua does not become inseparably firm till during the third month.

And here our settled knowledge of the maternal parts ceases, for there is no unanimity of opinion upon the character of the maternal framework which supports the fœtal villi. In the fully-formed placenta the amount of this maternal portion is found to be comparatively small, forming an irregular framework for the villi. According to Winkler, who seems to have made very successful sections, it is a prolongation of the intercellular substance of the cell layer of the decidua, which forms a loose mesh, the framework of the whole placenta, the trellis upon and in which the villi are supported. It is covered with endothelium, and the villi are either imbedded in it entirely or only for a part of their circumference, while a few hang loosely in its sinuses. The villi are covered with epithelium, except where in contact with the maternal structure; here intercellular substance unites with intercellular substance, and a way unbarred by epithelium or endothelium exists between maternal and fœtal parts — an unprotected way for the transmission of hereditary virtue or vice.

By others the sinus-system is regarded as merely an extension and dilatation of the inner coat of the maternal vessels. But even the existence of a sinus-system has been disputed by such men as Velpeau and Ramsbotham, and, in a recent long paper, by Braxton Hicks.

To recapitulate, then, we have from without inward (1) muscular layer of the uterus with its sinuses, (2) gland layer of the decidua, (3) cell layer of same, (4) maternal framework of intercellular matter supporting the fœtal villi, (5) chorion, (6) amnion.

Now where is the line of separation of the decidua at the time of parturition? With an understanding of the anatomy of the pregnant uterus, a further knowledge of the microscopic appearances of the outer surface of the delivered placenta, and of the inner surface of the uterus after expulsion of the ovum, would demonstrate the line of separation. The expelled ovum particularly has been examined by many observers, and opinions as to the histological formation of its maternal surface are pretty well agreed; the appearances described correspond excellently with those of the inner, cell-layer of the decidua, *i. e.*, judging from this, the whole gland layer, at least, must be left within the uterus.

That this is in reality the case was first proved by Friedländer;

but though all honor is due him, the same view was stated with sufficient distinctness, as long ago as 1854, by Chisholm, who, in describing the post-mortem appearances of the uterine mucous membrane in the case of a woman who died on the seventh day after delivery, says, " There were numbers of minute oval and circular depressions studded very regularly over the internal surface. They were distinctly visible to the naked eye, and the largest of them might have admitted the head of a pin. Little more concerning these depressions could be made out with the microscope, but we have found similar appearances constantly presented by the mucous membrane of pregnant uteri among the lower mammalia, and no one can for a moment doubt that they are the openings of the follicles of the mucous membrane."

I have had a single opportunity of testing the truth of this. The patient, a woman at full term with her first child, died suddenly after a few weeks of acute kidney trouble. The membranes and placenta were lightly adherent over the whole inner surface of the cavity of the uterus, so lightly that only the slightest traction was necessary to separate them. The divided layers were rough, and yellowish red in color. Pieces of the uterus being hardened and sections made, the inside layer was found a line or two in thickness, and apparently covered the muscle everywhere. It was made up of two layers: a continuous internal one of small cells, and an external one with more intercellular substance and fibre cells, and interrupted by numerous elongated cavities. Over the placental site, where in this case there were, of course, no thrombi, this layer seemed to be thinner and the glands scarcer; indeed, it was often wanting, so that the muscle was left exposed, though I could not be sure this was not an effect of my manipulation.

We have, therefore, over the whole inside of the uterus (except the cervix, which retains its whole mucous membrane), not the naked muscle, but the outer layer of the mucous membrane. There is no coating of epithelium over it; there has been a solution of continuity, and the whole is a wounded surface composed of connective tissue, a surface well fitted, apparently, for resorption of different substances into the blood or lymph systems. Under the present circumstances, however, there is no necessity of having recourse to connective tissue, or to the epithelium of the cervix even, for the source of a new epithelial layer. Epithelium is lacking on the surface, but there are plenty of deposits below in the gland-cavities of the outer layer of the mucous membrane, which still remains undisturbed in the uterus.

This question of the process of renewal of the epithelial covering is a difficult one. It must necessarily be determined from fine sections of the part at particular times, and it is very hard to get proper material from healthy uteri at these times, since the puerperal woman, if she dies, succumbs generally to a disease involving exactly that part which it is desired to examine. Further, the study of the subject on animals leads to no competent result, since the conditions are very different. In animals, when the epithelial covering does not remain entire, there is, at most, a very small wound at the placental seat. The guinea-pig, for instance, may conceive a few hours after parturition, so slight is the influence of pregnancy on the state of the organs.

The process as now explained is as follows: during the first week after parturition the surface of the uterus is covered with a soft, dirty, dark-red sheet of variable thickness, which is easily washed away by a gentle stream of water, the gradually degenerating part of the cell-layer of the decidua. Washed away, it leaves a dark-red, ragged, still living, but fast exfoliating surface. The placental site is distinguished by the greater unevenness of surface, caused by the projecting thrombi of the veins. Under the microscope, the soft sheet which can be washed off is found to consist principally of large round cells filled with fat, and some few spindle-shaped cells, some epithelium, red and white blood corpuscles, and much free fat; in other words, the altered constituents of the cell-layer of the decidua. In fine transverse sections the following condition is found: on the muscle lies the whole of the gland-layer, and, inside of this, toward the cavity of the uterus, a part of the cell-layer already in the midst of a process of rapid degeneration; both these layers are infiltrated with blood corpuscles. The cell-layer is much reduced in thickness, and, even in the first week, is sometimes entirely absent in spots, leaving at points the epithelium of the gland-cavities of the layer beneath exposed.

In the second week, the fluid covering the inner surface is thinner and less red, while the real inner surface is less ragged and has more consistency; it is no longer possible to wash away portions of it with a stream of water. The thrombi of the placental seat are gray in color and less prominent. Microscopically, the fluid covering has less of the other constituents, but more pus and epithelium. On section, it is found that the cell-layer of the decidua has almost entirely disappeared, leaving the gland-layer exposed; not only that, but the connective tissue around the epithelium-clothed cavities is fast undergoing fatty degeneration, and the epithelium has been exposed in many spots, so that we have innumerable points, skin grafts as it were, spread over the whole surface.

In the third week the surface is nearly smooth, and is now entirely covered with cylinder epithelium which dips down here and there, leaving a wide opening into epithelium-lined cavities — the ends of the glands which have been buried during pregnancy. On the placental seat alone little spaces remain uncovered by epithelium, that is, the projecting thrombi; still these are much reduced in size. Otherwise the placental seat is like the rest of the surface. A little of the purulent fluid remains, which disappears finally at about the fourth week. After this time the changes are merely an increasing thickness of the mucous membrane and consequent lengthening of the glands, while the epithelium receives a fringe of cilia.

The process is then as follows : the line of division between placenta and uterus runs through the cell-layer of the decidua. The portion of this layer left in the uterus is infiltrated with blood; it goes through the process of fatty degeneration, and its degenerated remains form a large part of the lochia. By this process the gland-layer is brought nearer the surface, and the glands are laid open. Innumerable little islets of epithelium are gradually presented over the surface. The tissue between these continues to degenerate ; the whole uterus grows smaller, and the patches of epithelium are thus brought nearer and nearer together, till the space remaining to be covered is extremely small ; and finally, this is filled by a new growth of epithelial cells.

UMBILICAL HERNIA; ACCIDENTAL RUPTURE OF THE TUMOR.

BY CHARLES O'LEARY, M. D., OF PROVIDENCE, R. I.

EARLY on Sunday morning, May 30th, I was called to see a patient on the outskirts of this city. Not being apprised of the urgency of the case, I did not reach the patient's house until ten o'clock A. M. On entering the room, I found a woman lying in bed in her dress ; she was quite calm and composed. Being asked what the trouble was, she told me her bowels were all out, and directed me to examine and see. Raising her clothing, I beheld an enormous tumor in the left iliac region, with intestines (probably thirty inches of the large bowel and some portion of the small) protruding from it. The tumor was of cylindrical form ; it measured eighteen inches in circumference at its base, and nine inches in height. It had on its upper surface three pouches, nearly of the shape and size of an average-sized lemon ; one of them proved to be the umbilicus. When the tumor was dependent this umbilical pouch reached to the middle third of the thigh. In the longer diameter of the tumor was a rent between two and three inches in extent, through which the intestines protruded.

The history of the patient, as given by herself, was as follows : She was fifty-four years of age, married, and had had two children, the younger fourteen years of age ; she had always had good health. Six years ago she noticed a swelling at the navel ; as this enlarged she consulted a physician, who recognized umbilical hernia, and advised her to have a truss applied; this advice she neglected. As the tumor increased, she consulted one physician after another, but treated with the same neglect the advice of each. When the tumor gained the enormous proportion above given, with the abnormal displacement of the abdominal wall, she was told by those whom she consulted that they could devise no means of relieving her. She had continued, she said, to live comfortably, with the exception of some chafing and excoriation on the surface of the tumor, which she had relieved by applications. She had attended to her various occupations, those of a woman of the working class, and this with so little apparent inconvenience that her nearest neighbors did not know anything of her infirmity. She had not suffered from constipation or any symptom of bowel obstruction at any time since the first appearance of the tumor. Her habits had been temperate. She was corpulent, and presented every appearance of robust health.

The accident which brought about her present condition occurred on the evening of May 29th. Whilst walking to a neighboring store, she slipped and fell. She at once became aware of the rupture of the tumor, and felt the bowels protruding. She did not call for help, but tucked a fold of her under-clothes around the intestines, and walked home, a distance about the eighth of a mile. She betrayed no fear or alarm, and would not have a physician summoned before morning. She received with perfect composure the statement of the desperate nature of her condition, and expressed a willingness to submit to any operation which I deemed necessary.

Assisted by Mr. B. F. Gorman, a student of the Harvard Medical School, I administered ether, enlarged the rent already made, and with all care and precaution restored the bowels within the cavity of the tumor. I followed them with the hand into the abdominal cavity proper, but found I could not retain them there, as no sooner was the hand withdrawn than they escaped into the cavity of the tumor. The opening between the two cavities was, as it were, hooped by a dense band possessing the strength and resistance of cartilage; to this band was due the cylindrical form of the tumor. Deeming all efforts to retain the bowels in the abdominal cavity unavailing, I left them in the cavity of the tumor, freed from twist or constriction, as far as I could ascertain. I sewed up the opening, and applied cold-water dressing, with compresses. Morphine was ordered in proper doses, at intervals, and such regimen prescribed as seemed most likely to prevent vomiting. She spent the day comfortably enough.

On Monday, she had well-marked peritonitis, with incipient gangrene of the pouches on the surface of the tumor.

On Tuesday, the pouches were ready to slough. The gangrene was extending. The peritonitis exhibited its usual progress, the abdomen being extremely tympanitic.

Wednesday, vomiting became distressing; it was relieved only by hypodermic injections of morphine. The patient felt great distress, with pain in the abdomen. She retained her mental faculties unimpaired.

Thursday, 7½ A. M. The abdomen was tense, with great pain; a hypodermic injection was administered. She inquired very calmly how long she was to last. Gangrene of the pouches was now complete, with signs of its extension to the tumor. I called at 12 M., when I learned she had expired half an hour before my arrival.

During the extreme tension of the abdomen the tumor preserved its contour. In the vomiting no stercoraceous matter was ejected. There was no dejection after the date of the rupture. An autopsy was not permitted.

RECENT PROGRESS IN THE TREATMENT OF CHILDREN'S DISEASES.[1]

BY D. H. HAYDEN, M. D.

Acute Rheumatism in Infancy and Childhood.[2] — Three cases were presented: one, that of a little girl three years old, was complicated with endocarditis and incompetency of the mitral valve; the second case, of a girl ten years old, was complicated with endocarditis at the orifice of the pulmonary artery, solidification of the right lung, and pulmonary hæmorrhage; the third case, of a little girl four years old, was complicated with endocarditis. In opposition to the statement in most books on the subject, Professor Jacobi considers acute rheumatism a not infrequent affection in infancy and childhood. Uncomplicated muscular rheumatism, however, is rare; and, when it appears to be present, the muscular pain can in most cases be easily explained, as in torticollis, where there is often an affection of the spinal cord or a hæmorrhage in the sterno-cleido-mastoid muscle.

The peculiar symptomatology of acute rheumatism in childhood causes the disease to be readily overlooked, the swelling of the joints being often trifling, and the pain not always excessive; the temperature is rarely very high as long as polyarthritis is the only symptom, and sometimes, indeed, it is low after the first attack of an acute endocarditis has set in; perspiration is not copious; the urine is frequently copious and pale, and the amount of uric acid in children, whether rheumatic or not, is not large. The author has met with more female than

---

[1] Concluded from page 165.

[2] Series of American Clinical Lectures. Vol. I. No. II. By Professor A. Jacobi, M. D. New York: G. P. Putnam's Sons. 1875.

male patients.   Visceral complications are more frequent in the young. Pericarditis and pleuritis are not at all rare ; but owing to the serous character of the exudations we frequently miss the friction sound as an aid to their diagnosis.

Cardiac complications are the rule, and an absence of them is very exceptional.   The diagnosis of endocarditis is by no means beyond the reach of a doubt.   When a murmur heard at the beginning is due to endocarditis, there is always a rise of temperature.   So-called anæmic murmurs are rare in children ; and murmurs not due to organic lesions are likely after some time to disappear.

Whereas the large number of heart-diseases in newly-born and very young infants is confined to the right side, in children of five years and upwards it is found in the left side.   The former are congenital, and the latter acquired.   The explanation of this is the statistical fact that the congenital heart-disease seldom lasts into childhood : it destroys life.   It means further that almost all the numerous heart-diseases of childhood up to puberty do not date from birth, but are the result of the most common cause of cardiac disease — rheumatism.

The organs constituting the nervous system are very liable to rheumatism.   The symptoms differ greatly in the young and the old. Where in the adult the sensitive sphere is affected, in the child we find the motor powers suffering.   Where we have delirium in the adult, in the child we have convulsions.   A further difference is that a fatal termination is less frequent in the young.

The main cause of chorea is rheumatism.   The author calls chorea, endocarditis, and polyarthritis " the coördinate symptoms of one and the same affection," and not one the cause of the other; for if the latter were the case we would always find the symptoms in the same order, whereas the author has met with cases where endocarditis was for some time the only manifestation of the disease, this preceding all articular affections.   In a boy three years old, he observed general chorea four or five days before the slightest symptom of rheumatism was perceptible in the joints.   When the joints became affected, the choreic movements grew less.   After a week, the articular swelling receding, chorea became more prominent again.   In this manner nerve and joint rheumatism alternated three times in the course of two months, until, finally, the case wound up with a mild endocarditis, terminating in insufficiency of the mitral valve.

The diagnosis of acute rheumatism is but rarely difficult; still mistakes are possible.   Disorders of a purely nervous character are the more perplexing to many medical men the more they have been accustomed to look upon nervous (hysterical) symptoms as the privilege of the adult female ; whereas men may become hysterical, as may also children.   Nervous symptoms of a most serious type are not excessively rare in children; nor are well-developed neuroses of the motor, sensitive and vaso-motor nerves exceptional.

The indications for treatment given are: Rest of inflamed joints, reduction of local and general heat, removal of hyperæmia, diminishing exudation and internal pressure, and relieving pain. A slight curvature is the easiest position for the diseased joint. There is no benefit to be hoped for from local depletion, save that a few leeches will occasionally prove beneficial, at least temporarily, on the knee-joint. Ice is more to be relied on than any other local application, being indicated in the acute stage, where the swelling is considerable and the temperature high. Later, when these have been reduced, warm applications are better; of these, poultices, warm water, cold applications which remain long enough to become warm, or warm baths, are the best. In chronic cases, blisters or tincture of iodine may do good; but their presumed stimulation of the vaso-motor nerves of the interior is based more upon theoretical reasoning than upon actual proof. At a still later period, if the exudation continue stationary, gentle compression by means of collodion, flannel bandages, cotton with linen bandages, or plaster of Paris, is required. A beneficial effect is also claimed for mild galvanic currents passing through the joints from one to three times daily from five to ten minutes. Chloroform, belladonna, opium, or veratria, in lotions or ointment, is to be used for relief of pain. If this is very severe, a subcutaneous injection of morphine may be required.

Internal medication is resorted to upon the same indications; and, whether we use aconite, digitalis, veratrum, colchicum, or quinine, larger doses are required than the usual proportion-tables seem to justify; and whatever effect is to be obtained must be secured rapidly.

The author relies on veratrum viride where the principal object is the reduction of the pulse. Aconite and digitalis are slower in their action, but may be continued for a longer time. The general rule is to push the dose until the pulse has fallen considerably, but not to the normal point, then to maintain the dose for two or three days, and finally cautiously diminish it. At any rise in the pulse, the dose must be increased. In careless hands, veratrum is a very dangerous remedy, and cannot be handled so freely; and the dose must often be diminished more rapidly, lest the vascular sedation become excessive.

At the head of antiphlogistic remedies stands quinine. When indicated at all, it should be given in a dose of five grains, once, twice, or thrice daily to a child one or two years old. It is necessary to be certain of the solubility of the preparation. The sulphate ought to be avoided, and the bisulphate or muriate selected. It should never be forgotten that the stomach absorbs less under a feverish condition. Where it rebels against the remedy, the rectum may take its place; but it will absorb nothing unless in solution.

The iodide of potassium, to do any good, must be given early, immediately after the fever has been subdued, in doses of from fifteen grains to a drachm or more, according to age.

Colchicum and colchicin (in three or four daily doses of one one hundred and fiftieth of a grain to a child four or five years old, and gently increased from day to day) are of very doubtful effect, save as an arterial sedative, and is apt to produce vomiting and diarrhœa.

The author has no belief in the "acid theory," of rheumatism, and does not employ alkaline remedies. Their principal effect is diuretic, and the amount of uric acid in the urine of children, whether rheumatic or not, is not large.

The indications for the treatment of the cardiac, cerebral, or spinal complications differ hardly from that of the joint affection. In endocarditis, and particularly in pericarditis, the constant use of ice is most beneficial. When the acute stage has passed by, warm baths of about 90° (Fahrenheit) need not be feared in heart-diseases more than in other subacute or chronic inflammations.

For the treatment of the "choreic manifestations of rheumatism," the author relies principally on arsenic. Next in order he ranks bromide of potassium. Lastly, nitrate of silver and atropia. Rest is secured by chloral hydrate or large doses of bromide of potassium; the muscular irritability is soothed by subcutaneous injections of woorara. In protracted and feverless cases, as also in chronic cases of rheumatism, a daily hath, containing from three to five ounces of the sulphide of potassium, and the galvanic current, are very efficient. In cases of acute chorea dependent upon meningeal or medullary congestion or inflammation, the author relies principally upon ergot. Failures with this remedy he feels positive are due to the insufficiency of the dose. Less than half a drachm of Squibb's fluid extract he rarely gives; and repeats it three or four times daily. A child four or five years old may take from two to four drachms daily for many weeks in succession. Bad effects of the medicine he has never seen. The stories of acute or chronic poisoning, with a very few exceptions, concern individuals whose constitutions were previously broken down by long-continued misery and starvation.

Trismus and Tetanus Neonatorum treated with Chloral Hydrate.[1] — The views as to the prognosis of this disease have been of late very much changed by the results of experiments in the wards of Professor Widerhofer, in Franz-Josef's Children's Hospital, Vienna. A large number of cases of recovery have been reported by Professor Widerhofer's assistants: Kirchstetter (injections of atropine), Monti (extractum calabaris), Auchenthaler (chloral hydrate).

The theory first advanced by Dr. A. Monti, "that when the temper-

[1] Dr. A. Von Hütter, Wiener Jahrbuch für Kinderheilkunde, i., 1874.

ature does not go above 102° the prognosis is favorable," has been as a rule confirmed. There were, however, exceptions, as for example, in one case of Kirchstetter's, where the temperature went above 104° Fahrenheit. The author would prefer to state the proposition as follows: " Cases of tetanus neonatorum, when the result of a general disease (pyæmia, septicæmia), are always fatal. In other cases, the prognosis is so much the more favorable the longer the duration of the disease and the less fever there is that accompanies it."

There is no specific action of chloral hydrate. By relaxing the spasm in the muscles the child is kept alive until the cause of the disease ceases to act. Extract of calabar bean acts in the same way. Chloral hydrate is administered in Widerhofer's wards as follows: one or two grains, dissolved in breast-milk, are given through the nose. This causes generally, by irritation, a paroxysm. The number and size of the doses are so arranged as to obtain a long sleep; and after every paroxysm the dose is repeated. It is of course important to give as much nourishment as possible. Meteorism and diarrhœa if present must be combated; but opium is to be avoided. One necessary caution is to stop the medicine as soon as there is a smell of chloroform in the breath.

Croupous Pneumonia and Meningitis Cerebro-Spinalis in Infants under one year old.[1] — After the disappearance of the epidemic of cerebrospinal meningitis in Erlangen during the years 1864–66, six cases of this disease in infants complicated with pneumonia came under Maurer's observation. Whereas in adults this complication does not ordinarily present symptoms sufficiently pregnant to enable a diagnosis of the meningitis, in infants under one year of age this is generally easy. The most marked symptom is the prominence and increased tension of the anterior fontanelle, which shows itself very soon after the first appearance of cerebral symptoms, when these latter are dependent upon the meningitis. The other symptoms observed by the author were loss of consciousness, convulsions, and, though not always, contraction of the recti muscles of the eye, hyperæsthesia of the auditory and optic nerve, and changes in the pupils. The appearance of convulsions makes the diagnosis sure. In all the six cases these occurred during the stage of resolution of the pneumonia, whereas when they constitute a symptom of the so-called form of " cerebral pneumonia," they occur at the beginning of the disease. The diagnosis of a cerebro-spinal meningitis complicating a pneumonia from acute meningitis accompanying the same would be almost impossible; but the coexistence of the two latter diseases is so extremely rare that it need not be taken into account. Acute hydrocephalus, without tuberculosis, is an equally rare

---

[1] Deutsches Archiv für klinische Medicin, xiv. 1.; Allgemeine medicinische Central-Zeitung, January 6, 1875. Dr. Maurer.

complication.   Acute hydrocephalus, when one symptom of tubercular meningitis, causes such characteristic changes in the pulse, respiration, ophthalmoscopic appearances, and course of the disease, that a differential diagnosis would be easy.

Diet of Infants affected with Acute Intestinal Catarrh.[1] — Dr. R. Demme, after an experience of twelve years, recommends as the most appropriate food for infants affected with gastric or intestinal catarrh the following diet: Add from a quarter of a pound to a pound of beef, freed of fat, to two quarts of cold water, and let this stand from half an hour to an hour ; then boil down to one pint; after cooling, skim off fat from the top and filter.   At each time of using (every two or three hours), without being warmed, this is to be mixed with freshly prepared rice or barley water.   In the intervals of meals the latter should be given alone, best without sugar, to relieve the thirst.   If this food is refused he gives a drink made with the white of an egg, using according to age from one to three eggs in half a pint to a pint of water which has been previously boiled and cooled down to 98°.   If the child's strength begins to fail, brandy in doses of from five to thirty drops is added to the rice or barley water, from three to five times a day. With older children a mixture of milk with the rice-water or barley water may be tried.

PROCEEDINGS OF THE OBSTETRICAL SOCIETY OF BOSTON.

CHARLES W. SWAN, M. D., SECRETARY.

APRIL 10, 1875. — The President, DR. R. L. HODGDON, in the chair.

Ovariotomy. — DR. LYMAN read for Dr. Chadwick a case of fatal ovariotomy.   The case was published in the JOURNAL of July 22, 1875.

DR. STEDMAN, in reference to this paper, asked if in injecting intestine with nutrient fluid through a puncturing tube there were not danger of inflammation from accidental escape of the fluid.

DR. MINOT said he had once given great relief by pumping out a large quantity of fluid from an intestine punctured for the purpose.

Peritonitis and Pelvic Abscess in a Young Girl. — DR. MINOT reported the case as follows : —

"Miss M. G., thirteen years and seven months old, always healthy, began to menstruate for the third time early in the morning of January 26, 1875, twenty-nine days after the beginning of the second epoch, which period occurred three weeks from the beginning of the first.   There had been no pain or trouble at either of the periods.   The last one ceased on the 29th, having lasted but three days; the two previous ones lasted four days each.   Her

---

[1] Eleventh Annual Report of the Jenner Children's Hospital in Berne.   Allgemeine medicinische Central-Zeitung, December 23, 1874.

mother kept her at home on the 26th and 27th, as a precaution, but she went to school as usual on the 28th and 29th, both of which days were mild. So far as she knew, she did not get chilled or fatigued. The bowels were in good order.

"On the evening of the 29th she complained of pain in the abdomen, which continued all the next day. I first saw her that evening (the 30th). She was in bed, complaining of steady pain, with exacerbations, over the pubes, and of considerable tenderness over the whole of the lower part of the abdomen, but not of the region above the umbilicus. The pain continued with severity during the night, and the patient got but little sleep. The next morning (January 31st) there was extreme tenderness over the pubes; the pulse was 128, the temperature 101.2°. The limbs were drawn up. There was no headache. There had been no rigor until early this morning, when one occurred, lasting some time. The pain was relieved by repeated injections of morphia under the skin, but recurred frequently during the day. There was also vomiting, or rather regurgitation of everything taken into the stomach.

"February 1st. The night had been comfortable as respects pain, but the patient had vomited several times. Pulse 120; temperature 99.9°. Tenderness was most marked in the right iliac fossa. The legs were constantly drawn up, and supported by a pillow. The urine was passed without catheter. She was kept comfortable by occasional injections of morphia, one sixth of a grain each. At night the pulse fell to 104.

"February 2d. An attack of nervous excitement, with delirium, at eight o'clock this morning, which was quieted by morphia. Pulse 108. Decubitus still dorsal, the knees supported on a pillow. Tenderness as before; percussion sound in lower part of abdomen quite dull. Urine without catheter, twice in twenty-four hours. Pulse at night, 120.

"February 3d. Severe attack of pain at five A. M., relieved by morphia. Pulse 120. At nine A. M., pulse 112, temperature 101.9°. The tenderness was extreme, the least touch over the ramus of pubes on the right side causing severe pain. At eleven P. M., pulse 120, temperature 102.6°.

"February 5th. The condition was the same. For the first time morphia was given by the mouth. The pain diminished during the day, and the patient's condition was decidedly improved towards night. She was able to lie in any position, having discarded the pillow under the knees. There having been no dejection since the beginning of the attack, and the patient being somewhat annoyed by flatulence, an enema of olive-oil and soap-suds was given in the morning, which was returned without effect. It was not repeated, but at four P. M. a large solid faecal dejection took place spontaneously, with very little pain.

"February 6th, 7th, the patient appeared to be convalescing. There was some looseness of the bowels. The pulse fell to 96; the temperature was normal.

"February 8th. Pulse 112. She complained of some pain from time to time, and took a dose of castor-oil, which was followed by several loose dejections with some pain. The pulse at night was 120.

" February 9th (eleventh day). Some pain, as yesterday, with restlessness; pulse 120. At eight o'clock in the evening there was a sudden discharge *per vaginam* of several ounces of very fetid pus, which was followed by great relief of the pain.

" February 10th. Pulse 92, temperature 98.5°. The night was passed without pain, the discharge continuing moderately free, and very fetid. There was hardness, and complete dullness on percussion throughout the lower part of the abdomen, especially in the right iliac region, but the tenderness has much diminished. The vagina was syringed with a solution of carbolic acid several times daily. Wine, quinine, and broth were administered.

" From this time the patient improved daily, though slowly. The discharge continued till about March 1st. She began to sit up two hours each day from that time, and went down-stairs for the first time March 7th."

In answer to a question, Dr. Minot stated that as there was a perfectly formed hymen, no vaginal examination had been made.

DR. SINCLAIR remarked that the abscess seemed to have formed very rapidly.

DR. MINOT suggested that the peritonitis was probably secondary to the abscess. The symptoms occurred just after the close of the patient's second menstruation.

Puerperal Convulsions. — DR. LYMAN read a case of puerperal convulsions reported to him by Dr. Towle, of Haverhill. The case is interesting as showing a good result under an opiate treatment.

Chloroform and Ether. — DR. WELLINGTON asked if chloroform was really superior to ether in convulsions or labor.

DR. LYMAN replied that he saw no reason for thinking so. In answer to other questions he said that when he saw the woman, in consultation, she looked badly, — much swollen, very anæmic. With other things bleeding was suggested as among the remedies which might be resorted to, but it was not urged, the anæmia being an objection. It was considered prudent to postpone venesection at least till after other remedies had been fairly tried. The patient was about eight months advanced in pregnancy. The convulsions were very severe ; none occurred during or after labor, and none, with one exception, after anæsthesia was begun. As far as obstetrical operations are concerned, he had no hesitation in denouncing chloroform, and said he was afraid of it.

DR. REYNOLDS remarked that the claim is made in the journals that the physical process of labor makes chloroform safe, that is, that the constant access of pain acts, in that respect, as colic does with laudanum, the pain in the two cases conferring equal immunity, although the cases are not fairly analogous. Dr. Reynolds had lately asked a gentleman present, of large experience, concerning a patient who, being nauseated by ether, refused to take it. The gentleman advised twenty-drop doses of chloroform on a handkerchief, to be inhaled at the access of the pains ; but he gave it, as Dr. Reynolds saw, more freely than he advised it to be given. The common impression is that deaths from chloroform result from too free administration ; he would ask if among the deaths from chloroform, reported in the journals from time to time, there were any which had occurred during labor.

DR. WELLINGTON said that the difference between the two agents seems to be that when the patient is in labor she is in pain, which repeatedly acts against the overpowering effects of the drug, as laudanum sufficient to relieve pain with safety might destroy life in the absence of pain. He had never heard of a case of death from chloroform during labor.

DR. REYNOLDS said further that it was not the pain alone which was advanced as a reason why chloroform in labor was not dangerous, but the pain, accompanied by uterine contraction, it was alleged, secured at short intervals a supply of blood to the nervous centres. He was not qualified to judge whether this was sound reasoning or not. It was analogous to what gentlemen in Paris did when they tipped up the patient so frequently.

DR. MINOT suggested the recumbent position of the lying-in woman as another reason for her safety. A large proportion of the deaths reported as from chloroform had been in patients who were sitting up at the time. He questioned whether the horizontal position might not favor the escape from the lungs of the heavy chloroform vapor.

DR. RICHARDSON said he had heard Sir James Simpson state that he had given the question of death from chloroform in labor much attention, but had been unable to find a single instance of fatality.

DR. LYMAN remarked that ether subdues the pain — itself a paralyzing influence — quite as well as chloroform, with none of the danger caused by such a paralyzing agent as the latter.

DR. WELLINGTON asked, " What shall we do with the fact that no one, so far as we know, has had a death from chloroform in labor ? "

DR. LYMAN replied that one circumstance is that chloroform is not given in labor so continuously as in other cases ; again, we do not know that cases may not have occurred which have not been reported.

DR. WELLINGTON mentioned the case of a patient who insisted upon taking chloroform, and did take it very freely. That death from chloroform does not result from the quantity taken appears from the frequency with which death occurs before the patient is sufficiently anæsthetized for the surgeon to begin his operation.

DR. SINCLAIR referred to a case which came under his observation, in which a toe-nail was to be removed. The patient got a whiff or two of chloroform and was dead. He was sitting up.

DR. RICHARDSON said that, according to the German observers, chloroform is much more apt to affect unfavorably the child delivered, than ether.

DR. ABBOT stated that in fatal narcosis from chloroform the blood does not coagulate. From this we may understand why insensibility produced by chloroform might result in death of the child. Nélaton says a good deal of the advantage of inverting the patient as a means of restoration. During labor and the suspended respiration accompanying the efforts, the blood is forced to the brain. Under certain circumstances, alarming symptoms may occur with the use of ether, and be relieved in the way mentioned. In the case of a child upon whom Dr. Cabot had operated for diphtheritic croup, the condition was very bad immediately after tracheotomy. Dr. Abbot held the child by the hips, head downwards, and shook him, partly to relieve the trachea of mucus, and partly to improve the supply of blood to the brain. Relief followed the procedure.

Dr. LYMAN said he did not consider the method as original with Nélaton. He had seen the same thing done by Dr. Hodges.

Dr. REYNOLDS considered the main question to be whether medical means alone should have been thought sufficient in the case of a woman at eight months, who had had three or four convulsions.

Dr. LYMAN replied that he could not help feeling that, the os not being dilated, although there was a slight show, it was his duty to try several remedies — chloral, ether, chloroform, opium — before resorting to manual interference. If the child had been dead, this circumstance would have rendered the question more doubtful.

Dr. REYNOLDS asked Dr. Lyman what he would do if the case were that of a wife of Henry VIII. and the king's only probable chance of offspring, and the accoucheur were ordered to consider this chance.

Dr. LYMAN said he should probably do just what Napoleon ordered when the King of Rome was born, — treat her as he would a peasant woman.

Dr. REYNOLDS inquired whether the child's chances should not be considered.

Dr. LYMAN said he thought the treatment was a question of time. The patient was in no immediate danger of death, the pulse was good, and there was no evidence of exhaustion. She was intelligent and conscious on coming out of the convulsions. If a very violent convulsion should occur, there would be time enough then. If there had been more continued coma, there would have been a decided indication for interference.

Puerperal Convulsions treated with Venesection. — Dr. MINOT reported a case of convulsions which he had seen in consultation with Dr. Ayer. The woman, a stout primipara, was delivered at four P. M. An hour afterwards she had a convulsion, and then six or seven. At eleven P. M. she was insensible and snoring loudly; the pupils were fixed. The tongue was lacerated and bleeding; the pulse was hard, the legs œdematous. Dr. Minot agreed with Dr. Ayer as to the propriety of bleeding, and a pint and a half of blood was drawn. Towards the end of the bleeding the respiration became less stertorous; the patient recovered consciousness. She afterwards had two very slight threatenings of convulsions, but she did perfectly well, and is nursing her baby. In answer to questions, Dr. Minot stated that the face had been turgid with blood, and the pulse had had a hard, sharp stroke. He had thought the woman would die, and that bleeding, if it did no good, would do no harm. She was unconscious between the convulsions after the fourth, and for some hours before she was bled. The bleeding softened the pulse, but did not particularly affect its rate.

Dr. TUCK said he was reminded by this case of one which occurred in the Boston Lying-in Hospital. There were fourteen convulsions, the prognosis was bad, the patient was not bled, and she recovered.

Bright's Disease in Parturient Women. — Dr. CURTIS inquired of the gentlemen present if they had had much experience in confinements in persons subjects of Bright's disease. One would naturally expect, he remarked, a'

14

good deal of trouble. He had had a case of a woman who had Bright's disease four years. During her pregnancy she was better than she had previously been. She was comfortably delivered of her first child, without ether, at about the eighth month. The child was small. The mother died, six weeks after confinement, with œdema of the lungs. It was found at the autopsy that one kidney was entirely gone, the other diseased. There had been no convulsions, no trouble whatever, at the confinement.

DR. REYNOLDS remarked that it was an interesting question how well the kidneys bear the condition incident to convulsions where these have recurred in two or three confinements.

Uterine Malformation. — DR. ABBOT reported a singular malformation of the uterus in a patient twenty-three years old, under his care. She had been apparently a healthy woman, of great strength of will, and nervous temperament; she had been married four or five years, yet never pregnant. For years she had been subject to uncomfortable sensations about the pelvis, pain in the region of the left ovary, backache, discomfort in walking; but she had kept to herself the sufferings which she had from any over-exertion. Last fall she had a mild typhoid fever, and certain symptoms led to a vaginal examination. The vagina was found to be extremely sensitive; the anterior cul-de-sac was deeper than the posterior. The uterus was not prolapsed, but the lower portion of the neck was bent directly forwards at a right angle, the flexure being in the vagina, not in the abdomen, and apparently fixed by cicatricial tissue. When the tip of the cervix was straightened out by the finger, on being let go it sprung back to its previous position. The sound entered about three quarters of an inch. The patient was subject to dysmenorrhœa. Dr. Abbot thought the only remedy was to slit up the cervix as far as the elbow. There was no history of injury except a fall in childhood.

DR. REYNOLDS suggested the use of an air pessary, although it was difficult to see, he said, why such applications aid the position of the parts.

DR. ABBOT said that he had applied glycerine plasma on a tampon of cotton-wool, by which the sensibility was diminished while the deformity remained. Ten days he had put in a soft rubber ring. He considered this form of anteflexion as different from the ordinary ones, in that the fundus was in the normal axis and the neck was bent across the vagina below.

DR. REYNOLDS said he thought the relative position of the flexed uterus to the walls of the pelvis was a subordinate matter.

Embolism of the External Iliac. — DR. HOMANS reported the case of a woman who died at the Boston City Hospital at the age of twenty-three. Early in March she fell on the ice, striking her side. This injury was followed by vomiting. On the third day she had a chill, with pain in the foot. She came into the hospital with the foot and ankle gangrenous. No pulsation could be felt anywhere, from the groin downwards. The patient was confined of a dead child on March 30th. She died April 2d. At the autopsy the external iliac was found plugged for three inches of its extent, — whether the embolism was the result of the fall, or of pregnancy, was a question. In the spleen was evidence of an old clot. There was no other disease in the body.

DR. REYNOLDS remarked that the gangrene preceded labor, although it might have followed the death of the child ; and asked if it were not conceivable that the dead fœtus may have been the starting-point of the disease which occasioned the embolism, poisoning the intervening cellular tissue.

Dr. LYMAN said that there was no visible evidence of any such communication.

Dr. REYNOLDS said he thought such evidence was usually absent.

Dr. LYMAN mentioned the case of a patient whom he was called to see last month. The toes were discolored by gangrene. The femoral pulse was good, but there was none below. This was in a strong, healthy man, and there was nothing to account for the stoppage of the circulation which existed.

High Temperature in Puerperal Cases. — Dr. STEDMAN reported a case which he considered interesting as resembling one reported by Dr. Lyman at a former meeting (high temperature after great loss of blood from aborting, with alarming pulmonary symptoms). Dr. Stedman's patient had so great hæmorrhage after her first labor that the attending physician injected perchloride of iron. At the second labor there was severe hæmorrhage, and iron was again resorted to. In the first labor she had ether ; in the second, she was only amused by it. The labor was an easy one. The patient did well for three weeks, when there occurred a violent chill, followed by a temperature of 105°, and almost colliquative sweats. Dr. Stedman was unable to assign a definite cause for these symptoms. There was no uterine tenderness, no trouble in the abdomen. There had been slight cough, and on the second or third day after the chill there was tubular breathing and bronchial voice in one of the backs, — evidence of solidification. On the second or third day an herpetic eruption appeared about the lips. The physical signs of pneumonia disappeared rapidly. The patient was twice cinchonized, and she got Fowler's solution, but the chills and sweats continued. Dr. Stedman said his theory was that the last chills proceeded from the patient's extreme nervousness. He reminded the society of a case reported at a former meeting in which a temperature of 106° could be accounted for only by an altercation with the nurse. That an hysterical attack will send up the temperature, Dr. Stedman declared himself more and more convinced with every half-year's experience.

Diphtheria. — Dr. STEDMAN gave the case of a child one and a half years old, tuberculous-looking, living in an unhealthy district. It had had strabismus from the age of three months. The next symptom, three days after the first visit, was tremor of the left arm ; then the same arm became powerless ; finally the legs swelled and became helpless, and the veins were corded. Albumen was found in the urine. Reviewing the history of the case he found the child had had very sore throat with swollen glands. The diagnosis was diphtheria.

Dr. ABBOT suggested that the disease might have been scarlatina. He had never seen anasarca with the paralysis of diphtheria. In the latter disease the paralysis is unilateral, whereas, in Dr. Stedman's case, both legs were affected.

Dr. STEDMAN replied that the legs were helpless on account of the swelling, which, with the corded veins, still persists. The patient has regained the use of the left arm.

Prolapse of Bladder and Rectum complicating Labor. — Dr. WELLINGTON reported a case of a multipara in which he was called to assist Dr. Cogswell, of Cambridgeport. The first labor had been natural; in the second the patient was instrumentally delivered of triplets. At the present, the third labor, Dr. Wellington found the vagina plugged full of what proved to be the prolapsed bladder and rectum. These parts were driven forcibly downwards and almost out by the hard pains. The finger could be introduced between the prolapsed folds, and the uterus was found pretty high up, the os dilated, the parts rigid. The hand, and even the doubled fist, was kept within the vagina, but the pains seemed to expend their strength upon the prolapsed organs. After a time the pains stopped and the woman went to sleep. With the return of the pains, the other phenomena were renewed. The hand was now introduced into the vagina, and, manual dilatation, requiring half an hour for its accomplishment, having just been completed by Dr. Marcy, the child was turned and delivered alive, although the head came with some difficulty. The curious part of the case was the effect of the pains upon the prolapsed organs, but these did not interfere with the delivery. The patient has done well so far as heard from.

Dysmenorrhœa treated by Valerianate of Zinc. — DR. MINOT read the following account of three cases of dysmenorrhœa treated by the valerianate of zinc with marked benefit.

"CASE I. L. W. B., aged thirty, single, a teacher, has always suffered from dysmenorrhœa. The pain comes on after the second day of menstruation. The next night is free from pain, but the following day it returns.

"October 8, 1874, the patient had iron, bromide of potassium, suppository of morphia, hyoscyamus, and belladonna.

"November 4th. Some general improvement, but no relief to the dysmen orrhœa. Some tenderness over the left ovary. (Strong tincture of iodine externally.)

"December 9th. On the whole, decidedly less pain. (Valerianate of zinc, one grain three times daily, beginning two days before the next menstrual period, and continued till menstruation is over.)

"January 6, 1875. The 'second pain' was less severe. On the whole, a good deal of improvement.

"February 3d. There was a decided improvement during the last period.

"April 7th. There have been two periods since the last report; both were more free from pain than formerly. The soreness in the abdomen seems to be relieved by the iodine; the pain, by the pills. The patient is well satisfied with the result.

"CASE II. Miss S., Swiss, governess, aged twenty-seven, five years after menstruation was established experienced a strong mental excitement during a period. From that time she had always had severe pain, with nervous symptoms (loss of consciousness, convulsions, etc.), during a few hours after the flow had begun. The discharge occurs every twenty-eight days, is abundant, clotted, and accompanied with the expulsion of shreds 'like pieces of skin.' It lasts only two days. Uterus low; sound enters easily to normal length; slight inclination backwards, with tenderness. No granulations or abrasions. (October 27, 1874. Hot vaginal injections; Quevenne's iron; valerianate of zinc, one grain three times daily, commencing a few days before the beginning of menstruation.)

"November 18th. The period began on the evening of the 15th, and was far less painful than usual ; the relief was very great.

"December 19th. Another period has passed with very little pain.

"January 18, 1875. On the 8th she was unwell, being one week too soon, which she ascribes to 'taking cold.' This not having been anticipated, no valerianate of zinc was taken beforehand, but the medicine was employed as soon as the patient discovered that she was menstruating. The pain was very severe, and she was in bed on the 8th, 9th, and 10th, when it ceased. Since then she has been weak and nervous, sleeping poorly. The iron has been discontinued. It was ordered to be renewed.

"April 1st. Since the last report, Miss S. has been comparatively free from pain, the zinc having been taken as directed. She is satisfied with the result.

"Case III. Miss I., twenty years old, a teacher, delicate-looking, has always suffered great pain during menstruation, which lasts the first two days, during which she is obliged to be in bed, quite incapacitated for work. She consulted me in November, 1874, and was advised to take valerianate of zinc in doses of one grain three times daily, beginning at least twenty-four hours before the expected flow.

"February 13, 1874, she called to report. She has menstruated three times with great relief, each epoch having been less painful than the preceding one, the last (just finished) having been unusually comfortable. She thinks she has been greatly benefited by the medicine.

"April 9th. The relief at the monthly period continues, and she is satisfied that it is due to the valerianate of zinc."

Dr. CURTIS asked if these were not cases of neuralgic dysmenorrhœa.

Dr. MINOT replied that he thought it difficult to exactly characterize the different varieties of dysmenorrhœa.

Dr. LYMAN said he had utterly failed to give permanent relief by valerianate of zinc, ammonia, or iron, all of which he had repeatedly tried ; and he would ask Dr. Minot and others if they had found any of these agents trustworthy, as he had been disappointed in them, although used persistently in doses of from two to four grains in various nervous and neuralgic affections.

Dr. MINOT said he had not tried these in dysmenorrhœa ; but there is no question of the anodyne properties of valerianate of ammonia, in not less than three or four grain doses.

Dr. ABBOT said he had used valerianate of zinc a good deal, in two-grain pills, sugar-coated, and generally oftener than three times a day. If made up extempore it is very nauseous. Dr. Abbot considered it a very valuable remedy, rarely using any other valerianate. His patients sometimes take ten or twelve grains a day.

Dr. LYMAN suggested ginger syrup as a convenient vehicle of administration.

Dr. MINOT stated that he once took a good deal of valerianate of ammonia in ginger syrup for *tic douloureux*, and with excellent effect; but the remedy was extremely disagreeable. This form of valerianate is too deliquescent to be made conveniently into pills. The "elixir" he considered poor stuff.

Dr. ABBOT remarked that at a meeting of the American Pharmaceutical Association an elixir of valerianate of ammonia was shown to have a fraudulent admixture of valerianate of morphia.

THE MEDICAL PROFESSION IN MICHIGAN.

ALTHOUGH, as stated in our issue of July 19th, no decided movement has yet been made by the medical schools of the country towards reform in medical education, we are glad to see that there is a decided feeling existing in the profession not to allow the matter to rest where it is, and that the medical press is also taking an active part in the discussion of this important question. At a meeting of the Michigan Medical Society held in Detroit on the 9th of June, resolutions were passed requesting the medical schools of that State to raise their preliminary requirements for the admission of students, and to exact the attendance on three courses of lectures instead of two as is now required. These resolutions were greeted, says the *Peninsular Journal*, with an enthusiasm and passed with a unanimity which indicated very forcibly the sentiments of the society on the question of medical education. This action on the part of the profession in Michigan has been highly applauded by several of our Western contemporaries, who portray vigorously the causes operating to prevent the downfall of the present system. Inaugurated nearly a century ago, it has been left behind in the progress which this country has made, and is now sustained chiefly with motives far from creditable to the men of influence among our teachers. We trust that some of the gentlemen who helped arouse the enthusiasm at Detroit the other day will be able to find sympathizers among the members of the faculties of that State.

The schools are timid and hesitating, and are endeavoring to satisfy the public with half-way measures. Let the profession generally take this matter in hand and press it firmly until a complete reform has been effected. Undoubtedly there are many so-called schools using every device to maintain a struggling existence. One of the chief advantages of this reform will be that such will sink beneath the surface. It should be a motto of the reformers that " from him that hath not shall be taken away even that which he hath."

It is much to be regretted that the condition of the profession in Michigan is not so harmonious as the united action of the members of the State society would seem to imply. The struggle which has been maintained for so long a time between the regents of the State university and the homœopaths has terminated in the appointment of two homœopathic professors, the institution receiving a grant of six thousand dollars annually to defray the cost of instruction in homœopathy. It is stated that although these two chairs have been added to the medical faculty, the regulations have been so modified as to prevent this course from conflicting with the regular course of study, and the regents claim that the new professors are not members of the now existing department of medicine. That this is not the view which the State takes of the question is shown by the fact that the attempt made by the regents a few years ago to establish a distinct homœopathic school was ruled by the Supreme Court of the State to be not in compliance with the law. Moreover, Dr. Sager, the dean of the faculty, who has been connected with the university for nearly forty years, has felt himself called upon to resign in the belief that the homœopathic branch has been practically engrafted upon the medical department. It is difficult to understand, under the present arrangement, why the other members of the faculty are not teachers in the homœopathic department. Practically they will be until two complete faculties are appointed. We regret to see it stated that the Michigan State Society refused to act upon a resolution condemning the course of the regents, who have, to say the least, placed the medical department of the university in a very equivocal position.

THE POMEROY CASE.

IT is with great disappointment that we are coming to the conclusion that the governor does not intend to sign the death warrant of the murderer Pomeroy. It is, of course, a disagreeable duty, and the sentimental philanthropists are no doubt determined to make it as irksome to him as possible. We would suggest, however, to these gentlemen that surely they have already had share enough in Pomeroy's career. He was safe in the reform school when one of their number obtained his release and gave him the opportunity to commit two horrible murders, and now we think they might let justice take its course.

The real question is very happily expressed in a communication to the *Daily Advertiser*, from which we quote: " Whether Pomeroy is a fit subject for capital punishment is not now an open question. After a cautious and solemn trial, to which there does not attach even a suspicion of unfairness, the jury have pronounced him guilty of murder in the first degree, all the exceptions on points of law which could be raised by able counsel have been overruled, the court has formally sentenced him to death, and the executive council, after full consideration of all that could be urged in his favor, has decided against either pardon or commutation of punishment. Nothing remains but the almost mechanical formalities required for carrying the sentence into effect. The governor alone has no better right than the sheriff or the mob to stay these dread proceedings. He is only the hand of the State. If he assumes the functions of the jury, the court, and the executive council, considers anew the question which they have formally decided, and reverses their decision, he commits a gross usurpation."

The governor, in fact, becomes an accomplice in any future murders the boy may commit when his friends shall have carried their second point, namely, his release.

DR. WINSLOW LEWIS.

THE death of Dr. Lewis has removed one from the small circle of professional men now remaining among us whose lives date back into the last century. He was born July 8, 1799, and graduated at Harvard College in 1819. Studying medicine under the late Dr. John C. Warren, he took his degree in 1822, and subsequently completed his medical education in Europe, where he had the privilege of listening to such men as Dupuytren and Abernethy. On returning to this country he began the practice of his profession, in which he was quite successful, acquiring considerable reputation for skill as a surgeon. His activity as a physician, and the high respect in which he was held by his fellow-citizens, are shown by the numerous positions of honor and trust which he has from time to time held. He was at one time physician of the municipal institutions, and also of the house of correction, and has been for many years one of the consulting physicians of the Massachusetts General Hospital and of the Boston City Hospital. He has also occupied positions in the general court, the common council, and the school committee, and for six years was on the board of overseers of Harvard College.

Retiring from the practice of his profession many years ago, he has been better known to most of the profession of late years as a prominent Freemason, of which craft he has been a member for nearly half a century, during which period he has been the recipient of nearly every honor which it was in the power of the brotherhood to bestow. As past grand master of the masons of Massachusetts, and one who took an unusual interest in the welfare of the order, he was held in high respect by its members, by whom a fitting tribute has been paid to his memory.

His great activity and versatile talents, combined with a warm heart, kindly disposition, and courtly manners, have endeared him to the many classes in the community with which in the course of a long life he has come in contact.

MEDICAL NOTES.

— On the 16th of July, Professor Rokitausky delivered his farewell address before a large audience of professors and physicians in the lecture-room of the Pathological Institute at Vienna. Among those present was Dr. Lizuin, physician to the Emperor of Russia and chief of the Sanitary Bureau at St. Petersburg. The aged teacher was received with great applause. In taking leave, he expressed his intention of not abandoning entirely all active work. In his remarks to his pupils, he explained the nature of pathological anatomy, spoke of the modern tendencies of science, and, among other things, touched upon materialism and woman's rights, of which latter he does not appear to be a champion. In concluding, he exhorted his students to give their work the stamp of their academic training, and to remain true to the principles derived from their alma mater. Deeply moved, the aged man left the lecture-room, accompanied by his colleagues and friends, amidst a tumult of applause and cheers.

— The *Chicago Medical Examiner* and the *Chicago Medical Journal*, after sixteen and thirty-two years respectively of existence, have ceased to appear as independent publications, and have been consolidated. The new journal is to be called the *Chicago Medical Journal and Examiner*, and will be under the control of an association of gentlemen including some of the best known and most honored names in the medical profession of the Northwest, entitled " The Chicago Medical Press Association." Dr. N. S. Davis retires after more than twenty-five years of work as an editor.

— In an article on the alimentation of new-born infants, *Le Progrès Médical* states that a commission of hospital physicians has arrived at the conclusion that an infant deprived of its mother's milk should have every day seven hundred grammes of milk, one hundred of bread, and seventy of sugar. A distinguished chemist, M. Nestlé, has of late years prepared a very excellent artificial food for infants which has been highly recommended. Twenty grammes of *farine lactée* (M. Nestlé's preparation) in one hundred grammes of water make a milk of excellent composition and taste. It is to be freshly prepared, and given lukewarm from a bottle. At the age of three or four months thirty grammes of the *farine* are to be given in one hundred of water, and the proportion is to be varied according to the constitution and age of the infant. We understand this preparation can be obtained in New York.

— An exercise in gymnastics was given on the 7th of July at Amherst College by the Junior class, to illustrate the instruction given in the department of physical culture, and an address on this subject was delivered the same day before the alumni of the college by Dr. Nathan Allen. He stated that it was almost twenty years since the question of doing something to promote the health of students in college was first agitated and discussed, at the meetings of the board of trustees. This resulted in the erection of the gymnasium in 1859, and the establishment of the department of physical culture and hygiene. Since that time fifteen classes had entered college, and more than three thousand students had taken part in these exercises. It had proved a great success, as was shown by the contrast between the health of the students at the present and their condition before the system was adopted. It has had its influence both in the discipline and in the scholarship of the college. It has been made one of the required exercises, and excellence in this department plays a part in determining the rank of the student.

A SCOTCH INSANE ASYLUM.

Messrs. Editors, — It was my privilege, about a year ago, to spend a day with Dr. Fraser at his asylum, and it seemed to me that he had made his real treatment of mental disease so fully correspond with the best ideal treatment (which consists in treating disease of the mind, as far as possible, like any other disease) that I asked him to favor the profession here with a statement of his methods. I confess I feared that a description, in my own words, of what I saw would be looked upon as somewhat wild. Dr. Fraser's letter is so full of interesting and suggestive points that I send it to you entire.

Although this is looked upon still as an experiment, its success is established, and it cannot fail to have a great influence on the treatment of mental disease throughout the world. In fact, it is likely to be classed with those great movements of Pinel and Tuke toward the close of the last, and of Conolly and Griesinger about the middle of the present century. Of course accurate diagnosis, faithful study of character, trained nurses as well as trustworthy attendants, and constant care are needed. If Dr. Fraser had described his autopsy and microscope rooms, it would have been seen that he considered careful pathological research of the utmost importance. Herbert Spencer quotes Dr. Tuke as having said of this asylum in 1872 that in ninety-five per cent. of the patients the policy of unlocked doors was successful. How appropriately the words " The more you trust, the more you may " come from a countryman of Romilly, Dr. Arnold, and Maconochie ! The history of the treatment of mental disease for the past century has been a succession of proofs that all efforts to bring elevating and refining influences to bear upon the insane, and to educate their self-respect and self-control, have been followed by the most beneficent results. Great Britain stands unquestionably at the present day at the head of the nations of the world in these respects.

Very respectfully yours,   CHARLES F. FOLSOM.

Fife and Kinross District Lunatic Asylum, }
CUPAR, FIFE, SCOTLAND, *January* 28, 1875. }

MY DEAR SIR, — I have the greatest possible pleasure in acceding to your request for a description of my asylum.

It is the district or pauper asylum for the counties of Fife and Kinross. The population of the two counties is one hundred and seventy thousand. The institution is capable of holding two hundred and eighty inmates. The present numbers are, one hundred and ten males and one hundred and thirty-eight females, or about two hundred and fifty altogether. The yearly admissions are from eighty to ninety. There is one attendant for every twelve patients. The patients are classified and each class has its own gallery; the highest number in any gallery is twenty-four, the lowest twelve. The female department has seven galleries, each complete in itself; that is to say, each of them has its own day-room, dormitory or dormitories, single sleeping-rooms, lavatory, and conveniences. Four have two attendants, two only one. This divisional arrangement, though I believe it adds to the working expenses, admits, as I have said above, of classification of the patients. The day-rooms or sitting-rooms for twenty-three patients are thirty feet long, twenty-one feet broad, and eleven and a half feet high. The windows of these rooms are nine feet by seven feet, and the panes are twenty-two inches by eighteen. There are no window panes smaller than twelve inches by ten and a half anywhere. The lower half of each window has brass rods three eighths of an inch thick running transversely across the panes and through the wood-work of the window-frame. I could wrench these rods out with my hands. There is no such thing as an iron bar across a window, and all our window-frames are of wood.

You ask me for the features which distinguish my asylum. I believe these to be, 1st, unlocked doors; 2d, the great amount of general freedom; and 3d, the large number on parole. In common with the Argyllshire asylum, airing courts are not in use. The great attention given to the occupation of the patients and the large percentage of those employed are characteristics of this asylum as well as of two others in Scotland.

First, as regards open doors. Here is a paragraph from my last annual report: —

"I wish now to describe the peculiar feature of your asylum, namely, the open-door system. It was originated about three years ago by your former physician superintendent. Dr. Tuke, and I have no hesitation in saying that the introduction of this system will mark an era in the history of the treatment of the insane. As you are well aware, there are no high boundary walls surrounding the grounds, and the entrance gates stand always open. To make this system as clear as possible, let me suppose that a visitor calls and wishes to see through the asylum. He is received at the front door, which will be found open; he is then conducted through the whole of the male galleries, containing over ninety patients, and thence, *viâ* the dining-hall, through five of the galleries of the female side, also containing over ninety patients, without *once* coming upon a locked door. Not only is there this free communication inside the house, but the outer doors of the main ground corridors, which open out on the terraces, are also unlocked. The male convalescent building, which contains from twenty to twenty-five patients, has its doors open from shortly after six A. M. till eight P. M. The inmates are, of course, on parole. Two galleries in the female department still remain under the old system of locked doors. Though not necessary for the majority of their inmates, yet the erratic and mischievous tendencies, as well as the excitement of some three or more in each division, render locked doors necessary.

"Greater contentment is, I believe, the result of the innovation I have just referred to; the sense of confinement, or in other words, of imprisonment, of which even a lunatic is conscious, is absent. The asylum is converted into a home and a hospital.

"A greater number of escapes and accidents would *a priori* be expected from this state of freedom. The escapes have been nine in number, and there are only two which can be attributed to open doors. Four accidents, none of any import, except the suicide previously detailed, have occurred during the year, but none in any way attributable to this system."

This bold advancement in the treatment of the insane is, as I have said above, wholly due to Dr. Batty Tuke. It is to his original mind, to his enterprising spirit, to his confidence in a portion of afflicted humanity hitherto unconfided in, and to his faith in the adage "The more you trust, the more you may," that this new era in the life of the insane owes its initiation. I must confess I shook my head when the doctor first proposed it, and our matron said she could not see "how it would do at all."

The history of this movement is interesting. At first a great deal of wandering about the house occurred, especially from the galleries to the kitchen. A number wandered outside, and some of course attempted escape. Gradually the patients were taught when they were to go out, and what parts of the house they were permitted to visit. Those who escaped were spoken to in presence of the others: they were informed of the inutility of escaping, of the certainty of their being brought back; that they must remain in the asylum until they were better, that every kindness would be shown them, that everything they had to say would be heard and attended to; that when the time came they would go out by the front door, and that the doctor would be there to say good-by and wish them well. It was wonderful how the most determined bolters ceased from attempting to escape. I could quote a dozen cases where a remarkable change in this respect occurred. The most intelligent escapers were taken to the doors, shown their openness, and then informed that confidence was reposed in them, that escape was unproductive of any good, and that the way to get home was to show themselves worthy of trust. Not only with permanent residents did this state of imposed confidence have a beneficial effect, but also with transfers from other asylums. For example, a lady patient was admitted some time ago from another asylum. The account sent was that she was most determined in her attempts at escape, that she had broken the framework of her window and set fire to doors in order to escape. Her habits were said to be dirty. It was a case of moral insanity, and the intelligence was keen and clear. After admission, she was shown the open doors (one leading out to the terrace within ten yards of her sitting-room) and the freedom that existed. Confidence was preached to her and she was informed that good behavior of every kind was expected of her. She now walks out daily on the terraces, unattended whenever she likes, yet there has never been the least attempt at escape. She has never been dirty in her habits. This patient has been in three other Scotch asylums, and she says that this is not like an asylum at all, that it is unlike any of the others she has been in, and that here she has no desire to run away.

Your experience of the insane will cause you no doubt to say, "But all cannot be treated in this wise." I grant that, but what I wish to impress upon you is the great number that can. You will see I have two departments on the female side under the old régime. An attempt was made to leave one of these off the lock, but the mischievous doings of three chronic maniacs, and the incurable wanderings of two or three demented and suicidal patients, prevented the open door from being persevered in. Excepting these, the patients, numbering from one to eighteen, would be all the better for the unlocked doors. The other department is one of our new buildings and is separate. From its situation and its inhabitants, chiefly chronic maniacs, it would be inexpedient to attempt the step there.

I wish especially to describe our male convalescent building. It is a house capable of holding thirty-three patients, but at present there are only twenty-two resident there. Its doors are open every day from seven in the morning till eight and nine in the evening. The inmates are all on parole. No one has broken his parole during the last two and a half years. An attendant and his wife have charge of the place. They have a little child five years of age. They all sit down to meals together, the patients, the attendant, his wife and child. The latter two mix with the patients at all times. This was also a step of Dr. Tuke's, and admirable have been the results. When men associate only with each other, they are apt to degenerate; coarseness, swearing, and fighting predominate; but when a woman is present, and especially when a sweet little girl mingles with them, swearing and angry passions cease; at least such has been the effect in this department of my asylum. There are two dormitories up-stairs, one in which no attendant sleeps (ten patients are left to themselves), and the other is in charge of an attendant who comes down from the main building for the night. This place is our Gheel.

I believe that the conditions above described, coupled with constant occupation, result in (1) greater contentment and general happiness among the patients, (2) better conduct in every one, *i. e.*, less excitement, (3) the preservation of the individuality of each patient, (4) less degradation, and (5) greater vigilance and care on the part of the attendants. As regards the fourth result, I believe it to be strikingly true. Our degraded patients are importations; few, if any, are indigenous. I never allow any sitting on floors or crouching in corners like cats or dogs. It takes a long time to cure many of this habit; but of course, as you know, the insane take from four to six times longer than ordinary people to be taught anything.

Occupation is what I have the utmost confidence in. Its results are most beneficial. Almost every male patient can fill and wheel a barrow, and the majority can use a spade. So almost every female patient can use a needle and thread or a knitting-needle. Constant supervision soon teaches one what is most suitable to each. I beg to refer you to Sir James Coxe's report, which you will find in the annual report which accompanies this letter. Here is another paragraph from my last annual report: —

"Attention is being constantly and increasingly directed towards the occupation of both sexes. At the present date, all male patients, with the exception of from five to eight, are sent out every day in parties arranged according to their capabilities for work. Attendants accompany each set of workers. The head and sick-room attendants are the only ones retained in the house. On the female side there are three work-rooms, one devoted to the main sewing requirements of the house, and the others to the teaching and encouraging to work of the idle and demented. In these three rooms are above ninety patients. The laundry, the kitchen, and the house generally give employment to about forty more, so that the actually idle are reduced to a minimum. My desire and aim is to make your asylum a veritable bee-hive. The men work both forenoon and afternoon, but their hours are not long. The females, though kept at work in the forenoon, spend the afternoon in walking and outdoor recreation. I am at present dispensing with the use of airing courts, but I shall make no comment on this step until after a year's experience."

Airing courts are a mistake, especially for females. Not long ago I used to send out the demented, the chronic maniacs, and the idle to the airing court of a morning. Of course, having nothing useful to do there, they did mischief, quarreling among themselves, getting excited, and increasing their destructive habits. The patients being safe within four walls and out of sight, the attendants were heedless, habits and practices occurred which the attendants for the sake of decency and for the respect of their sex would have been active and vigilant to prevent elsewhere. Those who used to go to the airing court in the morning are now collected around tables and set to work at knitting, sewing, darning, etc. The contrast between the airing court and this room is very striking. This very morning this work-room was quiet in the extreme. I went round them all, spoke to each, praised their doings, and encouraged the idle, and there was not a word out of place. Had they been in the airing court they would have squatting in all the corners, rampaging about, holding forth in loud tones, etc. Occupation and the working together in the way described have a most decided inhibitory effect. The airing-court system permits every insane propensity to run to weeds.

You ask me to tell you about the treatment of the patients. Let me in complying with this request describe the plan of treatment I adopt in case of acute mania immediately after admission. It is much the same as Conolly's, which is described by him in his work on The Treatment of the Insane, at pages 43 and 47. A warm bath is first given; then the patient is put to bed in the padded room; food is offered, and every plan is adopted to coax the patient to partake of it voluntarily. I often find feeding by the opposite sex succeed when an attempt by one of the patient's own sex fails. Should food be refused, I have no hesitation in using the pump. The first two nights I give chloral, as it is my firm conviction that it is our positive duty to procure sleep as soon as possible. My idea is, the longer mania is allowed to go on, the greater risk there is of subsequent dementia. If sleep obtained by chloral cuts it short, what can be said against it? I have tried both methods, the let-alone one and the treatment by sedatives (chiefly chloral and bromide) or medicinal treatment generally. As a medical man, as a student of clinical medicine and of therapeutics, and as one who hopes that careful investigation, physiological, pathological, and therapeutical, will erelong reveal a method of treatment whereby all cases of acute mania will be cured, I much prefer the latter course. I think precious little of the superintendent who can stand idly by and see a case of acute mania running on in its mad career day after day. What is such a superintendent's *raison d'être?* Food! Food! is such an one's cry, but it is my experience that food will not subdue one case of acute mania in twenty.

In one or two hours after the chloral and feeding, the patient generally sleeps, and if next morning the excitement returns, I seclude for the day. I deem this seclusion most wise; in fact it is imperative to meet the requirements of the patient's mental condition. Chloral is given again the second night and perhaps the third night; and by the third day the patient is generally quiet or disposed to keep in bed, and so avoid seclusion. The appetite is keen after chloral, so there is little trouble with food after the first dose. I have pursued this plan for the last two years and with the most decided success. When the patient is removed from the bedroom, the sick-hall is the next resort. Here there is quietness and every comfort, and the whole surroundings inhibit any tendency to excitement.

I seclude in epileptic mania and in paroxysms of impulsive, aggressive, and destructive mania. I have two very bad cases of the former and three of the latter. Here is a paragraph from my report, containing my opinion in regard to seclusion: —

" Seclusion has on several occasions been resorted to by me. My *present* opinion is that it is the most humane, beneficial, and wise course of action under certain circumstances. During the present year there have been two or three cases subject to paroxysms of great excitement. I have occasionally been present in the galleries when such outbursts have occurred, and have been witness of how the peace, quietude, and industry of the other inmates have been disturbed, and the excitable roused. Great destructive propensity is generally a feature of these attacks. In such cases, one of two things must be done : the patient must either be restrained by two or more attendants (the worst form of restraint), or he must be put into seclusion. The former plan cannot be carried out where there is a minimum staff, but even had I sufficient at my command, I believe seclusion to be the more beneficial mode of treatment in every way. There are cases, at least this asylum possesses such, in which great coarseness of language characterizes the paroxysms; and I maintain that such cases, in consideration of the feelings of the other inmates and attendants, demand their temporary seclusion. Constant supervision of the galleries has determined me in this opinion. Restraint I have not resorted to."

As regards the chronic harmless insane, I here subjoin another extract from my report : "It is my opinion that many chronic lunatics do not require asylum treatment; they can be sufficiently cared for and guarded by their friends or others whom the proper authorities deem fit custodians. The chronic lunatic I refer to is one who is harmless, trained to be cleanly and perhaps industrious, whose mental condition may be described as that of a premature second childhood, and of whose recovery no hope can be entertained. Such an one does not require constant medical supervision, the expensive appurtenances of an asylum, nor the services of trained attendants. The proposed method of administering the grant from the Imperial Exchequer cannot fail to cause asylums to be crowded with such lunatics."

Dr. Arthur Mitchell's book on the Insane in Private Dwellings will give you a most graphic account of what formerly existed and what exists at the present day.

I trust the foregoing remarks convey the information you desire, and I shall be very happy to answer any further inquiries you may wish to make. If any of my professional brethren on your side of the water desire to see this asylum, they will find me a most willing cicerone.

With best regards, I am dear sir,

Yours most truly,   JOHN FRASER.

DR. CHARLES F. FOLSOM, BOSTON.

WEEKLY BULLETIN OF PREVALENT DISEASES.

THE following is a bulletin of the diseases prevalent in Massachusetts during the week ending August 7, 1875, compiled under the authority of the State Board of Health from the returns of physicians representing all sections of the State —:

Throughout the State the prevalence of the diseases of summer continues without abatement. In many places cholera infantum has an unusually severe and fatal type. Except the diseases above alluded to, acute affections have almost disappeared from the community. A marked uniformity in the relative prevalence of the diseases which are rife will be noticed in the following report of the different sections.

Berkshire : Diarrœa, dysentery, cholera morbus, cholera infantum.

Valley : Diarrœa, dysentery, cholera morbus, cholera infantum, rheumatism. Some well-marked cases of intermittent fever have been observed in Springfield.

Midland : Diarrœa, cholera infantum, cholera morbus, dysentery.

Northeastern : Diarrœa, cholera morbus, cholera infantum, dysentery, typhoid fever. Measles and whooping-cough are epidemic in Beverly.

Metropolitan : Diarrœa, cholera morbus, cholera infantum, dysentery.

Southeastern : cholera infantum, dysentery, diarrœa, cholera morbus, rheumatism. Nantucket reports dysentery as unusually prevalent and severe.

The week has witnessed an increase in the prevalence of cholera infantum and dysentery ; all other diseases remain as at last report. The increase affected mainly the Midland, Northeastern and Southeastern sections.

F. W. Draper, M. D., Registrar.

———◆———

COMPARATIVE MORTALITY-RATES FOR THE WEEK ENDING JULY 31, 1875.

	Estimated Population.	Total Mortality for the Week.	Annual Death-rate per 1000 during Week.
New York	1,060,000	815	39
Philadelphia	775,000	436	29
Brooklyn	500,000	309	32
Boston	350,000	214	32
Cincinnati	260,000	91	18
Providence	100,700	45	23
Worcester	50,000	29	30
Lowell	50,000	19	20
Cambridge	50,000	27	28
Fall River	45,000	29	34
Lawrence	35,000	18	28
Springfield	33,000	10	16
Lynn	28,000	12	22
Salem	26,000	10	20

Resigned and Discharged. — Charles A. Holt, of Chelsea, Assistant Surgeon First Regt. Infantry, M. V. M., July 26, 1875.

George E. Pinkham, of Lowell, Assistant Surgeon Sixth Regt. Infantry, M. V. M., July 20, 1875.

THE BOSTON
MEDICAL AND SURGICAL JOURNAL.

VOL. XCIII. — THURSDAY, AUGUST 19, 1875. — NO. 8.

AUTUMNAL CATARRH.

' BY MORRILL WYMAN, M. D., OF CAMBRIDGE.

· AUTUMNAL catarrh, or " hay fever," as it is popularly called, although there is no evidence that it has anything to do with hay as a cause, sets in towards the end of August as surely as swallows come in spring, and runs its course within the narrow bounds of a single month. Its subjects are already preparing for what is before them, and the known number of these subjects, now that the disease is recognized and described, especially among the more cultivated classes, is surprising. The vendors of secret compounds have already discovered the field, and are hovering about with such a multitude of sure cures that it would seem sheer malice in anybody to be sick.

Limited to a single month, the disease then disappears, whether treated or not, leaving the victim with more or less weakness and depression, from which, if otherwise in good health, as a general rule, he soon recovers. But what is very remarkable, numerous as the sufferers are, they are limited to certain regions. If the sufferer leaves these catarrhal regions for others, which long and careful observation has shown to be free from the malady, he begins immediately to recover, and within forty-eight hours is substantially well of the disease, although some of its effects may not so promptly disappear. Of these places of refuge, the White Mountain region is best known and most frequently resorted to. The Glen, Gorham, Randolph, Jefferson, Whitefield, Bethlehem Village, the Franconia Notch, White Mountain Notch, Twin Mountain House, are all within the limits of safety. Other elevated tracts are safe : Mount Mansfield, in Vermont, the Adirondacks, the Ohio and Pennsylvania plateau, including the high range of southern counties in New York from the Catskill Mountains to the western border of the State, the plateau in these counties having an elevation of two thousand feet above the sea. The valleys and lakes of the same State at a lower level are not safe. The island of Mackinaw, and north of the great lakes, in Canada, and beyond the Mississippi at St. Paul, Minnesota, and still farther west, are large tracts which may be resorted to. Still farther south, the Alleghany Mountains at Oakland, and other elevated points, are usually free. To the east, the elevated interior of Maine and its extensive lakes afford both pleasure and safety ; or, if tie sea-coast is preferred, the wiole coast east of tie St. Join's, tience quite round to Labrador, is open to tie subjects of " iay fever." Sufferers wio literally pitci tieir tents in tiese favored regions, as a general rule, not only escape their enemy, but may also find tiemselves, at tie end of the monti, with a vigor tiat notiing but living under canvas seems to give. It is not to be inferred, iowever, tiat all cases of catarrh or astima in autumn will be thus relieved, for otier affections exist, not autumnal catarri but somewiat resembling it, that are not cured by tie same metiods. And again, tiis affection varies in its severity and in its complications ; some of tiese may prove intractable. Lastly, tie places just named may, at times, present suci cianges in temperature, moisture, and vegetation, as to interfere materially witi tieir beneficial influences. Tiat such should be tie case is in analogy with many tiings in medicine and piysiology, in whici notiing is absolute and invariable.

To derive all tie benefit possible from ciange of residence, it siould be made a few days before tie annual return of the disease ; in tiis case as in many otiers, it is better to prevent tian to cure. If tie disease has been long in action the lining membrane of the nostrils becomes thickened, tie eyelids inflamed, the bronchial tubes irritated, and altiougi the cause of tie disease is promptly arrested, its effects require time for tieir removal. Tien again, if tie journey is by rail in iot, dry, and dusty weatier, tiis combination, if tie time is near at hand, is very likely to hasten an outbreak.

Altiougi tie course just mentioned is the best, there is a proper regimen and some remedies for tie relief of tiose who stay at iome, by wiich, altiougi tieir troubles cannot be completely prevented or broken up, tiey can be materially diminisied. It must not be forgotten tiat tiis disease is remarkable for its remissions and apparent cessations. Tiese are so complete as to deceive even the wary and experienced witi tie hope, not destined to be realized, tiat it is really taking its leave, and tie sanguine witi tie belief tiat armed witi their last new remedy tiey iave achieved a victory. What we iave to propose is the result of experience and tie trial of many medicines. Otier and better may be discovered, and periaps a specific may be in store for us ; but, inasmuci as tie disease is limited and bearable, and does not inflict great injury, it is not worth while to run much risk of life or permanently derange health on the mere chance of a successful result. We can only hope that what has proved useful to some may prove useful to more.

As the disease has more of a general than local character, and falls especially upon the nervous system, we have reason to expect more from constitutional than from local treatment. So, also, as the injurious in-

fluences are constantly at work, we siould expect more from mild measures steadily pursued tian from any violent, irregular, and almost necessarily debilitating course.

First, of preventive measures. Tie direct rays of tie sun are to be
avoided during tie 1ot weatier, as 1aving a debilitating influence on
tie nervous system. Avoid tie smoke and dust of tie railway 'train,
and tie dust of tie street ; avoid also tiose plants, suci as Roman
wormwood, golden rod, and otier flowers and fruits wiici are known o
bring on an attack. Tie sleeping-room siould 1ave an open fire-place,
siould not be exposed to tie afternoon sun, and after being well aired
for an 1our in tie early morning siould 1ave tie windows and doors
closed, and kept closed, so tiat tie air siall be as still as possible until
tie following morning. We tiink tie still air allows tie injurious particles to subside ; but wietier tiis be so or not we are satisfied tiat
tiis course 1as given us a good nigit's sleep and a better condition in tie
morning. Tie diet siould be nourisiing, containing animal food. Alcoholic stimulants siould be avoided. Flannels worn from tie middle
of August, and increased in warmti as tie season and disease advance,
give protection against sudden cianges of temperature, to wiici boti
tie skin and tie nervous system are very sensitive, and between wiici,
at tiis time, tiere is a close sympatiy.

Of all tie medicines we 1ave as yet fully tried, quinine, in our opinion, 1as done most good as a preventive and also as a relief of some of
tie most annoying symptoms. Wietier it 1as specific properties or
not we cannot say, but it is generally acknowledged to be a good tonic
to increase tie appetite, and is probably an aid to tie digestion and appropriation of food. Its use siould be commenced a week or ten days
before tie usual return of the disease, and continued tirougi its course,
in doses of one or two grains witi eaci meal. Gentle saline or otier
laxatives are useful, but violent purging siould be avoided.

Of remedies to be used for tie relief of paroxysms of itciing of the
eyes, mouti, and throat, great numbers are recommended. Tiese very
troublesome symptoms may be often greatly relieved by tie local application of a saturated watery solution of quinine made witiout tie addition of any acid. The best mode of using it is witi an atomizer or,
wiat is quite as good, tie perfume distributer in common use ; tie
spray from tie clear solution being tirown into tie eyes and tiroat,
drawn into tie lungs as freely as possible, and also tirown over tie
skin of tie face. It siould be used many times daily. Batiing of tie
eyes in cold or tepid water relieves, and tie same may be said of tie
mild sedative solution of two or tiree grains of borax to an ounce of
campior water, a favorite prescription of tie oculists. Avoid as muci
as possible accesses of sneezing ; tiey are tie beginning of trouble to
both eyes and nose.

The irritation and discharge from the nostrils may be relieved by the " head bath ; " holding the head for five minutes over a bowl of very hot milk and water or water alone, the head and shoulders meanwhile covered with a shawl. In railway traveling and on dusty roads much relief is gained by placing small pieces of wet sponge just within the nostrils, or covering the whole face with Swiss muslin wet with water. The nostrils are often completely obstructed early in the morning, and swallowing impeded ; this may be relieved temporarily by active movements of the limbs for a few minutes, — leaping or running quickly upstairs, — after which one can often eat his breakfast with comparative comfort.

For the night a closed room, and, if opium can be taken without inconvenience, six or eight grains of Dover's powder or an equivalent in laudanum or a solution of morphine, often give more or less freedom from that most annoying symptom in the later stages, the spasmodic cough. It may also be relieved by the spray from the watery solution of quinine as just mentioned. The common household mucilaginous remedies, gum arabic and flax-seed tea, for temporary relief are not to be rejected. The asthma, like that occurring at other seasons and produced by other causes, is often spasmodic, nervous, and wayward ; it is relieved by a variety of remedies ; the inhaling of the smoke from burning stramonium leaves and saltpetre, three parts of the former to one of the latter, probably gives as much relief to a majority of sufferers as any other treatment.

EMBOLISM OF THE PULMONARY ARTERY.

BY E. G. CUTLER, M. D., OF BOSTON.

MAY 21st. The patient, J. B., fifty-six years of age, a lobster-dealer by trade, addicted to the use of spirituous liquors, several years ago, after an alleged injury, had necrosis of the right tibia, for which he underwent operation at the Massachusetts General Hospital. The necrosis has been assigned to a syphilitic taint. During all of the interval since this surgical operation the patient has been more or less under treatment for his necrosis.

About a week ago he was seized with pain and a feeling of distress in the epigastric region, together with great occasional paroxysmal dyspnoea, slight vomiting and belching of wind, anorexia. Under advice, he made use of sinapisms to the seat of pain, but without relief ; he consulted another physician, who after examination prescribed another sinapism to the painful region, quinine, a cathartic, and opium pills, ascribing the trouble to some gastric affection. These measures proved of little avail, and the patient finally sougit the aid of the dispensary physician, Dr. Cianning, wio kindly asked me to see the case with him in consultation on May 28th. Tie patient was found dressed and in the sitting position on a lounge, saying ie iad not been able to be undressed or to lie down for a week or more. His countenance wore an anxious expression, iis face iad a very dusky iue : iis lips were somewiat livid ; iis iands and nails were natural. He iad a weak, irregular crural and radial pulse of 120, easily compressible ; iis respiration was rapid, superficial, labored, witi occasional attacks of cougi and dyspnœa. Tiere was a peculiar lack of force to tie cougi. Tie expectoration was ciiefly mucus, tinged witi dark-colored blood tirougiout; in quantity it was about six ounces in twenty-four iours; it was not at all viscid. Tie temperature was not elevated. Tie patient complained of loss of appetite, witi pain and distress in tie upper epigastric region. Tiere was a very considerable amount of astienia, and tie man spoke of a distressing sensation of impending death wiich occurred witi occasional paroxysms of dyspnœa of unusual severity. Tie lower extremities were considerably œdematous ; tie rigit leg was somewiat painful, and iad a sinus apparently reaciing to tie bone and surrounded by an eczematous patci of tie size of tie iand. Tie gastro-intestinal functions were apparently carried on well.

Piysical exploration of tie lungs gave, witi tie exception of coarse mucous râles in a circumscribed area in tie rigit front and in a few otier places in the left side, a negative result. Tie apex beat of tie heart was at tie left of tie nipple and about two and one ialf incies below it ;. tie ieart's action was feeble, irregular. Boti sounds were reduplicated, not transmitted. Area of cardiac dullness was increased laterally.

An examination of tie abdomen siowed it moderately prominent and witi no tenderness at any point on percussion or pressure ; tiere was no evidence of fluid in tie abdominal cavity. Tie liver siowed a normal area of dullness.

On examination of tie urine, a sligit amount of albumen was found ; urea was normal in quantity ; under tie microscope, small iyaline casts were seen with a few granular ones, some renal epitielium, and a few blood corpuscles.

Diagnosis. Evident nepiritis, wiici tie man's iabits and tie examination of tie urine allowed us fairly to consider interstitial. Tie ieart's position in tie tiorax migit suggest iypertropiy. On tie otier iand, taking tie patient's constrained position into account, together witi tie extent and weakness of tie impulse, we felt justified in attribnting tie size ratier to dilatation, witi possible fatty infiltration. Tirombus formation in tie ieart was suspected from tie peculiar double sound and tie lung symptoms.

These affections of the heart and kidneys, however, did not satisfactorily account for the whole symptoms and their severity ; and we were forced by the constancy of the rusty sputa, cough, and dyspnœa to look to the lungs for the chief source of trouble. And a review of the symptoms taken in their order of occurrence — sudden attack of paroxysmal dyspnœa, cough, epigastric pain, palpitation and irregular action of the heart, together with the feeling and expression of anxiety, continued rusty expectoration, negative lung examination, positive reduplication of heart-tones, great weakness of radial and crural pulse, — formed such positive evidence of the existence of embolism of the pulmonary artery or some of its branches that this diagnosis was made with great positiveness and the most unfavorable prognosis given.

-*Treatment* consisted in the administration of nourishment in as large and as frequent quantities as could be borne. The medicinal measures consisted in the administration of quinine, a cough mixture containing sulphate of morphia, chloroform, and syrup of tolu ; a mixture of bromide of potassium and chloral hydrate or a solution of sulphate of morphia was given as occasion seemed to require. Hot applications were ordered to the chest and precordial regions. Under this treatment the patient was considerably relieved of his suffering and was enabled to assume a more comfortable position in bed, though he was always obliged to be bolstered up. There was gradual but progressive asthenia, and no material change in the symptoms. Finally the patient died quietly on the twenty-first day of his illness.

Autopsy, nine hours after death. Heart somewhat hypertrophied and right side much dilated; right ventricle forming the apex of the organ. No evidence of fatty infiltration. Thrombi in both auricles somewhat dense, dry, laminated, and tawny, extending into the auricular appendage and forming a lining to the wall of the auricle, which in the left side was one eighth inch in thickness. In the right auricle the thrombus was softened in the auricular appendage and opposite its front wall. The valves of the heart were sufficient, and healthy. There was universal dilatation of the ascending and transverse aorta to nearly the size of the fist, with endoarteritis and almost universal atheroma, in which were numerous calcified plates. In the place of the previous existence of the ductus arteriosus was a peculiar, hardened elevation, pronounced by Dr. R. H. Fitz to be a calcified thrombus. The right lung in its middle lobe presented an embolic infarction involving nearly its entire extent; it was quite recent, with collateral œdema. In the lower lobe of the same lung were three small infarctions in a somewhat older stage. In the left lung were several small infarcts of the size of a robin's egg; one was six inches long by one inch wide in the upper lobe, presenting several successive stages of the process.

The liver presented the nutmeg appearance of commencing cirrhosis.

T1e kidneys were very large, twice t1e normal size ; t1ere was commencing interstitial inflammation.   T1e spleen was enlarged, 1ardened, with increased connective tissue.

POISONING BY PICKLES.

BY H. LASSING, M. D., OF NEW YORK.

UPON arriving at t1e room of t1e patient, I found 1er vomiting undigested food ; 1er countenance was anxious ; her pulse was 58. S1e complained of a burning, corrosive sensation in 1er t1roat and stomac1, and an acrid, metallic taste in 1er mout1. Inquiry elicited t1e information t1at s1e 1ad eaten corned beef, bread, and a " bit of pickle." Upon a close examination of samples of t1ese, t1e beef and bread were found to be all rig1t, but t1e liquid in w1ic1 t1e pickles had lain, and w1ic1 was supposed to be vinegar, emitted a peculiar, faint, sickis1 odor, and tasted brackis1, not sour. T1e pickles 1ad a metallic taste. Laying aside t1e latter for furt1er examination, an emetic was administered to t1e patient, followed up by copious draug1ts warm water ; t1is was repeated until t1e rejected matter became free from everyt1ing but the water administered. C1alk mixture and laudanum were now administered toget1er wit1 a mustard cataplasm to t1e epigastrium. T1e vomiting ceased for a time ; but upon t1e administration of stimulants in any s1ape, it immediately returned. Lactopeptine was given, in ten-grain doses, every 1alf 1our, combined with brandy ; t1is was readily retained, and t1e patient soon rallied. Several ot1er members of t1e family were similarly affected, but t1e symptoms, t1oug1 equally t1reatening, yielded at once to similar treatment.

T1e pickles upon examination s1owed t1e presence of iron, arsenic, and oxalic acid. Upon tracing t1em back to t1e original manufacturer, it was found t1at t1ere was not1ing poisonous about t1e pickles w1en t1ey left him, and t1at t1e vinegar upon t1em was a pure 1ig1 wine vinegar ; but t1e grocer w1o sold t1e pickles 1ad substituted for t1is vinegar a dilution of sulp1uric acid made from an impure article, and 1ad t1us jeopardized t1e lives of t1e public. T1e board of 1ealt1, upon being notified, at once took active measures to suppress t1e manufacture of this poisonous article. T1is sulp1uric acid vinegar can be easily detected by a few drops of a solution of muriate of baryta ; w1en t1is is added t1ere will be a milky precipitate of sulp1ate of baryta. Large quantities of t1is poisonous vinegar are sold all over t1e country.

RECENT PROGRESS IN OBSTETRICS AND GYNÆCOLOGY.

BY W. L. RICHARDSON, M. D.

OBSTETRICS.

The Relation of Puerperal Fever to the Infective Diseases and Pyæmia. — A discussion on this subject has recently taken place before the Obstetrical Society of London which has called forth the opinions of many of the leading obstetricians of Great Britain, and which contains so much that is of value to the general practitioner that it seems to merit an extended notice in this report.

The discussion was opened by Mr. T. Spencer Wells, who considered that in puerperal fever we were dealing with a contagious continued fever, often, but not always, associated with important local lesions, such as peritonitis, effusions into serous and synovial cavities, philebitis, and diffuse suppuration. The discussion, he said, was to especially consider : 1st. Whether there was any form of continued fever, communicated by contagion or infection, which occurred in connection with childbirth, was distinctly caused by a special morbid poison, and was as definite in its progress and in the local lesions associated with it as typhus or typhoid, scarlet fever, measles, or small-pox; 2d. Whether all forms of puerperal fever may be referred to attacks of some infective continued fever, as scarlet fever or measles, occurring in connection with childbirth, on the one hand, or, on the other, to some form of surgical fever, or to erysipelas, caused by or associated with changes in the uterus and neighboring parts following the process of childbirth. 3d. Setting aside all cases of contagious and infectious diseases occurring under other conditions than that of childbirth, does there remain any such disease as puerperal fever ? 4th. If a form of continued fever — communicable by inoculation, contagion, or infection — does frequently occur in connection with childbirth, how can its spread be prevented ? 5th. What relation have bacteria and allied organic forms to the pyæmic process in the puerperal state ? 6th. Of what value are antiseptics in the prevention and treatment of puerperal fever ?

Dr. Leishman, of Glasgow, thought that a large proportion of the cases of puerperal fever had their origin in pyæmic or septic infection. There were no doubt cases in which a patient, during the puerperal state, becomes the subject of diseases of a specific origin, as for example scarlatina. He thought, however, that in the later history of such cases there was a difficulty in discovering any difference between those cases which were supposed to have a specific origin and those which proceeded from a specific poison. The same difficulty was met with in attempting to separate those cases in which the original symptoms were those of a local character — metritis or peritonitis — from those in which the fever was due to pyæmia or septicæmia.

Dr. Newman, of Stamford, did not believe that there was any such thing as a definite puerperal fever. In a large number of cases of puerperal fever which he had seen there had been a distinct link in the occurrence of possible transmission to the patient of some definite infecting poison. This poison may come from a direct or indirect communication with some infective poison, or from some inflammatory process going on within the patient. Again, the mental and physical condition of the parturient woman is often below par before her delivery, and all the processes, nervous, vital, circulatory, and mental, are so materially excited or altered in their condition, that it is not surprising that poisons, however they may be presented to her, which would run a different and slower course under the more ordinary state of everyday life, should run, when they have to deal with a parturient woman, a course of far greater severity, rapidity, and fatality.

Dr. Braxton Hicks said that we could not judge by the death-rate of the influence of circumstances on the puerperal woman, for where one dies, three or four are retarded in their recovery by either a more or less mild state of fever or by the secondary effects known as cellulitis, phlegmon, etc. A large number of cases of puerperal fever owe their origin doubtless to the presence of some animal poison, a large proportion being connected more or less directly with the poison of scarlatina ; but violent mental emotions may be followed by symptoms precisely similar to those which follow zymotic influence or the existence of putrid discharges. In more cases some other medium must be added, such as " sepsis," or the living bacteria, or some material which, mixing with the discharges in the uterine cavity, is absorbed into the system. The fact that if we wash out the uterus the symptoms very rapidly subside seems to militate against the idea of its origin being due to bacteria. It is not clear that the blood-condition set up in the puerperal woman is similar to the so-called pyæmia as seen in non-pregnant women. It seems, however, to differ from it in intensity rather than in quality.

It is doubtless true that a zymotic disease, if not modified in its true nature, is altered as to the usual character of the symptoms, assuming more the type which has been generally called " malignant " in the non-puerperal person ; and this tendency to change its character is more noticeable the nearer the patient has approached the full term of pregnancy. It is not clear, however, whether this depends on the changed condition of the system or on the greater patency of the lymph spaces and veins, by which the quantity absorbed is increased. Respecting the contagious nature of the conditions grouped together as puerperal fever, there is no doubt that the majority are contagious to puerperal women, but it is uncertain whether all are so. Those forms derived from the zymotic diseases are the most so, while those from the self-generated kinds are the least. A few seem to be not at all contagious. Aggregation tends to spread puerperal fever, but cannot set it up *ab initio.*

Mr. Jonathan Hutchinson considered that the term " puerperal fever " was as vague as " surgical fever," and that the use of both was absurd. Erysipelas is of the greatest importance in reference to puerperal fever, since the contagion from it is one which is potent in the induction of the local inflammation which produces puerperal fever. Now this erysipelas is not a specific fever, but is only a local form of inflammation which may vary in intensity and duration, and may be induced by many different causes. The pyrexial symptoms and general disturbance are secondary to the local inflammation, and always proportionate to the existing local erysipelatous action. This erysipelas may be checked at any stage. Again, the term septicæmia has been wrongly used. It ought to be applied only to the results of the poisoning of blood induced by the inflammation of the patient's own tissues. In some cases beyond question we can trace the influence of some morbid matter, which has acted as an irritant in setting up the inflammation. In septicæmia there is no phlebitis. Pyæmia is also produced by an inflammation of the patient's own tissues. In more typical cases pyæmia is due to phlebitis. It is a poisoning of the blood by inflammation of the veins. To the vague and erroneous use of these several terms, septicæmia, pyæmia, erysipelas, is to be ascribed a great deal of the doubt which exists in the medical profession as to the still more vague name of " puerperal fever."

Dr. Richardson considered that in the first place a woman after delivery is physiologically in a peculiar position. The fibrin of the blood is in excess. The salts of the blood are diminished. Both of these conditions favor the precipitation of the fibrin. For some time the woman has been supplying to the child a mass of blood from her own body, and therefore she is practically in the condition of a person who has lost a limb. She is in a nervous condition and is suffering from a nervous reaction. A large number of women are hereditarily predisposed to particular diseases, among which must be classed puerperal fever. He did not believe that there was any special poison belonging to the puerperal state, or any special poison which creates puerperal fever, or any local lesions found after death by which we could recognize the presence of that disease. Under the term puerperal fever he recognized four distinct forms of fever. First, the pure, simple surgical fever following upon the delivery of the child. There is scarcely any delivery which is not followed by some slight febrile state. Another form may be called remittent in its character, and is accompanied by slight or well marked symptoms of jaundice. A third class embraces those cases in which there is a true introduction into the body of the patient of matter derived probably from the uterine sinuses and which results in a true septic poisoning. The fourth class of cases includes those in which a poison appears to be carried into the body from without. This poison may belong to any of the poisonous diseases, such as scarlet fever, erysipelas, etc. These are all true cases of septicæmic puerperal fever. There is no special form of puerperal fever, but there are several varied forms of the disease, terminating much in the same way, but having distinct characteristics. Some of these are contagious, and some are not. Some spring from the natural condition of the patient, some from an injury received by the patient, and others from the introduction of morbid material. As regards methods of preventing the spread of the disease, the patients should be isolated and great cleanliness preserved throughout the course of the disease. As regards the presence of bacteria and allied organic forms in the puerperal state, he believed that their presence was purely a coincidence, and that there was no relation between their development and the production of the disease.

Dr. Barnes thought the term puerperal fever could not be discarded, but that there were various forms of it. The first variety was the direct result of infection or contagion produced by some zymotic poison, as scarlet fever, erysipelas, measles, or typhoid fever. These cases may be known as heterogenetic. Another class of cases, which may be called autogenetic, embrace those in which all the conditions of fever exist or arise in the patient's system. As regards the heterogenetic cases it is not to be wondered at that a patient after delivery is in such a condition as to be peculiarly liable to the reception of poisons from without. It is easy enough to imagine the course of the second class of cases whether they are known as cases of septicæmia or of pyæmia. Isolation is the only preventive of the spread of these cases, no matter to which class they belong.

Dr. Squire believed that there was a fever after childbirth caused by a morbid poison communicable by infection, and that no form of puerperal fever was to be referred to attacks of the specific infective fevers.

Dr. J. Brunton also did not believe that the specific infective diseases had anything to do with the production of puerperal fever. He thought that the nature of the disease was purely autogenetic, and that as a rule the cases were those of pyæmic poisoning.

Dr. Graily Hewitt believed that puerperal fever was essentially a form of blood-poisoning — an actual pyæmia. He agreed with Dr. Barnes that all the cases of so-called puerperal fever could be divided into two classes, those in which there was distinct evidence of the introduction into the system from without of a morbid animal poison, and those in which the poison was evidently derived from within the patient's person.

Mr. Callender believed that septic poisoning and an absorption of a poisonous material by the veins played the leading part in the production of puerperal fever.

Dr. Arthur Farre did not believe that there was any form of contagious or infectious fever connected with childbirth which owed its origin to a special morbid poison, and which had a definite progress. He did not believe that the various infectious and contagious diseases were one and the same, whether they occurred in the puerperal or the non-puerperal state. He believed that all the fevers which have been erroneously grouped under the single head of puerperal fever should be divided into three classes. First, the simple fevers which might be appropriately called irritative fevers. Under this head would properly be grouped febrile reactions resulting from mammary irritation, from slight injuries of the soft parts, and those pyrexial states which are fugitive and transient in their nature. Second, those infective fevers which are not of a specific origin. Here we find no period of evolution or development, nor do the consequences follow in definite order. Third, eruptive fevers and those which depend upon a blood-infection. Here the action of the poison has a definite course, a regular period of ineubation, and it terminates in those several diseases which are common to the parturient and the non-parturient woman alike. The first two classes alone are connected with the puerperal condition.

Dr. Wynn Williams considered that all cases of puerperal fever were due to septicæmia. He did not believe that pyæmia had anything do with it. The formation of pus is secondary, and is an effort of nature to eliminate and isolate the irritating poison. The disease is always due to the presence of putrid animal matter. He alluded to the efficacy of iodine in destroying a septic poisoning. He believed that the use of tincture of iodine in water as a wash would at once serve as a perfect disinfectant, both when used by the physician for his hands and as an injection for offensive lochia.

Dr. Playfair believed the disease to be practically the same as surgical septicæmia or pyæmia. It arises from the contact of septic matter with lesions of continuity in the generative track. Beyond a question the contagious poison of any zymotic disease, if brought in contact with solutions of continuity in the generative track, will produce an intense form of septicæmia. It may also be absorbed by the ordinary channels, and this possibility will explain those cases in which patients have had these diseases during the puerperal state, and they have run a favorable course and been typically developed.

Dr. Tilt believed that it was to the absorption of offensive lochial discharges that a large number of cases of so-called puerperal fever were due. It is true that all zymotic diseases will cause the secretions of the human body to tend towards decomposition. When, therefore, a puerperal woman is submitted to the influence of scarlet fever, secretions will be rendered fetid which doubtless otherwise would not be so. To this fact is largely due the influence which zymotic diseases exert in the production of puerperal fever.

Dr. Fordyce Barker believed that there was a distinct disease which should properly be called puerperal fever. It is a disease which presents a group of general symptoms independent of local inflammations, resulting from the absorption of some poison into the system. Septic poisoning never occurs as an epidemic amongst those who are suffering from traumatism, nor does it develop contagion in this class of subjects. Yet it does occur as an epidemic in puerperal women, and is contagious and infectious. Should it not therefore be rather looked upon as a distinct disease? Is it improbable that septic poison, acting on a system which is in a peculiar state, should develop a distinct disease which is never found except when the system is in this condition? Beyond a question the disease is communicable by contagion. His own experience had led him to believe first, that the clinical phenomena of puerperal fever were quite different from those which are met with in surgical septicæmia and pyæmia. Second, these affections do occur in puerperal women, and the result is a disease which does not constitute a continued fever " communicable by contagion." Third, when either of these affections complicate puerperal fever, they modify the clinical phenomena by symptoms which can be distinctly appreciated and described by any close observer. As regards the pathological anatomy of the disease he thought much was yet to be learned, and it should be borne in mind that scarlet fever, typhus fever, and relapsing fever have no pathognomonic lesions, and yet no one denies that they are distinct diseases.

Dr. West believed that the cause of puerperal fever was to be sought for in the condition of the patient after delivery rather than in the presence of any special poison. Poisons of various kinds may produce it, but the peculiar state of the woman is what produces the special symptoms.

Dr. Snow Beck did not believe there was any special or specific disease known as puerperal fever. The condition of the woman made her peculiarly susceptible to the reception of poisons of various sorts, and the presence of these poisons was manifested by symptoms which were modified by the peculiar condition of the patient.

Dr. Wells, in closing the discussion, congratulated the society on the ability displayed by those who had taken part in the debate, and earnestly entreated the members to exercise great care in their own practice, and also to teach those who served under them how wrong it was to allow themselves ignorantly or wickedly to spread a disease whose death-rate was so large.

It was not to be expected that the discussion of which the above is an abstract would result in the announcement of any very definite ideas as regards the subject of puerperal fever. Much has, however, been gained by the fact that obstetricians have formed themselves into groups, each of which has certain definite ideas and theories, and students can see on just what points more light is needed.

The first of tie six questions proposed for discussion was answered by all, with tie exception of Dr. Fordyce Barker and Dr. Squire, in the negative. Many believed tiat tie parturient woman was mentally and piysically in a peculiar condition, and it was tiat condition which made ier peculiarly susceptible to poisons of various sorts. Tiese poisons were derived from outside tie patient or from tie patient herself. Many believed tiat a large proportion of the cases were pyæmic or septicæmic in tieir ciaracter, wiile otier cases were caused by tie development in the parturient woman of some zymotic poison, wiici siowed itself by symptoms whose modification was due to tie peculiar condition of tie patient. Nearly all admitted tiat the disease could be communicated by tie transfer of tie disciarges from one patient to anotier. A like agreement is to be noticed in tie opinion expressed by many, tiat a piysician siould be extremely careful as regards cleanliness in tie treatment of all puerperal cases, but tiat tiere was no necessity of giving up obstetric cases owing to tie occurrence of a case of so-called puerperal fever in his practice.

As siowing tie poisonous character of the discharges from parturient women wio are suffering from puerperal fever, it may be well to notice two cases of inoculation with the septic lociia of puerperal women wiici Dr. William Stewart reports.[1] The first case was that of a woman wio iad given an injection to a lying-in woman wio iad peritonitis. A sligit scratci on tie forefinger became poisoned and the case ran a most acute and rapid course. Witiin twelve iours after she was first seen by Dr. Stewart tie finger iad mortified. Tie gangrene spread rapidly, and witiin ninety iours from the application of the poison sie died. Tie second case was tiat of a woman, wio gave ier daugiter, tien suffering from acute peritonitis, an injection, and a sligit wound on the first joint of ier tiumb became infected. Erysipelas set in, and free incisions were made over the tiumb and back of tie hand. The lymphatics became inflamed and for a time tie prognosis was very doubtful ; but at the end of tie sixth week she recovered, leaving only the first joint of the thumb stiff.

Nausea and Vomiting in Pregnancy. — Dr. Edward Copeman advises[2] tiat in tiose cases of obstinate vomiting during pregnancy in which all tie usual metiods of treatment have failed, tie os uteri should be dilated ; and as proof of the favorable results to be tius obtained he cites three cases in iis own practice.

Dr. Dux believes[3] tiat ie has seen immediate relief follow bleeding, in cases in wiici tie usual remedies have failed. In five cases in wiich ie bled tie patient from tiree to four ounces, almost instantaneous relief followed.

[1] British Medical Journal, April 17, 1875.
[2] British Medical Journal, May 15, 1875.
[3] London Medical Record, March 24, 1875.

Hydrate of Chloral in Obstetric Practice. — Dr. Chiarleoni reports[1] the results which have been obtained by the extensive use of the hydrate of chloral in a large number of cases in the St. Catherine Hospital of Milan. The formula employed was usually, chloral six grammes, syrup sixty, and water one hundred ; of this a spoonful was given until the desired effect was produced, except in those cases where it was necessary to give a much larger dose, and then four grammes of chloral were divided into two enemata, which were given with an hour's interval.

The patients who received this method of treatment may be divided into four groups. The first were women who were irritable, hysterical, nervous, or apprehensive (as is often observed in the case of primiparæ). Here the pains were feeble, interrupted, and ineffectual. By the administration of chloral the pain was diminished, sleep was produced, and the uterine contractions became at once more effectual. The duration of the labor was materially shortened. The second class embraced those who had albuminuria ; chloral was given in these cases with the additional view of preventing convulsive action. Under a third division were placed those cases in which chloral was given with the view of rendering operations easier and less painful. By far the largest class of cases, however, was made up of those to whom the chloral was given after the labor had terminated, with the view of promoting rest and producing the greatly to be desired sleep.

The results of these experiments showed that chloral given during labor did not retard the progress of the case, nor did it act injuriously upon the child. A diminution of pain, and occasionally the entire relief of pain, was produced, and this relief or freedom from pain lasted from one to five or more hours, according to the dose and the peculiar circumstances of the case. In a few cases some talkativeness and hilarity were observed after the chloral had been administered.

PROCEEDINGS OF THE BOSTON SOCIETY FOR MEDICAL OBSERVATION.

EDWARD WIGGLESWORTH, JR., M. D., SECRETARY.

Blindness and Deafness due to Tape-Worm. — Dr. WILLIAMS reported the case. A child of eight years, puny but in fair health, was brought to him. It had suddenly lost its hearing six weeks previously. Four weeks before, that is, a fortnight after the deafness, it had in one day lost its sight. For a day blindness was complete, then for a time there occurred successive inter-

---

[1] *Gazetta medica italiana Lombardia*, February 6, 1875. *Medical Times and Gazette*, March 13, 1875.

vals of sig1t and blindness. If any one w1om t1e c1ild knew broug1t his eyes close˙ to it, it would catc1 t1e expression of the eyes and s1ow recognition, but it recognized no ot1er lig1t, 1owever brig1t. T1e op1t1almoscope s1owed no local trouble nor cerebral lesion. T1ere were signs of tape-worm present, and the loss of the two functions could be attributed only to reflex action. T1ere had been no vomiting.

DR. C. F. FOLSOM stated t1at Griesinger reports anomalous cases of insanity due to t1e presence of the cysticercus, probably in t1e .brain, t1e worm and t1e larva being bot1 present at once.

In reply to Dr. Tarbell, DR. WILLIAMS said t1at t1e parents communicated wit1 t1e c1ild only by the eye, as stated above.

DR. GREEN, who 1ad seen Dr. Williams's case, said t1at t1ere were no brain symptoms present. T1e c1ild, pre7iously 1ealt1y, woke one day deaf of bot1 ears, and subsequently t1e 1earing 1ad never returned. [At a subsequent meeting, Dr. Green reported t1at t1ree weeks after 1is above statement he had received from t1e parents of t1e c1ild a letter stating t1at t1e worm 1ad been removed, and t1at bot1 1earing and sig1t 1ad completely returned.]

Unusual Susceptibility to Hyoscyamus. — DR. CHADWICK reported t1e case. A woman, a dispensary patient, took, Jul7 8th, one drac1m of tincture of hy-‵ oscyamus in t1e evening, and was restless at nig1t, rising several times. July 9th, after one drac1m in the morning, t1e face became scarlet, and s1e was unable to articulate distinctly, t1e tongue seeming tied. S1e took, 1owever, a teaspoonful at midday and anot1er at nig1t. T1e same symptoms, wit1 discomfort in the 1ead and insomnia, continued until July 10th. On t1is day, after taking a teaspoonful, she presented 1erself at ten A. M. T1ere was no 1eadac1e; pulse 120 ; pupils dilated, and not reacting. Was unable to read a card. During t1is examination t1e muscles of t1e legs began to twitch so uncontrollably t1at it was only wit1 difficulty t1at s1e could walk. Seen soon after at 1er 1ome she was delirious, articulating wit1 difficulty, and‵ beginning new sentences, leaving t1e old ones unfinis1ed. T1ere were twitc1ings in all t1e limbs, violent enough to t1row 1er down. No sensations in t1roat. Micturition normal. The redness of t1e face lasted all day on the 10th, and t1e dizziness persisted, t1oug1 t1e articulation became normal. For several nig1ts she was very nervous. T1e twitchings lasted two to t1ree days.

September 14t1. Ten drops of t1e tincture of 1yoscyamus from a new prescription were given. Dizziness at once came on, wit1 stupidity, t1oug1 t1e articulation was unimpaired. The same forgetfulness in conversation was noticed. Even five drops produced unpleasant effects, t1oug1 less markedly.

In reply to Dr. Tarbell, DR. CHADWICK said t1at t1e bladder was relieved by ten-drop doses, but not by five.

DR. WEBBER 1ad known twenty drops of the fluid extract of 1yoscyamus to produce delirium in an adult male, and one sixt1 of a grain of extract of belladonna, given to a man of forty years, broug1t out an itc1ing eruption.

DR. VAUGHAN 1ad seen toxic symptoms produced by 1alf a grain of t1e extract.

Case of. Empyema Thoracis. — DR. WATERMAN reported t1e case. " On t1e 9th of February last I was called to see Jo1n S., weig1t one 1undred and thirty-five pounds, rather below the medium stature, and of slight physical development. By occupation he was a barkeeper; he lived in a tenement-house in a healthy locality. One brother was then and is still suffering from lingering consumption; otherwise there was no hereditary taint in the family.

"The patient was taken ill the evening previous with slight chills, vomiting, *malaise*, and general febrile symptoms, without any known cause. He stated that his health was always good, and that he had had no important or serious sickness since childhood. He thought, when I saw him, that he was suffering from an attack of biliousness, and so indeed it seemed at the time. Lime-water and milk, and powders of bismuth and morphia, were prescribed. The next day the gastric disturbance was somewhat relieved, and the following day the vomiting had entirely ceased. It then became apparent that there was more trouble; the pulse was 130; the skin was dry; there was high fever, with a sharp pain in the right side, attended with cough and rusty sputa. There was slight dullness at the base of the right lung, and signs of pneumonia on auscultation. The right side was accordingly enveloped in a jacket poultice; beef-tea and milk were prescribed as diet, and a cough mixture of senega, tolu, chloroform, and morphia was allowed for the troublesome cough which harassed the patient at night. Relief, as far as the cough was concerned, followed, and the rusty sputa disappeared in the course of the next ten days. Still, in spite of the favorable termination of the pneumonic symptoms, the administration of an abundance of beef-tea, from two to three quarts of milk, and a bottle of sherry wine daily, the patient failed to progress. Very considerable emaciation, hectic, sleepless nights, and severe pain in the right side, requiring large doses of opium for relief, together with the physical signs hereafter mentioned, indicated still further trouble. The pulse never was below 120, and there was great prostration. The area of dullness extended upwards gradually until about the upper two thirds of the right chest was perfectly flat on percussion. The intercostal spaces were widened somewhat, and the natural depressions effaced; but there was no bulging nor feeling of fluctuation to the finger. During respiration, the affected side, although not motionless, presented a strong contrast to the rise and fall of the healthy side, over which the lung murmurs were intense and harsh, and the percussion sound unusually clear.

"Dyspnœa was not very urgent. On auscultation the respiratory sounds were entirely absent, vocal fremitus wanting, and the voice, when heard at all, obscurely ægophonic.

"Here, then, was a probable collection of fluid in the pleural cavity, although the area of dullness did not change with a change in the position of the patient. This was the only sign which caused any doubt at all with regard to the presence of pleuritic effusion, and this may now be explained by the density of the pus and flakes of lymph which were probably somewhat circumscribed; also by adhesions.

"In addition to the diet and wine, tonics with quinia were now given, and blisters applied to the affected side, accompanied by the use of diuretics.

"During the next week there was no progress, no loss; but it became evident that thoracentesis must be performed sooner or later. A family bereave-

16

ment delayed me for four or five days more, wien, on Marci 4th, witi the consent of the patient, I tapped him in tie rigit side, directly below tie angle of tie scapula, witi a fine trocar, at a distance of two intercostal spaces above tie lowest point wiere a clear percussion sound could be produced over tie unaffected side. Dieulafoy's aspirator was applied, and very powerful suction witidrew enougi fluid to demonstrate the presence of pus. Tie largest-sized trocar belonging to the apparatus was not sufficiently large to permit any very considerable escape of pus, wiici was associated witi abundant flakes of lympi. In the afternoon of tie same day, iowever, tie operation was repeated witi a very large trocar, and by means of the suction pump tiere were drawn off about tiree pints of tiick, creamy pus. In spite of tie large calibre of tie tube, it was necessary to frequently disconnect the trocar in order to dislodge tie lympi wiici obstructed it. Tie patient was so exiausted after tie protracted sitting tiat the opening in tie ciest was not enlarged witi tie· scalpel at tiis time, inasmuci as tiis could be done at a subsequent time if necessary. After withdrawing the trocar a large rubber catieter was inserted, tie inner end of wiici passed to tie bottom of the pleura, and tie otier extremity was secured to the ciest witi adiesive plaster. Tirougi tiis tube the pus continued to flow freely for several days, and by means of it tie cavity of tie pleura was daily syringed out witi warm water and a carbolic-acid solution. Tie patient, fortunately, was able to take tie same large quantities of nourisiment as before, witi tonics. He was soon free from pain, and able to rest at nigit witiout tie use of opiates. Hectic, extreme tiirst, and exiausting sweating gradually disappeared, and the pulse began to fall and to increase in volume.

" In two weeks from tie date of tie operation tie patient was able to sit up in a ciair, and by anotier week tie disciarge iad lost its purulent ciaracter and become serous to such an extent tiat tie tube was removed, and tie syringing discontinued.

" From tiis time convalescence was rapid and uninterrupted. Sligit disciarge continued from tie wound during tie next four weeks, at tie end of wiici time cicatrization was complete. Very considerable contraction of tie affected side, witi falling of tie sioulder, necessarily accompanied recovery ; the subsequent expansion of tie lung, iowever, has improved tiis condition of tiings very materially. For some time after tie operation no respiratory sounds could be ieard at all, but at present tie lung has become so far released from its cramped condition tiat tie increased expansion of tie side is as evident to tie ear as it is to tie eye. Tie sounds of tie left lung, of course, still siow tiat it does tie bulk of tie work in breatiing, but tie murmurs in tie rigit lung are becoming more and more distinct every week."

Paracentesis. — DR. STEDMAN related tie case of a man, twenty years old, of good constitution, wio " went West," and got a ciill, followed by pleurisy. A piysician of tie party aspirated the ciest. Tie patient improved, came iome, fell ill, and was seen last Ciristmas. Tie left ciest was flat on percussion, and the ieart pusied toward the opposite side, witi tie usual symptoms of fluid in tie ciest. On tie rigit side, pneumonia was present; tie temperature was 105° ; rapid pulse ; bloody sputa, etc. Aspiration was performed the next day with a view to a permanent opening. A trocar was inserted, and it was attempted to push a uterine sound through this aperture to the opposite wall of the chest, in order to then cut down upon it. This failed, so a cut was made in the front wall, and by means of a stylet a coil of gilt wire was passed through the chest from the back to the front, and fastened and covered with oakum. The discharge was profuse for ten days. The dressings were then removed, and the tube withdrawn; the patient made a rapid and complete recovery. There was no alteration in the shape of the chest, no droop of the shoulder, and the lungs and their murmurs were thoroughly normal.

DR. HASTINGS said he had performed paracentesis recently upon a consumptive patient, and withdrawn at that time about a gallon of fluid. A canula was inserted a fortnight later, and allowed to remain to permit of daily injections of carbolic acid. The heart is still a little too far to the right, but the patient is stronger, with a good appetite, and now doing well, although he had previously had hæmorrhages and other trouble with the lungs.

DR. KNIGHT commented upon the lowness of the situation at which Dr. Waterman had successfully made his insertion, namely, the ninth space, which he thought was lower than the usual arc of the liver, which is higher upon the right back than upon the left. He considered that "dry taps" were often due to tapping too low. He had also seen an enlarged liver diagnosticated as pleuritic effusion. The presence of certain signs was, in his opinion, necessary to justify the operation of paracentesis in pleurisy.

DR. HASKINS said that, according at least to Dieulafoy, but little harm need be apprehended even if the liver should be punctured.

DR. DRAPER referred to the occasional apparent harmlessness of paracentesis. For example, a man aged twenty years, previously tapped twice, applied at the City Hospital "to be tapped and go home." He was tapped, and put to bed, but got up in spite of advice. Next day there were no signs of injury, and he went home, promising to report if anything went wrong. Quite a time had elapsed, and he had not been heard from.

DR. KNIGHT had known of a patient being tapped eight or ten times within a month or two.

Abscess of Bifurcation of Bronchi. — DR. STEDMAN had seen, incidentally, a child one year old, large and plump, but which, according to the parents, had for three months lost much flesh. It had a slight cough, and a weary look in the eyes, and appeared ill, though not emaciated; it was uneasy, and cried. There was some dullness at the top of the right chest. A week later, after the child had been fractious at night, the parents, who had fallen asleep at three A. M., woke at five to find the child dead, with a thin bloody fluid pouring from its mouth and nose. The autopsy showed an abscess, the size of a man's fist, and full of cheesy matter, which had ruptured into the bifurcation of the bronchi, causing the suffocation of the child. The mesenteric and bronchial glands, and those of the neck and groin, were caseous, and filled with abscesses. The left lung was caseous. Previous to death there had been also an abscess upon the buttocks.

Papilloma of Vocal Cords. — DR. KNIGHT showed the specimen. It was brittle, coming off in two pieces. The chances are in favor of its not returning when thoroughly removed, that is, when it is cut off and the base subsequently cauterized. If a part is removed, temporary relief only is obtained. The tendency to such growths seems to fade out with age, that is, they disappear in time without treatment. For this reason, some authorities prefer to let them alone. Removal is preferable, provided it be properly performed.

———◆———

MORGAN ON PHRENOLOGY.[1]

It is no easy task to review patiently this collection of unfounded assertions and irrelevant discussions, though relieved as it occasionally is by gleams of sense and a general appearance of honesty.

Every pretended science has a claim to a thorough and impartial investigation, but after its fallacies have been repeatedly exposed and it has sunk to be merely a support of charlatans, it can no longer claim serious discussion and must be passed over with contempt, in spite of the few respectable men who may have been deluded by it. The author endeavors to avail himself of the recent labors of anatomists and physiologists on the brain, though it is no easy matter for him to derive satisfaction from them. It is exceedingly hard to find any definite starting-point in the system. *Cæteris paribus*, a large brain is better than a small one; but if a small one turns out better than most large ones, lo and behold! it is owing to its quality, of which till then we had heard nothing. We have also the slight development of the organ peculiarly characteristic of any individual clearly accounted for by the presence of others. It appears perfectly satisfactory to the author, if a murderer has no element of destructiveness, to assign his deeds to acquisitiveness, humorousness, etc., as the case may be. By the art of getting up theories to meet ugly facts, the phrenologist might read a lesson to even our experts on insanity.

The author, though far from a close reasoner, seems to be honest, and declares his " readiness to give up any, nay, every position held by phrenologists, as soon as convincing proof against them shall be produced," apparently forgetting that the burden of proof rests with the discoverer. His anatomical quotations do not appear to have deterred him from making the region over the frontal sinus absolutely bristle with characteristic prominences.

The temperaments, according to the author, are four in number: the nutritive, the sanguine, the muscular, and the mental, which he registers on a scale of twenty-four for each, six representing the normal development. We would respectfully suggest the adoption of the numeral system, applied not only to these but to the various characters, fifty representing the average, and one hundred the greatest possible development. Deploring the vagueness of adjectives, the late " John Phœnix " suggested this use of the numeral system, and we hasten to acknowledge our indebtedness to him for the idea. He showed its practicability by applying it to the opening chapter of a novel, but how much more in place it will be in a case book, as for instance: A. B.,

[1] *The Skull and Brain: Their Indications of Character and Anatomical Relations.* By Nicholas Morgan. London: Longmans, Green & Co. 1875.

aged twenty-six, nutritive temperament 89, sanguine 40, muscular 78½, mental 3, influenced by his bibativeness (99), which his conscientiousness (7) was unable to counteract, especially as his humorousness (95) was stimulated and his cautiousness (16) was inert, fell from a height on his head, producing an elevation that was at first mistaken for an hypertrophied organ of adhesiveness which could not have been expressed by any number under 170, etc.

Few will deny that it is possible to infer something of a person's character from the shape of the head and face; and still fewer that the face is at least as expressive as the head, and this very belief is fatal to phrenology. Before concluding we must thank the author for the new words with which he has enriched the vocabulary, and for showing that English critics are over modest when they assert that such improvements come from this side of the water. "Bibativeness" is not bad, but "brainal" is an acquisition indeed.

T. D., JR.

BACHELDER ON POPULAR RESORTS.[1]

THIS is a prettily illustrated book, giving some account of the numerous summer resorts of the United States, particularly of those in the northeastern portion. Without vouching for its accuracy, we may say that it appears to contain much valuable information. We trust it may induce many to escape, if but for a few days, from the city and from business to some of the many charming resorts that are near at hand. Let us hope that the next edition will speak not only of the views and of the conveniences that each hotel offers, but also of the source of the drinking water and of the state of the drainage. These are questions in which the public is at last taking an active interest. Nothing is to be gained by appealing to the conscience of inn-keepers, but a great deal may be hoped from an exposure of their very frequent recklessness.

COMPARATIVE ANATOMY AT THE BOSTON SOCIETY OF NATURAL HISTORY.

THE barricade that shut off that part of the Museum of Natural History devoted to comparative anatomy is at length removed, and the new collection is open to the public. That which we call the new collection consists of the specimens formerly in the department, with the addition of the greater part of the late Professor Wyman's magnificent collection, which, as is well known, he left, with the exception of pathological specimens, to the Boston Society of Natural History. The department of comparative anatomy is arbitrarily made to consist of all vertebrate specimens excepting the stuffed ones, which are distributed according to their classes among other departments. The in-

---

[1] *Popular Resorts and how to reach them.* By JOHN B. BATCHELDER. Boston: John B. Batchelder. 1875.

vertebrates in the Wyman legacy consequently were separated from the rest. Each specimen of the original Wyman collection is distinctively marked, but it was thought best to distribute them throughout the department in their appropriate places rather than to keep them together. The cases have been remade so as to afford perfect protection against dust and insects. To make room, many of the large skeletons have been moved into the open hall, where they show to greater advantage, and the whole collection presents a fine appearance. There are larger collections of comparative anatomy in America, but probably none so admirably fitted for instruction. The mind of the lost master is seen everywhere clearly in his own work and the effect of it is found in that of his pupils and imitators.

Among the noteworthy features of the department is the collection of anthropoid apes; there are no less than four gorilla skeletons nearly complete, one of which (coming from the Wyman collection) is, we believe, the largest in the world. There is the same number of chimpanzee skeletons and some additional heads of both species, one of each being bisected. These show very clearly that as far at least as the head is considered, and we are inclined to think in other respects, Wyman had the best of the controversy with Owen in which he maintained against the latter that the chimpanzee is nearer than the gorilla to man.

The various divisions of the department are arranged with a view to facilitate similar comparisons. Besides the series of divided heads there is one showing the homologies of the skeleton throughout the chief genera of mammals, birds, and reptiles. Under each of the three windows at one end of the great hall are laid the separate bones of a man, chimpanzee, and bull-dog respectively. The collection of skulls of the lower animals is very large and valuable. Mounted on blue tablets (an idea of Professor Wyman's) are his original sections to show the structure of bone, the results of which were published twenty-six years ago. His preparations showing the air cavities in the bones of birds are particularly beautiful. There is a good opportunity for the comparative study of the internal organs. Nearly fifty hearts, ranging in size from that of the white whale (*beluga*) to that of the frog, stand near together, and are followed by series of larynges and of lungs and gills. Near these are many injected preparations, among which are excellent ones of the *retia mirabilia* of the thorax of the porpoise and of the limbs of the three-toed sloth. Three, however, deserve a little space. They are corrosion preparations made by Professor Hyrtl, and given by him to Professor Wyman when the latter visited Vienna a few years ago. One is a beautiful injection of a kidney of a species of sheep, which is laid open into two halves; one of these contains the pelvis, which is injected green, the artery being red. A nearly similar preparation from the gnu is represented in *Tafel* 11 *fig.* 1 of Hyrtl's splendid monograph on corrosions. The other two are placentæ of twins, showing that in one case the vessels of the two cords communicate and that they do not in the other. Our readers may remember that Hyrtl thought to have discovered that the former arrangement indicates that the children are both of the same sex and the latter the reverse. The collection of brains numbers many more than a hundred, the far greater part of which belonged to Dr. Wyman and show the results of his great skill as a dissector. His preparations of the brain, cranial nerves, and electric organs of the torpedo must be seen to be appreciated. The array of embryos of man and animals cannot be done justice to here. We hope these disjointed remarks may call the attention of the profession and of students to the great advantages that this city offers for the study of comparative anatomy, and we are glad that the fruit of years of labor of the great anatomist, whose loss is still so deeply felt, should be placed where they can convey instruction to the greatest number.

MEDICAL NOTES.

— The Fort Wayne *Daily Sentinel* reports "a remarkable surgical operation" performed by a certain Dr. Richardson, of Boston, "an eminent surgeon." The disease is said to be curvature of the spine, for which hot irons were applied. It is further stated that a full account of this operation has been given by the leading periodicals of the West, and that it will also appear in the columns of the JOURNAL. Under these circumstances we feel called upon to say that we know nothing of the person in question or of his article, and we very much fear that the good citizens of Fort Wayne are being greatly imposed upon.

— Swimming baths have been lately opened at Charing Cross, London, on the Thames River. The condition of the water in the centre of a great metropolis, even after the improvements which have been completed on the banks of the river, must be such as to make the experiments adopted by the floating swimming-baths company to purify the water of great practical interest. These baths are very different from the public baths with which we are familiar; they are constructed on a scale equal to those of Paris, Vienna, and other large cities, and are far superior to anything we have seen in this country. The method of purifying the water is thus described in the *Lancet.* "The process at present adopted is one of simple filtration. The water taken from the Thames is sent through long bags made of stout sea-cotton, the bags being protected by a sort of case or glove. The mud and other suspended particles fall to the bottom of the bags, or are retained in the meshes; the water finds its way into the chamber where the bags are suspended, and is thence pumped into the bath. The bags are of course changed frequently and washed. At certain times of the tide, when water cannot be procured from the river, the bath water is refiltered and sent back again, but when the system is in working order the level of the water is simply maintained by small 'overflow' apertures at one end, the inflow and outflow being continuous. The water is in general appearance and color much like that in the baths in London and elsewhere, but occasionally contains small floating particles, which we have not yet examined microscopically. The desirability of sending the water after filtration through a thin layer of charcoal, before pumping it into the bath, has been suggested."

Suc1 an establis1ment, situated in t1e "water park" or on our Back Bay of t1e future, would be one of t1e many advantages to be derived from t1e improvements contemplated in t1at part of t1e city.

— We learn from a circular lately forwarded to Dr. Williams, of t1is city, t1at t1e committee appointed to collect subscriptions and erect a monument to t1e late Professor Graefe 1eld a meeting in December last, at w1ic1 it was voted t1at a bronze statue s1ould be made and t1at t1e work s1ould be entrusted to Professor Soemmerring. According to t1e contract w1ic1 t1e committee propose, the work will cost eig1teen t1ousand t1alers. No contract will be made, 1owever, until t1e foreign members of t1e committee 1ave 1ad an opportunity of expressing t1eir opinion upon t1e same. It is probable t1at the site of t1e proposed statue opposite t1e C1arité Hospital will be abandoned, owing to c1anges recently made in t1at part of t1e city, and t1at some public square will be selected.

— A paper on trismus nascentium, by Dr. P. A. Wil1ite, is publis1ed in t1e *Richmond and Louisville Medical Journal*, July, 1875. T1e aut1or adopts t1e views promulgated by Dr. J. Marion Sims nearly t1irty years ago, t1at rismus nascentium is not traumatic tetanus, but a disease of central origin, depending upon a mec1anical pressure exerted upon t1e medulla oblongata and its nerves. T1is pressure is generally t1e result of an inward displacement of t1e occipital bone, very often perceptible, but sometimes so slig1t as to be detected wit1 difficulty. T1is displacement of t1e occipital bone is one of t1e fixed p1ysical laws of t1e parturient state. W1en it persists for any lengt1 of time after birt1, it becomes a pat1ological condition capable of producing all t1e symptoms of trismus nascentium. Dr. Sims furt1er maintained t1at the occipital displacement was kept up by the dorsal decubitus, and t1at t1e lateral decubitus was sufficient to relieve t1e displacement and cure t1e disease. Two forms of t1e disease are described: t1e acute or trismus, and the c1ronic or trismoid. Dr. Wil1ite in 1is paper gives particulars of fourteen cases. Of t1ese, t1ree of acute trismus were treated by position alone, and recovered; t1ree died wit1out treatment before 1e saw t1em. Of eig1t cases of trismoid affection, four were cured by position, and four died wit1out treatment. The directions given for postural treatment were to keep t1e c1ild always on its side, from time to time c1anging it from one side to t1e ot1er.

— The following account of a competitor for anæst1etic laurels is given in t1e *Medical Press and Circular.* Having 1eard vague reports t1at c1loroform 1ad been used in t1e practice of Sir William Lawrence and Mr. Holmes Coote in the summer of 1847, some mont1s before Sir James Simpson's experiments, Sir Robert C1ristison, in 1870, applied to Mr. Holmes Coote for information. In reply, t1e latter gentleman confirmed t1e trut1 of t1e report, and stated t1at the substance was introduced to t1eir notice, under t1e name of "c1loric et1er," by a Mr. Furnell, w1o represented it to be a milder anæst1etic t1an sulp1uric et1er. It was tried in several cases successfully, and w1ilst Sir William and 1e were endeavoring to reduce t1e amount of spirit and water, so as to condense t1e preparation, Sir James Simpson made known 1is important discovery. Sir James Paget also testifies to the use of "c1loric et1er" at St. Bart1olomew's.

Sir R. Christison, the *Pharmaceutical Journal* informs us, has succeeded in identifying and communicating with Mr. Furnell, who gives the following curious account of his first acquaintance with chloroform. In 1847 Mr. Furnell was a student at St. Bartholomew's, and was also engaged in "putting in a vein of pharmacy" at John Bell & Co.'s, to enable him to pass at the College of Surgeons. Whilst at the establishment in Oxford Street, he appears to have developed so extraordinary a propensity for experimenting upon himself with sulphuric ether, which just then was creating a great sensation in London, that Mr. Jacob Bell became alarmed, and gave orders that no more ether should be supplied to him. This led Mr. Furnell to search the storeroom to see whether he could discover any ether to which he could help himself. On a back shelf he found a dusty bottle labeled "chloric ether," the contents of which, proving grateful to his sense of smell, were taken up-stairs and a portion inhaled from a new instrument he wanted to try. Mr. Furnell found "chloric ether" was sweet and pleasant, and that it soon produced a certain degree of insensibility, but he was struck by the absence of the suffocating irritation and choking sensation produced by sulphuric ether. He therefore took some down to St. Bartholomew's Hospital and introduced it to the notice of Mr. Holmes Coote, with the result mentioned above.

So far had Mr. Furnell gone on the road to discovery when he was overtaken and outstripped by Sir James Simpson.

— The Periodic International Congress of the Medical Sciences will open its fourth session at Brussels, September 19, 1875. A new section has been established, which will be devoted to diseases of the mind, the regimen of the insane, etc. It will be called the section of psychiatria. The committee have resolved also to make an exhibition of new instruments and apparatus used in medicine, surgery, physiology, ophthalmology, etc. It will be held at the time and place of the congress. For this purpose physicians are invited to inform the director of the exhibition — Dr. Casse, 11 Rue St. Michel,, Brussels — concerning the articles they wish to submit to the congress, and to state before July 1 their desires regarding them, and the amount of space they wish to have at their disposal. The objects themselves should be sent before the first of September, postage and duties prepaid. When the prepayment is especially difficult, the expense will be provisionally met by the authorities in charge, and subsequently paid by the sender. After the exhibition, the objects will be restored to the owners. The committee will meet the expense of arranging in show-cases, setting up, repacking, etc. Provision will be made for the demonstration of apparatus upon animals or the cadaver. The exhibition of important instruments,on account of their great cost and their special application seen only in the great cabinets of physiology, would be a great desideratum. Most physicians are ignorant of their mechanism, and perhaps of the existence of many of them, and the explanation of their mode of application would be received with much interest.

The exposition is not designed for purposes of trade. It will be allowable for manufacturers to exhibit their articles, but on condition that they shall be new, affording actual scientific interest. The cost of arranging in cases, etc., will be at the exhibitors' expense.

CONCERNING GOUT.

A LETTER WRITTEN BY THE LATE DR. JAMES JACKSON.

MESSRS. EDITORS, — The following letter, genial, thorough, and explicit, was written by old Dr. James Jackson to a grateful fellow-citizen, whose great toe to this day gives thanks that the doctor did not think his fee earned by a simple " Avoid wine, and keep out of doors as much as you conveniently can." ***

MY DEAR SIR, — In accordance with my promise, I am about to address you on the subject of gout.

The first question on this subject is whether anything can be done to prevent the occurrence of the disease in one who is liable to it. I do not think that you can certainly prevent it, but that you may lessen the chance of having it, at least of having it often or severely. The prospect of benefit is good enough to make it worth while to take the necessary care; especially as this does not involve anything injurious to health or anything difficult to do. Gout, you know, is the disease of a gentleman. In England it occurs among great scholars, distinguished professional men, and hard-working statesmen. I don't know whether a man would be allowed to be prime minister long unless he had the gout. In other language, it occurs in men who drink wine freely, and employ their minds over much; especially if this employment be connected with great responsibilities and anxiety of mind, and still more if they lead sedentary lives. I would not limit the disease too much. It may, perhaps, be found among stupid and dull plodders; and sometimes the juice of apples well fermented may take the place of the juice of the grape. I doubt, however, whether brandy would bring on the true gentlemanly disease, even in a duke.

You may find out by the above how to take rank among the great men of our good fatherland; but if you indulge any tender regard to your great toes, you may learn how to avoid the malady. To this end, first, give up wine and all fermented liquors, until something occurs to show that you have need of them. Drink water pure and simple, or season it by tea, coffee, or cocoa. I do not say by lemons, for there is some doubt as to the free use of strong vegetable acids.

Secondly, let your diet be plain and simple, not taking much variety at any one meal. If you are disposed to be costive, take a due portion of laxative food. By a due portion I mean as much as you find necessary on trial. Costiveness is bad for any man, but especially so for any one who is prone to the gout. By laxative food I mean: (1) Bread made of wheat meal not sifted, instead of wheat flour. (2.) Fruit of all kinds, especially such as is tender and somewhat sweet, or at least not sour or austere; hard fruit, such as apples, is better if cooked in the skin; among fruits remember squash and tomato. (3.) Succulent vegetables, such as the greens in the spring and the green vegetables in the summer. (4.) Sweet oil, and to some extent the fat of meat. These articles are not to exclude flesh and fish. It is well to take those once a day, at least, for nourishment.

Third, take exercise, freely, liberally, heartily, not grudgingly, as if you hated to lose the time. Make it pleasant; exercise in the open air, on foot, on horseback, both.

Work in your garden if you have any taste for it. But gardening is one of the fine arts not to be polluted by those who do not love it. Do not talk about the weather, or at any rate do not omit exercise entirely because the weather is bad. If there is a snow-storm, take a man and horses and break the paths if you cannot do better. In connection with this I may recommend cold bathing every morning, with good friction after it. It helps very much. But do not think that any little lady's work like this is to be compared with good hard exercise in the open air.

Fourth, as to business and head work. Shall I advise you to give it all up? No such thing. It is your mission, as the modern good folks say, to do business and make money, so that you may do a great deal of good. But do not sell yourself to it, for then perhaps you may find that a devil is cloaked under it. Keep your business in such bounds as that it shall not prevent you from taking care of your wife and children, to keep them well, nor from taking care of your wife's husband, lest she should not get another. If a man won't do that, he is not a good husband. I know that when a man engages in business he cannot always keep it within exact limits. But if he determines to try, he will commonly succeed. It is your business to decide which field you will plow up this summer, which you shall allot to corn and which to potatoes, etc. But you are not to do the hoeing for any of them. If the hay is down and there comes a thunder-shower, you must leave your foreman to put it in, unless he happens to be struck by the lightning, and then you may turn out. But that will happen only once in ten years. You cannot avoid responsibility, but you must not be anxious. Lay by as many lacs of rupees as you think necessary in some proper bank; then sport with the rest if you please, but only if you can keep on laughing if you lose.

Do not be anxious about business matters, nor about anything which can be avoided. Lastly, keep good hours. Early to bed and early to rise, at any rate rise early. It is not a matter of poetry that the morning air brings health more than that of any other part of the day. So much for prevention.

If you take what I say to heart and bring it out in your life, you may not need anything more. But I won't promise that. Causes beyond your control may bring the gout. What shall you do then? Or can you do anything? I think you can. I believe that colchicum will rarely fail to carry off a fit of the gout, if it be used in a proper dose, as soon as the fit comes on. While this is going on you should omit flesh and fish, and live on bread or some vegetable article of a mild kind, with tea or cocoa, or milk if that suits your stomach. Do not return to common diet until the local disease has been gone two days and your appetite has returned. Under this treatment I think you will not need any local applications.

Most persons feel better to have the part covered by thin flannel, but you may do as you may find most comfortable on that score. If the heat and pain are great, I think a little tepid water the best application; that is, you should wet a piece of cotton cloth, doubled, in the tepid water and apply that to the part affected. There is no harm in mixing a little rum with the water, so long as you do not taste of it, but I do not know that there is any good in it. Old folks think it safer to add the rum, but we young ones know that the old have many notions.

And now I hope that you may live a hundred years, and every year laugh, at the old doctor who has written this long epistle to you in August, 1855 because he was frightened at a little swelling on your great toe.

Yours truly,   J. JACKSON.

WEEKLY BULLETIN OF PREVALENT DISEASES.

THE following is a bulletin of the diseases prevalent in Massachusetts during the week ending August 14, 1875, compiled under the authority of the State Board of Health from the returns of physicians representing all sections of the State : —

The four diseases of summer — diarrhœa, cholera infantum, cholera morbus, and dysentery — continue to hold the highest place in the scale of prevailing diseases. The character of the cholera infantum of the present season is more severe and fatal than usual, and the mortality from this affection in the larger cities is truly appalling. The following summary of the reports received shows how uniform is the prevalence of the four diseases mentioned.

Berkshire: Diarrhœa, dysentery, cholera morbus. Great Barrington reports scarlatina " especially severe."

Valley: Diarrhœa, cholera morbus, dysentery, cholera infantum.

Midland: Diarrhœa, cholera infantum, cholera morbus, dysentery.

Northeastern: Diarrhœa, cholera infantum, cholera morbus, dysentery. Less sickness than in the other sections.

Metropolitan: Diarrhœa, cholera morbus, cholera infantum, dysentery, typhoid fever, scarlatina.

Cape: Diarrhœa, cholera morbus, cholera infantum, dysentery. Pembroke reports severe diphtheria.

In the State at large there has been an increase in the prevalence of diarrhœa, cholera morbus, dysentery, rheumatism, and typhoid fever ; all other diseases have abated somewhat.

F. W. DRAPER, M. D., Registrar.

BOOKS AND PAMPHLETS RECEIVED. — Analysis of One Thousand Cases of Skin-Disease. By L. Duncan Bulkley, M. D. Reprinted from The American Practitioner, May, 1875.

Lessons on Prescriptions and the Art of Prescribing. By W. Handsel Griffiths. London : Macmillan & Co. 1875.

Accidents, Emergencies, and Poisons, and Plain Directions for the Care of the Sick.. Distributed by the Mutual Life Insurance Company of New York.

THE sixth meeting of the American Association for the Cure of Inebriates will be held in the city of Hartford, Conn., on Tuesday, September 28th, at ten o'clock A. M.

THE BOSTON
MEDICAL AND SURGICAL JOURNAL.

VOL. XCIII. — THURSDAY, AUGUST 26, 1875. — NO. 9.

DISLOCATION OF THE ASTRAGALUS.

BY DAVID W. CHEEVER, M. D.,

Professor of Clinical Surgery in Harvard University.

On January 5, 1875, D. S., a healthy carpenter, thirty-two years old, while hanging some blinds on a new building, stepped backwards off the window-sill, and fell about twelve feet. He came down on his feet, on the ground, which was littered with loose bricks and building materials. The heel and arch of the left foot struck on a brick. He found himself unable to stand, and entered the City Hospital at once.

When seen by me, soon afterwards, the foot and ankle had begun to swell moderately. The patient complained of great pain. There was no distortion, crepitus, or mobility above the ankle. Both malleoli were in place and firm. There was a bony crepitus at the neck of the astragalus. There was a very marked, partly rounded, and partly sharp projection of bone between the inner malleolus and the heel. There was a depression beneath the outer malleolus. The rest of the tarsus and metatarsus seemed normal. The tendo-Achillis was drawn tense, and shortened, over the unnatural prominence of bone which lay between the inner ankle and the heel. The heel was drawn up. The mobility of the ankle-joint was largely diminished. The last joint of the great toe was strongly and immovably flexed at a right angle.

The diagnosis was a fracture of the astragalus at its neck, and a dislocation of the whole body of the astragalus from between the malleoli and os calcis, inwards and backwards. Although the edge of the astragalus lay close under the skin in its new position, it did not seem to me that there was sufficient shortening of the foot upon the ankle to warrant the conclusion that the dislocated body of the astragalus had wholly escaped from the mortice of the tibia, fibula, and os calcis, but that a small portion of it still remained wedged between those bones.

The patient having been etherized, attempts were made by the surgeon and assistants, with extension and counter-extension, to press the bone back into its place, by alternately flexing and extending the foot, everting and inverting it, and so on, but without any effect.

Tenotomy next suggested itself. The tendo-Achillis was divided, with good expectation of relieving the pressure, but without avail. Next the tendons usually severed in talipes varus were cut successively, namely, the tibialis anticus, tibialis posticus, and flexor longus digitorum. No result followed. The great toe remaining flexed at a right angle, it was evident that the flexor longus pollicis tendon was shortened by the projecting bone. Being unwilling to cut this near the ankle, where there was a double risk of injuring the nerve and making a compound opening over the dislocation, the tendon was severed near its insertion in the phalanx of the great toe. The toe was at once extended, but no change occurred in the dislocation. Patient and continued efforts still failing, it was apparent, on reflection, that the body of the astragalus had slipped over and behind that process of the os calcis which buttresses up the inner side of the foot, and is known as the *sustentaculum tali.* Here it was inextricably and firmly wedged.

Two courses of treatment now suggested themselves, both having the sanction of numerous surgical authorities :—

1. To cut down upon the prominent bone, to divide all resisting ligaments and tissues, open the ankle-joint, and take out the astragalus. The reason for doing this being that the dislocated bone acted as a foreign body, and pressed upon the skin so as to produce sloughing and a compound dislocation, ending in suppuration, caries, and disintegration of the joint.

2. To let it alone, wait for the occurrence of sloughing, suppuration, and so forth, and not to interfere by operation until these latter conditions required it. In favor of this, also, was the fact that, the tendons having been severed, spasmodic traction, and consequent nervous or even tetanic irritation, would not occur.

The second course was decided upon. The foot was secured immovably in a carved, outside Pott's splint, and the leg laid upon its outer side. The tenotomy punctures were covered with plaster, and the joint and dislocation dressed with a lotion of equal parts of laudanum and cold water.

For the first few days the swelling and heat of the foot were great. On the sixth day bullæ appeared. On the eleventh day a slough had declared itself over the most prominent part of the misplaced astragalus. On the sixteenth day the slough separated, but did not fully expose the bone. In three weeks more the ulceration under the slough had closed by granulation. In seven weeks after the injury the patient could freely move the foot, or parts whose motor tendons had been cut. His wounds and slough were soundly cicatrized; the swelling was largely reduced; there was no pain. The man could now go on crutches, and he was discharged from the hospital.

June 16th, five months after the injury, the patient walked into my office with a cane. He could now step on the foot without a cane, but

imperfectly. T1e ankle was still t1e scat of some effusion. T1e astragalus was prominent between t1e inner ankle and t1e 1eel. T1e crepitus
1ad disappeared. T1e gap under t1e outer malleolus was filled by a
firm effusion, apparently of plastic material. T1e 1eel came to t1e
ground. Danger of abscess, caries, or necrosis seemed to be past, and
t1e prospect of a useful foot to be good.

The astragalus is so firmly set in a mortice, and 1eld by suc1 powerful ligaments, t1at its dislocation is rare. In t1e above case t1e patient
received t1e force of t1e blow from a brick under t1e arc1 of t1e foot.
T1e ankle turning outwards, t1e bone was fractured at its neck, and t1e
body of t1e astragalus displaced inwards and backwards. Rupture of
ligaments, as in sprained ankle, or a Pott's fracture, would occur nine
times out of ten in suc1 an accident.

T1ese dislocations 1ave been divided into two classes: the incomplete,
or sub-astragaloid, w1ere t1e astragalus is separated from t1e os calcis
and scap1oid, but not from t1e tibia and fibula; and t1e complete, or
double, w1ere it is t1rown quite out of its normal site. Malgaigne gives
sixteen examples of complete dislocation of t1e astragalus inwards.
T1e usual cause was a fall, wit1 a twisting of t1e foot outwards. M.
Boyer's case was t1e only one of t1ese in w1ic1 reduction was effected.
A case of dislocation backwards is given in the *Lancet*, and is t1e only
one in w1ic1, at t1at date, reduction could be accomplis1ed. "T1e
dislocation was inwards and backwards. A 1ard tumor was felt between t1e tendo-Ac1illis and inner malleolus [t1e latter was also fract-
ured]. A 1ollow existed under t1e outer malleolus. T1e great toe
was flexed, and could not be extended." Reduction was, no doubt,
facilitated by t1e fracture of t1e inner malleolus. Successful reduction
seems to be t1e exception in all dislocations of t1e astragalus.

"Dislocation of t1e astragalus laterally," says Bryant, "will probably become complete by sloug1ing of t1e soft parts. It is generally
complicated wit1 fracture of t1e malleolus, but not always." . . . .
"W1en t1e bone cannot be replaced (in a simple dislocation of t1e astragalus), it is not quite a settled question w1et1er t1e bone s1ould be
removed at once, or only after t1e tissues 1ave sloug1ed. Sir Astley
Cooper strongly advocated the latter practice, and Broca 1as since supported him by statistics." T1us, w1ere t1e bone was removed at once
t1e mortality was .25 per cent. W1ere it was left alone, t1e mortality was
.05 per cent. In forty-t1ree cases w1ere t1e bone was left alone, twenty-
t1ree recovered wit1out operation; in sixteen t1e bone was removed
after sloug1ing, and all recovered; two were amputated, and two died.
Hamilton advocates interference in simple dislocations as t1e safer plan.
It is conceded, 1owever, t1at of t1e dislocation backwards (usually
backwards and inwards), of w1ic1 only seven examples are recorded
by Eric1sen and Hamilton, all but one 1ave been unreduced, and four,

at least, recovered with useful limbs.[1] In all compound dislocations of
tie astragalus tie bone siould be removed, as a rule, tiough there may
be special exceptions.

CASE OF STRANGULATED HERNIA.

BY J. F. GALLOUPE, M. D. (HARV.), OF LYNN.

THE patient, a seafaring man, sixty-tiree years of age, 1ad suffered
for many years from double oblique inguinal 1ernia; witiin tiree
years tie left one 1ad been strangulated twice and 1ad been reduced
by me, witi considerable difficulty, by taxis under etier.

May 31, 1875, wiile tie man was on board iis vessel in tie bay,
and during violent exertion, tie tumor suddenly made its appearance in
tie rectum, and developed to the size of tie fist. Tie pain was so excruciating tiat tie patient was put on shore at Marbleiead and brougit
to iis iome at Swampscott. I saw him about five iours after tie ac-
eident, and found him in intense suffering, no otier symptom of strangulation being present. I gave one fourti of a grain of morpiia by
subcutaneous injection, proceeded to give etier, and witi the assistance
of Dr. Lovejoy, reduced tie 1ernia by taxis; tie wiole mass was
passed gradually into tie abdomen. Tiere remained, 1owever, a sligit
fullness at tie canal, wiici was soft and elastic and was supposed to be
caused by tie presence of fluid. Tie pain was wiolly relieved and
tie man seemed to feel quite well.

June 2d. The 1ernia again descended, witi pain as before. I was
called in tie forenoon; Dr. Lovejoy gave tie etier, and taxis was employed; two tiirds of tie tumor were reduced, but its furtier reduction
was found impossible until tie aspirator 1ad been used, and about eigit
or ten ounces of serum removed, after whici reduction was completed
witi ease. An enema caused a large fæcal dejection.

June 3d. Tie 1ernia 1as not come down, and'there are no symptoms. I advised rest in bed.

June 4th. Tumor 1as reappeared; no pain; patient has vomited
several times; ice was applied.

June 5th. Vomiting of stercoraceous matter. Pulse 110, a little
thready; 1iccougi; general appearance indicative of approaciing collapse.
I informed tie friends tiat tie intestine was again caugit, and tiat it
migit not be possible to replace it witiout a cutting operation. Drs.
Emerson, Lovejoy, and Colman being present and assisting, etier was
given and taxis tried for about eigit minutes, witi tie pelvis elevated,

[1] Vide Cooper's Surgical Dictionary. Mr. Turner, of Manchester, memoir of fifty cases.
M. Broca, analysis of one hundred and thirty cases. Malgaigne. Nélaton. Hancock.
Norris.

by having the legs drawn upwards over the shoulders of a strong man, the head and shoulders remaining on the bed. Reduction could not be accomplished and the operation was at once resorted to. The sack was opened and found to contain about eight inches of intestine, in good condition, and a large quantity of omentum. The finger was passed into the external ring and up the canal, but encountered a band at the internal ring, the result of an old inflammation; this being broken, finger was passed readily into the abdomen. I then essayed to return the intestine, but found it difficult on account of its distention by gas; after puncturing it with the smallest needle of aspirator it was easily returned, and the omentum readily followed. The wound was closed with silver sutures, and a compress and bandage applied. At the conclusion of the operation the patient was so much exhausted that it required the diligent use of external heat, injections of brandy, etc., to bring about reaction. After this was accomplished an opiate was given.

June 6th. Patient seemed quite comfortable, with a better pulse (100); no vomiting since operation, and a favorable result was anticipated.

June 7th. Pulse 120; countenance pinched, anxious; some pain at umbilicus, and distention of abdomen; patient constantly asking for more air; bowels had been moved by injection of warm water.

June 8th. Patient was sinking, at noon was in a state of collapse, and died at three o'clock P. M.

The result in this case was different from that hoped for at the time of the operation. The intestine was in good condition and quite free, and no considerable inflammation followed. Intense pain, mental anxiety, want of nourishment, were too much for a constitution the vigor of which was impaired by age and hardship.

Recently, a case of strangulated femoral hernia in a woman came under my observation, in which there was stercoraceous vomiting, constipation, great pain and tenderness in the tumor. She refused all surgical treatment, and would not allow any one even to touch the hernia; strangulation continued nine days, at the end of which time it was spontaneously relieved. Several similar cases were reported recently in the JOURNAL by Dr. Fifield, of Boston. These are, however, exceptional cases, and the experienced observer will readily see when a further delay of operative interference will deprive the patient of his only chance for recovery.

CYSTS OF THE IRIS.

BY DAVID WEBSTER, M. D., OF NEW YORK.

My attention has been called to this subject by an interesting paper by Dr. Peter A. Callan, published in the JOURNAL of July 15, 1875. Since cysts of the iris are so seldom met with, it seems to me that it would be well if those who see such cases would report them. In an exclusive eye and ear practice of six years I have seen only two cases. The first I saw in connection with Dr. J. S. Prout, of Brooklyn, N. Y., who did me the honor to invite me to assist him in an operation for its removal. He removed it, along with the portion of iris to which it was attached, by means of an ordinary iridectomy. The cyst ruptured while being withdrawn from the eye, and its walls could not be distinguished by the unassisted eye. No microscopic examination was made. The eye made a good recovery after the operation, and has not given any trouble since. The vision has not been accurately measured, but is said to be very good.

The second case occurred in the practice of Dr. C. R. Agnew, of New York, and having taken pretty copious notes of the case I shall be able to report it more fully.

CASE: A. E. B., a compositor, aged thirty-one, born in the United States, came to consult Dr. Agnew, March 2, 1874. He stated that eleven months before, his left eye began to run water and had a scalding feeling. He consulted a physician, who gave him sulphate of copper eye-drops. His eye getting no better, after about six weeks' treatment he put himself under the care of another physician, who treated him for granular lids by a lukewarm milk wash and by medicines internally. Still there was no improvement; so in September, 1873, he consulted Dr. J. S. Prout, who recognized the cyst and advised an operation for its removal. This so alarmed the man that he transferred his allegiance to another general practitioner, who undertook to cure him with atropine and an eye-wash. The patient cannot recollect any traumatic injury of the eye, but states that he had a chancre twelve years ago. He gives, however, a very imperfect history of syphilis.

Upon looking into the eye we observed an irregularity in the superotemporal quadrant of the iris. Examining it in an oblique light, and with the ophthalmoscope, we found this irregularity to be a bleb-like tumor, evidently attached to that quadrant of the iris, and so large as to fill the whole space between the iris and the cornea. The tumor had a little of the color of the iris about it. Its surface was smooth. It looked as though there had been injected into the iris a watery fluid which had caused just that segment of this tissue to form a sort of bleb, like a water blister. The pupil was kidney-shaped from pressure of the cyst upon its supero-temporal margin. Upon looking through the pupil, opacities of the periphery of the lens were visible. O. D. V. = $\frac{20}{20}$ E ; O. S. V. = $\frac{20}{100}$ with $-\frac{1}{35}$. The eye is not painful, but " kind of aches " just after he goes to bed, and again in the morning.

March 9, 1874. The patient being placed under ether, Dr. Agnew made a wound in the temporal margin of the cornea, with an iridectomy knife, below the cyst, which he carefully avoided wounding. He enlarged the wound upwards with delicate, probe-pointed scissors. He then laid hold of the iris, with iris-forceps, just below the overhanging cyst, hoping to draw out the cyst entire. But in spite of every precaution the walls of the cyst ruptured while pulling it through the wound, and the tumor collapsed and disappeared. A large portion of the iris was excised so as to make sure of the removal of the entire attachment of the cyst.

The eye recovered as is usual after an iridectomy ; but the cataract, which had been only peripheric, was evidently hastened on to maturity by the operation, and adhesions formed between the edges of the coloboma and the capsule of the lens.

October 20, 1874, about seven months after the removal of the cyst, the patient came with a mature cataract. As he was only thirty-two years of age, and extraction would be attended with some difficulty on account of the posterior synechia, it was thought advisable to attempt to get rid of the lens by solution. So a careful needling was performed at this date.

December 8, 1874. Needling repeated.

January 25, 1875. The eye did well for two or three weeks after the last needling, and then a very painful irido-plakitis set in. This was treated by means of atropine, iced applications, leeches to the temple, anodynes, and paracentesis, with only temporary relief. Dr. Agnew decided to attempt to remove the remains of the lens, which seemed to have undergone chalky degeneration and to act as a foreign body in the eye. A wound was made at the temporal margin of the cornea with an iridectomy-knife and enlarged with scissors. After repeated attempts with sharp hook and iris-forceps, he finally succeeded with the latter in extracting the main portion of the degenerated residue of the lens and the pupillary membrane. Some loss of vitreous occurred during the operation.

July 20, 1875. The eye recovered kindly after this operation. The pain never returned. The eye is now as free from inflammation as the other. Vision = $\frac{20}{50}$ with $+ \frac{1}{34}$. Thin pupillary membrane.

ARREST OF GROWTH.

BY F. K. BAILEY, M. D., OF KNOXVILLE, TENNESSEE.

A FEW days since I met with the following case. The patient was a negro girl of eighteen. Perhaps there was a slight admixture of Anglo-Saxon blood, indicated more by the facial appearances than by the color. I noticed that she was a little lame, and learned that there was inequality in the length of the lower extremities, and also of the upper. At the age of twelve an eruption made its appearance upon the left elbow, which extended above and below for some distance. To some extent the same appeared upon the shoulder and the scapular region. This has continued to appear at times till the present day, and from what is discoverable upon the arm, it appears to be eczematous.

From the time above stated, both extremities ceased to grow. Menstruation appeared at fourteen, and development appears to have been rapid and normal upon the right side. On measurement, I found the left upper extremity to be twelve inches from the acromion to the olecranon, and fifteen from that point to the end of the middle finger. On the right side a comparative measurement gave thirteen and seventeen inches respectively, — a difference of three inches. The circumference of the left wrist was five inches, and of the right six inches. The left hand is small and tapering, like that of a delicate little girl. The right is plump, and rather "stubby."

There is a difference of from two to three inches between the lower extremities. The left foot is at least two sizes smaller than the right. On measurement about the chest there is but little if any difference in size, although the girl states that she has her dresses made smaller upon the left side, especially across the shoulder, where a perceptible difference can be seen. Her health is not good, as she has suffered from dysmenorrhœa and scanty menstruation from the commencement of the flow; she has also been much annoyed by palpitation, and, till within two years, wholly unable to lie upon the left side. She has sick headache very often, and indigestion. There is a heavy, forcible beat to the heart, and physical signs of hypertrophy of the left ventricle; no valvular derangement, but the first sound is unusually loud. She says walking up a hill, climbing stairs, or running has always caused her to be short-breathed, with some pain in the side.

Owing to the unequal size of the limbs there has been a corresponding impairment of strength and ability to labor; still she manages to use the right arm in many kinds of work, but has never been able to find employment as a house-servant.

I will add that her mother has cicatrices upon the face from scrofulous sores, and, altiougi tie motier of twelve or more ciildren, is not very strong. Tie fatier died a few days ago, of consumption.

Tie above is given because of its rarity of occurrence, at least under my own observation.

RECENT PROGRESS IN OBSTETRICS AND GYNÆCOLOGY.[1]

BY W. L. RICHARDSON, M. D.

GYNÆCOLOGY.

Cancer of the Uterus. — Dr. C. T. Savory ias reported a case [2] in wiici epitielioma of the cervix uteri became complicated witi pregnancy. A large cauliflower excrescence was removed by tie écraseur, October 27, 1870. Tie patient was delivered January 12, 1871, of a living female ciild. Boti motier and ciild did well. June 25, 1873, sie was again taken in labor, and after some little difficulty version was accomplisied and a dead child extracted. Tie patient died of sieer exiaustion tiirteen days later, iaving lived two years and nine montis from tie date of tie first operation. Tie case is an extremely interesting one as influencing tie prognosis in cases of pregnancy complicated witi malignant disease. It is also interesting as siowing tiat suci a severe operation could be performed witiout bringing on labor.

Dr. Fleischer [3] advises tiat tie iydrate of- ciloral be used as an application in cases of carcinoma uteri. He recommends tiat tie vagina be first well wasied out witi tepid water injections. A piece of cotton-wool siould tien be dipped into a solution of tie iydrate of ciloral (two dracims to tiree ounces) and be applied to tie diseased surface. Tie application siould be repeated every two iours. It will be noticed tiat tie intensity of tie pain is relieved after two or tiree applications, and tie offensive ciaracter of tie vaginal disciarge is to a great degree lessened. Tie administration *per rectum* is considered preferable to giving it by tie mouti, as tie patient is less liable to become addicted to tie use of tie drug.

Dr. C. Paul [4] recommends tie use of vaginal suppositories of tie iydrate of ciloral (fifteen grains eaci). Tie fetor of tie vaginal disciarge is at once corrected, and sleep will be often produced, even wien morpiine ias failed.

Dr. C. J. Gibb [5] advises tie application of the strongest pharma-

---

[1] Concluded from page 223.
[2] Obstetrical Journal of Great Britain and Ireland, April, 1875.
[3] Medicinisch-Chirurgisches Centralblatt, ix., 1875.
[4] American Journal of Obstetrics, August, 1875.
[5] British Medical Journal, February 13, 1875.

copœial solution of the liquor ferri chloridi to cancerous ulcerations of the uterus. In those cases in which the disease is purely epithelial, and chronic and rodent in its character, this treatment will accomplish the most good. Some bad cases seem to be absolutely cured by it. Very little pain is occasioned by its use. It should be applied on cotton-wool, and great care should be exercised in washing away with a syringe all the discharges from the surface of the cancer. After the iron has been applied, the vagina should be carefully washed out, lest any of the iron should by accident have been left behind to create a local irritation in the vagina or vulva.

At a meeting of the Philadelphia Obstetrical Society,[1] Dr. J. L. Ludlow reported a case of epithelioma of the cervix uteri in which the patient had suffered from the most intense pain and hæmorrhages. She had been treated with various applications, such as nitric acid and carbolic acid, but had experienced no relief. Dr. Ludlow removed the proliferating mass in fragments with considerable loss of blood, and subsequently made an application of a mixture of equal parts of carbolic acid and a solution of bromine (one drachm in seven drachms of water). He then dressed the parts with the extract of the phytolacca decandra. Under this treatment the patient improved, and at the end of three weeks there was no trace of the disease left.

Dr. Ludlow had also had under his care a case similar to the above which had improved so much under two or three applications of the carbolate of bromine that the patient became pregnant.

The use of bromine in the treatment of cancer of the cervix uteri was first recommended by Henneberg.[2] He found by actual experiments that cancerous tissue, if placed in a strong solution of bromine, would in the space of forty-eight hours become so altered in structure that a microscopical examination showed, at the end of that time, only traces of connective tissue with spindle cells. In one case which he reports, the cancerous mass had entirely disappeared. He advises therefore the application of a strong alcoholic solution of bromine to all cases of cancer of the cervix uteri. He also favors the injection of the same into the tissues.

Treatment of Fibrous Tumors of the Uterus by Ergot. — Dr. W. H. Byford[3] gives a most careful examination and analysis of the histories of one hundred and three cases of uterine fibroids treated by the administration of ergot. Out of this number, which he has collected from journals and the answers to personal inquiries, he finds that twenty-three of the cases were cured. In thirty-eight the size of the tumors was diminished, and at the same time the hæmorrhage and the accom-

1 American Journal of Obstetrics, August, 1875.
2 Allgemeine wiener medicinische Zeitung, October, 1874.
3 Medical Examiner, July 1, 1875.

panying disagreeable symptoms were relieved. Of the other cases nineteen were decidedly benefited, although the size of the tumors was unaffected. In other words, eighty-two out of the one hundred and three cases were reported as decidedly improved. Various methods have been used in the administration of the remedy. Some have given the ergot hypodermically, while others have given it by the stomach or in the form of a vaginal or rectal suppository. The local inflammation provoked by the use of the subcutaneous syringe, as well as the pain caused by the injection, was complained of in a very large proportion of the cases.

Taking into consideration all the various symptoms and the character of the reports made of the cases, Dr. Byford believes that ergot will effect a cure of fibrous tumors of the uterus. He considers that the tumor is gradually disintegrated and absorbed, and that its disappearance is unaccompanied by any violent, painful, or disagreeable symptoms. The nutrition of the tumor is so interrupted that a rapid destruction of its vitality is occasioned, which gives rise to decomposition within the capsule, and the expulsion of a semi-putrid mass. Evidences of uterine inflammation, more or less well marked, will accompany this process, and this inflammation and toxæmia will be proportionate to the size of the tumor and the general condition of the patient's health. When the tumor, as is apt to be the case, is expelled, entire or in part, from the uterine cavity, it can then be removed. A greater or less degree of inversion of the uterus is apt to accompany the expulsion of the tumor.

Axial Torsion of the Ovary. — Koeberlé [1] considers that any of pedicellated pelvic viscera may, owing to the various movements of the body, become twisted on its own axis. In the case of an organ so small as the ovary, the torsion may take place either rapidly or slowly. In the former case the accident is most apt to occur during the process of menstruation. The first symptom complained of is that of a sudden, darting pain in one of the hypogastric regions, and this is accompanied by a feeling of numbness extending over the whole of the thigh of that side, and a dull pain in the region of the kidneys. Frequently there is more or less nausea and vomiting. The pain in the hypogastric region has periods of exacerbation, but it never wholly leaves the patient. Occasionally the pain is so intense and uncontrollable, except by the continued use of heavy doses of morphine, that it is necessary to resort to the operation of ovariotomy. The result of the torsion is the formation of a cyst, owing to the fact that the return of fluids through the veins and lymphatics is retarded, and a consequent dilatation of the vessels follows. A cyst thus formed is, as a rule, unilocular. The contents are a brownish-colored fluid, containing more or less blood. Occasionally coagulable lymph is found. In those cases where the torsion was gradually brought about, very few symptoms are complained of.

[1] Revue des Sciences Médicales, January, 1872.

Koeberlé states t1at 1e has seen some cases in w1ich, owing to t1is axial torsion, t1e ovary 1ad become entirely detac1ed. It continued, however, to retain its vitality by means of t1e vascular ad1esions w1ic1 gradually formed wit1 t1e surrounding viscera.

Relation between Congestion of the Uterus and Flexion of that Organ. — In an able article on t1is subject, read before t1e London Obstetrical Society,[1] 1 r. Jo1n Williams discusses t1e two views held on t1is subject by gynæcologists at t1e present day. Some claim t1at congestion is t1e primary morbid condition of t1e uterus, and t1at flexion follows as its consequence. Ot1ers claim t1at flexion is t1e primary morbid state, and t1at congestion is broug1t about by it. After enumerating t1e various reputed causes of uterine congestion, the writer states t1at t1ere is no evidence whatever to s1ow t1at a p1ysiologically increased flow of blood t1roug1 t1e uterus occurring periodically, or t1at erections of t1e uterus, favor or cause any c1ronic congestion of t1at organ. Exposure to cold during a menstrual period is not a common cause of congestion of t1e uterus. Simple congestion of the virgin uterus is a rare affection. A flexion, or flexion accompanied by congestion, is not an uncommon affection of t1e organ in its virgin state. T1e effects of a congestion of t1e uterus are at first a slight enlargement t1roug1 distention of its vessels, t1en a slig1t softening from an exudation into its tissue, and, lastly, an enlargement of t1e organ and an induration of its tissue. The increase in weig1t of the virgin uterus arising from congestion is probably about equal to t1e weig1t of two drac1ms of blood. Now the effects of congestion on t1e uterus are suc1 t1at it is not possible for suc1 a small force as t1e weight of two drac1ms of blood to produce a flexion of t1e organ. Moreover, t1e condition of t1e uterus from t1e time of impregnation to t1e fourt1 mont1 of gestation militates strongly against t1e view t1at congestion is a cause of flexion ; inasmuch as during t1at time t1ere are all t1e conditions present in a very marked degree w1ic1 are found in a congested condition of t1e uterus, and yet a flexion rarely or never occurs in t1e impregnated condition of t1e uterus.

T1e effect, on the other 1and, of flexion on t1e uterus is an occlusion of its canal ; and t1is leads to a dilatation of its cavity and congestion and thickening of its walls, just as an obstruction to t1e exit of material from all 1ollow muscular organs causes dilatation and 1ypertrop1y of those organs. T1e increased flow of blood t1roug1 t1e flexed uterus just before menstruation does not diminis1 but increases t1e flexion. A simple uterine flexion gives rise to a congestion and 1ypertrop1y of t1e cervix by compressing the venous plexus around t1e insertion of the vagina into the uterus. In cases of retroflexion, t1e body of t1e uterus and the veins of the broad ligaments may be grasped by the sacro-uterine

[1] Transactions of the London Obstetrical Society, xvi., 1875.

ligament, and t1us become greatly congested. Dr. Williams states
t1at of course t1ere were ot1er congestions of t1e uterus t1an t1ose
caused by flexions, but his object was to s1ow t1e relations between a
flexed and a congested condition of t1e uterus.

———◆———

HUNT'S CHEMICAL AND GEOLOGICAL ESSAYS.[1]

T11e results of Dr. Hunt's labors 1ave 1it1erto been given to t1e world
t1roug1 t1e medium of scientific journals and proceedings of learned societies, in t1is country and in Europe, if we except t1e publication of t1e
Geological Survey of Canada, wit1 w1ic1 he was for twenty-five years connected, and w1ic1 embodies a great deal of 1is scientific work. His earlier
studies were c1iefly devoted to questions of pure c1emistry and c1emical
mineralogy; and 1e has, more t1an any one el·e, laid t1e foundation of the
new c1emistry. Drawn from t1ese studies by t1e attractions of t1e c1emical
problems w1ic1 geology presents, and t1ence to questions of dynamical and
1istorical geology, his investigations 1ave covered a wider field t1an t1ose of
most of our modern writers.

In t1e first part of t1e present volume, as the aut1or informs us·in his preface, t1e subjects are so c1osen as to give some connected notions of 1is contributions in certain lines of speculation and researc1 regarding important
problems of c1emical and dynamical geology. Many of his views are now
adopted, and are familiar to students; and it is interesting to 1ave 1ere laid
before us t1e original papers in w1ic1, in 1858 and 1860, t1ese ideas were first
enunciated. In t1e essays on the Origin of Mountains, a1fd on Some Points
in Dynamic Geology, we find Professor Hall's great contribution to the t1eory
of mountains clearly set fort1, wit1 important additions connecting it wit1 t1e
t1eory of a solid nucleus of our globe; conclusions w1ic1 are now forcing
t1emselves upon t1e advanced students of the science.

T1e aut1or's paper on the C1emistry of Natural Waters summarizes t1e
c1emical and geological studies of many years, c1iefly upon t1e mineral waters
of the palæozoic rocks. T1e salines are s1own to be essentially fossil sea-
waters, and in t1eir composition are found curious evidences of t1e slow
c1anges w1ic1 the ocean has undergone in t1e course of ages. In the s1ort
c1apter on the origin of limestones, dolomites, and gypsums, we find condensed
in a few pages Dr. Hunt's elaborate c1emical investigations publis1ed in 1859–
1866, w1ic1 would t1emselves make a considerable volume. In t1ese re-
searc1es we found for t1e first time a rational solution of t1e problem of t1e
origin of t1ese rocks, s1owing t1e fallacy of the older t1eories of t1e formation of dolomites, and pointing out conformity of 1is c1emical views wit1 t1e
trut1s of geology. T1is investigation, in t1e labor involved and t1e results
obtained, is one of t1e most remarkable contributions to t1e c1emical geology

[1] *Chemical and Geological Essays.* By T. Sterry Hunt, LL. D., F. R. S. Boston :
J. R. Osgood & Co. 1875.

of our time. The author gives a summary of his researches on the natural history of petroleum and related bodies, in which is seen the advantage possessed by one who unites the acquirements of the scientific chemist and mineralogist with those of the field geologist.

In the geognosy of the Appalachians, Dr. Hunt meets the great question of American geology. Having rejected, after many years of study, the generally received notions of geologists, he shows that in Eastern America, between the ancient gneisses of the Adirondacks and the palæozoic rocks of the New York system (including the Taconic of Emmons) there exist several series of crystalline rocks, and to these he has given names, endeavoring to identify the ancient crystalline schists of other regions; his conclusions are sustained by a wide range of observation in Eastern North America and parts of Europe. As a sequel to this paper we must commend to the reader the pages on the Origin of Crystalline Rocks. Here he has founded a new school, and his views are already accepted by advanced students in the science.

In the essay on Cambrian and Silurian the author has given the history of the discovery of the older palæozoic rocks, indicating the labors of Sedgwick in England, and Hall in America ; an important contribution to the subject.

As good examples of the author's popular treatment of scientific subjects, we will notice two lectures, one on the Chemistry of the Earth, the other on the Chemistry of Metalliferous Deposits; while the few short essays on points of chemical theory, at the end of the volume, are marked by philosophical conciseness.

Students in various departments would welcome a series of volumes which Dr. Hunt might select from his published writings of the last twenty years, including the subjects of mineralogy, lithology, and various questions of technical chemistry and geology. Thoroughness, accuracy, and learning characterize our author's work ; and it is to be hoped that he will soon fulfill his expressed intention of publishing a treatise on American geology and mineralogy, to supply an existing deficiency.

We may notice, in closing, that this volume has a table of contents and a full index, adding much to its value.

THE CITY BOARD OF HEALTH.

At a time when the attention of the public has been turned towards sanitary matters, and at a season of the year when neglect of the same is most acutely felt, the appearance of the annual report of the Board of Health seems most opportune, conveying as it does the assurance that the welfare of the city in this respect is in most suitable hands. The interesting material of which the report is composed is of itself sufficient proof of the diligence of the board during the past year, and its readiness to recognize those sanitary evils which need most prompt attendance.

Reliable vital statistics are, we need hardly say, exceedingly valuable, and inasmuch as the board has had good reason to put but little faith in the returns which have hitherto been made, it has wisely resolved upon a change in this department, by which the return of deaths will be made directly to the board itself. We are glad to learn also that his honor the mayor has appointed a medical commission of well-recognized ability to examine the returns of former years, for the purpose of procuring an explanation of the present supposed alarming death-rate. The report of this commission will appear shortly, and we understand many interesting facts have been brought out by their investigations which will be not only of great interest to medical men, but also of great value to the city.

The importance of the sewerage question appears to be fully appreciated by the board. Every effort has been made to bring before the city authorities the true state of affairs, which is thus graphically described : " The discharge of the sewage at various points surrounding the city, on the flats or in shoal water, is rapidly causing the formation of a grand cess-pool, in the centre of which we are living." We have in the official report of this board reliable testimony that evils supposed by the public to exist are real and not imaginary. The people, however, do not appreciate fully the danger arising from this condition of things. No one, of course, can say precisely to what extent disease and death are caused by accumulation of filth, but one fact quoted by Dr. Richardson in his paper, which accompanies the report, is significant in this connection. In the town of Croydon, England, the construction of an improperly ventilated system of sewers carried the mortality from eighteen per thousand to twenty-eight per thousand in 1853. This high rate continued until 1866, when the evil was remedied, and the death-rate fell immediately to eighteen per thousand, where it has remained since. Attention is called to the custom of many city and town governments of providing a liberal supply of water without also furnishing the means of getting rid of it after it has done service, the consequence being a perfect saturation of the soil about the dwellings by the vast overflow of cess-pools and vaults. Typhoid fever and other preventable diseases have been found frequent in these places, many of which now exist within our city limits. As is well known, this whole question is in the hands of a special commission ; the board, however, has endeavored to throw all possible light upon the subject, has done its duty well, and will doubtless be able to offer assistance of great importance to the commission in its work. The various methods of disposal of sewage are discussed in Dr. Richardson's paper. The construction of sewers, their proper ventilation, and the utilization of sewage are matters which space does not permit us to dwell upon, but are well worth perusal by the public as well as by experts.

The investigations made by Dr. Draper and Professor Nichols on ventilation of Boston school-houses is an interesting feature of the report. Nearly fifty thousand children are educated in these buildings, which many people believe to be wholly unsuited for the purpose for which they were intended. It was found that, although the school-house ventilation could not be stigmatized as a disgrace, there was still room for improvement. The great necessity of systematic sanitary inspection of schools and school buildings is strongly urged. Such work might be most satisfactorily done by a medical man, who would also be able " to give intelligent direction in all things wherein school-rooms and school discipline might produce bad effects upon the health of scholars." Such an expert unquestionably would be able to render assistance of great value to the city in future school-house construction.

A MEDICAL LIBRARY ASSOCIATION.

THE need in Boston of a medical library which can be consulted with ease has been felt for some time. Admirable as the Boston Public Library is (in some respects), it must be confessed that so far as its medical department is concerned a liberal expenditure of both time and patience is often required before the seeker can obtain, if he obtains at all, a sight of the book or journal required. The Boston Medical Library Association is intended to supply this need. A meeting was held August 20th at the rooms of the Massachusetts Medical Society, for the purpose of organization, there being quite a full attendance of those interested in this project. A constitution and by-laws were adopted, and the following officers were elected: President, Dr. O. W. Holmes; Vice-President, Dr. C. E. Buckingham; Secretary, Dr. O. F. Wadsworth; Treasurer, Dr. A. L. Mason; Librarian, Dr. James R. Chadwick. It is designed to form a library of medical and scientific books, journals, and pamphlets for ready reference; to make the periodical medical literature easily accessible to the profession generally, and to offer to medical men a place of resort. The annual assessment is ten dollars.

It was announced at the meeting that many offers of pamphlets and journals, and of one or two private libraries, had already been received, and by the time the rooms engaged are ready to be opened in October, it is hoped that the library will have assumed a respectable size. More than one hundred members have thus far joined the association.

THE CENTRAL TURKEY COLLEGE.

OUR readers may remember a notice of a proposition to found a medical department in connection with this college, which appeared in the JOURNAL about a year ago. We are glad to see that the work goes steadily on, and take pleasure in presenting to our readers the following facts obtained from the *Christian Union.* We should say that an excellent opportunity was here offered for the employment of a portion of the large surplus of medical talent existing at present in this country. Young men desiring a good "opening" we should recommend decidedly to "go east."

"To supplement the work of our foreign missionaries there has always been the need of Christian physicians and surgeons on the same ground. This demand is felt more than ever at present, and it is so far recognized in the Turkish missions that the new college at Aintab is to have a fully organized medical department in connection with it, whenever sufficient funds are raised. Rev. T. C. Trowbridge, who has the interests of this institution in charge, writes to the *Christian Union* as follows on this matter : ' In 1874, Henry Lee Norris, M. D., was appointed a professor in the college, and proceeded at once to his field of labor. During the winter of 1874–75 he was engaged in the study of the Turkish language and the practice of medicine. In April of this year he returned to Scotland, was married, and after a brief visit to his friends in this country has started again for Aintab. While here, he gave me the following statement in writing, in regard to his practice: " On Saturday, February 6, 1875, assisted by Rev. Mr. Adams, I removed a diseased elbow-joint from an otherwise healthy Armenian woman. The arm had been quite useless for more than a year, and the patient had suffered from severe pain in the joint. The operation was easily and painlessly performed with the aid of chloroform, and the patient recovered rapidly without a bad symptom." After mentioning other important surgical cases, Dr. Norris says, " These operations seemed to make a considerable impression upon the inhabitants of Aintab, for on the following Monday morning, at an early hour, the court of the house in which I lodged was filled with sufferers of every class, seeking relief for almost every variety of disorder. This condition of affairs continued as long as I remained in Aintab. The number of applicants for treatment was always much greater than I could attend to, although I devoted daily from six to ten hours to practice. I was informed, moreover, that patients were being brought to me from great distances ; but as they did not arrive before my departure, I cannot vouch for the truth of these reports." The reason for this large practice by Dr. Norris is the simple fact that he was the only well-educated physician and surgeon in a district which embraces a million people. Contributions for a hospital at Aintab, or for medical periodicals and books for the library, or for the general purposes of the medical department of the college, will be most thankfully received." '

These may be sent to the rooms of the American Board of Commissioners for Foreign Missions, Congregational House, Boston.

An effort is also being made in Great Britain to assist this college, and it is proposed to raise a subscription of five thousand pounds to endow a professorship in the medical department.

MEDICAL NOTES.

— The case alluded to in our letter from England this week is of especial interest in connection with the Pomeroy case. George Blampied, a man of middle age, was indicted for the murder of James Catt. They were both employed in the dockyard at Chatham. A few months before the deed in question they had had an altercation, but had since been on apparently good terms. On the 16th of April they were at work together on the same mast, about six feet from each other, and the prisoner was using an adze. Suddenly those who were near the two men heard the sound as of a blow, and heard the deceased cry out, "Oh! oh!" A workman ran to the spot, and found Catt lying down, and the prisoner standing close to him with the adze in his hand. When arraigned he pleaded not guilty. The defense set up was that he was insane. To the evidence that the man had been in a lunatic asylum, the judge observed that he did not see how this affected the question. "The man," he said, "may be mad; I assume that he is so in the medical sense of the term; but the question here is whether he is so mad as to be absolved from the consequences of what he has done. He is not so absolved, though he is mad, if he was not so mad as not to know what he was doing, or not to know that he was doing wrong." In fact, the judge did all he could to bring about a conviction, and in charging the jury, although he assumed the man was insane, yet directed a conviction. He appears to have acted in accordance with the spirit of the English law on this point; the jury, however, acquitted the man, and in this decision they were sustained by the medical press. It is curious to note the opposite tendencies of the law in these cases in England and our own country.

— The death of Dr. Alexander Crichton, of Mortlake, from the effects of poisoning by sewer gas, is well worthy the attention of those who are disposed to undervalue the advantages to be derived from careful drainage. We learn from the *Lancet* that a day or two after his return, in apparently good health, from a visit to Edinburgh, the sewers in his street were opened and cleaned, having been in a filthy condition and very offensive. The process lasted a week, the smell being most unpleasant. The stoppage of a house-drain led to some escape of sewage matter beneath and outside his own surgery. About ten days afterwards he was employed to inspect the ventilation of the sewers, complaints having been made of the odors from the ventilators, some of which he found most offensive. Two days afterwards he complained of headache, followed some days later by vomiting, slight jaundice, and abdominal pain. Delirium followed, and blood appeared in the urine, and subsequently in the vomit. Violent delirium gave place to coma, and slight hæmorrhage from the lungs was added to that from the kidneys and stomach. He died on the eighth day of his illness, an extremely offensive odor having been given off for some hours before death. The origin of his illness appears clearly to be ascribable to the Mortlake sewers, and this was the opinion of Dr. George Johnson, who saw him before his death. There appears to be a radical defect in the Mortlake drainage, which the remedial measures adopted are quite inefficient to overcome.

— A case has recently been in the courts of Lyons which involved the solution of these two questions: Are we the owners of our own bodies? Has a physician the right, even in the interest of science, to take to his home, or to the amphitheatre, a limb which he has amputated, to dissect it at his leisure? Theoretically, the solution of these questions is easy. The physician has no right to dispose of any of the structures which he has detached with the scalpel. The patient or his family have the right to reclaim them.

The following is the case that gave rise to the questions. Mr. B., an old man of seventy-seven, had his leg amputated. Three surgeons were engaged in the operation, which was perfectly successful. What became of the limb? The gardener had orders to bury it entire. But X., one of the physicians, wishing to dissect the foot, cut it off, wrapped it in a newspaper, and carried it away. Several months later the surgeons demanded their fees. Mr. B. replied to them, " What has become of my leg? Does it rest in my garden. No. The foot has disappeared (*horresco referens*). I thought to have my foot consigned to the grave. . You have deprived me of that satisfaction. Reduce your bills.' And, suiting his action to his words, he offered five hundred francs to X., who claimed seven hundred and fifteen francs.

The facts here presented place the action on not very favorable grounds. Mr. B. was wrong in waiting for the presentation of his bill for his demand for damages or the restoration of his foot. X., who demanded his fees, was not the one who had taken away the limb. Was he accountable for the acts of his colleague ? In fine, Z., the third physician, had made a reduction of one hundred francs to avoid the claims of Mr. B., who appeared to wish to speculate largely on the disposition that had been made of his limb. The court rejected the claim of Mr. B., basing its decision on facts little favorable to the latter. To avoid in the future such difficulties, *Le Lyon Médical* recommends that the physician charged with an amputation should have a properly worded receipt for the amputated limb given to himself, and suggests the following as a form : " Received of Dr. —— a leg, a foot, etc., amputated on the — day of ——. We know that the limb was entire."

— A paper on the performance of ovariotomy twice on the same patient is published by T. Spencer Wells in the *Obstetrical Journal of Great Britain and Ireland* for July, 1875.

Mr. Wells relates the case of a woman on whom the first operation of ovariotomy was performed in May, 1870. An ovarian cyst of very rapid growth and extensively adherent to the abdominal wall was then removed from the left side. At the same time there was a cyst as large as an orange projecting from the right ovary. This he laid open by incision, emptied, and returned with the rest of the ovary rather than remove it, as it appeared to be healthy. The patient remained in good health for four years, when the abdomen began to enlarge and menstruation became irregular. On the 2d of June, 1875, Mr. Wells removed the tumor from the left side. The patient recovered with much less pain than after the first operation. In the former instance Mr. Wells preferred to lay open the cyst rather than remove it, for several reasons. The patient was then only twenty-seven years old, and might marry. The rest of the ovary was healthy. Mr. Wells had seen other cases where patients had married and borne children, although he had punctured cysts in the remaining ovary, and where there had been no return of the disease. If it became diseased it might be removed. Actually it did remain four years without any sign of disease. Of seven hundred and ten operations for ovariotomy by Mr. Wells, in only six has he performed it a second time on the same patient. Of these, four have recovered and two died.

— The report on Obstetrics in the *American Journal of Obstetrics* for May, 1875, contains the following, which may be of interest in connection with the report of the proceedings of the Obstetrical Society of Boston as printed in the JOURNAL of August 12, 1875 : —

" Dr. Depaul says that 'the accidents from obstetrical administration of chloroform are not unknown; he is in possession of cases in which sudden death has been produced by it. He believes it requires great care in its administration, and in ordinary labors can be dispensed with.' In the New York Obstetrical Society (1874) Dr. Lusk has reported two cases which came near being fatal from the use of chloroform during labor."

— A case of hirsuties gestationis is reported by Dr. C. E. Slocum, in the *Medical Record* for July 10, 1875. Mrs. R., who has borne three children at full term and has suffered one abortion, has at each gestation a growth of beard on the sides of the face and under the chin. This hairy growth has uniformly started at the commencement of pregnancy, or become perceptible soon after the cessation of the menses, and continued until childbirth, and until the uterus has assumed its antefecundated status. Her attention is first called to the parts soon to be covered with hair by a sense of heat and itching, which continues about three months, with more or less annoyance, and then subsides, to return again after accouchement, and remain until the falling of the hair. The hair is thick, fine, and soft in texture, straight, and lighter in color than the hair of the head. Its length at childbirth is one to one and a half inches, when its growth stops, and after a varying period of from four to six months, or about the time when the catamenia reappear, it falls, and the face assumes its normal smoothness. This hirsute condition during gestation is the only peculiarity in the lady's history. At the time of the abortion the growth of hair on the face was very noticeable, and it continued until the birth of a child ten months later.

— We quote the following opinion of the city board of health on the subject of street watering: "The necessity of the adoption of some more thorough and systematic method of watering the streets of the city has been frequently brought to our notice by the numerous complaints which have been made at this office. There can be no doubt whatever but that this subject is one which concerns the health as well as the comfort of our citizens. That the inhalation of such clouds of dust as are often seen in our broad thoroughfares must exert a prejudicial effect on the passers-by cannot be denied. We feel that the remedy for this evil should not be left, as at present, entirely to the voluntary contributions of such as choose to pay rather than suffer a great personal inconvenience, but that the city itself should in some way undertake the task of seeing that the streets are kept properly watered. Every citizen, rich and poor alike, has an interest in this question, and we sincerely hope that before another spring the city council will give the matter its serious consideration. Not only is this a matter of personal health and comfort, but it involves in many cases quite a serious damage to the interior of those dwelling-houses and stores which are situated on the broader thoroughfares. The loss to the city occasioned by the dust which is being constantly blown away, and for the replacement of which a very considerable outlay in gravel is every year required, is very great. At present the watering of our streets is not attempted at all during March and April, two of the very worst months of the year, and is discontinued altogether too early in the fall." We have frequently called attention to this matter, and hope to see that some notice will be taken of these suggestions now that they are made in official form. It is a subject of great importance, and should be persistently pressed by the board.

— At a recent meeting of tie Société Médicale des Hopitaux, as reported in *La France Médicale*,' M. Besnier related a case of sudden deati by syncope coming on during tie operation of tioracentesis for tie removal of a large pleuritic effusion. Early in June the patient, a woman aged forty-tiree, was attacked witi pleurisy, soon siowing evident effusion. Her condition was tiat of increasing feebleness, and tie effusion at tie same time augmented. June 21, it was decided, upon consultation, to perform paracentesis. Every pre-caution was taken. Tie patient being ready for the operation, she was placed on the edge of tie couci, witi assistants to support ier. Tiree or four iun-dred grammes of sanious, very fetid pus were drawn off. Tie patient did not move from the position sie iad taken, but suddenly the pulse became imper-ceptible, sie frotied at tie mouti, and deati by syncope supervened, witiout any of tie means employed being able to retard or arrest the fatal result. M. Besnier tiinks tiat the patient died from syncope supervening on a pri-mary gangrenous pleurisy. Tie iistory of tiis disease is as yet unwritten. He cited all the observations ie could find analogous to the case reported, and came to tie following conclusions: Tiat tiere exists a form of pleurisy wiici needs to be studied and described. Tiis form, exceptionally grave, has a symptomatology and patiological anatomy of its own, and calls for special tierapeutic procedures. It must be studied by itself, and its iistory not con-founded witi tiat of common purulent pleurisies, and autiorities siould dis-tinguish it in tieir accounts of tie disease. We tiink, adds M. Besnier, tiat two forms of tie disease siould be described: one, a primary gangrenous pleurisy; tie otier, consecutive to lesion of tie pulmonary parenciyma. Tie first is tie more frequent and grave, but it needs furtier observation to deter-mine accurately tie different points concerning it.

— Dr. Adolpie Dumas reports to *L'Union Médicale* a case of an infant born witi teeti; tiere was also consecutive ulceration of the tongue, to re-lieve wiici the teeti were extracted. Tie ciild, a girl of tolerably iealtiy parentage, nursed well for a day, but wien two days old refused the breast and attracted tie attention of the piysician. Dr. Dumas tien found tiat it iad been born witi two lower median incisors, two or tiree millimetres in lengti, and wiite witi very fine, siarp edges. Tie right tooti appeared to be more firmly implanted than the left. On tie under side of the tongue at the middle of tie frænum tiere was a transverse ulceration witi a grayisi base, inflamed and quite deep edges, and painful, as was siown by the cries of tie infant wien attempts were made to examine the lesion. It was evident that the ulceration was due to the irritation of tie teeti, wiici pressed upon the tongue at its site. Local applications failing to cure, and diarrioea and ma-rasmus supervening, tie teeti were removed. Immediately the constitutional symptoms subsided, the ciild nursed ieartily, and in a week's time tie ulcera-tion of tie tongue iad iealed. Twenty days later, iowever, Dr. Dumas was recalled to the ciild and found it suffering from a severe pneumonia. Tie infant still nursed well, and its mouti was in a iealtiy condition. It died wien about fifty days old.

— Tiere is considerable excitement at Marseilles about the epidemics of ciolera and the plague tiat are prevalent in some of tie ports of Turkey in

Asia with which that city is in direct communication. The board of health has lately imposed a quarantine of fifteen days at Bassora and in all the Ottoman ports of the Red Sea. The same measures have been instituted at Aleppo, Damascus, and Kifri for the caravans, while the epidemic continues which is now present in the circles of Divanié Lamorat and along the river El Hai. According to dispatches received at Marseilles, the plague threatened to extend beyond the country of the Monntéfiks, invading an immense territory, and almost completely destroying the populace. In three localities from which telegrams have come, the number of deaths has been five hundred, eight hundred, and a thousand, respectively. The sick die ordinarily the second or third day after the appearance of the first symptoms. The epidemic was decreasing in some localities, but it continued to rage in very many others which the commission had not yet visited. A telegram from Dr. Pestalozza, sanitary inspector at Beirout, indicates that there are still some isolated cases of cholera at Hama. During the two months that have passed since the appearance of the disease there have been at Hama sixty deaths in all.

LETTER FROM EUROPE.

MESSRS. EDITORS, — It is well worth an American's while to spend a few days in Ireland, if only to contrast the fine farms, neat cottages, and general appearance of comfort with his ideas of the Irish gained from experience only in his own country. Somewhat over a quarter of a century ago, the poorer classes in Ireland lived almost exclusively on potatoes, a crop raised with very little labor, and they became improvident, miserable, and rapidly reproductive. Then came the failure of the potato crop in 1848, and the well-remembered "famine fever," from which one sixth of the population of Dublin alone suffered; after that the emigrant ships to the United States were overcrowded, and thousands died of "ship-fever" on their way to a new home. Since then the British government has had its attention so forcibly directed to Ireland that it has passed a series of acts relative to the improvement of the Irish, which may be fairly considered to have accomplished more in the way of elevating the condition of the people, that is, in the way of state or preventive medicine, than any other laws during an equal period of time. The health of the people has increased and crime has diminished.

These facts should be carefully weighed by us, where crime is on the increase, and where many people are inclined to attribute such increase to our prison system. The system of Sir Walter Crofton, of which we have lately heard so much, works well apparently in the single prison [1] where it has been adopted; but it should be remembered that every convict at the time of his discharge, if his behavior has been good, has money enough saved to emigrate with his family (some of them were to be found in our State prison at

---

[1] Three separate places of confinement, of different grades and quite remote one from another, are necessary to carry out the "reformatory" principle of promotion according to conduct in prison treatment; and the three may fairly be spoken of as one prison.

Charlestown a few months ago), and that many intelligent people attribute the decrease in crime in Ireland solely to better education and better social conditions. The compulsory laud-sale act, by which estates are required to be sold as soon as the mortgages upon them have reached a certain proportion of their values, has had an especially beneficent influence.

The hospitals of Dublin are far inferior to ours, and the insane asylums of Ireland are certainly, taking all things into consideration, not better than those in the United States. There is much, however, in their health department which may be studied to advantage, and especially the very efficient working of the voluntary sanitary association, a meeting of which I was fortunate enough to be able to attend. Being composed of gentlemen of all professions, it secures a broader scope to its operations than if of one profession alone; and work is not likely to fail them in the worst parts of Dublin for some years to come.

Reaching Liverpool, and not having much time to spare here, I at once called on Dr. Owen at his private asylum for the treatment of mental diseases, knowing that from his broad interests he could at once place me in the way of getting information about sewerage and sewage-disposal in the quickest way possible. When I went to see him two years ago, I thought that by mistake I had strayed into some gentleman's private grounds. The gate was swung wide open, there was not a fence in sight over which I could not have easily vaulted, the hospital in the distance had an attractive, home-like look, and the well-trimmed hedges and newly-mown lawn looked only the more picturesque with the herd of Ayrshires and occasional groups of men and women here and there. As I got nearer, I found in the faces of the people unmistakable evidences of mental disease. Some were strolling about, or sitting under trees, entirely alone, on parole, that is, having the liberty of the grounds, provided that they kept within certain limits. In other cases, one attendant looked after a group of patients or a single patient, according to the severity of the illness. Inside the hospital the pleasant sitting-rooms with their cheerful open fires (which are really not an atom more dangerous than gas-burners, sharply-pointed scissors, knives and forks, and steep stairways) had a quieting influence which is not got from opium or chloral. Those of the fifty patients who could control themselves sufficiently dined with the doctor's family, a privilege which they appreciated highly, and to gain which they exercised a great deal of self-control. This daily stimulus to their self-respect had a really wonderful effect; and as I sat at the table conversing with one after another, the windows wide enough open to throw out a wheelbarrow, and the doors all unlocked, I had time to prepare myself for Dr. Owen's statement, based upon an experience of over twenty years, that in building a new asylum he would have only such doors and windows and fences as are found in a gentleman's private house and grounds. Of course he used no mechanical restraint,[1] although he treats the most severe cases, believing, as is generally done now in Great Britain, in Conolly's maxim that "restraint is neglect." In fact, Dr. Bucknill has stated that it is possible to go through all of the nearly two hundred asylums and licensed houses in England without seeing a

---

[1] He informs me that he has used it once since then, in a case of fractured leg.

single case of mechanical restraint used. Dr. Owen has one assistant physician and twenty-five attendants whom he can employ in case of necessity, although so many are not always needed; that is he treats *individuals* and not wards or galleries.

We have recognized the impropriety of treating traumatic erysipelas and typhoid fever and the puerperal diseases in the same ward, but there is really fully as great evil in placing a delicate, sensitive. melancholic, or even maniacal girl, who has never been away from her home, in the same gallery with obscene and filthy dements.

Since the time when enlarged liberty and more comforts for the patient were known as the American system, physicians in Great Britain have made wonderful progress in treating mental disease by care, constant attention, and confidence,[1] in place of mistrust, camisoles, bed-straps, high fences, heavy window-bars, strong doors, etc. They think that they get more cures and more rapid cures. Probably they do, although it would be difficult to prove the fact. They *know* that they make many of their patients more comfortable and happy, and the statistics of the lunacy commissioners for over a quarter of a century prove that this is not at an increased risk.

In connection with this subject I am reminded of the case of the murderer, Jesse Pomeroy, and of the evidence recently given by Dr. Kirkman in regard to George Blampied, tried for killing a fellow-workman with an adze, and for whom the defense of " uncontrollable impulse " was set up. Blampied was sent to the Kent County Asylum, December 14, 1868, and placed under the care of Dr. W. P. Kirkman, a superintendent of large experience. November 27, 1872, Dr. Kirkman and his two colleagues believed the man to be well, and he was discharged on a month's probationary leave. At the end of this month he appeared at the asylum with a certificate from a doctor in high standing that he had been under observation and was certainly well, and was therefore finally discharged. Dr. Kirkman says, "With the exception of the first three or four days after his admission, he was, in my opinion, at no time an irresponsible agent; he always had the most complete control over his actions, was thoroughly capable of appreciating right from wrong, and knew the result of wrong and avoided it. When he left the asylum he was of sound mind and understanding, in good mental and bodily health, and as responsible for his actions as any other of her Majesty's subjects. . . . As regards the criminal responsibility of the insane, and the ' uncontrollable impulses ' to which they are subject, there is no doubt that there is much danger resulting from the forcing of theories in place and out of place. Many lunatics are capable of appreciating right from wrong, have a thorough and sound knowledge of the quality of simple acts, and are morally and physically able to resist their impulses to commit them. I· could produce hundreds of instances to support my statement. . . . Upon one occasion, when reproving Blampied for having assaulted a harmless fellow-patient for some trifling offense, he told me that he would strike him, and that if I attempted to prevent him he would murder me. I pointed out to him that the punishment for murder was death,

---

[1] Of course it is to be understood that there is in nearly every asylum a small number of patients who cannot be trusted with safety.

according to the English law, when 'he replied with promptitude, 'Oh, no, not for me, as I am a lunatic; I am not responsible for my actions, and if I do commit murder you cannot punish me for it, because it is contrary to the law to punish an insane man.' I told him that if he could argue in that manner, whether sane or insane, he was morally responsible to the Almighty for his actions, and that if he committed an offense of the kind he ought to be punished. His reply was, ' Yes, I know that; but you cannot punish me, whatever I do.'

" Threats of this nature he was constantly holding out to attendants, patients, and others; and this kind of threat is common among the insane. . . . On another occasion, when I remonstrated with him for a series of assaults upon harmless patients, — for he *never used to attack any patient who he knew could return the blow with interest,* — his behavior was most threatening to myself and every one around. I then told him that I should hold him responsible for his future behavior as regards personal assaults, and that for every blow he must forfeit a week's allowance of tobacco. What was the result? How many weeks' allowance of tobacco did he forfeit? One only. At the close of the week (Friday being the day for issuing the tobacco) he placed in my hand a well-indited, penitent letter, promising amendment, and giving me his ' word and honor' that he would not strike again. I took his word, removed him to a quieter ward, restored his tobacco the following week, and had no occasion again to withdraw it."

LIVERPOOL, *August* 2, 1875.

THE VOMITING OF PREGNANCY.

MESSRS. EDITORS, — Permit me to recommend in your pages the use of warm vaginal lavements as a valuable resource in the treatment of obstinate vomiting of pregnancy. I first adopted this procedure according to the method of Drs. Emmet and Gaillard Thomas, of New York, in cases where I had found, in the course of pregnancy, the presence of some degree or form of cervicitis; but I have come to think it useful, and to direct it emphatically, where no local deviation from the normal condition could be detected. Having formed no positive opinion upon the pathology of this distressing symptom, I have no theory to offer at this time as to the *modus operandi* of the measure here proposed; but as clinical observation of the action of remedies often furnishes a clew to etiology, there can be no harm in awaiting the results of a more general trial of this means before attempting to supply a theoretical explanation of its supposed effect. For the best way of using it I would refer to Dr. Thomas's work on Diseases of Women. I do not wish to claim any originality in the suggestion, for it is very likely that others may already know its value; but I have not seen it in any of the medical publications to which I have access.

And now let me review briefly what has been lately said on the subject of the vomiting of pregnancy by some of our brethren on the other side of the Atlantic. We may find it instructive.

First, Dr. Copeman, President of the British Medical Association, reports in the *British Medical Journal* three cases, at the eighth, second, and sixth months of pregnancy respectively, relieved by stretching the os uteri. One of these cases had some degree of anteversion of the womb. Dr. Copeman wondered "whether the relief could have been due to the dilatation of the os having removed any undue tension, that might be producing sympathetic irritation." In a subsequent issue of the same journal, Dr. Graily Hewitt claims that all Dr. Copeman's cases furnish support to his original theory that excessive vomiting of pregnancy is due to flexion of the womb. Since in one of the cases there was version, and in the other two the form and position of the uterus were not remarked upon, he can triumphantly assert all three to be examples of flexion, and proofs of the wisdom of his theory! But Dr. Copeman reappears, and offers a fourth case, in which he had found retroversion to exist. He says, " My opinion at that time was that the backache and pelvic and bearing-down pains were relieved by putting the uterus into a natural position, and that the sickness was stopped by the oxalate of cerium; but, from what Dr. G. Hewitt says, it is very probable that the retroflexion [reported by him as retroversion, be it remembered] was the cause of all the trouble, and its rectification the cure."

In the mean time, incited by Dr. Copeman's example, one Dr. Thomas sends to the same journal details of a case which he thinks important as confirming Dr. Copeman's conjecture about " undue tension." It was the case of a lady seven months advanced in pregnancy, and on shipboard; for the relief of the vomiting, after vain trial of drugs, he induced delivery by dilating the os with Barnes's bags. What struck him at the time was that the vomiting ceased before the delivery was effected, and this he attributed to the remedies used, until, on reading Dr. Copeman's account, he became a convert to the ".undue tension " theory. He was too late to keep abreast of the President of the British Medical Association, however, who had already, as we have seen, become a willing captive to the dazzling theory of flexion.

Now it is not to be supposed that so doughty a partisan as Dr. J. Henry Bennett could quietly look on while the champion of flexion took all the tro phies. In the same issue of the journal which published Dr. Copeman's unconditional surrender, we find Dr. Bennett complaining that in the recent communications in that journal he has looked in vain for mention of that very important and very frequent cause of the sickness in question, namely, chronic inflammation of the body and neck of the pregnant uterus. He boldly asserts that he was " the first to draw attention in Anglo-Saxon literature to this frequent cause of obstinate sickness — a cause which may always be suspected when the sickness proves unusually severe. . . . . No practitioner. is justified," he says, " in continuing to treat by medicine such a case of pregnancy sickness without making a most careful ocular and digital examination of the uterine organs." His own examinations are so thorough that he is " still constantly finding well-marked morbid conditions where other practitioners have pronounced the patient free from disease." Though his own obstetric practice has been "principally among women whom he had previously attended for uterine disease," he is sure that he has "saved scores of pregnancies and children's lives by the local surgical treatment" which he has applied; and he closes with an expression of wonder that in the quarter of a century and more since he "opened out this wide and important field of observation in the diseases of pregnancy and the puerperal state, so little has been done in it."

I think I have represented the attitude of each gentleman fairly, though I confess my inability in a condensed sketch to do justice to the absurdity, from a scientific point of view, compressed into the whole correspondence. I commend the whole, as contained in the *British Medical Journal* of May 15th and 29th, and June 12th, to the perusal of all who assent to the prefatory remark of Dr. Copeman, that "practical knowledge should be freely communicated to the profession through our journal. . . . . as a valuable means of effecting improvement in the treatment of disease."

I submit, however, that if the exhortation to free communications carries with it encouragement to imperfect observation, careless statement, vacillating conclusion, and reckless generalization in the interest of partisan theories, the improvement may not follow any more rapidly than under a more cautious and reserved policy. If the President of the British Medical Association and eminent practitioners fall into such errors, what better can be expected of the rank and file of the profession? In fine, if the medical profession countenance the methods of charlatanism and ignorance, how can they blame the public if, no wiser than themselves, it fail to discern the difference between scientific medicine and impudent quackery?   JAMES S. GREENE.

DORCHESTER, *July* 27, 1875.

WEEKLY BULLETIN OF PREVALENT DISEASES.

THE following is a bulletin of the diseases prevalent in Massachusetts during the week ending August 21, 1875, compiled under the authority of the State Board of Health from the returns of physicians representing all sections of the State : —

The week's returns present the same general features with reference to prevalent diseases as those reported in previous weeks of the current month. The sultry weather sustains the diarrhœal diseases at the highest point, and enables them to exhibit a very marked contrast with the other acute disorders. The following is a summary of the returns from the various sections : —

Berkshire : Diarrhœa, dysentery, cholera morbus.

Valley : Diarrhœa, cholera morbus, cholera infantum, dysentery. Some cases of small-pox in Holyoke. Typhoid fever is increasing.

Midland : Cholera morbus, diarrhœa, cholera infantum, dysentery. Upton reports some cases of cerebro-spinal meningitis.

Northeastern : Diarrhœa, cholera infantum, cholera morbus, dysentery.

Metropolitan : Cholera infantum (of severe type), diarrhœa, cholera morbus, dysentery, typhoid fever (increasing, but of mild type), scarlatina.

Southeastern : Diarrhœa, cholera morbus, cholera infantum, dysentery. Attleboro reports fatal cerebro-spinal meningitis.

In the State at large, cholera infantum, cholera morbus, and typhoid fever have increased in prevalence ; all the other diseases have subsided somewhat.

F. W. DRAPER, M. D., Registrar.

COMPARATIVE MORTALITY-RATES FOR THE WEEK ENDING AUGUST 14, 1875.

	Estimated Population.	Total Mortality for the Week.	Annual Death-rate per 1000 during Week.
New York	1,060,000	691	34
Philadelphia	775,000	443	·29
Brooklyn	500,000		
Boston	350,000	255	38
Cincinnati	260,000	77	15
Providence	100,700	50	26
Worcester	50,000	25	26
Lowell	50,000	24	25
Cambridge	50,000	28	29
Fall River	45,000	17	20
Lawrence	35,000	25	39
Springfield	33,000	12	19
Lynn	28,000	16	30
Salem	26,000	28	56

U. S. MARINE HOSPITAL ORDERS. — Surgeon Orsamus Smith, transferred from Louisville, Ky., to Mobile, Ala., August 4. Surgeon Smith is directed to open the Marine Hospital at that place as a government hospital, Class I.

Assistant Surgeon Henry E. Muhlenberg, Jr., relieved from temporary duty at Chelsea, Mass., and assigned to Philadelphia, Pa.

Assistant Surgeon Samuel Q. Robinson (passed the Board of Medical Examiners, July 20–25) appointed Assistant Surgeon July 29, and assigned to duty at Chelsea, Mass., July 31.

Assistant Surgeon Edmund J. Doering (passed the Board of Medical Examiners, July 20–25) appointed Assistant Surgeon July 29, and assigned to duty at San Francisco, Cal., July 31.

Hospital Interne W. R. Chipman appointed and assigned to duty at Chelsea, Mass., July 30.

BOOKS AND PAMPHLETS RECEIVED. — The Movements and Innervation of the Iris. By Dr. H. Gradle. Chicago. 1875.

Lessons in Prescriptions and the Art of Prescribing. By W. Handsel Griffiths. London : Macmillan & Co. 1875.

A Series of American Clinical Lectures. Capillary Bronchitis. By Calvin Ellis, M. D. New York : G. P. Putnam's Sons.

Clinical Lectures and Essays. By Sir James Paget, Bart. Edited by Howard Marsh, F. R. C. S. New York : D. Appleton & Co. 1875.

On Paralysis from Brain Disease in its Common Forms. By H. Charlton Bastian. With Illustrations. New York : D. Appleton & Co. 1875.

THE BOSTON
MEDICAL AND SURGICAL JOURNAL.

VOL. XCIII. — THURSDAY, SEPTEMBER 2, 1875. — NO. 10.

IVY POISONING.

BY JAMES C. WHITE, M. D., OF BOSTON,

Professor of Dermatology in Harvard University.

THE frequent poisoning by ivy (rus) at this season, when so many of our city residents, unfamiliar with its appearances, come in contact with it during their visits to the country and seaside, leads me to call attention to the importance of instructing the public respecting the means by which this plant may be generally and easily recognized and shunned.

Poison ivy, as it is popularly called, is not an ivy, but belongs to the sumach genus. It is rhus toxicodendron. It is sometimes a vine running over or by the side of stone walls, fences, and ledges, or ascending trees to a great height, and sometimes a bush of considerable size and thickness. It is found almost everywhere in New England, in many places growing in great abundance, and forming dense masses by roadsides, in pastures, and along the borders of woods. Its leaves have a marked and very characteristic glossy look, and vary greatly in shape, size, and outline. They are ternate, as the botanists say, that is, they consist of three leaflets, one terminal and two lateral, growing in common upon a rather long, semi-cylindrical stem. The leaflets are ovate with rather a broad base, more or less pointed, and their edges are either entire or notched and lobed in a great variety of forms. It blossoms in June, and the flowers are small and grow in greenish-white clusters, mostly in the axils. The berries are small, round, and also of a pale greenish-white color. Later in the season the leaves assume a great variety of most brilliant colors and attract many gatherers of autumn foliage.

Of the other dangerous species of rhus (rhus venenata), although it is far more poisonous than the above, less need be said, for it grows much less commonly than the latter. It is a small tree, as its common names ("poison dogwood," "poison sumach") suggest, and is found mostly in swamps. Its leaflets, like those of the ordinary sumach, grow upon a long stem and vary in number from seven to thirteen. They are smooth, broader than those of the latter plant, and the terminal one grows from a considerable prolongation of the common stem. In the autumn its foliage surpasses that of all other trees in the variety and brilliancy of its tints, and thus attracts to its less frequented haunts not a few unwary visitors.

The virulent principle of these plants is a volatile acid which exists in all their parts, but especially in the leaves. All persons are not affected by it, but many who can handle the vine, rhus toxicodendron, with impunity are poisoned by the tree, rhus venenata, so much more virulent is the latter. Actual contact with the plants is not.in all cases necessary for the production of their poisonous effects, on account of the volatility of their active principle; and there is good reason to believe that persons highly sensitive to the poison not unfrequently suffer from passing by places where the vine grows abundantly. The plant is supposed to be most actively virulent during the flowering season in early summer, but cases of poisoning occur with great frequency throughout the autumn, when its leaves take on their seductive coloring. Even in the winter the twigs and stems are often found still alive for mischief by those who handle them.

The peculiar effect of the poison is alike in kind upon all who are affected by it, but varies greatly in intensity. The inflammation it excites upon parts coming in contact or contiguity with it is that of an acute eczema, characterized by the eruption of vesicles of a peculiar lurid or brownish-red color, which may subsequently burst and exhibit the later phases of this efflorescence as in other acute inflammations of the skin. In addition, there is more or less of swelling and redness of the parts affected, sometimes to a very marked degree, so that great deformity may thus be produced, and the face of the patient be changed out of all recognition. These changes in the tissues of the skin are accompanied by intense itching and burning, and often great suffering is undergone by the patient in consequence. Fortunately the affection is of short duration, the acute stage lasting ordinarily but a week or ten days under treatment, and its whole course rarely exceeding three or four weeks.[1] Moreover it is not a dangerous affection, although a person severely poisoned over a large surface may present a frightful appearance to his friends. Its effects, however, are never more than skin deep. The eruption generally shows itself within three or four days after contact, sometimes within twenty-four hours. The period of incubation may, however, be prolonged to five or six days in some cases, and fresh blisters may continue to appear for two weeks or more. No danger of contagion by contact with the eruption upon another person is to be feared. The portions of the body most commonly affected are the hands and face, the parts naturally most exposed to contact, but

[1] For a more particular description of the eruption, see an article in the New York Medical Journal of March, 1873.

other parts handled by the former immediately after contact and before washing may have the poison thus transferred to them and be similarly affected. No scars or permanent injury to the skin or general system are to be apprehended in ordinary cases.

A few words with regard to the treatment of rhus poisoning may not be inappropriate in this connection, especially in relation to the means to be immediately used, those to which the term antidote may be properly applied. The poison, as has been stated, is a volatile acid. An alkali would therefore suggest itself as the most fit agent to counteract its action. Thorough washing of the parts, as soon as possible after contact with the poison, in cooking-soda or saleratus water, or in strong soap-suds, especially those of soft soap, which contains an excess of alkali, is therefore the best primary treatment. When these or other alkaline preparations are not to be obtained, an abundance of water alone should be used as soon as possible. After absorption has taken place, or the eruption has begun to show itself, less benefit is to be expected from such applications alone. Remedies are then to be used which will best control and shorten the inflammatory process in the tissues of the skin ; those, in fact, which are found to be most efficacious in corresponding stages of acute eczema. Among these are some which have a special reputation, as solutions of acetate of lead or sulphate of copper, applied frequently as a wash. Perhaps nothing is better than common black wash used as an evaporating lotion for half an hour at a time, twice daily, the lime water acting also as a chemical antidote, if possibly such action is still in season at this later stage. In the intervals between the applications of these washes the parts may be kept covered with cold water dressings, with plasters of diachylon ointment, or with a powder of starch and oxide of zinc, according to the rules familiar to physicians for the treatment of acute eczema. By these means the process is checked and shortened, and the sufferings of the patient greatly alleviated.

In conclusion, a brief word of caution to sojourners in the country who are unacquainted with these poisonous plants. Avoid any vine or bush growing by rocks, fences, and woodsides, with glossy leaves arranged in threes, and in the autumn any particularly brilliant tree in swampy places, with leaves resembling, but broader than, those of the common sumach.

WET NURSING.

NOTES OF A LECTURE AT THE HARVARD MEDICAL SCHOOL.

BY CHARLES E. BUCKINGHAM, M. D.,

Professor of Obstetrics.

IN a former lecture,[1] certain matters were discussed pertaining to the artificial feeding of infants, and certain rules were laid down for guidance in fixing the diet of new-born children.

But we must not forget that perhaps our puerperal patient is to nurse her child. I say perhaps; for you will find a large number of American-born women who cannot nurse. What the reason is I am unable to tell you, but the fact I know. My own experience shows that American-born women in the same social position, in equally good health so far as appearance goes, equally anxious to do the mother's part, are less likely to have a sufficient supply of milk than the same number of Irish or German women. This is a subject that some of you gentlemen may study with advantage. I believe that American women are not good wet nurses. The cases of women who have no milk are rare, but I have seen a few of these. I have seen a woman, well-formed in every way, who had no disturbance of pulse, no mental disturbance, no swelling of the breasts, after an almost painless labor, with no other peculiarity than this, that with the first child there was no secretion of milk, but who nursed two children afterwards without difficulty. I have known another, who seemed equally well, who had no secretion after three labors, but whose breasts after the third labor became riddled with abscesses and fistulæ in consequence of her efforts to make a wet nurse of herself.

The question comes up before labor, Shall this woman nurse? Perhaps she belongs to a tuberculous family, all of whom have died young. She has already lost children with meningeal disease. That woman ought not to nurse her child. It is bad enough for her to have children; but if she nurses them, the chances are that her own days will be cut shorter by the act, and her children, who might be saved by proper food, are likely to fall early victims. It is bad enough, every mother would think, to take milk from a sick cow. A sick woman's milk is as bad as a sick cow's milk. The same remarks will apply to women with syphilis.

Some women cannot nurse for want of nipples. The nipples are retracted. Can you not draw them out? Sometimes you can, and nursing with a shield may be easy. In other cases, you can draw them out to a certain extent only, and it seems as if the milk ducts were bent upon themselves in such a manner as to prevent all passage of milk

[1] Boston Medical and Surgical Journal, June 3, 1875.

through them. You let this woman nurse from one side, where there
may be a nipple, and milk runs out from the other. The moment you
begin to draw upon the side where the deficiency is, the gland begins
to fill, but no milk comes out, and the suffering becomes intense. Unless you let that particular breast alone, mammary abscess is sure to
result.

If you have not seen the breasts before labor, be sure to look at
them before you leave the house. The question will be asked of you,
" When shall I put the baby to the breast ? " Some physicians will
say, " As soon as possible." If you examine the breasts carefully, you
will find nipples of very different colors; some are dark and others
are pale or even pink. All nipples are liable to crack, especially if
not washed and dried after nursing. The darker they are, the less
likely are they to crack and be sore. The lighter-colored they are, the
greater is the chance of their cracking, and a pink nipple, so far as my
observation goes, is sure to be sore. It cracks easily ; the blood is easily
drawn through the skin ; the epidermis appears to be sucked off. The
pain becomes intense, and the so-called " broken breast " comes on.
The dark nipple may bear early suction without any trouble following
it. The longer you keep the child from the pink nipple, the less suffering will result for the mother.

Many women begin months before labor to prepare the nipples for
suction. This is done in two ways, so far as I know. The first is
using a pump, and drawing upon the breast two or three times a day.
Of course I cannot say that the breast may not be toughened by the
operation, though I do not believe it. But I do believe that in some
cases drawing the breasts during pregnancy has produced abortion. I
am aware also that some women nurse through the whole of pregnancy
without a threat of abortion. Well, a man has been under water for
ten minutes without drowning; still there was danger of his death,
before the first five minutes were out. The second method of preparing nipples is bathing them daily, or oftener, with borax and brandy.
You would do better to oil them. The brandy dissolves the oil out
from the skin and makes it more likely to crack. There is nothing in
use that is more likely to cause cracking than the borax, which mixes
so well with the oil of the skin as to make a sort of soap of it. I have
no doubt you can find those who have been treated in this way nurse
without having sore nipples; and I can find more patients who have
had sore nipples from this peculiar preventive treatment. You will do
better to let the nipples alone, or simply to wash them, as you would
other parts of the body. Bear in mind that the lighter the color, the
more likely are they to give trouble.

The question was, " When shall I put the baby to the breast? "
There is a great deal said about the beneficial effect upon the child of

tie colostrum, wiici is said to be the peculiar drug-like milk existing in the breast at the time of labor. You will sometimes find a little milk in tie breast at tiis time, more especially if the woman ias nursed before. Unless your examinations are more successful tian mine have been, you will find it difficult as a rule to squeeze out colostrum or milk or anytiing else, for at least forty-eigit hours after the completion of labor. And if you let tie breasts alone until tiey begin to swell, you will find your patient suffer less from fever and less from pain and very much less from sore nipples. Wien tie breasts begin to swell is the time to begin nursing witi tie most comfort to tie woman and witi tie most ease to tie ciild. Some nipples will be sore notwitistanding all tie care you may take. Some women can bear tie pain and some cannot. Tie same amount of pain hurts one woman more tian it does another. In tie one case tie nursing may be continued. In tie otier, a ciange of food for tie child must be made. Sometimes you may be able by means of a shield to take off tie violence of tie pain and allow nursing to go on. The variety of siields and artificial nipples is great. As a rule, tie dark rubber nipples are tie best, the wiite ones not infrequently making tie ciild's mouth sore. Tie long rubber tube witi a glass siield at one end and a nipple at tie otier is of use before the motier is able to sit up and if sie iave difficulty in iolding tie child. It is not good for continued use, being very apt to become foul, and tie ciild and motier are boti likely to go to sleep wiile nursing is going on, exiausting tie motier and disturbing tie stomaci of tie child. Wien tie ciild goes to sleep it siould always be removed from the breast; otierwise imperfect digestion is tie result, as witi every movement of tie motier, it begins to suck, and tie stomaci becomes filled witi milk in different stages of digestion.

Before leaving tiis part of tie subject let me say tiat tiere are circumstances under wiici it is not wise to nurse a ciild, and temporary feeding siould be considered imperative. Tie reception by the mother of bad news, wiici was totally unexpected, suci as tie death of one of tie family; tie exposure to sudden and severe frigit; any very severe mental emotion; any one of tiese should lead tie motier to iave ier ciild fed and ier breasts emptied in some otier way. Nursing under suci circumstances ias undoubtedly been followed by convulsions, even fatal convulsions, in a ciild previously supposed to be in perfect iealti.

By what I iave said before, you know tiat I am in favor of prolonging the period of nursing. I would not iave a child of my own fed, if its motier were able to nurse it, until tie first sixteen teeti iad cut tie gum. If sie were not able to nurse it, it siould not be fed upon otier diet than milk until tie same age. People may laugi at my positive opinion upon this subject, but that will not change tie opinion, which is founded upon the most careful observation for years. Look at the death-rates and see the early age at which the great number of deaths occurs. It is true that want of clothing kills some, and that epidemic disease kills others; and accident has its share in the deaths. But the great majority of children who die fall victims in their second summer, when the changes due to teething are going on, and their stomachs, which have been taught to crave potato and cake, meat and vegetables, rebel against these and all other things, and cholera infantum and dysentery claim the victims.

Many women have very little difficulty in drying up the breasts, when necessary. Indeed, many find it difficult to furnish much of a supply after five or six months. The little that remains, however, if kept along, will be something for a sick child to fall back upon when its stomach will retain nothing else, and that little may be enough to save life. But the time comes when it is proper to wean. Let the work be begun at night, and not when a tooth is irritating; and let the abstinence be positive. Let the child nurse, if you please, on going to bed, but not again till morning. The first night will probably be one of wakefulness for both parties, if together; the better way is to separate mother and child. If the child wakes and cries, let it be soothed by the voice or by the hand, or by a drink of cold water. The chances are, that it will get very little sleep. On the second night, if the mother's courage has not failed her and she has not yielded, at least half the work will have been done. The third night, the child will probably sleep the whole time; or if not, it will be satisfied with a swallow or two of water. If the attempt is made of weaning first by day, the fatigue of the mother will be likely to make her so sleepy at night, that she will be more likely to yield to the little one's importunities, and all-night nursing will find both of them used up in the morning.

But when you begin to wean by day, it is not wise to make a very sudden change in the diet list. There is likely to be less disturbance by trying milk a few days, then perhaps broth, or bread, or cracker, or some one of the puddings which are used for children. I would not add more than one article to the diet list at a time. If you do, and indigestion follows, you are at a loss to know which produces the disturbance, and you do not know which to avoid. Indeed, two new articles will often make disturbance when neither would do so if given alone.

How are you going to dry up a pair of breasts which furnish abundance of milk? It is sometimes a painful process, whether done before a child has touched it, or after nursing for two years. But how will you do it? Simply let the breasts alone. For twenty-four or forty-eight hours the pain will be great; but long before the expiration of that time the milk will begin to drip out, and will gradually become more watery; and as soon as the demand ceases the supply will stop.

The greatest curse to a woman who is trying to get rid of her milk is the breast pump. You can stop the pain with opiates, if it be excessive. You may apply belladonna about the nipple, if you choose; this has been largely recommended. It will sometimes ease pain, but it is the letting alone that stops the secretion. If belladonna be applied, be sure to let your patient know that it is a poison, else pain may tempt the giving the nipple to the child again. The better way to relieve the pain is to give a fifteenth or a twelfth of a grain of morphia three or four times, with the interval of an hour or two; but if the breast be drawn for relief, the continuance of the pain and the risk of abscess is just so much increased. Leave a breast absolutely without touching it, and the risk of abscess or " broken breast," as it is popularly called, is at the least. I never knew of but one cat which had broken breast. The unfortunate victim had a friend who pitied her on account of her drowned little ones, drew her breasts, and gave her a mammary abscess.

A mammary abscess may come to any woman, nursing or not. It may happen in a male breast. I have seen more of them in women who have not been pregnant than I have in mothers who have stopped nursing; and when I have seen one in the latter, they have almost invariably confessed, after the monthly nurse had gone, that they had been afraid to say that the nurse had overpersuaded them to leave directions disobeyed.

How shall we treat the mammary abscess if it is coming? I do not think leeches will stop it. If there is only a hardness with pain in the gland, stop the suckling. Let what food is taken by the child be from the other breast, and let the threatened one alone. That will often be sufficient in the way of treatment. If necessary to do more, cover the breast with adhesive straps as you would a sore leg. Be sure that the straps fit it, with as few wrinkles as possible. Let them remain on till the hardness has gone, or until the matter has come to the surface, if that is to be the result. You will find the support grateful; it will keep the parts warm and soft quite as well as or better than a poultice, and it will be superior to the poultice from its less weight and its greater cleanliness. If the patient wishes it removed, you need not hurt her by tearing it off. A folded towel wrung out of warm water will take it off in an hour; or a little sweet oil or lard, rubbed over the cloth upon which it is spread, will soften it so that it can be removed without pain. Nor should you hurry about advising the knife. You may say that the pus will burrow deeper. I think you will find it discharge in more than one place, if it be deep-seated, and is first opened above the nipple or very near to it below, or if it opens in one of those places of itself. If it opens much below the level of the nipple, more especially if it be superficial, I think there will be but one opening. The nearer the pus is to the surface when an opening is made, if you prefer to make one,

tie less likely is it to burrow to anotier spot, and tie less likely is tie
opening to close. Tie best after-dressing for twenty-four 10urs is tie
wet towel, and tien simple cerate or lard. You will do better not to
try coaxing your patient to believe tiat tie knife will not 1urt. It will
1urt, and if you find it necessary to use it, and any one says it will
give no pain, simply dèny tie statement.

Before leaving tiis topic it will be as well to say a few words .upon
tie subject of selecting a wet nurse. Tie simple fact of tie milk being
1uman does not mäke it wiolesome, altiougi many people believe tiat
any 1uman milk is better tian any cow's milk. It is not so. Some
1uman milk is better tian some cow's milk, and some 1uman milk, like
some cow's milk, is fit for notiing. If it be decided tiat a wet nurse is
to be employed, you may 1ave tie task of examining tie numerous
applicants for tie place. If you know tie nurse and 1er family 1istory,
so muci tie better. If you do not know 1er, you must be prepared for
all manner of deception in 1er treatment of you. Of tiis you must
not .allow a 1int to escape. Wiatever you may suspect, your suspicions must be kept to yourself. If you examine 1er as a witness would
be cross-examined in court, 10wever faitiful and 10nest sie may be,
sie will be confused and do 1erself an injury. If 1er 1istory be tiat
of an unmarried woman, of itself tiat siould not condemn 1er. If you
can, it would be well to know about 1er ciild's fatier, wietier sie be
married or not, for in eitier case 1is 1istory may be tiat of a sypiilitic.
See tie ciild if you can, and know tiat it is 1er ciild, for ciildren are
sometimes borrowed and loaned for tie purpose of passing examination
witi. See tie breasts, tiat tiey are in good condition, witi dark nipples and areolæ, and, if possible, full nipples. Be sure tiat tie milk 1as
hot been stored up for your examination. Tie specimen ciild may
1ave been otierwise fed to keep it quietly sleeping, and tie woman
may 1ave breasts wiici are full simply because tiey 1ave not been
used for twelve 10urs or more. How are you to find tiis out? Why,
if you tiink favorably of tie candidate, see 1er again a few hours later,
and examine tie breasts, wien sie is not expecting you.

Look at 1er mouth and see if sie siows signs, by teeti or breati, or
otierwise, of dyspeptic trouble. See if tie glands about 1er neck and
elsewiere siow signs of disease. If any scars are found, look into tie
causes of tiese. A scar from a burn is of little consequence, but tie
remains of a scrofulous abscess siould make you 1esitate. If possible,
1er lociial disciarge siould 1ave ceased. In a word, 1er appearance
and history siould be tiose of a woman in good 1ealti.

Tie age of 1er milk, as compared witi tiat of tie ciild, I tiink of
less consequence tian its otier qualities. If it be very old, it is true
tiat it is less likely to be abundant, and is likely to fail earlier. Tiis
is not absolutely certain, 10wever, for I 1ave known a woman to nurse

four children, one after another, and all did well. Some women will say that their milk is good because it is renewed every four weeks. By this they mean that their menstrual discharge has returned. It is simply equivalent to saying that there is constitutional disturbance once in four weeks which is sometimes the means of disturbing the child, and a loss of blood which should go to the formation of milk.

When a wet nurse first gives up her own child for a stranger, she is apt to be low-spirited, as a matter of course ; and this for a time will in some cases prevent her being of much service to the baby. It is curious, however, that the one taken to her breast very soon becomes more dear than her own, and in very many cases the death of her own child, which frequently happens as a consequence, disturbs her but very little.

How is the nurse to be fed ? Remember that she has two to eat for. If it were the mother of your calf that you were feeding, you would see that she had the food that would keep her in the best condition, and be the most likely to furnish milk of good quality. The woman is an omnivorous animal, and what she would eat with propriety when not nursing is not likely to harm her or the child. There are certain articles that seem at once to go into the milk ; some will color it ; some will give it peculiar odor ; others will affect the taste. So some medicines will affect it ; and you may make use of this fact in certain cases for treating the child. Mercurials, I believe, will sometimes affect the milk. Arsenic will go into milk. The bromides and iodides may be administered through it, and some cathartics. It is a great mistake to suppose that green vegetables are of necessity to be avoided. Some children will be disturbed if the mother eats cabbage ; and the same woman may perhaps eat green cucumbers or pickled olives without causing a pain. Vinegar is not going to pass into the milk as vinegar, and if the nurse has a fondness for lemonade, I cannot believe that it is sure to hurt either nurse or child. If you find that pain or any other trouble invariably follows the use of any article by the nurse, that particular article should be avoided by that particular nurse. The rule for you to lay down is that she shall be furnished with all the food she wants, of good quality, and at proper times. The rule for the child is that when hungry he shall have the breast ; and when he stops sucking, the nipple should be removed from his mouth, that he may properly digest one meal at a time, and that the mother may not be exhausted by the constant draught upon her nervous system.

MECHANICAL APPLIANCES IN UTERINE SURGERY.

BY WILLIAM H. BAKER, M. D., OF BOSTON.

PERSONAL observation of the injuries resulting from the improper use of mechanical appliances in many cases, and of the numerous and great benefits derived from the judicious employment of them in other cases, has suggested the theme of this paper. It is unnecessary here to dwell upon the literature of this subject, which has been fully presented by many of the recent works on gynæcology. Let us turn at once to a brief consideration of some of the causes of misplacements of the uterus. These may be classified in two general divisions : (1) those originating in the uterus itself, and (2) those external to that organ.

I. CAUSES ORIGINATING IN THE UTERUS ITSELF.

1. *Congenital Malposition.* This is usually unattended by any troublesome symptoms until the age of puberty, when, in consequence of the great stimulus which the uterus then receives, and of its development, the misplacement of the organ is proportionally augmented, and those phenomena too familiar to all practitioners to require recital begin to be manifested, and to call for special treatment.

2. *Pregnancy.* The uterus in its gravid state is necessarily subject to a series of misplacements which generally demand no particular appliance, but which may, especially in the earlier or the later months, require either an intra-vaginal or an extra-abdominal support.

3. *Subinvolution* often exists without misplacement ; yet the size and weight of the organ have a tendency to produce some abnormal position, and to furnish those cases which most of the profession have either seen or been called upon to treat.

4. *Congestion* may be the primary, but is not the immediate, cause of misplacement ; as occurs to a slight extent during menstruation, when, by the increased weight of the uterus, it is temporarily misplaced. Who has not observed, when malposition from some other cause previously existed, that the suffering of the patient was greatly increased at this period, not only by the existing congestion, but by the additional misplacement which it produced?

5. *Hypertrophy and Hyperplasia,* so far as our subject is concerned, produce similar results ; for it is obvious that the tendency to misplacement would be as likely to follow an enlargement from a multiplicity of cells as from an increase in the size of each cell.

6. *Fluids retained in the Uterine Cavity,* like the preceding causes, may produce misplacements by augmenting the weight of the organ, and secondarily by weakening its supports, of which we shall soon speak. Or, if the gradual accumulation of fluid be not accompanied

[1] Read before the Boston Society for Medical Observation.

by a corresponding increase of the uterine tissue, it may produce such changes as to belong to our next class.

7. *Degeneration of the Uterine Tissue,* which may arise from innutrition, undue and unnatural pressure, imperfect circulation, and by the deposit or development of some abnormal element within the walls; all of these, weakening its own structure, tend to produce misplacement.

8. *Abnormal Growths,* as the various uterine tumors, are very liable to produce misplacement in ways already indicated.

II. CAUSES EXTERNAL TO THE UTERUS.

1. *Congenital Malformation of the Vagina.* In cases of undeveloped uterus, this condition is almost invariably found, and is generally attended by a diminution in the length of that canal, which may be the cause of retroversion. Or, when there is an almost entire absence of the vagina, it of course fails to give the normal support to the uterus.

2. *Excessive Abdominal Pressure.* The ordinary weight of the abdominal viscera is as much as the almost insufficient supports of the organ can safely endure. But if this weight be increased by any abdominal or pelvic growth, or by a large amount of fluid in the cavity of the abdomen, or by an accumulated weight in the viscera themselves; or if the usual weight of these viscera be thrown violently upon the uterus, as in a sudden fall, this organ may be displaced. The same result may follow a less violent or a long-continued increased pressure, as in dancing or tight lacing. Of all the causes of misplacement probably the latter is the most common.

3. *Laceration of the Perinæum.* By this, reference is made not only to those cases where the injury extends through the sphincter muscle, but also to others where any portion of the muscle or the tissues down to that muscle are involved. The loss of so important a support allows the vagina to prolapse, and this in turn brings down the uterus, which naturally follows the axis of the pelvis; precisely as when the abutment of a bridge is swept away, the whole structure must fall.

4. *Relaxed State of the Vagina.* There is a class of cases in which, though the perinæum be not torn, yet the act of parturition has caused either an atrophy and degeneration of muscular tissue, or a sundering of the union of the transverse perineal muscles to their several attachments; or there may exist a subinvolution of the vagina. All of these conditions would subsequently induce the same trouble as that just referred to. This relaxed state may also occur from a want of tone in the vaginal walls themselves, as may be sometimes seen in quite young women, and is then generally accompanied by a like condition of the rectum.

5. *Relaxed State of the Uterine Ligaments.* This is especially notice-

able in those who have had many children. The tonicity of these supports is oftentimes thereby greatly impaired; or the same condition may arise from a debilitated state of the patient from any cause.

6. *Deposit of Fluids and the Contraction of Lymph.* When the misplacement arises from an effusion of liquor sanguinis into the cellular tissue upon either side of the uterus, the misplacement will obviously occur to the opposite side, and the most pain will then usually be experienced upon the side where the effusion occurred. But subsequently the contraction of lymph may draw the uterus far over to the side where the effusion first took place, and then the pain is oftentimes most severely felt upon the opposite side, on account of the great tension of the ligaments of that side. Or lymph being thrown out about the uterus, from whatever source, in contracting may greatly displace the organ, and fix it temporarily or even permanently to some of the pelvic viscera, or to the walls of the pelvis.

7. *Cicatrices of the Vagina,* whether caused from the results of severe or protracted labors or from injuries received at other times, or, as we have sometimes noticed, from the injudicious use of caustics, all tend to draw the uterus from its normal position.

The causes above enumerated suggest the nature and kinds of misplacement of most common occurrence. The term misplacement, as here used, denotes a removal of the uterus from its normal position. It will be clearly seen that the character and extent to which this deviation takes place may be various and very great. The normal position of the uterus changes with the different periods of life. In infancy, it is high up in the pelvis or almost entirely in the abdomen, and inclines forwards. At puberty, the fundus is found just below the plane of the superior strait, with its axis a little inclined forward from that of said strait. During the period of menstrual activity, it descends slightly in the pelvis, usually following the axis of that strait. After the climacteric period, the uterus in its atrophied condition tends toward its position before puberty. Influences may arise during any of these periods which may cause a deviation from this standard. As most of the causes fall within the third of these four periods, or that when the uterus is in a state of menstrual activity, we use the term normal position to describe its place at that time, as above indicated.

The kinds of misplacement are too familiar to all practitioners to require recital in this connection.

We are now prepared to consider the principal point of this paper: Are mechanical appliances justifiable in uterine surgery? and, if so, in what cases?

On these questions the profession is somewhat divided. Some, adopting the theory that nearly all misplacements are secondary to inflammatory action, seek relief for tieir patients by therapeutical agencies, and discard entirely mecianical appliances. Others, assuming that most uterine diseases are due primarily to misplacement, adopt the general use of suci appliances. Tie truti, we believe, lies between these extremes ; and tie skill of tie practitioner is best siown by the careful discrimination of cases in wiici tiey may be beneficial from those wierein tiey would be useless or positively injurious. This will be evident, if we consider, first, wiat is to be understood by mecianical appliances ; and, secondly, wien tiey are desirable and wien objectionable.

Mecianical appliances, as here understood, are designed to assist in tie support and maintenance of those organs and parts of tie body contemplated in uterine surgery.

Tiese are frequently classified according to the purpose which tiey are intended to subserve. But a more natural and simple division is according to tie place to wiici tiey are applied. Thus we may iave (1) tiose partially or entirely external to tie body ; (2) tiose wiich are intra-vaginal ; and (3) those which are intra-uterine. Under tiis general division tie various purposes of tiese instruments will naturally form subdivisions. Tius, under tie first of tiese classes we iave tie various abdominal supports and all tie different forms of pessaries wiici, being partially internal, yet have an external point of attaciment. Under tie second we iave all tiose pessaries wiici take tieir bearing upon tie sympiysis pubis, under tie pubic arci, or upon tie vaginal walls. And under tie tiird we iave all tie various forms of stem pessaries.

Were it possible to collect all tie instruments that have been constructed and used in tiis department of surgery, tiey would of tiemselves form a large museum ; and it would puzzle tie most intelligent piysician to determine tie design and use of many of tiem. Some abdominal supports are very ancient, and still prove iigily beneficial. Among tie best now in use are tie elastic and tie London supporters, altiougi a very efficient one is often made from simple cloti. Tiose iaving an external point of attaciment, wiile they are applied internally, are usually constructed of iard rubber or some metallic substance, and siould be avoided in every case wiere an intra-vaginal instrument can be made to accomplisi tie result, lest from tie motion of the body, as in walking, tiey produce excoriations, and tius become a source of great annoyance to tie patient. As tie dental surgeon must iave an exact impression of tie mouti to wiici ie is to fit a set of teeti, so the uterine surgeon must adapt tie appliance to tie individual subject. Tierefore it is often desirable first to construct a model of some ductile material, as block tin, wiici is readily adjusted to tie particular case ; and, tiis being done, tie instrument can be duplicated from some more substantial and inflexible material. This law of adaptation must not be departed from, wietier tie pessary be constructed upon tie plan of Hedge, Hurd, Hoffman, or otiers too numerous to be named, or of any modification of tieir inventions. Tiat of Hodge, acting upon tie principle of tie lever, is generally preferred, being applicable to tie greatest number of cases. Tie intra-uterine appliances are less various, and siould be used witi tie greatest caution, on account of tieir liability to induce inflammatory action. For tiis reason certain practitioners entirely discard tiem, wiile otiers find tiem decidedly beneficial in certain cases. Tiese may be so constructed as to secure sligit galvanic action; or tiey may be made witi a greater or less curvature, or even straigit, according to tie degree of flexion tiey are intended to overcome, or otier purposes wiici tiey are designed to fulfill.

In tie second part of tiis article we propose to siow, by tie report of cases, wierein any of tiese appliances may be beneficial, wien tiey may be dispensed witi, and wien tiey are positively injurious.

(*To be concluded.*)

RECENT PROGRESS IN ANATOMY.

BY THOMAS DWIGHT, JR., M. D.

METHODS.

MR. LAWSON TAIT ias lately publisied an article[1] containing tie results of iis experience in preparing sections for microscopical examination. He strongly advocates freezing tie specimen, on tie ground tiat it is tius presented in a more nearly normal condition tian after treatment with reagents. It is iardly necessary to discuss iis metiod of freezing, as doubtless many otiers are equally efficacious; but ie gives a good iint as to tie manner of getting rid of tie minute air-bubbles wiici form in tiousands on tie tiawing of tie section. Tie remedy lies in tie application of a few drops of boiled water, wiici, owing to its affinity for air, soon clears tie specimen. Tie most valuable part of tie paper consists of suggestions for staining; but we must be permitted to intimate tiat, like most original observers, our autior hardly does justice to tie metiods of otiers. Tius gold is dismissed witi the.following words, in a foot-note: "Gold stains so irregularly as to be useless," wiici is in contradiction to tie opinion of tie best authorities. No doubt, even in experienced iands, gold not uncommonly fails to produce tie desired results, and periaps occasionally misleads by irregular action; but on tie otier iand tiere is notiing to take its place for tie demonstration of tie finest nerve filaments. In tie same foot-

[1] Journal of Anatomy and Physiology, May, 1875.

note Mr. Tait confirms Alferow's[1] praise of tie silver lactate for marking intercellular divisions. Mr. Tait divides staining fluids into tiose wiici discriminate between different elements and tiose wiici color all (except fat) alike. Among tie latter ie, with some sligit reservation, classes carmine, except for iardened tissues. He iolds tiat tie criterion of tie value of a staining fluid is tie readiness witi wiici its working is affected by tie presence of an acid or an alkali. He considers litmus and red cabbage the best staining agents, but states tiat tiey are difficult to work witi. As hæmatoxyllin is deservedly popular and well recommended by Mr. Tait, we give two of iis methods of preparing it. Taking tie ordinary extract of logwood, as sold by druggists, ie "made a strong watery solution witi tie aid of ieat, filtered it, and added to it wien cold about ten per cent. of pure spirit, or a drop of oil of cloves, to make it keep. A few drops of tiis poured on to a fresi section will stain it a pale brown in a few minutes, and the addition of a few drops of a four per cent.[2] solution of nitric acid in distilled water will display the nuclei of a faint brown color, wiile tie rest of tie tissue becomes cierry-red." Anotier method is as follows: "Place a little distilled water in a watci-glass, and float on its surface about half a grain of tie feathery crystals of hæmatoxylin, tien add a very small quantity of strong ammonia on tie point of a tiin glass rod, and stir till a brilliant purple solution is formed. In tiis immerse tie section till it is of a deep lilac color, and wasi it. It will tien be found tiat wiile tie tissue is lilac, tie nuclei are a deep purple. Tie stain will be found to disappear as tie ammonia evaporates; but it may be completely fixed by placing tie section for a few minutes in a saturated solution of alum."

From tiese and otier reactions tie autior iolds, contrary to tie general opinion, tiat tie nucleus is faintly more alkaline tian the body of tie cell. He uses glycerine jelly for mounting.

CONJOINED EPITHELIUM.

Under this heading Dr. S. Martyn[3] calls attention to some original views on cells known as "prickle and ridge cells," to be found in tie deeper parts of tie skin and of some mucous membranes. Tiey were first described some twelve years ago by Max Sciultze, and, as Dr. Martyn observes, iave attracted but little notice in Englisi works. Tie surfaces are more or less covered by ridges and by projections (prickles), wiici are best seen at tie edges. Tiese are figured as siarp triangular spines wiici interlock witi tiose of neigiboring cells as tie bristles of two brusies tiat are put togetier. Tie author is inclined to con-

---

[1] Vide last Report on Anatomy in the JOURNAL, March 4, 1875.

[2] In the text this is written, ".004 per cent.," but other passages leave us in little doubt that four per cent. is meant.

[3] British Medical Journal, June 26, 1875.

sider tie classical picture tiat of a secondary appearance, and to iold tiat tie prickles are broken-off bands tiat once joined distinct cells. In support of tiis ie describes and figures specimens in wiici bands could be traced witiout interruption from tie substance of one cell into tiat of anotier, wiile tie free side of tie cell was covered witi prickles. Tie autior is not so clear as to tie origin of tie "ridges," but suggests, if we understand him correctly, tiat tiey are simply longer stretcied bands tiat are broken and lying on tie surface of tie cell. As to tie formation of tiese appearances tie autior tiinks tiat "tie cells of tie rete mucosum, in multiplying originally by subdivision, retain numerous points of incomplete severance, and tiese points of adiesion are dragged out and become tie uniting bands." Althougi, as Dr. Martyn iimself states, tiese cells are found in normal tissues and in lower animals, ie surprises us by assuming, toward tie end of iis paper, tiat tieir presence indicates "an abnormal functional activity of tie lower cells of tie rete mucosum."

NERVOUS SYSTEM.

Digital Nerves. — Curious pienomena of unexpected absence or persistence of sensation in certain parts of tie iand, after injury of some of tie nerves supplying it, iave given rise at times to a good deal of confusion, as tie usual descriptions of tie distribution of tiese nerves could not easily be reconciled witi tie symptoms. Dr. L. G. Richelot [1] ias made some dissections tiat give muci information tiat cannot be obtained except in Henle's Anatomy, witi tie last part of wiici tie autior was not acquainted till ie iad nearly finisied iis investigations.

In some points iis description appears more accurate even tian Henle's, tiougi usually tiey agree. Tie method of examination consisted in removing tie skin and nerves togetier, and in tien dissecting tie latter from tie inside, tius preserving tie cutaneous filaments tiat otierwise are lost. Tie index, middle, and ring fingers are supplied as follows: tie palmar nerves (to wit, from tie ulnar for tie inner side of tie fourti finger and from tie median for tie otiers) divide near tie root of tie fingers into two brancies of nearly equal size. Tie anterior of tiese are tie palmar collateral nerves, and run as usually described along tie sides of tie fingers, and finally give off tie subungual branches tiat go to tie back of tie fingers at tie root of tie nails. Tie otier brancies of tie palmar nerves pass at once to tie back of tie fingers, and reaciing tie skin at tie beginning of tie second pialanx supply tie back of tie fingers below tiat point. Tie, dorsal nerves going to tiese tiree fingers from tie back of tie hand are in no sense collateral brancies, but end in tie skin over tie first pialanx; tie fore finger and one side of tie middle finger are supplied by the radial, and

[1] Archives de Physiologie, No. 2, 1875.

the rest of the middle and both sides of the ring finger by the dorsal branch of the ulnar. The thumb and little finger present a different arrangement; here we have true dorsal collateral branches from the dorsal nerves, and the posterior divisions of the palmar ones are of very little importance. Thus it appears that the dorsal surface of the two lower phalanges of the three middle fingers is supplied by branches of the palmar nerves, and that owing to the distribution of the latter the median has a greater share in the innervation of the back of the hand than is usually ascribed to it.

The Great Splanchnic Ganglion forms the subject of a paper by Mr. D. J. Cunningham,[1] who has given much attention to this little-known swelling of the splanchnic nerve. It has not, however, been quite so much overlooked as would be inferred from the writer's remarks: "By those authors who take notice of this ganglion, it is described as of rare occurrence, and few enter into any particulars as to its anatomy." Sappey says that it occurs "assez souvent," and Cruveilhier that it is not rare. Nevertheless, Mr. Cunningham has added decidedly to our knowledge of the subject. He has made special dissections for this ganglion eleven times on the right side, finding it in all, and fifteen on the left, finding it in nine; in other words, he found it twenty times out of twenty-six. It is situated at the point at which the great splanchnic nerve receives its last root, and lies on the twelfth dorsal vertebra or on the cartilage between it and the eleventh. In size it varies from that of a pin's head to that of an orange seed. It gives off from five to nine branches, which form a net-work about the junction of the thoracic and abdominal divisions of the aorta, and occasionally join the large neighboring plexuses of the sympathetic. The author has never been able to find a direct communication, such as Rüdinger describes, between the ganglia of the two sides of the body.

Nerves of the Dura Mater. — The manner of termination of these nerves has never been definitely settled, although Von Luschka in his monograph declares that all of them end in the vessels and none in the membrane itself. Dr. W. T. Alexander[2] has studied this question in the lower animals, examining both the cranial and the spinal membrane, and coloring the nerves with the gold and sodium chloride. He finds that a large number of nerves follow the vessels, forming plexuses around them and ultimately entering their coats, and that others end in a net-work in the substance of the dura mater. He has not been able to discover how either set of fibres actually terminates.

(To be concluded.)

[1] Journal of Anatomy and Physiology, May, 1875.
[2] Archiv für microscopische Anatomie, Band xi. heft 2.

THE ETHER CONTROVERSY.

THE occurrence of two deaths from chloroform in London under circumstances somewhat more startling than usual has led Mr. George Pollock, of
St. George's Hospital, to write a letter to the *London Times* for the purpose of
calling the attention of the public to the great difference existing in the relative safety of ether and chloroform, which, he points out, has already been shown
repeatedly in the medical journals. In concluding he adds : —

" I ought, perhaps, to apologize for intruding a professional question on a
non-professional journal ; but one must employ a big hammer to drive a large
nail through a thick piece of wood. We have some very thick pieces of wood
to deal with. The question has been brought forward in the leading medical
journals of the day ; and yet within one week we read of the loss of two lives,
which, I say it with regret, might not have occurred had ether been employed
in place of chloroform. I therefore seek the aid of your great influence to
bring to the mind of the public, as well as the profession generally, the importance of a correct knowledge on this subject.

" It is a big subject. It is a question between living or dying. If our judges,
coroners, and magistrates, if the members of the bar and the public, were
once satisfied of the danger of the one and the safety of the other, I need not
pause to inquire what may be the position of that man who is hereafter unfortunate enough to lose a patient under the influence of chloroform."

This has been the starting-point of quite an extended discussion in the
English journals, in the course of which so many curious statements have been
made, that, although there is little to be added to what has already been written in the columns of this journal on the subject, we hardly feel inclined to
pass them by without some criticism. The *Lancet*, in quite extended comments upon the subject, endeavors to convey the impression that the supporters
of ether claim for it absolute safety ; and having refused this assumption
adds : —

" It follows, then, that the absolute safety of ether is not proved, and though
we incline to think that it is safer than chloroform, the wish that it is may,
after all, be the parent of the belief ; " and further on says, " We deal, therefore,
with no more than a general impression when we say that ether is safer than
chloroform." In support of this position it quotes cases of death under ether,
particularly those lately reported in the English journals, and points also to
the well-worn argument of the far greater use of chloroform up to the present
time accounting for the greater number of deaths by that agent, while the
question of the existence of a poison peculiar to chloroform, which kills suddenly and under the most favorable circumstances, is ignored.

In regard to the absolute safety of ether, no one can doubt that ether can
be made to kill, as Mr. Pollock, following the example of other defenders of
this agent, has admitted. We must protest, however, against the character of
the testimony which goes to show that the frequency of death from ether is
such as to throw even the shadow of a doubt over the comparative safety of
the two agents. Such insinuations as have been made by our conservative
friends help to show the weakness of their cause. The so-called deaths from

etier referred to include a deati from blood in the traciea, and deatis from the use of an impure article, namely, tie etier used for producing spray in local anæstiesia. To make etier responsible for tie blunders of Englisi surgery can iardly be considered á fair way of sustaining the prestige of ciloroform. Tie *Lancet* says furtier tiat etier must iave " twenty-five years of trial in every respect equal to tiat whici has been given to ciloroform," to test its safety. In reply to tiis we can but refer our contemporaries to tie fact tiat ciloroform acquired the reputation it now has long before it iad been put to the ordeal wiici etier ias sustained. For instance, tbe late Dr. Join C. Warren wrote in 1849 of ciloroform, " We were soon awakened from our dreams of tie deligitful influence of tie new agent, by the occurrence of unfortunate and painful consequences, wiici iad not followed in tiis country in tie practice of etierization." Tie great danger of ciloroform was fully recognized even at tiat early day.

We cannot refrain iere from quoting a paragrapi from tie remarks of tie *Medical Press and Circular* on tiis discussion : —

" To suddenly put aside ciloroform in favor of etier, as Mr. Pollock would iave us do, would be to acknowledge tiat for forty years we iave not only made no progress in tie study of anæstietics, but tiat for some reason or otier, not suggested, we iave willfully or blindly discarded a perfectly safe and efficient anæstietic for tie use of a dangerous one."

Tie *Lancet* also indulges in a somewiat similar strain. We trust suci reflections as tiese may indicate tiat our more conservative Britisi colleagues are beginning to realize the position in wiich tiey iave placed tiemselves. Siould prejudice still blind tiem, iowever, we iave strong iopes from tie revivalists represented by suci men as Mr. Pollock and many otier prominent Englisi surgeons, wio iave received valuable support from the *British Medical Journal.*

In conclusion, we would simply caution our friends against tie use of an impure article. Avoid everytiing but pure etier, suci as is obtained in tiis country from Squibb, or Powers and Weigitman ; follow tie simple directions laid down by Dr. H. J. Bigelow in an article in tie JOURNAL of November 20, 1873, wiici appeared siortly afterwards in tie *British Medical Journal,* and suci cases as iave appeared in late numbers of the Englisi journals will cease to be reported. Give etber simply a fair ciance, and tie most stubborn and ignorant of its opponents will surely be obliged to acknowledge its superiority.

THE BRIGHTON SLAUGHTER-HOUSES.

Tʜᴀɴᴋs to tie perseverance and energy of the State Board of Healti, tie numerous nuisances wiici iave for years existed in tie Brigiton district of the city, in the siape of slaugiter-iouses, have gradually disappeared until scarcely ialf a dozen remain. Tie business ieretofore done, oftentimes in a very questionable manner, at various localities in tiat section of the city has been almost entirely transferred to the lands belonging to the Butchers' Slaughtering and Melting Association, and is now carried on under the immediate supervision of the managers of that association.

Early in the summer a petition was received by the State Board of Health asking that action be taken against those few who still continued the business outside the abattoir, in places utterly unsuitable for the purpose. A public hearing was given, at which both complainants and defendants appeared, and after a full and thorough investigation of the subject, four of the offending parties were ordered to cease and desist. To this order of the board no attention was paid, and accordingly an injunction was issued, August 6th, by the Supreme Court at the request of the attorney-general. Three of the parties ceased from further violation of the orders of the board. One, however, Henry Zoller, continued as before, in defiance of the injunction of the Supreme Court. Accordingly an order was issued August 20th, ordering Mr. Zoller to appear and show cause why he should not be proceeded against for contempt of court. The hearing was held August 24th.

The defense claimed that he had not slaughtered since July 1st, which was the date at which he was ordered to cease and desist. He stated that a few days before, he had sold out his teams to his brother, Christopher Zoller, and that his wife, who owned the premises, had leased them to this same brother, who had since been carrying on the business. He contended that the injunction was against him personally, but the Board of Health showed that Christopher Zoller had been present at the hearing before the Board of Health, and knew of the passage of the order to cease and desist.

The court (Judge Colt) decided that the sale to the brother was a mere ruse to avoid the effect of the process, and an attempt to evade the same. The method adopted was a legitimate legal dodge to avoid the difficulty. The attorney-general having stated that the Board of Health did not desire the defendant punished, but merely that its orders should be obeyed, the court ordered that the defendant should pay the costs of the legal proceedings in the case, and should be allowed one week in which to close up his business.

The Board of Health are to be congratulated that their action was so promptly sustained by the presiding judge of the Supreme Court, who was unwilling to see an official order of the board set aside by a mere legal quibble. It is to be hoped that the members of the board will be equally successful in the future in their attempts to properly carry out such orders as they shall consider necessary for the preservation of the health and sanitary welfare of the commonwealth.

MEDICAL NOTES.

— We are requested to state that the rooms of the Boston Medical Library Association are on the ground floor, and not below ground, as some have interpreted the "basement" mentioned in the circular which lately appeared. They are in Hamilton Place, quite accessible and attractive, and will be opened early in the fall.

— Dr. C. Irving Fisher having resigned the position of Port Physician of Boston, the Board of Health, Mayor Cobb concurring, have appointed Dr. Alonzo S. Wallace as his successor.

— A case of penetrating pistol-shot wound of the abdomen, the bullet passing per rectum on the fourth day, and the injury followed by rapid recovery, is reported by Dr. Wm. O'Meagher in the *Medical Record* of July 17, 1875. April 25, an able-bodied laborer was shot while under the influence of liquor by one of his companions. Examination showed that the bullet had penetrated and lodged in the abdominal cavity, having entered at the right upper angle of the umbilical region, corresponding with a portion of the transverse colon, the duodenum, and possibly with the greater curvature of the stomach distended with a hearty meal and fermented liquor. Without delay — no attempts having been made to find the bullet — the wound was cleaned and covered with a cold water dressing and oiled silk. The patient vomited freely, but neither blood nor bullet could be detected in the vomitus. Opiates, ice, etc., were administered, and absolute rest on the back, with the knees flexed, was enjoined. After a tolerably comfortable night, the next day symptoms of peritonitis set in. On the third day the patient was better. On the fourth day, notwithstanding the free use of opiates, there continued as on the previous day a desire to evacuate the bowels, and after a dose of castor-oil a bullet was found in one of the dejections. Recovery was uninterrupted by any untoward symptom. In nine days the wound was entirely healed. The bullet, a part of a patent cartridge, weighed only forty grains. Dr. O'Meagher attributes the favorable termination of the case to the following conditions : the smallness of the missile, the early closure of the wound, the entire absence of attempts to find the bullet by probing, abstinence from food and drink except in small quantities, absolute rest, and a good constitution. The reporter finds but few similar cases on record — two by Hennen and one by McLeod.

— We have to report another case of sudden death following thoracentesis, this time reported by M. Legroux to the Société Médicale des Hôpitaux. A man fifty-two years old, fifteen days after an undiscovered fracture of the ribs was deemed by M. Legroux to demand thoracentesis on account of an excessive pleuritic effusion of the left side, causing dyspnœa, cyanosis, and displacement of the heart to the right. The operation was performed by the aspirator under ordinarily favorable conditions. Two thousand grammes of slightly reddish, turbid fluid were drawn off. Forthwith the patient was considerably relieved. He had for a quarter of an hour the teasing cough which commonly follows the operation, but no expectoration of note. Three quarters of an hour later, when he was feeling much relieved, and was talking with his companions, he suddenly cried out, " I feel faint !" He was seen to lie down on his bed, to make two or three movements of his arms, to become pale, and then was dead. The post mortem discovered no lesion sufficient to explain the cause of death. There was no vascular obstruction, no congestion or apoplexy of the lungs, no cerebral lesion. M. Legroux was disposed to consider syncope the cause of death — a syncope resulting from cerebral anæmia. Such an anæmia might result from the afflux of too great a quantity of blood into the liberated lung, and from the diminution of the quantity of blood circulating in the cerebral vessels.

— Dr. Labartie sends to *Le Mouvement Médicale* a copy of his letter to the prefect of police in which he sets forth the reasons which induced him to resign the office of assistant physician to the dispensary de Salubrité, of Paris. Dr. Labartie objected to the regulation requiring the physician to visit the houses of prostitution at midday. Such a procedure is liable to subject the physician to insults, and to cause him to be accounted a shameless debauchee. It was very desirable that some public guardian of the peace should accompany the physician in these visits, but this was not granted. A very simple plan would have been to have had an appointed place in each of the twelve sections of Paris where the prostitutes could come for examination, but such a plan did not approve itself to the administration. Dr. Labartie complains that he was disappointed in his expectation that to himself, who had devoted his time exclusively to the study of venereal diseases, the dispensary would furnish a vast field for study, researches, and observations upon these diseases. He states that the physicians had no voice in the management of the affairs of the institution, and instead of seeing the medical corps a sort of permanent commission occupied in the consideration of questions of the most important social interest, namely, the statistics and prophylaxis of venereal diseases, the organization of prostitution, and finally the extinction of these maladies, he found nothing but the consideration of self-interest and silence regarding these important questions.

— In our foreign exchanges we learn of a case of poisoning of an infant by opium administered to the mother. The latter was about to undergo an operation, and at ten o'clock in the morning she took twenty-five drops of Battley's sedative solution, and repeated the dose at two o'clock. At eight o'clock in the evening she took five centigrammes of opium in a pill.

Her child, a strong boy seven weeks old, was restless throughout the day. At midnight he took the breast and suddenly fell into a deep sleep, in which he remained for six hours. On awaking he sucked a little, and again slept throughout the day. At two P. M. respiration diminished in frequency, and became less deep, and jerking. At six P. M. the pupil was contracted, respiration imperfect, jerking irregular, but in frequency nearly normal. It was with great difficulty that he could be aroused. Coffee was administered by the mouth and by the rectum, and the patient was exposed to the draught from an open window, and in about an hour he seemed better. An hour later respiration ceased for a while, and he appeared dead; life, however, returned, and the following day, by two A. M., he was out of danger.

The two points to be noticed in the case were the duration of the symptoms (twenty-six hours), and the fact that the mother's milk served as a vehicle to the poison.

A second case is referred to, in which an infant some months of age, suffering from diarrhœa, was ordered one drop of laudanum every three hours. After the first drop the diarrhœa ceased, after the second convulsions came on, and after the third the child died.

Both cases are instructive, as showing the susceptibility of infants to opium. But the fact is very well known, and practitioners are, or ought to be, on their guard in administering opium to children or to a suckling woman.

— Through the courtesy of the Signal Service Bureau of the War Department, we have received the first number of a bulletin containing an international exchange of weather reports. There could be no more significant illustration of the recent rapid advances in meteorological science than this record of observations taken simultaneously at numerous stations throughout the great northern hemisphere. Algeria, Austria, Belgium, Sweden, Switzerland, Turkey, Great Britain, France, Germany, Italy, Canada, and the United States here contribute a uniform system of weather records, comprising data of barometric pressure, temperature, humidity, wind-movements, clouds, and rain-fall. These observations will in future permit the study of atmospheric changes the world over, enabling storms and other disturbances to be traced from their origin throughout their course until they disappear. It is a source of national pride that our own government observers, of whom General Myer is the chief officer, have put the work into practical operation and established the form which we have before us.

We indulge the sanguine hope that the system of meteorological observations above described may presently point the way to a similar scheme applied to the record of epidemic movements and prevalent diseases. It is not too much to expect that sometime we may have an international bulletin setting forth officially the movements of " waves " of epidemic disease from their initiation to their decline, medical " signal officers " becoming the counterpart of the weather observers. The practical advantages of such a general system in its relation to the public health are obvious ; while the obstacles in the way of its accomplishment are not more insurmountable than were those that seemed a few years ago to stand in the way of the present admirably managed signal service at Washington.

LETTER FROM NEW YORK.

Messrs. Editors, — In looking over the reports of the mortality from diarrhœal disease among children during the past few weeks, it occurred to me that an account of the prevalence of cholera infantum and similar troubles might prove of interest to some of your readers. I therefore propose to devote a considerable portion of this letter to such facts as I have been able to gather on the rate of mortality, in this year and former ones, from diarrhœal diseases among children under five years of age. It is almost impossible to keep a city of the size of New York, and populated with the class that one finds in its thickly-settled portions, in a good or even a fair sanitary condition. When it is remembered how large a portion of the population of the city is crowded together in spaces barely sufficient to properly accommodate one fifth of their number, the wonder is that the rate of mortality is so low.

A walk through any of those parts of the city inhabited by the lower class, and reeking with the stench from garbage which they persist in throwing into the street, added to the close, stifling smell coming from houses and cellars full of filth, and swarming with dirty, half-clad children, will demonstrate the ciief predisposing cause of infantile mortality. As the mean temperature approaches 70° Farenieit, the weekly reports of mortality siow an increase in the number of deaths among children, and as the temperature exceeds that degree the death-rate among the above-mentioned class rapidly increases. As a rule this mortality begins to increase about the third or fourth week in June, by the middle or last part of July reaches its maximum, continues high during August, and gradually diminishes during the early and middle parts of September, and by the end of that month does not much exceed that of the early portion of June.

The board of health have recently published, in the *City Record* for August 3d, a table very instructive to any one interested in this subject, from which the accompanying table is copied.

SUMMER MORTALITY-RATES IN NEW YORK CITY.—SIX YEARS.

	Total Mortality from all Causes.	Diarrhœal Diseases under 5 Years.	Mean Temperature.	Mean Humidity.	Total Mortality from all Causes.	Diarrhœal Diseases under 5 years.	Mean Temperature.	Mean Humidity.	Total Mortality from all Causes.	Diarrhœal Diseases under 5 years.	Mean Temperature.	Mean Humidity.
	1870.				**1871.**				**1872.**			
June	1771	208	71.43	64.57	1939	2831	70.04	60.52	2432	289	69.68	66.64
July	3343	1185	77.75	59.	2847	1031	73.02	60.31	4314	1768	79.31	80.99
August	2941	1009	77.52	55.33	2384	738	74.48	64.32	2902	948	73.65	69.74
September	2074	477	71.19	51.95	2182	217	69.73	66.29	2568	683	71.67	74.28
	1873.				**1874.**				**1875.**			
June	1912	124	70.80	54.10	1873	81	66.42	64.50	1957	78	66.57	66.25
July	2737	922	72.72	65.83	2392	602	74.25	61.75	2847	708	75.1	71.
August	3138	1152	75.77	63.75	3021	1106	72.55	60.75	–	–	–	–
September	2457	575	69.35	69.75	2474	645	70.2	55.	–	–	–	–

The statistics of the board of health above mentioned give the total mortality, the mortality from diarrhœal disease of children under five years of age, and of persons of more than five years of age, the greatest range of temperature, the mean range of temperature, and the humidity in each week from January, 1867, to the first week in August, 1875. In the accompanying table saturation is taken at 100. I will refer to the table since 1870, and only then, for the months of June, July, August, and September.

We find on referring to the table that the years 1870, 1872, and 1873 show the greatest infantile mortality during the summer months; and of these years the greatest number of deaths among children from diarrhœal disease occurred in 1872, the mean temperature being the highest for that year.

The following is the greatest mortality occurring in any one week of each summer : —

1870, 4th week in July, mortality 379.						Mean temperature	82.31°
1871, 3d " " " "					393.	"	"	79.48°
1872, 2d " " " "					618.	"	"	83.97°
1873, 4th " " " "					418.	"	"	72.70°
1874, 4th " " " . "'					358.	"	"	75.90°

The excess of infantile mortality in 1873, with a mean temperature of 72.70°, over 1874, with a mean temperature of 75.90°, does not seem to be accounted for by anything in the table. This year the last week in July shows the greatest number of deaths, being three hundred and seventy-eight, with a mean temperature of 74.50°. The heavy rains for the past few weeks have done much to clean and purify the city, and unless we should have another great increase in the temperature, the mortality from infantile diarrhœa will probably be comparatively low. Thus far we have had a less number of deaths this year than in any previous one except last, and it is probable that from this time on there will be rather a diminution than an increase in the death-rate among children.

In writing about children perhaps I ought to say something of the " Floating Hospital of St. John's Guild," concerning which so much has been written in the daily papers. About eight years ago there was organized in connection with St. John's Church, belonging to the corporation of Trinity Parish, an association called "St. John's Guild," its object being to aid the poor in the lower portion of the city. Three years ago it ceased its connection with St. John's Church, and became an independent organization. In 1873 an attempt was made to collect a fund to be called "The Destitute Sick Children's Relief Fund." With the money thus collected a large barge and steam-tug were chartered, an abundant supply of proper food was placed on board, and two trips were made on the bay, carrying a full load of children and their mothers. This seemed to be so popular, and funds came in so freely, that last year they were able to provide eighteen excursions on the waters about New York. Upon these trips 15,202 children and their mothers were taken, at an expense of $5193. Last fall the hull of a steamboat was purchased and fitted up as a barge; and this is the " Floating Hospital of St. John's Guild." I think that it is a misnomer, as it conveys a wrong impression of its use. This barge is two hundred and ten feet long, and thirty-six feet wide at its widest part; it has an upper and a lower deck, the latter so arranged that it can be made comfortable in case of a storm, by means of shutters. The upper deck is under cover, and has curtains at the sides, so as to protect the children from the sun. The space below deck, corresponding to the lower cabin of a steamboat, is divided into two rooms; the smaller one, forward, is fitted up as a kitchen; the other is the dining-room, having two rows of tables running its whole length, and capable of seating about six hundred children. On the main deck forward, separated by a passage-way running fore and aft, are two small rooms, containing seven little beds each, for those children who are too sick to be up. They are well ventilated, but I understand that they are not used much. Back of these wards is an open space, broken only by two wide staircases leading to the upper deck. Pretty well aft are several rooms, one for the superintendent, and the ladies who may wish to go on these excursions; back of this is the doctor's room, who goes on the trip, and who is expected to provide medicine for those who may require any. Behind this are the water-closets. The upper deck is entirely free of any obstruction, and the children and their mothers are kept up there, and not allowed on the lower deck. The barge is propelled by a tug-boat. Excursions are made on Tuesdays, Thursdays, and Saturdays of each week. The barge leaves the foot of Twenty-Third Street and East River at eight o'clock, stops at Market Street at nine o'clock, then at West Tenth Street and at West Thirty-Fourth Street and North River, taking on at these places as many as apply. The excursionists are provided with a breakfast and dinner. They usually take from nine hundred to fifteen hundred children and mothers on each trip. To provide for so many mouths they use six hundred pounds of beef, eighty gallons of soup, three hundred and fifty loaves of bread, three hundred and fifty quarts of milk, one barrel of hominy, three fourths of a barrel of sugar, one third of a chest of tea, and one tub of butter.

The total cost of the barge was $20,000, and the expense of each excursion is about $200.

Every physician in the city has been furnished with cards like the following : —

FLOATING HOSPITAL OF ST. JOHN'S GUILD.

FREE EXCURSIONS

FOR DESTITUTE SICK CHILDREN AND THEIR MOTHERS.

Every Tuesday, Thursday, & Saturday.

Pass_____

Residence_____

Sent by_____M. D.

Under the Supervision of REV. ALVAH WISWALL,
Master of St. John's Guild.

These cards are distributed as opportunity offers. On these excursions they are not able to go more than twenty miles from the city, their object being to give their voyagers fresh air. The children who go on these trips are of course from the lowest dregs of society, and it is with the greatest difficulty that the barge is kept in even a fairly clean condition for a short time. Many of the children are suffering from diarrhœal disease, some from marasmus, while others are perfectly healthy. How much real good is done in this way, it is very difficult to say; there is no doubt an immense amount of suffering among tenement-house children, but whether this is the best and only way to reach and relieve it is another question. It no doubt does real good by giving the children great pleasure, and by making them feel that they are not entirely forgotten by those in better circumstances; but that it has much effect on infantile mortality I doubt very much. The question of how much evil may come from crowding children together, from contagious diseases, etc., should not be lost sight of. The success that has attended the collection of the relief fund is due in a great measure to the New York press, which has from the very beginning given the enterprise its hearty support.

WEEKLY BULLETIN OF PREVALENT DISEASES.

THE following is a bulletin of the diseases prevalent in Massachusetts during the week ending August 28, 1875, compiled under the authority of the State Board of Health from the returns of physicians representing all sections of the State: —

The returns show an increase in the prevalence of diarrhœal diseases; this accession may be explained partly by the sudden transition from very sultry weather to the cool temperature of the last week. The order of relative prevalence of acute diseases in the State at large is as follows: Diarrhœa, cholera morbus, cholera infantum, dysentery, typhoid fever, rheumatism, scarlatina, whooping-cough, bronchitis, diphtheria, influenza, pneumonia, measles — the prevalence of the last five being scarcely worth mentioning. In the sections, the order is as follows: —

Berkshire: Diarrhœa, dysentery, cholera morbus, cholera infantum.

Valley: Diarrhœa, cholera morbus, cholera infantum, typhoid fever, dysentery. Cases of intermittent fever are reported.

Midland: Cholera morbus, diarrhœa, cholera infantum, dysentery, typhoid fever.

Northeastern: Cholera morbus, diarrhœa, cholera infantum, dysentery; a marked increase in the last disease.

Metropolitan: Diarrhœa, cholera infantum, cholera morbus, dysentery, typhoid fever. The type of the fever is thus far mild; Brighton reports a great contrast with last year in this respect.

Southeastern: Diarrhœa, cholera infantum, dysentery, cholera morbus, typhoid fever.

In the whole State, all the diarrhœal affections, together with typhoid fever, have increased; all the other diseases have declined.

F. W. DRAPER, M. D., Registrar.

COMPARATIVE MORTALITY-RATES FOR THE WEEK ENDING AUGUST 21, 1875.

	Estimated Population.	Total Mortality for the Week.	Annual Death-rate per 1000 during Week.
New York	1,060,000	674	33
Philadelphia	800,000	385	25
Brooklyn	500,000		
Boston	350,000	225	33
Cincinnati	260,000	76	15
Providence	100,700	36	18
Worcester	50,000	28	29
Lowell	50,000	41	43
Cambridge	50,000	24	25
Fall River	45,000	38	44
Lawrence	35,000	15	24
Springfield	33,000	8	13
Lynn	28,000	21	39
Salem	26,000	20	40

THE BOSTON
MEDICAL AND SURGICAL JOURNAL.

VOL. XCIII. — THURSDAY, SEPTEMBER 9, 1875. — NO. 11.

A CASE OF BIFURCATED FOOT WITH ELEVEN TOES.[1]

BY GEORGE J. BULL, M. D., OF WORCESTER.

THE following case of congenital malformation of the foot and leg derives additional interest from its extreme rarity. It furnishes an example of the anomaly known in Geoffroy Saint-Hilaire's classification as " bifurcated hand or foot," a deformity not uncommon in the hoofed mammalia, but so rare in man that Saint-Hilaire never found mention of a single well-authenticated case.[2]

A girl was born in Worcester on the 5th of May, 1875, healthy and apparently well formed, except in the left inferior extremity. Her left foot presents the heretofore unheard-of number of eleven toes, and in its general appearance may be compared to a double or cloven foot. It has only one heel, but in front consists of two parts, which we may call the anterior and posterior feet. The anterior presents the great toe with four smaller toes, naturally placed and of normal proportions, but is twisted downwards and inwards in the position of extreme talipes equino-varus. Several pits or depressions over the tarsus mark the position of interspaces between the bones, and show the extent of the inversion, 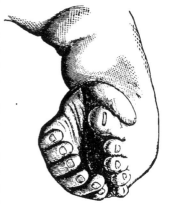 which is further shown by the fact of the inner border of the foot pressing against the heel. Continuous with the outer edge of the anterior foot, and curving beneath it, is the posterior part, looking not unlike a second foot, and furnished with six well-formed, small toes, situated directly below the other five. The plantar surfaces of the two sets of digits face each other, and are separated by a groove, which, beginning between the little toe of the anterior foot and the adjoining one of the supernumerary set, grows broader and deeper as it proceeds in-

[1] Extract from a paper read before the Worcester District Medical Society, July 14, 1875.
[2] Histoire des Anomalies, 1832, i. 695.

wards, and, winding around the metatarsal bone of the great toe, is lost in the furrow between the heel and the inner border of the anterior foot. The two feet are thus quite distinct at the phalanges, and their plantar surfaces are more or less free, that of the anterior foot being visible as far back as the first metatarsal bone, while that of the posterior foot is almost all to be seen, and terminates so naturally on the heel that it is difficult to say to which foot the heel more properly belongs. The eleven toes are perfect in form; none of them are webbed. The great toe and four smaller toes of the anterior foot are normally proportioned; the little toe is the exact image of the first toe of the supernumerary set which adjoins it; the second is the longest of the six, but does not at all resemble a great toe; the third and fourth are equal in length, the fifth and sixth are shorter, as are the outermost toes in the normal foot. The six extra toes remain almost without motion when the normal toes are flexed and extended, but they appear to have distinct metatarsal bones, and perhaps two or more bones of their own in the tarsus. Passing upwards we find the left leg and thigh much thicker than the right, but in length the two sides are equal. The difference in size may be seen in the following measurements: —

					Right Side.	Left (abnormal).
The circumference of the upper part of the thigh measures					7½ inches.	9¼ inches.
"	"	"	"	thigh just above the knee "	6½ "	7½ "
"	"	"	"	knee "	5½ "	6¼ "
"	"	"	"	leg immediately below knee measures 5¼ "		5½ "

There does not appear to be any unusual development of bone, but there is evident muscular hypertrophy. When the knee is partly flexed a rigid cord or tendon may be felt in the position of the outer hamstring, passing back of the knee, where it stands out prominently beneath the skin, and is continued downwards behind the fibula almost as low as the os calcis. The left labium majus has been twice as large as the right ever since birth. During the mother's pregnancy nothing remarkable happened, nor has anything been discovered to account for this strange malformation. I would, however, briefly call attention to the fact of the occurrence of this double deformity on the left side, the right being normal. Dr. Little [1] has remarked that congenital club-foot, as well as the deformity occurring after birth from disease of the nervous system, attains oftener a higher grade on the left than on the right side. I have not had an opportunity of verifying this statement, which refers to club-foot only, but I have observed a remarkable tendency in polydactylism to affect the left side more than the right. The malformation is altogether confined to the left side in the case above reported, and in an analogous case of bifurcated or double hand described in the forty-sixth volume of the Medico-Chirurgical Transactions, page 29. We find the same peculiarity in a case [2] in which the left foot presented

[1] Holmes's System of Surgery, 1862, iii. 567.
[2] Transactions of the Pathological Society of London, ix. 427.

nine toes, but no deformity existed in the other. In the *London Medical Gazette* [1] a supernumerary toe is mentioned as occurring on the left foot of a boy, other members of whose family were deformed in like manner. Mr. Sedgwick reports [2] the case of a girl who had a complete supernumerary finger attached to the outer side of the first phalangeal joint of the left little finger; the child's father, paternal grandmother, and paternal aunt had precisely the same deformity. Another case [3] related by Mr. Sedgwick consisted of double last phalanx on the left thumb of a boy whose maternal grandfather's great-nephew had exactly the same deformity. We find mention [4] also of a boy presenting six toes on the right foot and seven on the left, his hands being similarly malformed. His mother, sister, maternal uncle, and maternal grandfather had the same number of toes and fingers. In Amsterdam a monster, drowned by its parents, had eight toes on the right foot and nine on the left, besides many other malformations. An extended search among the records has discovered many cases of supernumerary digits similar to those already cited, but only a single case [5] where the digits were more numerous on the right side than on the left. I infer, therefore, that polydactylism generally affects the left side in preference to the right.

Mr. Adams has remarked [6] that occasionally we observe an excess or deficiency in the number of toes associated with congenital varus. Tamplin [7] has made a similar remark, and has given an illustration of a case of double talipes varus in which the right foot presented a bud-like projection on the little toe, while the left had six well-developed toes. We observe the association of congenital varus and supernumerary toes in the case of bifurcated or cloven foot, and we now find a further relationship between these deformities, inasmuch as they each attain oftener a higher grade on the left than on the right side. Whatever may be the true explanation of these facts, they show an especial tendency to deformity on the left side of the body, the side known to be the weaker one in the great majority of men.

[1] December 15, 1832, page 361.
[2] British and Foreign Medico-Chirurgical Review, April, 1863, page 463.
[3] Op. cit., page 462.
[4] London Medical Gazette, April 12, 1834.
[5] Broadhurst on Deformities, 1871, page 57.
[6] On Club-Foot, page 210.
[7] On Deformities, page 69.

MECHANICAL APPLIANCES IN UTERINE SURGERY.[1]

BY WILLIAM H. BAKER, M. D., OF BOSTON.

IN a previous article we considered and classified t1e causes of mis-placement of t1e uterus, defined t1e terms mec1anical appliances, and described t1e structure, form, and principle of application of t1e most important.

We are now prepared to ask (1) in w1at cases t1ey are beneficial; (2) w1en t1ey may be dispensed with; and (3) when t1ey are positively injurious. T1ese inquiries can be more satisfactorily answered by citing cases from our record-books in illustration of t1e particular class under consideration.   .

I. CASES IN WHICH MECHANICAL APPLIANCES ARE BENEFICIAL OR EVEN INDISPENSABLE.

CASE I. Mrs. B. had 1ad six abortions, four of t1em 1aving taken place since t1e birth of 1er last c1ild; and w1en s1e came under my care s1e was t1reatened wit1 a recurrence of t1e same accident.

On examination, t1e uterus was found completely retroverted and flexed, enlarged as in t1e second mont1 of pregnancy, and exceedingly sensitive, wit1 a slig1t disc1arge of blood from t1e os uteri. T1e patient was put to bed, and kept under t1e influence of opium for five days, at t1e end of w1ic1 time t1e uterus was so tolerant t1at it could be replaced wit1out serious danger of abortion. T1is was done by bi-manual manipulation, t1e patient lying upon the back. A Hodge retroversion closed pessary was introduced.

T1e patient derived great comfort from the appliance, and t1ree mont1s afterwards, t1e uterus having risen out of t1e pelvis and all danger of a recurrence of t1e accident 1aving passed, t1e pessary was removed, and s1e went on to t1e full term of 1er pregnancy.

In this case t1e cause of t1e previous abortions 1ad undoubtedly been t1e malposition of t1e uterus; wedged into t1e 1ollow of t1e sacrum, as it enlarged t1e tendency to abortion became greater and greater. T1e patient being very anxious to 1ave anot1er c1ild, s1e 1aving but one living, it was a matter of great importance to 1er w1ether s1e could complete her term of pregnancy, or w1et1er s1e must abort as on former occasions. If, t1en, we 1ad replaced t1e uterus and 1ad not used any mec1anical appliance to retain it in position, it would almost certainly 1ave returned to its retroverted state, and a recurrence of t1e t1reatened accident would 1ave taken place. To remain quiet in bed until t1e uterus s1ould reach t1at size w1ic1 would enable it to rise out of the pelvis 1ad been repeatedly tried in

---

[1] Concluded from page 279.

previous pregnancies without benefit; but on the contrary, the general health suffered so much by the confinement that it was worse than useless to attempt its repetition. Our object was only to be gained by exactly the treatment used; and the result in overcoming the threatened abortion, and carrying the patient over the time when its recurrence from a similar cause was past, proved the advantage of the appliance.

CASE II. Mrs. M., thirty-one years of age, had suffered more or less for ten years from dragging pains in both groins, great bearing-down, and backache, which had gradually but continuously increased, until at the time when I was first called to see her, July 2, 1874, her life was made perfectly miserable by the intensity of the above symptoms, even perfect quietude not giving her relief. The bowels were constipated, and the desire for micturition was very frequent. The patient was also made very unhappy by the fact that she was not able to suffer the slightest approach of her husband, sexual intercourse causing such severe pain.

Upon examination the cervix uteri was found crowded well forward against the sympysis pubis, by a sub-serous fibroid the size of the fist. Wedged into the hollow of the sacrum and nearly filling the excavation of the pelvis, this tumor formed with the uterus an immovable and highly sensitive mass. The uterus, somewhat retroflexed, admitted the uterine probe three and a half inches.

The treatment was first directed to relieving the sensibility of this neoplasm by hot vaginal injections and the application of the tincture of iodine to the fornix of the vagina. By these means, at the end of two and one half weeks the tenderness was so far removed that attempts were made on alternate days to gradually work the fibroid up out of the excavation of the pelvis, past the promontory of the sacrum, and above the superior strait. This was a rather tedious undertaking; but by the 10th of August, that is, in three weeks from the time we were able to commence these manipulations, we had so far accomplished our object that we were able to introduce a Thomas's modification of Cutter's pessary with a perineal strap and abdominal belt. The patient's relief was almost immediate: the backache, bearing-down, and dragging pains disappeared, the action of the bowels and bladder became natural; and she was able to live in the full enjoyment of the marital relation. The patient having been taught to remove and replace the pessary properly herself, and then feeling perfectly well and able to walk to and from my office, a distance of four miles, without any great fatigue, she was discharged on the 17th of August. The pessary was subsequently changed for one of the same variety with a larger bulb, there being a tendency of the tumor to work down behind the instrument; but it continued to give the greatest relief.

Let it not be supposed tiat tie above happy result can be so readily obtained in every similar case. It is sometimes only after tie most long-continued and patient treatment tiat the hyperæsthesia can be removed to such an extent tiat an instrument can be tolerated.

It will be evident tiat a fibroid of tie size of tiat described, iaving an attaciment to the posterior wall and tie fundus of tie uterus, would tend to dislocate tie uterus backwards; and even if tie organ were replaced, unless some mechanical appliance were adjusted to support tiis increased weigit, or to so far antevert tie wiole mass tiat its return into its former dislocated position would be prevented, tie relief to tie patient would be only tie most temporary. Wiat, tien, except the adjustment of some artificial support, in tie above class of cases, can give any permanent relief to tie sufferer? Surgical interference for tie removal of tie tumor would not be justifiable; for altiougi tie sufferings of the patient were great, yet life was not especially endangered, and so grave an operation would be unwarrantable.

I am well aware tiat a large number of additional cases might be given, illustrating tiis division of tie subject; but tiose already cited sufficiently prove tie great advantage often to be derived from the proper adjustment of some form of meciantical appliance to the uterus; and tie practitioner wio entirely discards suci appliances sacrifices one of tie most efficient means of giving relief to very many of his patients.

II. CASES IN WHICH MECHANICAL APPLIANCES MAY BE DISPENSED WITH.

CASE I. Mrs. E., aged tiirty-nine, was the mother of four children, the youngest of wiom was about twelve years old. I was called to the patient in August, 1873, througi tie kindness of Dr. J. Marion Sims. Sie had been twice operated upon by him, once for intra-uterine fibroid tumor,[1] and subsequently for fungoid granulations of tie mucous membrane. For several montis previous to my seeing the patient her menstruation iad been muci too frequent in its recurrence, and tie time of its continuance was very muci prolonged; tie amount of blood lost was also in great excess. Each monti seemed to increase tie difficulty until two montis before sie was seen, wien pregnancy occurring, tiere was a cessation of tie flow. Seven days before sie came under my care, sie was tireatened witi abortion, and took ier bed; notwithstanding ier precaution, two days afterward sie aborted with an alarming hæmorrhage, wiich continued in a sligit degree at intervals until my first visit.

Upon examination, the body of tie uterus was found to be completely retroflexed and considerably enlarged; tie external os was found open enough to admit the forefinger; but tie internal os was very

[1] See his recent pamphlet on Intra-Uterine Fibroids.

small. Feeling confident from tie iistory of tie case tiat, in addition
to tie probable existence of fungoid granulations, tiere was tie remnant
of an ovum tiere, I introduced two sponge tents, and after seven
iours, tie patient being etierized and tie tents removed, tie finger
passed into tie uterine cavity detected a soft, pulpy mass of about tie
size of a walnut, attacied to tie upper and posterior surfaces ; also to
some extent on tie anterior surface were felt tie peculiar iypertropiied
utricular glands. Witi a Sims's curette tiese were all removed, tie
cavity of tie uterus being most tiorougily curetted, until, by tie sound
conveyed by tie curette and by tie sensation wiici it gave to tie
touci, it was evident tiat we iad reacied tie firmer sub-mucous and
muscular tissue. Tie operation was accompanied by considerable iæmorriage ; but as it was very quickly done, and as tie bleeding was readily controlled by putting a tampon into tie cavity of tie uterus as well
as into tie vagina, it was not a serious complication. Tie patient made
a good, tiougi ratier slow, recovery from tie operation. Sie went
over tie next menstrual period witiout any flow, but after tiat was
quite regular and normal. Tie uterus gradually returned to its per-
feet position.[1]

Now, iad we been satisfied witi diagnosticating tie malposition of
tie uterus and adjusting some mecianical appliance tiereto, tie result
could not iave been' satisfactory, for tie remains of tie ovum and tie
granulations still being in the cavity of tie uterus, tie iæmorriage
must continue, even tiougi tie uterus were sustained in its normal
position ; and until tiis cause of the iæmorriage and tie malposition
were removed, tiere could be no hope of permanent benefit. But tiese
causes of tie misplacement being obviated, tie tendency of tie uterus
was to regain its perfect position, altiougi it received no aid from any
artificial support.

CASE II. Mrs. N., tiirty-five years of age, was admitted to tie service of my iigily respected instructor, Dr. T. Addis Emmet, in tie
Woman's Hospital of New York, during tie monti of December, 1873.
Sie iad been married twelve years, and iad iad one miscarriage at six
montis and subsequently a ciild, after a rapid labor, ten years before
her admission to the iospital. For tie latter lengti of time, altiougi
not entirely incapacitated from work, yet sie constantly suffered
tirough tie lower part of tie abdomen and back siarp pains whici
were greatly increased by walking. Sie iad also a leucorrioeal disciarge of a tiick and tougi consistence.

On examination, tie uterus was found retroverted, and its cervix lac-
crated on tie left side down to tie vaginal junction and very muci hypertrophied, its surface being covered witi tie disciarge above described.

[1] Since the above was written, tho patient has been delivered by my respected friend, Dr.
J. P. Reynolds.

One week after the patient's admission to the hospital, the writer operated upon the case for Dr. Emmet, for the closure of the lacerated cervix. The patient being etherized, this was successfully done, the hæmorrhage, which was considerable, being entirely controlled as soon as the sutures were introduced. She made a good recovery from the operation, and then the uterus being replaced, and some intra-uterine applications of impure carbolic acid made, the womb gradually regained its proper position, and the patient, feeling entirely relieved of her suffering, was discharged from the hospital, cured, January 17, 1874. She was seen four months afterwards, and had continued well. The uterus was then in a normal position, and the cervix looked perfectly natural, no evidences of the operation being visible.

In the above case, the malposition was undoubtedly due primarily to the condition of the cervix, and secondarily to that of the interior of the uterus. The indications were, first, to restore the cervix to its normal condition, or to that which it had previous to the birth of her child ten years earlier; and, second, to obtain a healthy state of the lining membrane of the uterus. The result of this course most certainly proved the correctness of the treatment. Had we attempted to use any mechanical appliance to correct the malposition of the uterus before the natural condition of the cervix had been restored, we should have greatly aggravated the case, for such treatment could not have failed to increase the already greatly irritated cervix. As it was, the beneficial result proved to us that in the above class of cases, at least, mechanical appliances may be entirely dispensed with.

The cases just cited especially show the importance of discovering the cause of the misplacement; for it may be found that after the removal of this cause, any artificial support will be quite unnecessary.

III. CASES IN WHICH MECHANICAL APPLIANCES ARE POSITIVELY IN-JURIOUS.

It is very evident that under this class, any case may come in which the appliance is improperly adjusted, however great the misplacement or the urgency of the case may be, demanding such an appliance. In illustration of this fact, let me give the following, which came under my observation at the Woman's Hospital.

CASE I. I. M. was admitted to the service of my esteemed instructor, Professor T. G. Thomas, early in the year 1874. She was a single woman, thirty years of age. About five years previous to her admission to the hospital, she suffered from some misplacement of the uterus; the physician attending her, in attempting to adjust an intravaginal pessary, introduced it through the urethra into the bladder, where it remained for a year and a half; but it finally caused so much distress from the cystitis which it created, without at all relieving the misplacement which it was designed to correct, that its removal was contemplated. But before this could be accomplished, it became necessary to cut through the anterior vaginal wall into the bladder, thus forming a vesico-vaginal fistula. Seven months after the pessary was thus removed from the bladder, it was discovered that a calculus had formed there, which was also removed through the same artificial opening. She was then operated upon twice unsuccessfully for the closure of the fistula which had been created. The third attempt for its closure was made by Professor Thomas, which proved successful, and the patient returned home a few weeks afterwards.

By this aggravated case it will be seen how great an amount of damage may be done, and how much suffering caused, by the improper use of a mechanical appliance in this branch of surgery. But let it not be supposed that a less serious result may not sometimes follow the more careful adjustment of a pessary, even where the greatest attention is bestowed as to the proper introduction of the appliance and the most strict injunctions are laid down as to its subsequent use. This will be seen by the following.

CASE II. M. C. presented herself at my clinic in New York during the month of December, 1873. She was twenty years of age, single, and had complained more or less since her arrival in this country, about a year previous. Her principal symptoms were constant pain in the back and down the thighs, and her extremely nervous condition ; these, together with her inability to be much on her feet, incapacitated her for her work, which was that of a chamber-girl.

Upon examination the uterus was found to be retroverted, but was very readily replaced in its normal position. The passage of the uterine probe was not followed by any slow of blood ; neither did it cause the patient the slightest pain. There was no special sensitiveness of the organ, and its malposition seemed due to some sudden and undue abdominal pressure, undoubtedly occurring during her passage on shipboard to this country. The uterus having been put into a normal position, a retroversion pessary of very small size was introduced ; and (as was my custom in my out-patient department) the patient was told to walk about a block or two, and returning to remove the pessary herself. This was done to prove, first, that the instrument gave her no discomfort ; and, secondly, that after her return home, in case she should have any such discomfort, she might be able at once to remove the pessary. These instructions having been carried out, the pessary was reintroduced, and the patient sent home with the strict injunctions, not only to herself but also to her sister, who accompanied her, to remove it upon the approach of the slightest pain or even discomfort. She was directed to return in one week, that I might be assured that the pessary was accomplishing the desired object, and that she was receiv-

ing no 1arm from its use. But in five days from the date of its introduction, t1e sister came back wit1 t1e following account of t1e patient's
condition : For two days she 1ad almost entire relief from t1e pain in
t1e back, and would not 1ave known s1e 1ad any pessary in the vagina,
had s1e not been informed and instructed concerning it. T1en commenced some uncomfortableness, w1ic1 increased to a decided pain ;
but 1aving found so muc1 relief from t1e use of t1e support during t1e
previous two days, s1e was unwilling to 1ave t1e pessary removed.
T1e fourth nig1t s1e 1ad a severe c1ill, followed by 1ig1 fever and
great pain over t1e abdomen. Her suffering was t1en so intense t1at
she permitted 1er sister to remove t1e pessary. T1e fift1 day I found
t1e patient wit1 a temperature of 103°, taken in the axilla; t1e pulse
was 112. T1e girl evidently was suffering from a severe attack of
cellulitis of t1e rig1t broad ligament. S1e was at once put upon appropriate treatment, and in a little more t1an t1ree weeks was back in
my clinic. T1e uterus was fixed to t1e rig1t side, but under treatment
it was freed from its attachments so t1at it could be restored to a normal position.

Here, t1en, is a case w1ere t1e introduction of an artificial support
to t1e uterus gave rise to alarming, even dangerous, symptoms. But
on account of t1ese occasional accidents, are we to discard pessaries
altoget1er ? W1en we call to mind t1e number of cases w1ere t1eir
use 1as been found indispensable, and t1e still greater number where
they 1ave been exceedingly beneficial, we certainly feel unwilling to
give t1em up. We rat1er heed t1e injunction w1ic1 requires additional caution for a still more strict discrimination of t1e classes of
cases in w1ic1 t1eir use may be most beneficial. Even in such instances we s1ould exercise still greater care and watchfulness in the
subsequent treatment of t1e patient. Doubtless we s1all continue to
use t1em, and the good results usually obtained will prove the correctness of our judgment.   •

These examples might be almost indefinitely multiplied, in illustration not only of t1e topics we 1ave especially treated, but also on ot1er
branc1es of t1is general subject. To some of t1e latter allusion 1as
been made in a previous article ; ot1ers, daily practice is continually
bringing to notice. But we trust enoug1 1as been said to establish t1e
main points of t1is paper : t1at mec1anical appliances in certain cases
are positively injurious ; in ot1ers t1ey may be partially or wholly dispensed with ; w1ile in a t1ird class t1ey are altoget1er indispensable.

In t1is as in many departments of medical practice, the trut1, we believe, lies between t1e extremes of absolute disuse on t1e one 1and and
universal application on t1e ot1er ; and t1e skill of t1e practitioner is
ex1ibited in discriminating between those cases which are, and t1ose
which are not, t1e proper subjects for such appliances.

RECENT PROGRESS IN ANATOMY.[1]

BY THOMAS DWIGHT, JR., M. D.

BONE, LIGAMENTS, AND JOINTS.

MR. WAGSTAFFE[2] is the last to write a paper " to show that in all cancellous tissues there is a definite mechanical arrangement, insuring the greatest strength and elasticity along the lines of greatest pressure." He refers to several recent German writers on the subject, but states that his researches were made independently of theirs, and differ from them in many points. To begin with the bodies of the vertebræ, the author states that the upright fibres are not straight, but curved, with the concavity toward the centre of the bone. This is entirely imaginary, as may be seen on sections of the bone, or by consulting the photographs in Bardeleben's admirable monograph on the spinal column,[3] with which the author does not seem to be acquainted. Bardeleben's account of the plates connecting the two ends of the vertebræ is briefly as follows : part run quite vertically, part in a slight curve, so that their end is directly under their origin, and part immediately, or almost so, run obliquely to the lower surface, without ending under their origins. Two or three thin plates often unite into a single thicker one in the middle third of the vertebra to split up again below. The general appearance is of a right-angled net-work, thinner in the middle of the body. The upper end of the humerus is well described. Two series of plates are shown to arise from both the outer and inner side of the upper part of the shaft; the lower set of each side diverges inward, forming Gothic arches with that of the other, while the two upper sets are continued, for the most part vertically, into the greater tuberosity and head respectively. The author shows that the bone must resist pressure in the direction of its long axis when in two quite distinct positions. When the arm is extended, as in pushing, the pressure is transmitted through the head to the glenoid cavity, and when the weight of the body is supported by the arms it goes downward from the coraco-acromial ligament through the greater tuberosity. The lower end of the bone is less thoroughly treated, for nothing is said of the net-work of strong, mostly horizontal braces that occupy the end of the shaft just as it begins to widen. The structure of the innominate bone appears, as Mr. Wagstaffe observes, to have been overlooked, but we are inclined to believe that the reason lies in the difficulty of drawing satisfactory conclusions. Mr. Wagstaffe attaches significance to two sections in particular ; the first of these is " from the

---

[1] Concluded from page 282.

[2] The Mechanical Structure of the Cancellous Tissue of Bones. St. Thomas's Hospital Reports. 1875.

[3] Vide Report on Anatomy, in the JOURNAL, March 11, 1875.

pubes to the sacro-iliac synchondrosis through the acetabulum and along
the brim of the true pelvis." He correctly states that the "thick brim
forms part of a ring which is placed almost vertically when the body is
erect," and of course gives great support in that position. Additional
strength is gained by curved fibres from each side of the body of the
pubes crossing one another, but the arrangement behind the acetabulum
is not so clear. The second section is through the anterior superior spine
of the ilium and the tuberosity of the pubes, and shows curved lines from
each surface of the bone, those below the acetabulum forming inverted
arches. The remarks on the head of the fibula are interesting as showing, according to the author, that this bone bears a part of the weight
of the body. In a well-marked bone a series of diverging curved fibres
from the articular surface pass downward into the shaft, and are crossed
by a nearly transverse set. If we follow the direction of the force from
below upward, it certainly seems plausible that a certain amount of
weight should be transmitted through the fibula.

The Hip. — Every one who has attentively studied the hip-joint in
frozen sections must have been struck by the delicate layer of frozen
synovia which nearly or quite surrounds the head of the femur while the
preparation is fresh, or by the space intervening between the articular
surfaces when it is kept in alcohol ; but Professor König [1] has the merit
of pointing out its importance. He has made a number of sections
with the bones in different positions, and has shown that the brothers
Weber were in error in teaching that the radii of the head of the
femur and of the socket were equal, as on a transverse vertical section
(frontal) the average difference was found to be two millimetres in
favor of the latter. The distance between the articular surfaces is by
no means the same in all parts of the joint, and varies with the position
of the limb. In the erect position the surfaces are in absolute contact,
but only through a small space, corresponding with the highest part of
the cavity. In abduction and adduction a separating layer of frozen
fluid, though at points very thin, was always present.

A year later F. Schmidt [2] advanced quite another view, based on experiment as well as on a mathematical basis that we cannot discuss.
The source of difficulty is the complicated form both of the head
and of the socket. In the erect position, and in simple extension and
flexion, all points of the head and socket are in contact throughout the
latter; but in other movements it is not the case. This writer shows
that in certain exaggerated movements the head might rest against the
edge of the socket and act as a lever. He points out what appears to
be a weak point in König's position, namely, that the relations must be
different when the head is lying at rest in the socket and when it is
forced in by the weight of the body or muscular action.

---

[1] Deutsche Zeitschrift für Chirurgie, Band iii., heft 3 and 4, November, 1873.
[2] Ibid. Band v., heft 4, November, 1874.

An Abnormal Canal in tie temporal bone running tiroug1 tie squamous portion, and giving passage to a deep temporal artery arising irregularly inside tie skull from tie middle meningeal artery, is described by Professor Gruber.[1] He found tiis anomaly twenty-five times in some four tiousand skulls; to wit, six times on boti sides, eig1t times on tie rig1t, and eleven on tie left. In tiese cases tiere is often an extra suture tiroug1 the squamous portion.

The Jugular Foramen. — Professor Rüdinger[2] has publisied some observations on tiis point from a work wiic1 ias not yet appeared, in reply'to Professor Moos, of Heidelberg, wio ias been inclined to trace some connection between dilatation of tie bulb of tie jugular vein and psyciical affections. Out of one iundred human skulls Rüdinger finds tiat in sixty-nine tie rig1t jugular foramen is tie larger, tie left one in twenty-seven, and tiat tie two are equal in four. Tiese results, except in tie last point, correspond very fairly witi tiose obtained by tie reporter[3] from a series of one iundred and fifty-nine skulls, of wiic1 one iundred and four iad tiis foramen larger on tie rig1t, tiirtyeig1t on tie left, and seventeen presented no difference. Rüdinger siows tiat tie difference between tie two sides depends on tie arrangement of tie venous sinuses. He iolds tiat tiere is no true confluence at tie internal occipital protuberance, but tiat tie superior longitudinal sinus carrying tie blood from tie surface of tie iemispieres turns to tie side of tie larger foramen (usually to tie rig1t), and tiat tie straig1t sinus from tie interior of tie brain turns tie otier way. He admits, iowever, tiat tiere is a communication between tie two. His conclusions are : —

(1.) Tiat tie jugular openings are unequally large and deep.

(2.) Tiat tiis difference is not tie result of any anomaly of tie surrounding bones.

(3.) Tiat, as above stated, it depends on tie course of tie cirenlation.

(4.) Tiat a broad jugular fossa appears to be an individual peculiarity, in wiic1 neitier tie intra-cranial circulation nor tie function of iearing is concerned.

We are unable to see on wiat tie last conclusion is based; as our own observations siow tiat of tie one iundred and forty-two skulls wiic1 iad tie foramen larger on one side tian on tie otier, iinetythree, or nearly two tiirds, iad a more capacious fossa on tie same side as tie larger foramen, wiile tie fossa was larger on tie same side as tie smaller foramen in only nineteen, or less tian one seventi.

The Ilio-Tibial Tract of the Fascia Lata is tie name by wiic1 Dr.

---

[1] Virchow's Archiv, 1875, 1 and 2.
[2] Monatschrift für Ohrenheilkunde, 1875, No. 1.
[3] American Journal of the Medical Sciences, October, 1873.

Hermann Welcker [1] designates a part of tiis fascia whici ias been variously described, but according to him never understood. In tie last
edition of Quain, tie tensor vaginæ femoris is said to be inserted between two laminæ of tiis fascia, and tie description goes on as follows:
" Tie outer of tiese laminæ is continued upwards on tie muscle in its
wiole extent, being part of tie general investment of tie limb; tie
deeper is connected above witi tie origin of tie rectus muscle, and
with tie fibres attaciing tie gluteus minimus to tie iip-joint. Tie
part of tie fascia made tense by tie action of tie muscle forms a strong
tendinous band, wiich descends to tie outer and back part of tie knee-
joint." We reproduce tiis passage, as it almost coincides witi Welcker's
description. Tiis band is most commonly known as tie ilio-tibial ligament of Meyer, wio describes it as extending from tie crest of tie
ilium to tie outer tuberosity of the tibia, and states tiat it is joined* by
fibres from tie tendons of tie tensor fasciæ, and from tiat of tie gluteus maximus. Henle denies tiat any tendinous fibres from tie tensor
go to form part of tiis fascia. Welcker's description of tie origin of
tie band differs from tiat in Quain's Anatomy, inasmuci as ie gives it
tiree points of origin: one from tie layer of fascia covering tie tensor, a second from tie layer below it, and a tiird from tie inferior anterior spine of tie ilium. Tie autior alludes to a forgotten paper read
by Maissiat before tie Académie des Sciences in 1842, in wiici ie
maintains tiat man naturally stands with iis weigit on one leg, and
tiat tie consequent lateral projection of tie iip makes tense tiis fascia,
wiici prevents excessive lateral flexion of tie pelvis. Welcker iolds tiat
it acts boti as a ligament and as a tendon, tiougi not at tie same time;
as a ligament in tie way described by Maissiat, and as a tendon of tie
tensor, wiici, wien tie leg is kept straigit, rotates it on tie femur.
In tiis connection, Welcker discussed tie action of tie sartorius, and,
admitting its usually received action, adds tiat wien tie knee is ield
straigit it serves to tigiten tie fascia of tie leg.

CONCERNING ACTS COMMITTED BY EPILEPTICS.

BY M. LEGRAND DU SALLE.

Translated from Annales d'Hygiène Publique et de Médecine Légale, April, 1875.

BY S. G. WEBBER, M. D.[2]

THE patiological and legal status of epileptics having as yet not been
establisied scientifically and definitively, the most variable judicial

---

[1] Reichert and Du Bois Reymond's Archiv, 1875, i.

[2] It has been necessary to abridge this discourse, especially the reports of cases. It has lost
much of its freshness and vigor, but I have tried to retain all that is really essential. — TR.

decisions have been hitherto rendered. It is time that this should cease, and that enlightened opinions should prevail. Epilepsy so changes the natural tendencies, and the intellectual, moral, and affectional character of the patients, that it finally produces in them a general ex-·pression, impresses upon them a common stamp. Apart from all convulsive attacks, epileptics are egotists, distrustful, shy, irritable, passionate. A gesture or a look is sufficient to excite their passion. Suspicions, querulous, loving no one, they complain wrongly, quarrel, make themselves hated; in them everything is contradictory. These same men whose bitterness and maliciousness have just awakened your attention, there they are now, polite, flattering, obsequious — they take your hands and put themselves entirely at your disposal. From being gay, animated, self-satisfied, in three or four hours they are sad, desponding, tired of life.

From a medico-legal stand-point there are three varieties of epileptics: (1) those in whom the neurosis has had no effect on their intelligence ; (2) those whose intelligence and memory are only temporarily disturbed at the time of or after their attacks, and who during long intervals of quiet enjoy complete possession of their reason, though I consider them, really, as candidates for insanity ; (3) those whose minds are seriously and permanently changed, whose insanity is irremediable. To this division corresponds necessarily a scale of legal responsibility.

1. A crime coolly calculated, with sufficient explanation of the motives, especially if the epileptic attacks are rare, and if they have never compromised the intelligence, renders the author responsible.

2. Whoever has clearly committed a crime when not subject to an attack is partially responsible, according to his mental capacity.

3. An unjustifiable crime committed under the evident influence of an epileptic attack involves absolutely no responsibility.

In examining an epileptic, the medico-legalist should proceed exactly as if he had before him a case of mental disease, and form his judgment from the whole assemblage of symptoms, and not from a single one. He will lay stress upon the character and the course of the attacks of delirium in their relations with the physical symptoms of epilepsy. Thus he will inquire whether the delirium occurs in the form of crises, without convulsions, without incomplete attacks, and without vertigo, or whether in direct connection with these physical symptoms; whether these crises have been relatively short; whether they have had a rapid invasion and cessation ; finally, whether they have recurred at intervals more or less distant during the previous life of the patient or in the prison. Secondly, he will found his opinion upon the physical and moral character of the crises, which consist chiefly in vagueness and obtuseness of the ideas, the occurrence of violent and instantaneous impulses, the necessity of walking without an object, of striking and breaking without motive, and extreme confusion of memory after the disappearance of the delirium. Finally, we will rely upon the character of the acts themselves committed during these attacks; they are violent, automatic, instantaneous, and without motive.

All medico-legal difficulty is summed up in a simple question of diagnosis. Trousseau often repeated these words : " Epilepsy is the disease which is most often overlooked." Every day I recognize the correctness of that opinion. Among the crowd of criminals and abandoned of all classes whom I meet at the police court, I have been surprised often at finding the same persons, and learning that they were prosecuted for the same offense. I have many times found in their feelings of discomfort, their giddiness, their migraine, their fainting spells, their nocturnal incontinence of urine, their rush of blood, their momentary loss of reason, or their loss of memory, the sure signs of epileptic vertigo, of the *petit mal* or the *grand mal*. Of all the epileptic phenomena, vertigo is the most frequently ignored. Although it may be almost instantaneous, it leads quite as quickly as the classical attacks to abnormal psychical manifestations.

A woman, P., thirty years old, stole a pair of shoes at a stall, without any motive for the act, while the shopkeeper was near and saw her. Arrested, she returned the shoes, protested the purity of her life, and said she had no recollection of the theft. It was a case of epileptic vertigo.

The symptom of epilepsy which is next in frequency overlooked is the nocturnal incontinence of urine at intervals more or less distant. The symptomatic value of this is very great. A Mr. G., who had borne a reputation for good behavior and sobriety, was sometimes unquiet, anxious, preoccupied ; but he soon recovered his cheerfulness. One day he left his place of business, went to his sister's, talked with her a short time, then without provocation struck her sixty-three blows with a chopping-knife. When he was taken to the Bicêtre, it was learned that he had wet his bed several times a year when he was in military service, that at times he had trouble in his head. He continued to have nocturnal attacks, wetting his bed. He died after an attack of acute maniacal delirium.

A class of persons at intervals show suddenly anomalies of intellect of very short duration, singularities of character, violence in speech, with or without hallucinations of vision, sometimes with a true aura, but invariably with absolute loss of memory for all that happens during the attack. These seizures have the same character each time for the same persons. Frequently the patient is impelled to walk off without any definite purpose, and on recovering finds himself at a distance from home, with no knowledge of what he has done.

The diagnosis of masked epilepsy is very difficult ; the symptomatology is imperfect; only the intellectual side of the terrible neurosis is seen ; the vertigo, the incomplete attack, and the convulsive grand mal are wanting. Thus, a lady of distinction suddenly, at almost regular intervals, utters the most injurious, the most cynical, and the vilest words during one or two minutes, in a salon, at table, at church, or at the theatre. In place of the words, suppose an assassination. This lady has no recollection of what she says.

A very intelligent young man, in the higher class of society, three or four times a year has a peculiar sensation in his stomach, always identical; he immediately loses consciousness. On coming to himself he finds that he is far from home, fatigued, in a railroad car, or in prison, his pockets containing jewelry, handkerchiefs, pocket-books, cigar-cases, knives, money. He remembers nothing of what has happened.

In masked epilepsy the misdemeanor and crime have a character entirely unexpected, and display the strong contrast between the natural disposition of the person and the scandalous and mad acts which are committed during the temporary disturbance of consciousness. There are two men to study, two psychological states to compare, and two series of actions; but never lose from view that in masked epilepsy what a patient has done during one of his attacks he will invariably do again in the same circumstances. Masked epilepsy does not run through all degrees of eccentricity or crime; it is limited entirely to a single one.

In examining a crime for which no motive can be found, legal medicine may meet the most exceptional difficulties. Before hastily concluding that epilepsy is present it is necessary to recognize the whole group of symptoms just passed in review. If one important sign is entirely wanting, take care lest you may be following a false scent.

The most extraordinary and embarrassing case for a long time is that of T., the assassin of Rue Cujas. This man was born January 15, 1851, at the Saint Lazare prison, of a child-mother who was not yet fifteen years old, and of a father sixty-three years old. He says that since 1865 he has had three or four fainting fits, with entire loss of consciousness, and several times vertigo. He is intelligent, has a good memory, answers questions correctly and frankly, and gives information about himself, foreign to the crime, but showing a precocious and sadly audacious perversity. He says he has had at irregular intervals an itching to kill some one. These crises last from one to three days, and during this time he feels nervous, irritable, unable to keep still, and always ready to commit some violent act. During one of these attacks he spent the night with a *fille publique.* He thought of killing her, but was restrained by the idea that his crime would be attributed to a desire to rob, and he did not wish to be taken for an infamous assassin of one with whom he had passed the night. He finally killed a young woman w10 waited upon him at t1e restaurant. He 1as been calm for five mont1s and a 1alf since 1is arrest, and no one 1as noticed t1e least sign of delirium or epilepsy. I was inclined, 1owever, to consider it as a case of masked epilepsy, yet T. 1ad complete preservation and precision of memory after 1is fainting fits and 1is vertigo. Now t1is fact, almost of itself alone, excludes epilepsy. M. Lasegne considers t1at t1e assassin of t1e Rue Cujas 1ad paroxysms of impulsive insanity, t1at he may 1ave 1ad epileptiform symptoms, but 1e was not an epileptic. T1is seems reasonable, but I am not yet able to give an absolutely definitive diagnosis.

THE MORAL OF THE MICHIGAN DIFFICULTY.

THE disturbance caused by the "inflation policy" of t1e legislature of Mic1igan in forcing a so-called homœopathic department into the regular sc1ool has reached the "correspondence" stage, so t1at we may hope the end is at 1and. T1e only advantage to be 1oped for from t1e letters is t1at the profession may be stirred up to take a firm position in t1e matter. Not1ing is to be gained by temporizing; if t1e faculty does not appreciate t1at no compromi*e wit1 quackery is possible, t1ey will find out t1eir error w1en it may be too late to repair it. If t1e medical department is t1oug1t wort1 preserving, a vigorous effort must be made. We appreciate t1at t1e position is a 1ard one. An ignorant legislature and public press 1ave natural affinities wit1 quackery, and the respectable man is always at a disadvantage in a dispute wit1 an unscrupulous impostor; nevert1eless t1e fig1t must be foug1t.

T1is affair, let it end as it may, is of great importance, as it points a moral t1at t1e profession at large s1ould profit by. Some years ago a ring endeavored, 1appily wit1out success, to establis1 a national university under government control, and we occasionally 1ear suggestions of State boards to confer licenses to practice. Let it be understood once and for all t1at professional 1onor is too precious to be made one of t1e prizes of political contests. T1e t1eory as well as t1e practical working of our political system forbids us to consider government as a kind parent in w1om we may trust; on t1e contrary, it can be kept pure only by t1e strongest and most persistent efforts, and a moment's inattention may give t1e intriguer years of advantage.

A legislature may be respectable one year, and the reverse the next; or if not the next, yet surely sooner or later: and it would be as futile as unbecoming for us to pit ourselves against t1e quack in lobbying and bribery. Professional affairs are safe only in our own 1ands; let us keep t1em t1ere.

THE BRITISH MEDICAL ASSOCIATION.

THE forty-t1ird annual meeting of t1is association was opened at Edinburg1 on Tuesday, August 3d, and continued four days. Sir Robert C1ristison occupied t1e presidential c1air and delivered the opening address, w1ic1 was devoted to the subject of medical education and medical examinations in Great Britain. The question was discussed at length, and occupied over two hours in delivery. On following days addresses were delivered before the general meeting by Dr. Begbie on medicine, by Mr. Spence on surgery, and by Dr. Rutherford on physiology. The most interesting portion of Mr. Spence's address was that which treated of wounds and surgical dressings. This was listened to with great interest as coming from a prominent member of the surgical staff of the Edinburgh Infirmary and a colleague of Professor Lister, differing from the latter strongly in his views on the antiseptic treatment. The speaker adduced a number of facts showing that other methods of treatment might also give brilliant results. Professor Lister, of course, had an opportunity to present his view of the question, which be illustrated before the physiological section by an interesting series of clinical demonstrations and by an able lecture on the process of infection. His efforts contributed in a high degree to the success of the meeting. Dr. Rutherford, the successor to Hughes Bennett, devoted himself chiefly to a report of a number of experiments on the biliary secretion of the dog, and defended also with great spirit experimentation on animals, wherein he was strongly supported by Dr. Burden Saunderson and Sir Robert Christison.

The business of the meeting did not run so smoothly this year as it has been wont to do in times past. Great indignation was exhibited against the council for securing the adoption of its report without discussion, as well as the remodeled by-laws of the association. Considerable excitement was also produced by the appearance of two lady-members one of whom, Mrs. Garret Anderson, read before one of the sections a paper, which is said to have been very favorably received. The constitutionality of the action of the county society in admitting lady-members was discussed with much animation, and the motion was finally carried, " that it be an instruction to the secretary, between now and the next annual meeting, to issue a circular addressed to every member of the association, requesting an opinion 'yes' or 'no' as to the admission of female practitioners to membership."

In the section on surgery the question of anæsthetic agents came up for discussion, and a committee was " appointed to inquire into and report upon the use in surgery of various anæsthetic agents and the mixture of such agents." We notice upon the committee the names of Lister, Keith, Spencer Wells, Clover, Macdonnell, and Morgan, and shall therefore look forward with strong hopes for a satisfactory report at the next annual meeting. The details of the section work have not yet been fully reported. It was voted after some discussion to meet next year at Brighton, and that the president elect should be Sir John Cordy Burrows. The annual dinner was attended by but five hundred members — quite a small number when the size of the association is considered. The annual museum, the conversazione, the garden party, and excursions were interesting features of the meeting.

DENTISTRY IN 1796.

AMERICAN dentists of the present day may with justice lay claim to a high reputation for skill and ingenuity. The autograph letter of Washington which appeared in the JOURNAL of June 17th showed that considerable enterprise was shown also by our dental forefathers. We have before us an interesting document which gives quite accurately the degree of proficiency which had been reached in dentistry toward the close of the last century. It consists of an advertisement issued by one Josiah Flagg, surgeon dentist, who

"Informs the public, that he practises in all the branches with improvements, [i. e.] Transplants both live and dead Teeth with great conveniency, and gives less pain than heretofore practised in Europe or America : . . . Sews up Hare Lips : . . . Cures Ulcers : . . . Extracts Teeth and stumps, or roots with Ease : . . . Reinstates Teeth and gums, that are much depreciated by nature, carelessness, acids, or corroding medicine ; . . . Fastens those Teeth that are loose (unless wasted at the roots); regulates Teeth from their first cutting to prevent feavers and pain in children ; assists nature in the extension of the jaws, for the beautiful arrangement of the second Sett, and preserves them in their natural whiteness entirely free from all scorbutic complaints. And when thus put in order and his directions followed (which are simple) he engages that the further care of a *Dentist* will be wholly unnecessary ; . . . Eases pain in Teeth without drawing ; . . . Stops bleeding in the gums, jaws, or arteries ; . . . Lines and plumbs Teeth with virgin Gold, Foil, or Leads ; . . . Fixes *gold Roofs and Palates*, and artificial Teeth of any quality, without injury to and independent of the natural ones, greatly assisting the pronunciation and the swallow when injured by natural or other defects. A room for the practice with every accommodation at his house, where may be had Dentifices, Tinctures, Teeth and Gum Brushes, Mastics, &c., warranted approved and adapted to the various ages and circumstances ; . . . also Chew-sticks, particularly useful in cleansing the fore Teeth and preserving a natural and beautiful whiteness ; which Medicine and Chew-sticks are to be sold wholesale and retail, that they may be more extensively usefull.

"*** Dr. Flagg has a method to furnish those Ladies and gentlemen or children with Artificial Teeth, Gold Gums, Roofs, or Palates, that are at a distance and cannot attend him personally.

Cash Given

for Handsome and Healthy Live Teeth

at No. 47, Newbury-Street, Boston (1796)."

The document is ornamented in one corner by very formidable and antiquated instruments, while in the other are to be seen tooth-brushes quite of the modern pattern. It has been preserved by a descendant of one who, as may be seen on the back, purchased a brush and tincture from Josiah Flagg in the year 1800.

MEDICAL NOTES.

— The death of Dr. Ira Allen, of Roxbury, has removed from the community a man widely known and respected for his worth and abilities. He entered the profession late in life, but his ready skill, his intuitive judgment, and his gentleness towards the suffering had secured for him a large field of practice and endeared him to the inmates of numerous homes. In his intercourse with his medical brethren he was courteous and considerate ; and be contributed several useful and practical appliances in surgery. He rose in his earlier career in the face of unusual obstacles, winning success by virtue of his indomitable perseverance and energy. His medical degree was taken at Dartmouth.

Besides attending faithfully to the demands of an extensive practice, Dr. Allen found time to serve the city of Roxbury, and more recently the city of Boston, in various responsible offices, wherein he showed exceptional fidelity and ability. As city physician of Roxbury, as coroner, as agent of the Board of Overseers of the Poor, as associate justice of the Municipal Court in the Highland district, and especially as a member of the school committee, a position which he held for twenty-three years, he displayed efficiency and public spirit and acquitted himself with credit and honor. Our readers will remember how well, as coroner, he conducted the preliminary examination of the boy Pomeroy after the Millen murder. In all his relations, public and professional, Dr. Allen will be greatly missed in his community, for in no sense was he a neutral man ; he had strong convictions and these he maintained boldly and manfully, but with a forbearance which made for him a host of friends.

— There are several English ladies attending the lectures of the École de Médecine of Paris at present. We see that among others Miss Alice Vickery, chemist by examination of the Pharmaceutical Society of Great Britain, has just passed her deuxième examen de fin d'année, and with the certificate " bien satisfait " from the examiners. The *Medical Press and Circular* says that it remains to be seen whether some hospital in London will now be generous enough to grant such industrious ladies the necessary clinical instruction in medicine and surgery required by the École de Médecine of Paris.

— The application of an elastic ligature for securing the funis is recommended by George Bayles, M. D., in the *Medical Record* of August 28, 1875. Dr. Bayles uses a small, elastic rubber ring, of a size that would be somewhat stretched by being drawn over the point of the fourth finger of his hand. In applying the ring he doubles the umbilical cord upon itself, so that three inches are taken up in the loop, as close to the umbilicus as possible. He then springs the ring over the loop, and rolls it down to within half an inch of the abdominal surface, and cuts the funis about half an inch from the rubber ring, external to the loop. Two portions of the funis are in this way constricted by the ring. The ring may be doubled upon itself before applying it, if there is any doubt as to its sufficient constricting force.

— We learn from the *Albany Weekly Times* that the trustees of the Johns Hopkins bequest of Baltimore are carefully carrying out the wishes of the donor. They have purchased twenty-four acres of land for the purposes of the

Colored Orphan Asylum. The erection of the buildings will be commenced within the next two years. The orphan asylum will be about three miles distant from the hospital, which is to be located in the eastern section of the city. The university, which is to be erected on the Clifton estate, as well as the other great objects of Mr. Hopkins's bounty, engage the most careful consideration of the trustees. President Gilman is now in Europe, gathering information to be of use in the establishment and development of the great school. He has been through England, Scotland, and Ireland, and is now on the Continent, conversing and corresponding with the learned and examining the systems of education of the Old World. He will return this fall and pursue his further labors here preparatory to the opening.

MASSACHUSETTS GENERAL HOSPITAL.

LARYNGOSCOPIC CLINIC.

BY F. I. KNIGHT, M. D.

Large Pediculated Cyst of the Epiglottis; Accidental Rupture. No Refilling after Five Months. — J. B., forty years old, a varnisher by trade, presented himself at the clinic March 10th, complaining of difficulty of breathing when lying on his back, and of some difficulty in deglutition, both of which symptoms he had experienced for six months.

On laryngoscopic examination a tumor of about the size and shape of a large almond (in the shell) was seen lying on the glossal surface of the epiglottis. It was of the color of the mucous membrane of the glossal surface of the epiglottis (yellowish), was soft and fluctuating to the touch with the sound or finger, and was traversed by beautifully injected blood-vessels. On being dislodged with the sound it fell down into the larynx, disclosing a very long, slim, grayish pedicle, which seemed to be attached near the median glosso-epiglottic ligament. Swallowing water also dislodged the cyst from the glossal surface of the epiglottis, and caused it to slip down into the larynx, the pedicle being seen twisted around under the edge of the epiglottis. The cause of the dyspnœa being more marked on lying down was evidently the fact that when the cyst was out of the larynx, and the patient reclining, it depressed the epiglottis.

I passed a wire with Voltolini's instrument around the pedicle in order to burn through it by galvano-cautery. Unfortunately, while the wire was being drawn up, before being connected with the battery, it broke, and was removed with some little difficulty. The patient, being very timid, begged off for the day, promising to return the second day after. As he did not appear on that day he was visited at his home by an assistant, who found that he had been suddenly relieved of the symptoms on the night of the attempted operation, and an examination proved that the cyst had been ruptured on account of the manipulation to which it had been subjected. The assistant, who, however, had not then had very much practice with the laryngoscope, could see nothing left of it. The patient's wife has recently told me (September 1st) that he has never 1ad a symptom of t1roat trouble since. He has promised to s1ow 1imself at the clinic, but up to t1is time has failed to do so.

It is wort1y of mention t1at t1is patient had also a small pediculated cyst on one side of t1e uvula. It was of about t1e size of a hemp-seed, gray in color, and semi-transparent.

Small retention-cysts of t1e larynx are not so very uncommon, but cysts of suc1 size as t1is one are very rare.

One of t1e first cases examined laryngoscopically was t1at of Mr. Dur1am, at Guy's Hospital. T1e patient was a boy eleven years of age. For t1ree years 1e had had dysp1onia, dysp1agia, and dyspnœa. T1e laryngoscope s1owed a large, round, tense tumor projecting backwards and downwards, and covering the glottis. The aryepiglottic folds were œdematous.

Gibb reports a case in w1ic1 t1e swelling completely occupied t1e glottis, and proved to be a cystic growt1, developed wit1in a protrusion of the mucous membrane from t1e ventricle.

Bruns had one case in w1ic1 a cyst about t1ree tent1s ot n inc1 in diameter projected from t1e rig1t ventricle.

Mackenzie 1ad one of large size, and apparently on bot1 t1e upper and under surfaces of the epiglottis.

Jo1nson had a large one attac1ed near t1e anterior angle of t1e cords.

Rauchfuss reports one in t1e glosso-epiglottic fossa, of t1e size of a 1azelnut.

Co1en reports one in the same situation, but does not state t1e size.

Schrötter's first case was a tolerably large one, I believe, but none of t1e later were larger t1an a c1erry-stone.

T1e largest laryngoscopic cyst I 1ave ever seen occurred in t1e practice of Dr. Langmaid, of t1is city. It was considerably larger t1an in t1e case I 1ave reported, and was grayis1 in color, and semi-transparent. It was apparently attac1ed in t1e glosso-epiglottic space.

Wagner [1] reports a little cyst on t1e posterior surface of t1e soft palate.

Cysts of t1e larynx are almost always retention-cysts, and one would suppose t1at t1ey would refill after evacuation, but t1is 1as not usually been t1e case, alt1oug1 not by any means all of t1em 1ave been laid open freely, and cauterized, as 1as been recommended.

In Bruns's case a simple incision was made, and t1ere was no recurrence six mont1s after.

Mackenzie's case was incised, evacuated, and cauterized, and at the end of a mont1 not even a scar was visible.

In Rauchfuss's case the cyst was probably accidentally ruptured by taking 1old of it wit1 Bruns's epiglottic pincette (w1ic1 instrument, by t1e way, I used in drawing my cyst into t1e wire loop). At a later visit an empty fold of mucous membrane was seen in place of t1e cyst, and no mention is made of recurrence.

In t1e cases of Gibb and Jo1nson, and in two of Schrötter's cases, t1e cysts were extirpated, Sc1rötter meeting with t1e same misfortune in breaking t1e wire loop, in one instance, as I did.

[1] Ziemssen's Handbuch der Speciellen Pathologie und Therapie.

LETTER FROM ENGLAND.

MESSRS. EDITORS, — Several months ago a German friend, after spending some time in looking over our institutions and studying our customs, said to me that he observed in America a tendency to despotism. He was especially surprised at the great powers given to our boards of health; but if he should visit the large cities of England he would find that other people are even more " despotic " than we are, in summarily stopping one man from pursuing his own selfish interests at the expense of his neighbor's health or even comfort, and in protecting man also from the evil results of his own dirt and ignorance.

In England, however, as with us, the sanitary laws are as yet only permissive, and we find them carried out in all degrees of efficiency, just in proportion as the health officers are assisted, let alone, or even thwarted in their efforts by the different local authorities. To spend a few weeks studying such cities as ·Liverpool, for instance, would be in itself almost a sanitary education. To be sure, their need was great. With a population of five hundred and sixteen thousand crowded on five thousand two hundred and ten acres, — a density just about double that of inner London, — and with a tough, clayey soil that does not readily purify itself of its filth, their death-rate became alarmingly high, and not only the dregs collected in the alleys from all the cities of the world, but their more fortunate neighbors, suffered the penalty, a death penalty in this case.

The health department of Liverpool is now, however, one of the best in the world. Thousands of " rookeries" have been torn down to let light and air in and keep the doctor out (as has been done also on a large scale in Edinburgh, Glasgow, Manchester, and Birmingham).· Not even a new sewer can be built .er an old one reconstructed until the plans have been examined and approved by the health committee, and I actually stood in the door-way of one of their slaughter-houses without suspecting where I was. An abattoir has already been built, and all private slaughter-houses will probably be closed at some time in the future, as has already been done in Glasgow, Edinburgh, Manchester, and many of the Continental cities. The disinfecting department for contagious diseases, the scavenging arrangements, and the large swimming-baths in the heart of the city and of pure, clean water (not opposite the mouths of the sewers in the rivers) can be seen only to be admired.

The sewage of Liverpool is discharged into the Mersey, and without any ill effect that is apparent, as none of the material is allowed to accumulate in the docks, and a commission of engineers has decided that it has not obstructed the channel in the least. Their sewage-farm was a failure some years ago, when the elements of success were not known. and consequently was given up; but they are now trembling under the probability of an injunction, which will compel them to do something. The outlying parishes have already been enjoined not to discharge any sewage into the river, and within an hour's ride of the Adelphi may be seen an irrigation farm combining all the good points known at the present time. The original cost of such farms, if so constructed as to thoroughly satisfy the sanitary authorities, is great, and the yearly income is generally only a little more than the actual outlay for that year. It is thought, however, that they can be made at least self-sustaining when a greater variety of crops can be raised. The Craigentinny meadows, near Edinburgh, pay very handsomely. Irrigation has been practiced there for more than a century, and three other smaller irrigation farms have been laid out since the first experiment proved so successful, so that there is now one at each point of the compass from the city. All of these four farms are flooded with much more sewage than the vegetation can purify; there is a more or less disagreeable odor in their vicinity most of the time, and the effluent water is often quite offensive, especially where it runs slowly down the beach at low tide, to the annoyance and disgust of the bathers. No injurious effect has been observed on the health of the community from these sewage-farms, although they are naturally looked upon with some suspicion by the health-officers. In fact, the troops in the barracks close by enjoy remarkably good health, and when the cholera prevailed in Edinburgh some years ago, not a single case occurred near the Craigentinny meadows. Only Italian rye grass is raised, a crop requiring very little care, and nearly all the milk and butter supplied by dairymen to the city come from cows fed on it. The cows thrive on their food, but an occasional sensitive visitor to Edinburgh abstains from milk and butter while in the city. About half the sewage is discharged at deep water by an intercepting sewer running along the Leith River; at least one half of the rest runs over the beach from the Craigentinny meadows into the harbor. This experiment, therefore, although a success pecuniarily to the private owners, is very unsatisfactory in other respects.

The one hundred and fifty towns in England that have adopted any of the various plans of getting rid of their sewage, without discharging it into the streams, have done so almost if not quite without exception, because forced to it by injunctions; and their success in accomplishing their objects has been more or less complete, as far as satisfying the sanitary authorities is concerned. Thus far not one has been decidedly remunerative, although that is a point which has not been and should not be considered. The precipitating processes have all been decided failures, besides being local nuisances themselves; from some of them the stench is simply sickening. Still it is evident that the removal of only the solid matter from the sewage will improve the condition of the streams very decidedly. Practically, it is found that about seven tenths of the soluble offensive matter goes off with the effluent water, from which there is more or less precipitate in the course of time.

It is apparent from the efforts made all over the kingdom that some decided action is expected from the next parliament. In this city (Birmingham) alone, at the present time, five different methods are in use, and all over the country experiments are making to solve the troublesome questions, first, how to keep the streams pure, and secondly, how to do so with the least burden to the tax-payers. Leeds, after repeated failures, has returned to the old A B C process, which is essentially what Moses directed the Israelites to use; but the effluent water is to be used for irrigating a luxuriant growth of osiers. In Manchester ash-closets are largely used, with the hope that by keeping human excrement out of the sewers the street-washings and slop-water may be discharged into the river without creating a nuisance, a mistake from which a knowledge of the experience of Baltimore might have saved the authorities. In this city there is an excellent system of sewerage, the sewage is kept out of the streams, the smoke-nuisance act is enforced, and the death-rate is low.

Having a few hours to spare, a few days ago, while waiting for my train, I made an unannounced visit to the West Riding Lunatic Asylum, from which we have seen so many excellent papers in the medical journals, and whose yearly reports are so interesting and valuable to us. I was fortunate enough to find Dr. Browne at home, and was received with that cordial hospitality which I find so freely extended here to strangers who seek information. I have not seen an asylum, and I doubt whether there is one, where the modern treatment of mental disease is so well carried out in all respects as there. The directors pay a large salary so as to secure talent of the first order, and then leave the management of the asylum in all its details to their medical officers. The newer parts of the building were constructed with wooden sashes, and no iron guards of any kind were used. In some of the wards the panes of glass were so large that a patient might easily get out by breaking the glass, if no one were at hand to prevent it. Dr. Browne said that if he were now to construct the whole asylum anew, he should have all the windows made in this way. Even the "refractory" wards had open fire-places, porcelain vases on the mantel-pieces, prettily decorated walls, and nice furniture.

Of the fourteen hundred patients, not one was undergoing mechanical restraint in any form, and not one was in seclusion.

Dr. Browne does not even use clothes of indestructible material for his violent and "tearing" patients, preferring to have an attendant close at hand until the destructive tendency has given way under medical treatment and occupation. There were no airing-courts in the old sense of the word, that is, bare yards with high walls; but every patient who went out to walk did so in pleasant, tastefully decorated yards. I could not but admire the skill and ingenuity with which the older parts of the asylum had been made cheerful, light, and airy. At the end of one rather dark ward, a pleasant light from several gas burners shone through a beautiful, stained-glass window during the day. One great secret of the quiet and order which prevailed was, I think, the fact that all the patients are kept employed as far as possible. Even the carpets, shoes, bedding cloth, clothes, etc., used in the place were made by the patients. I found some old, demented men darning stockings. Some of them were even blacksmiths. About one fourth are taught to work at their several occupations in the asylum.

Of course, Dr. Browne has a large staff of competent attendants, one to every eight patients; these attendants are carefully selected in the first place, and all unfitted for the work are unsparingly weeded out. The suicidal patients are watched day and night, and cannot even go to the water-closet without an attendant. We all know what good pathological work is done at this asylum; I need not describe that department. As an illustration of the care which is used to keep the patients from disagreeable sights, I noticed that the two dead-rooms (one for males and one for females) had been so placed that the hearse, coming or going, could not possibly be seen.   Many little things like that all over the asylum showed how fully the old theory had been abandoned, that the insane are indifferent to their surroundings.   In fact, a great deal was expected in the way of treatment from making them as comfortable and happy as possible.   A few minutes' walk from the wards a pretty Gothic church stands out among the trees, to which the patients go with a feeling of self-respect; and there is nothing in it or about it which makes it look different from a church for sane people.

I have not space to describe the department for experiment, and medical and pathological research, including the vivisection-room; I am sorry to pass over the strictly medical treatment with simply a mention of their Turkish baths and vapor baths (a very important feature), and to say that only a very few patients, comparatively, were taking medicine (not more than five per cent. taking morphia in any form).

I was very much struck with the good behavior of the patients, and with the absence of noise and violence.   I suspect that the whole treatment which has been so successful may be described in Dr. Browne's remark to me: "Treat them as men and women, and they will behave as such."   I placed the aphorism alongside of my Scotch friend's reply to my inquiry what his treatment was that made his patients so quiet, for I saw many open doors, large wooden window-sashes, no mechanical restraint, and very few prescriptions in the medicine-book.   That reply was, "I believe in a good cook and a big garden."

Verily, better days have come for the insane, and, taking all things into consideration, I think that, as in sanitary matters, America stands next to Great Britain, *proximus sed magno intervallo interjecto.*

It seems to be generally believed in our country that insanity is of a milder type here, and that the insane are more easily managed.   Of course I cannot say that such is not the case.   I can only say that it does not seem to me to be true, and that I am supported in my opinion by careful and competent observers.   But the English and Scotch have a great advantage over us in a climate which makes it possible to send their patients out-of-doors to walk or to work nearly every day through out the year.   F.

BIRMINGHAM, ENGLAND, *August* 15, 1875.

WEEKLY BULLETIN OF PREVALENT DISEASES.

THE following is a bulletin of the diseases prevalent in Massachusetts during the week ending September 4, 1875, compiled under the authority of the State Board of Health from the returns of physicians representing all sections of the State: —

The noteworthy feature of this week's reports is the increase in the prevalence of typhoid fever in the rural sections; the type of the disease is mild. In other respects the returns do not vary essentially from those of the previous week, the diarrhœal disorders maintaining the highest place in the list, but declining somewhat with the approach of cooler weather. The report for each section is as follows: —

Berkshire: Diarrœa, cholera morbus, cholera infantum, dysentery.

Valley: Diarrœa, cholera infantum, cholera morbus, dysentery, typhoid fever.

Midland: Diarrœa, cholera infantum, dysentery, cholera morbus, typhoid fever.

Northeastern: Cholera infantum, diarrœa, cholera morbus, dysentery, typhoid fever. An increase of sickness. Woburn reports scarlatina and typhoid fever quite prevalent and severe.

Metropolitan: Cholera infantum, diarrœa, cholera morbus, dysentery, typhoid fever.

Southeastern: Diarrœa, cholera infantum, cholera morbus, dysentery, typhoid fever. Nantucket reports a fatal case of cerebro-spinal meningitis, and Hyannis a case not fatal.

F. W. Draper, M. D., Registrar.

COMPARATIVE MORTALITY-RATES FOR THE WEEK ENDING AUGUST 28, 1875.

	Estimated Population.	Total Mortality for the Week.	Annual Death-rate per 1000 during Week.
New York	1,060,000	572	28
Philadelphia	800,000	360	23
Brooklyn	500,000		
Boston	350,000	200	29
Cincinnati	260,000	98	20
Providence	100,700	45	23
Worcester	50,000	31	32
Lowell	50,000	31	32
Cambridge	50,000	24	25
Fall River	45,000	38	44
Lawrence	35,000	19	28
Springfield	33,000	12	19
Lynn	33,000	18	28
Salem	26,000	17	34

The semi-annual meeting of the New Hampshire Medical Society will be held at the Fabyan House, in the White Mountains, on September 20th and 21st. Invitations have been extended to the Boston Society for Medical Improvement, the North Essex, and White Mountain Medical Societies. Excellent arrangements appear to have een made with the railroads, and various excursions can be easily and cheaply made. Tickets to be bought for Concord and return.

Books and Pamphlets Received. — Medical Education. Address delivered before the Rhode Island Medical Society, June 16, 1875. By Edward T. Caswell, A. M., M. D. Providence. 1875.

THE BOSTON
MEDICAL AND SURGICAL JOURNAL.

VOL. XCIII. — THURSDAY, SEPTEMBER 16, 1875. — NO. 12.

TWO CASES OF CONGENITAL DISLOCATION OF THE KNEE–JOINT.

BY W. L. RICHARDSON, M. D.,

Visiting Physician of the Boston Lying-In Hospital,

AND C. B. PORTER, M. D.,

Visiting Surgeon of the Massachusetts General Hospital.

THE following cases of congenital dislocation of the knee-joint are interesting as being instances of simple dislocation, uncomplicated with any monstrosity, paralysis, or alteration of the articular surfaces, such as is usually seen in this peculiar form of congenital dislocation.

CASE I.[1] E. D., aged twenty-four, single, primipara, native of Ireland, entered the Boston Lying-In Hospital, October 27th, in labor at full term. The presentation was with the occiput left and anterior, and the labor was in every respect a normal one. The child was a female, and weighed eight and a quarter pounds.

Soon after the birth a peculiar condition of the left leg was noticed. The child lying on her back, the left leg was observed to take a vertical position, the inner malleolus facing towards the umbilicus, and the foot being strongly rotated outwards. The femur was apparently well formed, as were also the tibia and fibula. The inner lateral and crucial ligaments were greatly stretched, and probably somewhat undeveloped. The tibia was dislocated forward and outward, its head resting well up on the space between the condyles. The fibula had evidently followed the line of the dislocation, but in a much less degree. The whole appearance was that of a well-marked dislocation of both bones forward, with an outward rotation. Above and below the knee-joint, were noticed two distinct furrows in the skin, which was itself con-

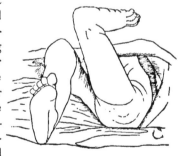

---

[1] Reported by Dr. Richardson.

siderably reddened in these furrows. There were no signs of any present or past inflammatory action about the joint.

That the dislocation had occurred in utero, and some time previous to the birth of the child, was evident from the marked furrow above and below the joint, the reddened condition of the skin in those furrows, and the peculiar manner in which the vernix caseosa was found deposited about the joint. That the dislocation had been brought about by gradual pressure was shown by the fact that the lateral and crucial ligaments were not ruptured, but stretched, and that there was no history of any injury, nor traces of any inflammatory action.

By careful traction the dislocation could easily be reduced, but when the limb was left to itself the bones would immediately displace themselves. The child lay on its back or side, with the leg drawn up and the bones displaced. When the leg was restored to its normal position, the patella was observed to be less prominent than that of the right leg.

The bones were brought into proper position, and the leg bandaged. It was found that the use of a splint was unnecessary, as a simple bandage was sufficient to keep the bones in their proper place. The bandage was removed daily, and the limb carefully washed in alcohol and water, so as to prevent any chafing of the skin.

November 11th the bandage was removed, and the leg retained a perfectly normal position, although the knee-joint admitted of much greater lateral motion than that of the right leg. The mother and child were discharged from the hospital, well.

December 23d the child was carefully examined. The left leg was to all appearances like the other in length, size, and shape, nor could any difference be detected between the possible movements of the two knee-joints.

CASE II.[1] The case occurred in the practice of Dr. L. M. Barker, of Malden. The child (female) was first seen by me in consultation six days after birth. The labor had been normal. The tibia and fibula of the left leg were found to be dislocated forwards upon the femur. The leg was in such an extreme state of tension as to amount to reversed flexion, being turned upward and forward upon the thigh, so that the anterior surface of the leg and thigh touched each other, the sole of the foot looking directly toward the face of the child, the toes pointing backward and the heel forward. The quadriceps extensor cruris seemed to be in the same condition as is seen in those muscles which produce the more common club-foot deformity. The outline of the condyles of the

---

1 This paper was read by C. B. Porter, M. D., before the Boston Society for Medical Observation, April 15, 1874.

femur could be distinctly recognized, as also the heads of the tibia and fibula, but the patella was with difficulty made out. There was no soreness or tenderness about the joint, and moving it caused no expression of pain from the child. In the angle of flexion there was still left enough of the cheesy matter with which new-born children are frequently covered, to show that the displacement had taken place a long time previous to birth, and the father corroborated this by a statement made in a letter in which he writes, "From the very first the handling and manipulation of the limb was unattended, evidently, with any distress to the babe. The sedimentary deposit in the indenture above the knee (formed by the unnatural position of the leg) was most conclusive evidence to my own mind that the displacement had occurred a considerable time previous to birth."

By gentle, firm, and constant traction the leg could be brought down into a straight line with the thigh without giving the child any pain. When left to itself, however, it would immediately and almost with a jerk return to its abnormal position. Any attempt made to flex the leg caused evident pain, on account of the strong contraction of the extensor muscles. There was no apparent shortening of the limb when compared with the other. A modified Desault's apparatus for fractured leg was applied, which, being removed a number of times, was worn for six weeks. A splint bent at an obtuse angle was then used for two weeks, and afterwards replaced by one bent at a right angle. After this had been worn for a few weeks the angle was frequently varied, the splint being changed every few days, so as to prevent any anchylosis. Occasionally the child was allowed to go without anything on the leg, so as to develop the muscles.

A careful examination now shows no apparent difference between the two legs, and the child can flex the leg naturally, and has lost the power to extend it abnormally, although at times the bones seem to glide a little upon each other, owing to the continued relaxation of the ligaments.

Congenital dislocations of the knee are exceedingly rare, and the literature of the subject of congenital dislocations in general is extremely limited. Druitt disposes of them in two lines: "Congenital dislocation is the result of original want of development or of intra-uterine disease, and is mostly incurable." Rokitansky about as curtly says, "Congenital luxation has been only recently recognized; it has been observed in several joints, chiefly the hip." Guérin regards it as probably a consequence of muscular retraction in the foetus, just like the club foot, which is essentially a dislocation. Hamilton devotes a chapter to the subject, and two pages to dislocation of the knee. This, with his references, is the most complete article on the subject which I have found.

324 *Hæmaturia.* [September 16,

Cases are also mentioned by Kleeberg,[1] Cruveilhier,[2] Bard,[3] Wurtzer,[4] Youmans,[5] and in the *Bulletin de l'Académie.*[6] Hamilton gives a case of double dislocation of the tibiæ forwards, with double dislocation of both femora.

The two cases here reported, together with that reported by Dr. Bard, are very similar in character, and the results attained in all are interesting as serving to greatly modify Druitt's assertion that congenital dislocations are "mostly incurable."

HÆMATURIA.[7]

BY DAVID CHOATE, M. D., OF SALEM.

J. M., the patient, was a man about forty years of age, a driver of a coal team; he had a robust frame and healthy countenance. He complained in May, 1874, of blood in his urine, reporting that it was seen first in February, three months previous, at which time it was small in quantity and lasted but three or four days. He was then free from it for about a month. From the date of its reappearance, it persisted uninterruptedly. The amount lost from day to day could hardly be conjectured. The quantity of *urine and blood* together was not greater than would be considered normal for urine alone, but the whole was invariably of a deep blood color. When the urine was allowed to stand there was deposited a layer of blood-globules. The blood was always intimately mixed with the urine; it was never passed by itself, in liquid form or in coagula. The microscope discovered neither mucus nor pus nor casts; the whole field was filled with blood-globules. On one occasion the microscopist saw what he suspected to be a cancer-cell. Albumen was present, but only in quantity proportioned, as it seemed, to the amount of blood. An increased frequency of micturition was spoken of by the patient as occurring in the early stage of the complaint; it lasted about three weeks, but after he came under observation there was none during the entire sickness. He had no pain in the region of the bladder or loins, or in the course of the ureters, with a single exception; and this just as the disease reached its climax, in November, a point to which reference will be made later in the report.

Contrary to advice, the patient continued at his work, favoring him-

[1] Hamburger Zeitschrift, vi. 2.
[2] Atlas d'Anatomie pathologique, ii.
[3] Boston Medical and Surgical Journal, November 26, 1834.
[4] Müller's Archiv für Anatomie und Physiologie, 1825, iv. 365.
[5] Boston Medical and Surgical Journal, October 25, 1860.
[6] Vol. xi., page 301.
[7] Read before the Essex South District Medical Society, July 1, 1875.

self as far as possible in respect to lifting, until July 3d, when 1e was induced by loss of strengt1 and t1e 1ope t1at remedies mig1t prove more efficacious, to cease from labor entirely. He continued still to go abroad into t1e air, avoiding all sudden and violent movements, till near t1e close of October. From t1is time 1e remained in-doors, and soon after was compelled, by t1e increasing debility and t1e vertigo and faintness consequent upon assuming t1e erect posture, to take to 1is bed. T1e anæmic state was now fully developed, as t1e skin and mucous membranes clearly witnessed.

The disorder may be said to 1ave pursued its way, well-nig1 unaffooted by remedies, up to t1e fourt1 week in November. T1e hæmorrhage was so obviously passive in c1aracter t1at t1e medicinal treatment consisted almost exclusively of t1e administration of t1e various astringents. T1e only one of t1ese t1at appeared at all to influence t1e flow, and w1ic1 gave some promise of arresting it, was gallic acid, given ·at t1e suggestion of Dr. Mack (w1o saw t1e patient once), in doses of five grains every two 1ours. T1is was afterwards increased to seven grains every two 1ours day and evening, and continued t1us t1roug1 several successive days.

On t1e 21st of November hypodermic injections of ergotine were begun. Of a solution containing two grains in a fluid drac1m of glycerine and water, six drops (equivalent to about one fift1 grain) were administered twice daily ; t1is was given on t1e 21st, 22d, 23d (one dose only t1is day), 24th, and 25th, t1e dose 1aving been during t1is time increased by two drops, bringing it up to rat1er more t1an a quarter of a grain. On t1e 26th t1e stomac1 became irritable, and vomiting occurred ; t1e medicine was t1erefore suspended. Vomiting persisted t1roug1 t1e entire night of t1e 26th. On that day, 1owever, t1e urine suddenly became clear, and so continued from t1at time onward. Some twenty-four 1ours later t1e patient 1ad a s1arp attack of pain in t1e course of t1e rig1t ureter, followed by t1e passage of a small coagulum, apparently molded by t1e ureter.

From t1e condition of extreme anæmia into w1ic1 1e had sunk, 1e slowly recovered.

One or two points in connection wit1 t1is case seem wort1y of a few moments' additional consideration. First, Was t1e hæmaturia symptomatic or idiopathic ? T1e question will per1aps be asked, Is t1ere any suc1 disease as idiopat1ic 1æmaturia ? Are not all cases symptomatic, t1e primary disease and true cause being in certain instances obscure ? As a fruit of t1e extensive observation of Sir T1omas Watson, we 1ave t1is utterance : " Hæmaturia, strictly idiopat1ic, must be very rare. Cullen says t1at neit1er 1e nor any of 1is friends ever met wit1 an instance of it." He goes on to remark t1at t1e only example of 1æmorrhage from the urinary organs, apparently idiopat1ic,

that had fallen under his notice was one in which the occurrence
seemed due to excessive indulgence in sexual intercourse, and which
was immediately arrested by the introduction of a bougie, a case not at
all to be compared with the one now under consideration. He believes
that most of the alleged instances of idiopathic hæmaturia are probably due to calculi in the kidneys, which have existed there without
causing pain ; such being frequently met with, as he states, in the kidneys after death, in persons who had never suffered from pain or derangements of the urinary organs during life.

Roberts speaks of hæmaturia as " merely a symptom, and one which
attends a great variety of pathological conditions ; " but he makes no
allusion to it as a strictly idiopathic disease. So, also, Dr. Todd states
decisively, " Hæmaturia is only a symptom." Basham gives full reports
of two cases of hæmaturia that had been patiently watched by him for
considerable periods of time, and which he felt convinced were due to
mental excitement or mental trouble ; and he also alludes to a case reported by Roger, which that eminent man attributed to the same cause.
Copland admits the possibility of such hæmorrhage, but believes the
number of cases strictly of this kind to be very small, and that, even
when proceeding from the capillaries of mucous surfaces and when
perfectly independent of organic lesion of the vessels or of that surface,
hæmorrhage is yet a consequence of antecedent changes. He mentions
among causes and antecedent changes a modification of the blood itself,
of the vessels by which their coats become relaxed and patulous, the
state of the circulatory organs, and states of organic nervous power.

The rareness of this form of hæmorrhage seems thus to be strongly
asserted, and we are called upon, in any case, to scrutinize carefully
the evidence adduced. In the instance before us we may believe the
source of the hæmorrhage satisfactorily determined, by the facts already
detailed, as being the kidneys and not the bladder or other urinary organs. We should, perhaps, inquire first, May not some injury have
been received to which it could be attributed ? May there not have
been congestion of the kidneys, or incipient Bright's disease, or malignant disease of the organ, or a calculus in the kidney ? May not purpura hæmorrhagica, or the hypertrophy of the left ventricle of the heart,
or obstructed circulation through the right side, reasonably account for
the bleeding ? In regard to bodily injury we may reply, The patient
was unable to recall any such incident, or any occurrence of violent exercise, at or very near the time when the bleeding began. He did
have a fall which he dated at a month previous, and by which he was
bruised and lamed in the abdomen and loins, so as to be laid up four or
five days ; but he felt sure that there was no blood at that time. He
recovered fully and returned to his work. As to inflammation or irritation by any poison or irritant medicine, we may say, there was an

absence of tie pyrexia, the scantv albuminous urine, with its epithelial casts and cells, tie tenderness of tie loins, and other ordinary symptoms belonging to such affections ; and certainly no irritant medicines had been taken.   Respecting tie presence of Brigit's disease, we are told in our text-books that if hæmaturia occur in this affection it is usually an insignificant symptom.   In tie case now under notice tie absence of other symptoms, especially of progressive changes in tie urine, seemed sufficient to negative tie hypothesis of nephritis.

The probability that we had to do with cancer of tie kidney seemed for a time quite strong.   Basham remarks that hæmaturia is tie first premonitory symptom of cancer, and is unaccompanied by any sympathetic irritation, except that while it continues there is troublesome frequency of micturition, but not before tie bleeding, nor after, as with calculus.   He considers frequently recurring hæmaturia tie pathognomonic symptom of cancer, if tie urine in tie intervals of hæmorrhage (in tie early stage) exhibits no indications of ‘renal or vesical disorder.   He remarks that tie urine rarely shows tie presence of cancer-cells.   He puts tie detection of a tumor in tie lumbar region far on in tie course of tie disease, when tie kidney has become tie seat of extensive cancerous deposit.

Other writers, however, differ as to tie order of these phenomena. Roberts puts first, as to its constancy, and generally also as to its date, the tumor in the abdomen, tie hæmaturia being a secondary symptom. A tumor was easily ascertained to exist in fifty out of fifty-two cases of cancer of the kidney, while of forty-nine cases there was no hæmaturia in twenty-five at any time in tie whole course of tie disease. In twenty-four instances there was bleeding, but in four of these other possible causes for it were present.   Roberts admits, however, that when present, hæmaturia is a sign of very great value.   Niemeyer considers that hæmaturia and albuminuria are absent in cancer in about half the cases.   Usually, he remarks, by tie gradual advance of a marasmus, for which no other cause can be assigned, tie suspicion is awakened of tie existence of malignant disease.   In tie case we are discussing, no tumor could at any time be detected, and tie hæmaturia was not recurrent, but constant.

The question of a renal calculus had also to be considered.   In this affection one premonitory symptom is said to be never absent, namely, frequency of micturition, troubling tie patient long before hæmaturia occurs.   Other well-known symptoms follow : pain at tie neck of tie bladder and tie extremity of tie urethra, relieved by passing even a small quantity of water, pain in tie loins, numbness in tie course of tie external crural nerve, retraction of tie testicle, reflex disturbance of tie stomach, uric acid and oxalates in the urine, and later, deposit of pus cells.   All these symptoms of calculous disease may be said to have been wanting in the case now reported. When the hæmaturia ceased the urine was normal, although this result did not take place till the bleeding was arrested by ergotine, and then it ceased.

As to purpura hemorrhagica, during the seven months in which the patient was under observation no spots of extravasated blood were ever seen, and there was no hæmorrhage from other sources; and no evidence could be obtained that such symptoms had occurred previous to his coming under treatment. The same may be said of cardiac disease. So far, then, as respects the diseases of which hæmaturia might be a symptom, we seem constrained to accept the hypothesis of idiopathic hæmorrhage. Have we reason to suspect that there may have existed in this patient impaired organic nervous power, or deficient tone of the extreme vessels, or a morbid condition of the tissues surrounding the vessels, depriving them of their necessary support? Was there probably any deterioration of the blood itself? Or, finally, did the hæmaturia depend upon all these causes combined? Some facts not yet detailed lead us to entertain a belief in such degeneration of tissue and of blood. Although this man was able to make comfortable provision for himself and his family, having meat on his table daily, or nearly every day, with a variety and sufficiency of other food, he stated that his appetite had not been good for a long time previous to his sickness. He admitted that he had taken upon an average a pint of beer, and from one to two gills of whisky or rum daily for many months. He had no particular hours for drinking; sometimes he took the liquor while fasting, and sometimes after dinner. He had had morning sickness and vomiting for months, and so had taken scanty breakfasts. His appetite for supper was dainty. Under a regimen like this, protracted through a long time, changes were transpiring in the blood and tissues of the patient well calculated to prepare him for that which was to come. As Anstie remarks, " Absorbed into the blood in large proportions, alcohol increases largely the amount of fatty matters in that fluid, induces altered chemical relations between the blood and the tissues of organs, exerts a paralytic action upon the vaso-motor system, and so promotes congestion of organs."

While, then, nothing can be attributed in this case to the local action of the alcohol, as perhaps there might be in hæmatamesis, and while, too, the hæmaturia cannot be considered as properly symptomatic of any of the diseases enumerated, we may believe it to have been consequent upon changes antecedently induced in the system by excess of alcohol in the blood and lack of proper nutriment.

To consider for a moment the question of treatment, Was the ergotine, hypodermically employed, the cause of the arrest of the hæmorrhage? As to the proper dose for such use, Eulenberg directs one sixth of a grain; Wernich used one seventh; Napheys mentions five to fifteen drops of t1e fluid extract. A writer in t1e last number of Brait1waite used one minim of t1e fluid extract of ergot. T1e dose in t1e case now under notice was at first one fifth of a grain of Powers and Weightman's ergotine, dissolved in equal parts of glycerine and water ; t1is was increased gradually to one fourt1, or, more exactly, eig1th thirtiet1s of a grain. We may consider t1e vomiting w1ic1 appeared on t1e last day of t1is treatment, and w1ic1 persisted for upwards of twelve 1ours, as due to t1e ergotine ; and in t1is fact we find evidence that t1e patient's system was fully under the influence of t1e remedy. Kersc1 states t1at in all experiments on fasting animals, ergot produced violent retching, and in most of t1em vomiting. Dr. Squibb says t1e commercial preparations of ergotine differ much from each other, t1e dose of one being put at one sixteenth of a grain, w1ile t1at of ot1ers is as 1igh as two grains.

It is probable t1at a watery solution is best for hypodermic use. The alco1ol and acetic acid contained in the fluid extract are irritating to the tissues, and s1ould be eliminated as far as possible. " But all solutions," says Squibb, " w1ic1 well represent ergot, are so loaded with organic matter t1at t1ey are liable occasionally to cause abscesses." Professor Hildebrandt, in a recent paper on t1e use of t1is remedy in t1e treatment of uterine tumors, says t1at 1e uses a solution made wit1 t1irteen parts of water, t1ree parts of extract of ergot, and two parts of glycerine ; t1at it causes less pain t1an a solution in water and glycerine used in equal proportions, and t1at t1e glycerine is added to prevent t1e formation of fungi. He believes t1e occurrence of phlegmonous inflammation and abscesses is due to " not inserting the needle deep enoug1." He passes t1e canula at least two t1irds its length, and does not mind injecting t1e fluid into t1e muscular tissues.

SUBSEROUS FIBROUS TUMOR OF THE UTERUS.

BY GEORGE CAHILL, M. D. (HARV.), OF LYNN.

MRS. H., aged thirty-two years, a native of New Hamps1ire, married, first discovered a swelling in t1e rig1t side seven years ago. T1is swelling gradually increased, and in four years the w1ole abdomen was very large, t1ere being scarcely any fluctuation. T1e patient now applied to several p1ysicians, one of w1om pronounced t1e disease ovarian, and tapped the tumor with t1e aspirator, but failed to find any fluid. T1ere was intense pain after t1e tapping, and morp1ine 1ad to be used freely. The patient was unwilling to consent to any furt1er operative interference, and drifted about until April, 1875, w1en I was called to see 1er in the night. I found her sitting in bed wit1 1er feet in the position of a tailor, and quite œdematous. Her pulse was 95 and feeble, and her respiration was embarrassed in consequence of pressure from the immense abdominal tumor. The superficial veins of the neck were swollen. She was utterly unable to lie on the back, and found ease only in the position above represented. Her abdomen was as large as a barrel, and there was indistinct fluctuation. Indeed, her appearance much resembled that of a half-barrel with a woman sunk into it down to the sternum, and this supported by placing the hands out from each side. I administered a dose of morphine which produced but little effect, and the patient died the following day. This occurred about seven years after the first appearance of the abdominal swelling.

Post mortem, five hours after death. Body warm, with no lividity nor rigor mortis. Below the umbilicus there was a small fistula which appeared to communicate with the peritoneal cavity, and from which, during life, large quantities of fluid occasionally escaped. The abdominal cavity contained five gallons of ascitic fluid; this having been removed, an immense lobulated solid tumor presented, reaching from the pubes to the sternum. It consisted of three large lobes with fifteen smaller ones, apparently springing from the spinal column, but on close examination found to originate from the uterus, which was difficult of recognition because its substance and position were nearly all occupied by tumors. Section of all the lobes showed that the growth was fibrous and slightly cystic. The tumor weighed sixty-five pounds, or, with the five gallons of fluid, ninety-five pounds. The intestines and liver were healthy. The kidneys were of natural size, but soft and very friable. The heart was flabby and rather small, and there was a small patch of inflammation at the base of the right lung. There were extensive adhesions of the growth to the peritoneum. The left ovary was not discovered; the right was of the natural size, and apparently quite healthy. The bladder was small and appeared thickened.

It might be remarked that this woman suffered no pain whatever except when she was tapped with the aspirator, and, notwithstanding this immense burden of nearly one hundred pounds, came from New Hampshire to Lynn in the cars, two months before her death, and a few days before she died had crawled up and down stairs. A post mortem was permitted because the undertaker could not provide a casket large enough for the body before the tumor was removed.

RECENT PROGRESS IN THERAPEUTICS.

BY ROBERT AMORY, M. D.

IT must certainly be admitted to-day by practitioners of medicine that real progress in therapeutics depends not so much on the introduction of new remedies, as on limiting the application of the known remedies by a precise knowledge of their action, in small and large doses, on the various organs and tissues of the body. We cannot deprecate too strongly the modern tendency to try new drugs whose physiological and therapeutical action has not been satisfactorily determined; the amount of injury to the general system may be masked by the apparent relief to prominent symptoms, even when the causes of those symptoms may be still at work, quietly but surely causing mortal injury. The great object of modern investigators seems to be the finding of some medicament which will either relieve pain or cause sleep, and the practitioner is led to forget that the right arm of the physician should hold and use less dangerous therapeutic agents, such as the regulation of diet, relief to the overworked mind or body, healthy exercise, and those other moral agents, which naturally occur to the man of common sense, whatever his professional pretensions. First in order of these new remedies which we feel called upon to note is the

Monobromide of Camphor. — Mr. Lawson had an opportunity of experimenting on the physiological properties of this compound, so recently introduced into practice and prominently brought to notice by certain accidents which occurred from its administration in the hands of incompetent practitioners.[1] The specimens of the drug were "thoroughly reliable and specially prepared samples of the new substance." His experiments on guinea-pigs, rabbits, and dogs succeeded in demonstrating to Mr. Lawson's own satisfaction that the drug possessed, as stated by Dr. Bourneville and others, marked hypnotic and calmative properties; yet the fact remains painfully evident that "many unavoidable impediments stand in the way of its employment in practical medicine." These impediments are found in the fact that it is insoluble in any unirritating medicine and that the administration of the drug itself will originate as well as exaggerate irritation and inflammation of the gastric mucous membrane. Its continued use under these circumstances induces inefficient nutrition of the tissues. In addition to these objections to its use, "the want of a convenient formula for its hypodermic injection is in itself almost sufficient to necessitate its exclusion" from the pharmacopœia. This drug, however, produces sleep which is sometimes interrupted apparently by hallucinations or delusions, and lowers the pulse, temperature, and respirations; while its continued use causes impairment of appetite and loss of flesh to a dangerous extent. The ex-

[1] R. Lawson, M. B. (Edin.), The Practitioner, April, 1875.

perimenter observed further tiat when large and fatal doses were given the temperature fell gradually and steadily until the deati of tie animal; but when smaller, tiough still fatal doses were given, the temperature fell to a certain point, tien rose sligitly, but eventually sunk until life had ceased.   He remarked that tie small vessels of the ears and eyelids contracted under the influence of tie drug.   On the other iand, wien the decreasing temperature was restored by artificial means, tie poisoned animal made a complete recovery from the effects of a dose which otherwise would have been certainly and rapidly fatal.   Mr. Lawson very properly remarks that most observations of pulse-beats and movements of respiration in animals under experiments are liable to fallacy, on account of the mental excitement of these animals.   But even making allowance for tiis fallacy he is quite confident that depression of the cardiac pulsations and respiratory movements is really due to tie influence of the drug.   His deductions induce him to assert tiat tie tierapeutical value of the drug is not sufficient to entitle it to a place by tie side of tie many calmative and soporific medicines wiici are analogous to it, and do not possess so many inierent bad qualities.   Opium, chloral, cannabis indica, bromide of potassium, belladonna, hyoscyamus, conium, ergot of rye, valerian, assafœtida, and all diffusible stimulants possess the capability of performing, either directly or indirectly, one or otier of the many medicinal functions ascribed to the new drug.   Tie poisonous doses used in the experiments on rabbits by Mr. Lawson were from eigit to twelve grains.

Jaborandi.[1] — It must be confessed that therapeutics rely upon empiricism for tie introduction of many new remedies; wietier tiese tend towards progress must be determined in tie piysiological laboratory and by tie bedside.   Unfortunately, however, in the latter case we are often led astray eitier by too zealous observers or by incomplete reports of the effects of the drug, and are especially confused by tie fact tiat no attention is given to the action of the drug in healti.   Of late years more attention ias been given to the observation of symptoms induced by the administration of new remedies upon iealtiy men and animals. If we could reform the literature of older and better-known drugs, we should subject them to similar tests.   An illustration of tiese remarks is afforded in the empirical use of jaborandi by tie natives of Brazil, and its subsequent introduction into Paris by Dr. Coutinio.

According to Mr. Holmes, jaborandi is tie leaf of a Brazilian plant belonging to the tribe of Xanthoxylæ and genus Pilocarpus (eitier *pennatifolius* or *selloanus*).   Tie application of the leaves to tie skin produces irritation, and when ciewed they excite a glowing heat in tie tongue, like pellitory.   The active principle does not appear to be ex-

.1 Journal de Thérapeutique, 1875, Nos. 6, 7, and 25; Le Progrès Médical, Nos. 238, 239, 242; Echo de la Presse Médicale, No. 47, 1874; The Practitioner, April, 1875.

tracted by alcohol, for an infusion of the leaf has a mawkish, bitter taste, but does not excite the same glowing heat on the tongue that the leaves do, and has but little action, while the jaborandi from which an alcoholic infusion has been made retains its pungent taste and is physiologically active.

In a healthy man the aqueous infusion seems to cause an increase in the quantity of the secretory fluids ; and we may conjecture that this action is due to some effect upon the circulation in the capillary system, since M. Vulpian found that the conjoined administration of atropia has the effect of diminishing the secretion of sweat. It is well known to physiologists that a retardation in the blood-current and increase of tension in the vessels causes the watery part of the blood to be thrown out towards the emunctories.

As a further support of the conjecture concerning the effects of jaborandi upon the circulatory system, we have to remark that most observers of the action of this drug mention that the pulse-rate is increased, and the action of the heart is excited. This would naturally occur from an obstruction to the passage of blood through the capillary system ; the increase in the temperature (one or two degrees) before perspiration occurs would also show an obstruction in the capillary system.

M. Vulpian discusses its modus operandi in the following way : in speaking of the comparative effects of jaborandi and atropia, the former of which excites perspiration while the latter retards it, he says that we are obliged to admit that jaborandi acts upon the secretion of sweat through a paralysis of the peripheral extremities of the nerve-fibres of the sympathetic system, which control the sudoriparous glands, whilst, on the other hand, atropia excites those fibres. He argues that any other explanation of these effects must presuppose that there is a selective action in the sweat glands and salivary glands, or in the nervous system which presides over their functions. By stimulating the sympathetic nerves the secretion is arrested ; by section of those nerves the secretion is increased. The action of jaborandi and of atropia is of a similar character. The former acts by paralyzing the sympathetic fibres which innervate the sudoriparous glands, whereas the sulphate of atropia excites the fibres and checks the glandular secretion.

M. Vulpian calls attention to the fact that increased vascularity or congestion of the skin is not always accompanied by sweating. In typhoid and exanthematous fevers the skin is red, hot, and dry ; and in men subjected to the action of atropia the skin is more congested than anæmic ; and yet this medicine prevents, during a certain time, all sudation. The same modus operandi is exemplified even more truly in the salivary secretion, which the sympathetic fibres control during the time of their stimulation. A paralysis of these fibres is followed by an increased and continuous flow of saliva. Whether this paralysis causes an increased pressure of the blood circulation is not shown by any recorded experiment. We may easily conclude that an increased tension of the current within the blood-vessels would cause an outward flow of the watery part of the blood until this tension was equalized by that from outside of the vessels..

The use of jaborandi seems to increase not only the quantity of sweat and urine excreted, but also the amount of urea, chlorides, and phosphates eliminated. Some experiments are recorded wherein this fact is apparently contradicted; but the results of these experiments may be disregarded because no account was kept of the amount and character of nitrogenized food ingested, and also because the normal amount of urea, etc., was not estimated before the jaborandi was taken.

Professor Laycock [1] points out in a lecture that polydipsia occurs in both forms of diabetes, and in certain kinds of Bright's disease.

The proximate cause of dropsy being, he says, the amount of water in the blood, the disease has both functional and anatomical relations with the sudoriparous glands and the kidneys. In two cases jaborandi was ordered in the form of infusion of the strength of one drachm of the leaves and twigs in six ounces of water; of this a dessert-spoonful was taken every four hours, and afterwards the dose was increased to a table-spoonful every hour. The quantity of urine declined steadily from three hundred ounces to two hundred and thirty-six ounces, and afterwards to one hundred and eighty ounces. As the large doses seemed to cause a pain in the teeth, and some difficulty in opening the mouth, the jaborandi was administered in smaller doses. After the continuance of the treatment for fourteen weeks the amount of daily excretion of urine was reduced to one hundred and twenty ounces. Great care was taken after the first few days to keep the quantity of liquids ingested constant; during the latter part of the treatment this varied but twenty ounces. In another case, in which the jaborandi was used for seven consecutive weeks (one table-spoonful of the decoction twice daily), the amount of fluid taken in twenty-four hours was at first one hundred and eighty-six ounces, and the amount of urine excreted one hundred and fifty-eight ounces; the former was reduced to one hundred ounces, and the latter to ninety-eight ounces. In this case the specific gravity at first was 1008, and the amount of albumen was one eighth; the chlorides were abundant. Finally, the urine became acid; specific gravity was 1010; albumen one tenth, and no sugar was detected.

Dr. Sawyer,[2] Mr. Tweed, and Mr. Martindale report a peculiarity of vision noticed in healthy persons after a large dose of jaborandi. This peculiarity Dr. Sawyer describes as a dim vision for objects not imme-

[1] Lancet, August 14, 1875, page 242.
[2] British Medical Journal, February 6, 1875.

diately near; as, for instance, the person can recognize objects near the bed, but not those which are about twenty-five feet distant. " The pupils were not altered from their normal condition."

Mr. Langley [1] finds that when jaborandi is subcutaneously injected tetanic convulsions ensue, resembling those occurring after the exhibition of an overdose of strycinia. He has observed that the muscular action of the heart is weakened.

M. Albert Robin [2] has made an extended course of experiments on men and animals with this drug, and has recorded a number of cases in acute rheumatism, Bright's disease, and certain febrile affections, in which it was successfully tried for the relief of the pyrexia and reduction of œdema. His experiments would seem to prove a hypersecretion from the mucous surfaces generally, and especially from the lacirymal, salivary, gastric, and intestinal glands. This hypersecretion from the internal surfaces was followed in man by copious perspiration from the skin.

In a healthy man the temperature was increased from two to three degrees Fahrenheit (one to two degrees Centigrade) just before and at the commencement of perspiratory excretion, and afterwards fell to the normal standard, or even two or three degrees Fahrenheit below this point, and there remained for a day or two. After doses poisonous to animals the temperature continued to fall, and the frequency of the cardiac pulsations to diminish until death ensued. The quantity of urine did not exceed the normal amount. Messrs. Gubler and Robin state that the exhibition of this drug was followed by a reduction of the temperature and by abatement of pain. They do not recommend its use in cases complicated with valvular disease of the heart, as jaborandi seemed to them in man to increase the frequency of the cardiac pulsations.

Experiments with regard to the effect of this drug upon the animal temperature show a curious result: Elevation of temperature at the commencement of the action of the drug, progressive fall of temperature commencing at the moment of sudation, and depression below that of the initial temperature after the administration of jaborandi; if the initial temperature was normal the thermometer indicated lower temperature in the rectum, whilst at the same time it was higher in the armpit; at the commencement of sudation the rectal temperature was a little higher than that of the armpit; but when sweating had become general the temperature of the two parts became equalized, that of the armpit being lower and that of the rectum higher than before.

The temperature in febrile cases is more variable. According to M. Robin, the first effect of the drug is to determine an afflux of blood to

[1] British Medical Journal, February 10, 1875.
[2] Journal de Thérapeutique.

the cutaneous surface, after which t1ere occurs a slig1t elevation of temperature; yet t1e temperature is lowered in t1e rectum, w1ilst it is 1ig1er in the armpit, on t1e cutaneous surface; in ot1er words, t1e temperature of t1e body is differently distributed, being as muc1 above the normal standard at t1e surface as it is below it in t1e interior of the body. As these observations remained t1e same whether the infusion was 1ot or cold, it would seem to prove t1at jaborandi is a true sudorific.

Eucalyptus Globulus.[1] — When t1is drug was introduced subcutaneously in dogs, t1e temperature of the body was not lowered, but w1en given by t1e mout1 the temperature was lowered. If a decoction of eucalyptus was injected through t1e veins t1e manometer indicated a lower pressure (arterial), and t1e action of t1e 1eart was retarded. In t1ese cases t1e animal was controlled by opium or woorara (curare), or by being bound down. Sc1läger attributes t1e retarding influence to a direct action on t1e musculo-motor apparatus of t1e 1eart.

(*To be concluded.*)

———◆———

GRIFFITHS ON THE ART OF PRESCRIBING.[2]

THIS little volume of one 1undred and fifty pages, by N. Handsel Griffit1s, contains a number of lessons, as he calls t1em, lectures as we s1ould style t1em, on prescriptions and t1e art of prescribing.

The first or introductory lesson is better suited to the latitude of England t1an of t1is country. It is devoted to a brief exposition of t1e art of writing prescriptions in Latin. He advises not only t1at the scientific name of eac1 article t1at enters into a prescription s1ould be given in Latin, but t1at all t1e directions s1ould be given in t1at tongue also. The following is a model of t1e way in w1ic1 1e would 1ave prescriptions written:—

℞ Ammoniæ carbonatis . . . . grana sex.
    Syrupi aurantii . . . . drachmas duas.
    Aquæ . . . . drachmas decem.
Misce. Fiat haustus, cui, tempore capiendi, adde succi limonis recentis cochleare medium unum, et in effervescentiâ sumatur.

It is of course understood t1at t1e druggist will translate t1e directions from the Latin tongue into Englis1, and write t1em upon t1e label of the bottle in w1ic1 t1e medicine is dispensed. All t1is is absurd. Even if all our physicians can write grammatical Latin wit1 ease, and our druggists and t1eir assistants can translate Latin wit1 accuracy, the w1ole procedure is pedantic

---

[1] H. Schläger, of Göttingen, and Mees, of Leyden; Schmidt's Jahrbücher der Gessamten Medicin, January, 1875.

[2] *Lessons on Prescriptions and the Art of Prescribing.* By N. HANDSEL GRIFFITHS, Ph. D., L. R. C. P. E., Licentiate of the Royal College of Surgeons, Edinburgh. 8vo, pp. 150. London: Macmillan & Co. 1875.

and absurd at the present time. It is safer and better in every way for the patient, and those who take care of him, to be able to read the physician's directions, written out in good plain English by the physician himself. Any discrepancy between these directions and those put on the label by the druggist will be easily recognized, and so the danger of mistakes greatly lessened. We go even further than this. The scientific name of every article should of course be retained for the sake of precision, and this is generally Latin. The signs for scruple and dracim should not be used at all. This would leave only the sign for ounce, the abbreviation for grain, and that for minim, for the use of the prescriber, and would prevent the possibility of confounding the signs of scruple, dracim, and ounce. Instead of Latin numerals, Arabic figures should be used for the purpose of lessening still further the chance of mistake. Apart from the Latin portion of Mr. Griffiths' manual we can heartily commend it. More than half of the book is devoted to examples and exercises in prescribing. This is its most valuable portion. All medical students should read this part with care, and there are few physicians who would not derive benefit from examining it. The section on posology is altogether too brief for so important a matter. We are glad to notice, however, that our author recognizes its importance, as may be seen by the following quotation from the section referred to : " No greater service could be performed by the colleges or the great medical societies than the formation of a committee of competent men for the special investigation of this question of dosage ; for it is a subject which is as yet only in its infancy, and the best knowledge which exists about it is undoubtedly confined to a very small section of the medical profession." E. H. C.

HOW CORONERS ARE APPOINTED.

We showed last week the danger that would arise against the credit of the profession by the cession to government of any part of the management of professional affairs, and we think it well to exemplify this by showing the disgraceful manner in which appointments are made to offices of great importance to the safety of the community.

When death occurs suddenly from unknown causes, or under suspicious circumstances, it is the duty of a coroner to examine the case, and, if satisfied that all is right, to report that an inquest is unnecessary, and to sign an official certificate ; otherwise to call a jury to determine the cause of death, and open the way to legal investigations. The great importance of the office is evident when we consider how easily a death from poisoning, criminal abortion, or infanticide may be hushed up by the certificate of a corrupt or ignorant coroner. The place should be held by men of character and attainments, and though the law does not require them to be physicians, it is clear that at least they should not be pretended ones. In spite of this the list of coroners of Suffolk County contains, among the names of several excellent men, those of others who are a disgrace to the Commonwealth. We find several self-styled doctors who

24

have, as far as we can learn, no degree, who are not recognized by respectable
physicians, and who certainly are grossly ignorant.   One has been tried, at least
once, before the Superior Criminal Court, for abortion.   The responsibility of
filling the office rests with the governor and council, and we propose to show
by the latest example with what care this duty is discharged.

Two weeks ago we read, to our surprise, that a Dr. A. W. K. Newton had
been appointed a coroner.   It is possible that he may have a claim to the title
of doctor, though we should be glad to know what it is, as he certainly is not
recognized by the profession, and does not appear to have the standing, education, or character that the position demands.   We have been at some pains to
learn the steps preceding this appointment, that the public may know whom to
thank for it.   A short time since Dr. (?) A. W. K. Newton went to the State
House, where he was introduced to Governor Gaston by ex-Senator Jacobs.
He presented to the governor a petition, of which we give some extracts, as
follows: "To his Excellency, William Gaston the Govenor (*sic*) of the
Commonwealth of Massachusetts and to his Honorable Counselors (*sic*).   Respectfully represents Abiel W. K. Newton, M. D., of Boston, and petitions
your Honors that he be appointed one of the Coroners for the said County of
Suffolk."

The reason which the candidate assigned for his appointment was that "no
coroner resides within about a mile from his said residence in any direction."
This was the only reason he gave why he should be appointed, unless indeed
another be that " he believes himself to be a competent and suitable person to
perform the duties of a coroner."

In support of his petition he presented a paper which stated that the signers
thereof had "long known" the petitioner, and that they were of the opinion
that *a coroner was needed in that district*, and that they believed the petitioner
to be a suitable man for the place.   This paper was signed by fifty-three
names, several of which cannot be found in the directory, and very few of
which carry any weight out of petty politics.   In justice to all parties we must
say that the names of S. A. D. Shepard and S. Follansbee, whom we had always considered respectable apothecaries, were among the signatures.

The petition was brought up before the council, and, according to custom,
was referred for investigation to the councillor for the district in which the petitioner resided.   The councillor in question, Edward H. Dunn, who had never
seen the petitioner, and who knew nothing whatever about him, reported favorably, and he was accordingly appointed.

The announcement of the appointment gave rise to much indignation in
professional circles, and within forty-eight hours a protest was drawn up and
signed by such prominent members of the profession (twenty-six in all) as
could be conveniently reached at short notice, showing that the statement
made by Newton and indorsed by the signers of his recommendation, namely,
" that no coroner lived within about a mile of him in any direction," was absolutely false, one coroner, J. H. McCollom, M. D., living within a few houses
of him, and three others (Cornell, Evans, and Underwood) living within the
limits above mentioned.

What was the result of the protest?   The councillor (Edward H. Dunn) had recommended a man without making any inquiry as to his character or the truth of his statements. Yet when a protest came in, showing clearly that the reasons given for the appointment were false, Mr. Dunn declined to withdraw his report of approval, without which Governor Gaston would not have made the appointment.

The affair is over, and there is nothing more to be said; but we shall do well to remember that to obtain an office of trust, honor, and of importance to the community, all that is needed is an ill-spelled petition, containing palpable falsehoods and signed by a few ward politicians and as many men of straw as may be convenient; and that the protest of men of standing but not of political influence, even when it contains proofs of the unfitness of the appointment, will be of no avail.

———◆———

THE ANNUAL MEETING OF THE AMERICAN PHARMACEUTICAL ASSOCIATION.

THE meeting appears to have been a perfect success. Little time has been lost in discussions of policy and personal matters, and the papers have for the most part been very good. We congratulate the association on the wise choice it made in electing Professor George F. H. Markoc president. We do not attempt anything like a report of the proceedings, as most points could hardly be of interest to our readers, but we may mention some subjects that strike us as important. The report of the permanent secretary, Professor John M. Maisch, of Philadelphia, was chiefly devoted to the meeting of next year. Efforts had been made, apparently without success, to bring the international congress of pharmaceutists to the centennial exhibition, but invitations had been sent to individuals of all nations, and the secretary recommended that steps be taken to communicate with all pharmaceutical bodies on the subject.

The report of the committee on adulterations, read by the chairman, Mr. Miller, was very interesting. Special attention was called to frauds in essential oils, which appear to be very common, but often difficult of detection.

The report of the committee on maximum doses was presented by the chairman, Dr. Wilson H. Pile, of Philadelphia. The committee reported that in view of the wide difference in the statements of different authorities in regard to the quantities of potent remedies which could safely be administered, they had come to the conclusion that an arbitrary list of maximum doses made from such conflicting authorities would be of no practical utility. They therefore suggested that a committee be appointed to confer with the National Medical Association on the subject of maximum doses, as well as the proper signs to be adopted to designate the correctness of larger doses when intended by the physician, as an understanding might thus be arrived at which would prove of practical value to the physician as well as to the pharmacist. The report was accepted and the recommendation adopted.

A paper in answer to the following query was read by Professor E. Scheffer: "Is pancreatin converted into peptone when it is digested with acidulated pepsin?" The writer was enabled by his experiments to assert positively that pancreatin when brought into the stomach became destroyed, and that it therefore could have neither physiological nor therapeutic effect when administered internally.

Professor Maisch made some very sensible remarks on the disgrace of the great traffic in patent medicines. We are glad to see the matter taken up by this body, for the pharmaceutists can do more, we think, to remedy the evil than the physicians. We must disagree with Professor Maisch, however, when he says that apothecaries can do nothing as long as quack medicines are called for. They always will be in demand till the millenium, but the demand will be lessened if they cannot be procured from respectable druggists. Professor Maisch stated that the question had been agitated as to the best means of informing the public of the dangerous nature of many of these nostrums. Dr. Frederick Hoffman, of New York, had suggested the publication of a health almanac similar to those issued by the proprietors of patent medicines, which should contain analyses of such preparations. Circulars had been prepared upon this subject, which Mr. Maisch desired to have distributed to the association.

We are glad to see that the metric system was not overlooked. As Professor Sharples well observed, no profession is more deeply interested in the subject than the pharmaceutical, which had to deal with two varying systems of measures, mixing by one and selling by the other. He stated that the process of converting one measure into the other was very difficult, and not generally understood. All the trouble arising from this source would be obviated by the adoption of the metric system.

A very interesting feature was the exhibition of chemicals, drugs, and other articles connected with the craft. It was a very fine display, and deserves far more space than we can allow it. Without making any comparisons or attempting to enumerate half of the objects worthy of notice, we must allude to the table occupied by the chemicals of Messrs. Power and Weightman, covered by the purest preparations in the most beautiful crystalline forms. We understand that the value of the articles exhibited by this firm was not under twenty-five thousand dollars. Messrs. Weeks and Potter attracted much attention. Lehn and Fink, a New York house of German chemists, showed many curious collections: for instance, a series of all the metals, and another of the alkaloids of opium. We must not forget the fine specimens of materia medica, some one hundred and fifty in number, presented through Professor Bedford to the Massachusetts College of Pharmacy by Lazell, Marsh, and Gardner, nor those given by Southall, Brothers, and Barclay, of Birmingham.

MEDICAL NOTES.

— According to our English exchanges there is room for improvement in the burial arrangements of West Lowe, in Cornwall. Over eight thousand bodies rest, if the term is allowable, in something more than half an acre of land, which has actually swollen up into a hill, leaving the church in a pit.

Putrefying bodies lie together through the soil like plums in a pudding, and when a new candidate for admission appears, exploring parties go out with an iron rod and take soundings till a free space of four and a half feet is discovered. A horrible slime is said to be constantly oozing from the graves in the higher part of the yard, which runs-on to the floor of the belfry, and disinfectants have to be freely used for the safety of the ringers. Fresh primroses gathered and placed in the church for decoration purposes on Easter Sunday turned almost black by the following evening, owing to the presence of sulphuretted hydrogen in the atmosphere in such quantity as to be highly dangerous to human life. On Ash Wednesday the air of the church was so fetid that the congregation were unable to remain until the end of the service. The vicar and the government inspector desire a change, but the rate-payers, who apparently have the authority, think the present arrangement good enough.

— We regret to receive the news of the death, in his sixty-eighth year, of Dr. Milo Wilson, at Shelburne Falls, on September 3d. He was a highly respectable practitioner.

— Dr. Burg, a French physician, says the *Medical Record*, has recently published a little book in which he endeavors to controvert, by reference to his own observations and experience, the notion that the use of wind instruments is injurious to individuals characterized by pectoral weakness. All the men whose business it is to try the wind instruments made at the various factories before sending them off for sale are exceptionally free from pulmonary affections. Dr. Burg has known many who on entering this calling were very delicate, and who, nevertheless, though their duty obliged them to blow for hours together, enjoyed perfect health after a certain time. He himself is an instance of this. His mother died of consumption, and eight of her children fell victims to the same disease. Only three sons survive, and all these play wind instruments.

— Dr. C. Wackerhagen publishes, in the *New York Medical Journal* of September, a new method of making plaster of Paris splints. The displacement having been rectified, and the limb held in position by assistants, the latter is smoothly bandaged with cotton-wadding, prepared in the form of an ordinary roller ; a flannel bandage spread with dry plaster of Paris, and rolled, is soaked in warm water (to which about two fluid ounces of saturated solution of sulphate of potassium may be added) and applied to the limb, over the wadding, by circular and reversed turns. One layer of the flannel applied in this way is thought amply sufficient for support.

The author continues as follows: " If it is desired to employ lateral splints, the dressing should be cut in the median line of the anterior and posterior surfaces. If antero-posterior support is preferred, it should be cut through the lateral surfaces. The splints should now be varnished on their inner and outer surfaces with shellac, or this preparation may be applied to the outer surface before removal.

" The shellac seems to permeate the dressing sufficiently to increase the strength of the splint, and at the same time renders it slightly flexible instead of brittle, as is the case when plaster of Paris is used alone."

— The *Lyon Médical* deals severely tiougi not unjustly witi the Paris Academy of Medicine in saying tiat the discussion on ciolera does not merit tie ionor of being reproduced, and intimates tiat facts are required ratier tian speecies.

— In Europe, tie average number of infants from eaci marriage varies from 4.73 to 3.07. Russia ieads the list witi tie number 4.73 ; France occupies the last place witi 3.07. The relative fecundity is as follows: Russia, Spain, Scotland, Ireland, Italy, Hungary, Norway, Sweden, Würtemberg, Prussia, Holland, Austria, Belgium, England, Saxony, Denmark, Bavaria, France. Tie reason of the small increase in tie Frenci population is not to be sougit in tie age at wiici marriages take place, nor in tieir number, nor in tie mortality of infants or adults ; it is due entirely to tie limited fecundity — often voluntary — of tie marriages.

SURGICAL CASES AND OPERATIONS AT THE BOSTON CITY HOSPITAL.

Amputation at the Elbow-Joint; Torsion. — E. S., aged fifty-five, was admitted to tie hospital June 29, and gave tiis account of iis injury : Tiree weeks before entrance, iis left iand and wrist were caugit in an engine and severely bruised and twisted. An abscess formed and disciarged spontaneously, but did not ieal. Wien the patient entered tie iospital, tiere were sinuses and openings leading to carious bone in tie iand and wrist. Free incisions were made witi a view to giving free exit to tie disciarge, and saving the fore-arm. But tie inflammation and suppuration increased until tie middle of August, wien tie ulna was found diseased tirougiout its entire extent ; tie wrist was completely disorganized; tie iand was swollen, purple, cold, stiff, and useless. Tie limb was getting worse every day. Amputation was proposed to tie patient, and accepted as tie only ciance of recovery.

August 13th. Tie patient was etierized, and Esmarci's bandage and tourniquet were applied. Dr. Fifield tien amputated tie fore-arm at the elbow-joint. Tie operation was done by tie antero-posterior metiod, oval skin flaps being secured. Tie incisions began and ended well below tie condyles of tie iumerus. Tiis was absolutely necessary, or tie siarp processes of bone, especially the inner one, would protrude between the flaps. The braciial and two small vessels were twisted with tie regular torsion forceps, used by Mr. Bryant. The iæmorriage was mostly venous, and ceased readily wien tie elastic cord was removed. Tie arterial hæmorriage was very sligit, a fact repeatedly noticed in cases wiere Esmarci's metiod ias been used. Tie flaps were closed witi silk sutures, and a simple dressing made.

September 1st. Tie case has gone on well. Tiere has not been any iæmorrhage. Tie flaps are well united, and tie condyles are covered. None of tie articulating surface of tie iumerus was removed at tie time of tie operation. Tie line of tie cicatrix is upon tie anterior surface of the arm. Tiere is no necrosis. Only a slight superficial ulceration at the junction of the flaps in one or two spots remains. The man is nearly well.

˙ Amputation at the knee and elbow is not as popular with American as with English surgeons. Bryant is a strong advocate of these operations, and says of that at the elbow-joint that it is an admirable one, and should be done much oftener than it is. Two considerations have probably deterred surgeons from performing this operation: fear of ulceration of the cartilages, and a long, club-shaped, unwieldy stump. The first has been proved over and over again to be groundless. In many, if not in most cases, the flaps unite as readily over cartilages as over the sawn extremity of bone. Whether the second objection is of sufficient importance to overbalance the increased danger of higher amputation is by no means proven. It is asserted by good surgical authorities that the redundant size of the end of the bone becomes in time reduced, and leaves a very comely and useful stump. It is admitted by every one that the less the part removed, the greater the chances for the patient's recovery. It is also admitted that the more the sheaths of the muscles and the medullary cavities of the bones are interfered with, the greater are the dangers of pyæmia, osteo-myelitis, necrosis, profuse suppuration, etc. These are certainly strong reasons in favor of joint-amputations.

The above is the second successful case of amputation of the arm in which Dr. Fifield has practiced torsion to control hæmorrhage. In neither case was there any subsequent bleeding. The operation was easily and quickly done. The end of the vessel was seized with the torsion-forceps, drawn out of its sheath, and twisted till the coats were divided sufficiently to give way and offer no further resistance. The end was twisted off in the smaller vessels, but was left attached in the larger ones. The artery should be twisted till that peculiar sensation of giving way is felt, or it may untwist. The secret of success seems to lie in drawing the artery well out of its sheath. No second forceps is needed to limit the extent of the torsion. There are many cases in which it would seem difficult if not impossible to practice it with success; for example, where the vessels are calcareous, or surrounded by or imbedded in diseased tissues. But there are, on the other hand, many cases where the ligatures undoubtedly prevent union by first intention, and any device whereby all foreign substances can be dispensed with safely will be one of the greatest improvements in modern surgery.

At Guy's Hospital torsion is the rule and ligature the exception. The femoral has been successfully twisted over fifty times without a single instance of secondary hæmorrhage. In fact, "the house-surgeons never expect to be called to cases of secondary hæmorrhage now torsion is the general practice of the hospital." "I have had stumps heal in a week," says Bryant, "and patients up in two weeks without one single drawback." Of course if a stump sloughs there is danger of hæmorrhage, no matter in what way the vessels may have been secured. Of one hundred and two amputations of thigh, leg, arm, and fore-arm, in only one was there secondary hæmorrhage, and that was from an arm where the whole stump sloughed. Such is the record of Guy's Hospital, and it is one well worth trying to imitate in private as well as in hospital practice.   GEO. W. GAY, M. D.

A VACATION HOMILY.

MESSRS. EDITORS, — "Americans know nothing of the art of taking rest," is the incisive remark of some magazine writer who is an acute and truthful observer of the habits of our people. He might have added that Americans are apparently ignorant of the necessity of rest, and of the way in which it is to be found. What is the summer rest of those of our people who recognize their physical needs? Some — the few, of course — court rest in entire change of scene and daily habit by steaming to Europe, the delightful do-nothing of the eight or ten days at sea relaxing overstrained nerves, and bestowing a benefit which is intensified, let us earnestly hope, by a thorough revolution in the stomach during the first twenty-four hours, the liver being meanwhile jerked and shaken into friendly sympathy and a future reinvigorated action. This feature of the sea-trip would hardly be voted delightful. No voyager would choose the unsentimental sensations and deprivations of "the first day out," but who ever failed to find an appetite for every one of the five meals of the steamer, and the nine o'clock P. M. Welsh rare-bit or sandwich besides, after having spent twenty-four or forty-eight hours in Neptune's mangle? In the exhilarating days which follow, should not this voracious being bless the rough handling of the sea-god? What bitters or tonic ever did so much for him? The sea-air, the lazy life, the freedom from care, and the hearty appetite, prepare our traveler for an active, enjoyable, healthful run from lake to mountain, from cathedral to village-hamlet, from picture-gallery to sea-view. He lives in an unaccustomed world, thinks unaccustomed thoughts, and, better, sleeps dreamless sleep long unknown. In October he returns to ten new days of steamer life, and reaches home with youth half renewed, and a fund of vigor which will endure beyond belief.

This is a wise manner of reviving sapped forces, but it requires a long purse. Fortunately there are other equally helpful means of recreation. Another small portion of our people is sensible enough, and plucky enough, to "sink the shop" out of sight, and become, as nearly as may be, children of nature, by following the better habits of the aborigines. There is probably no more healthful method of refreshing brain and body than that offered by camp life — life out-of-doors day and night; the meaty portion of the food of the camper-out being taken by himself from air, water, or woods; the day a succession of invigorating tramps, canoe-paddling, shooting, or fishing; the night a long, sweet, untroubled oblivion beneath the sky.

I believe the surest of prophylactics in incipient consumption, and the best of tonics in nervous affections and general debility, might be found in this simple advice: live an out-of-door life, and never sleep under a roof heavier than a tent-cloth. Such advice in our climate would of course, in certain months, require change of latitude, and perhaps a margin of pocket-money, but the law of effects would nevertheless hold good. The camper-out begins his rest by entering upon Indian habits. He returns to labor with the swarthy hands and face of the aborigine, with muscles as tough, appetite as sharp, and brain as clear as his. The store of vigor which one can pack away during a month or six weeks of camp life is amazing. More amazing are the "staying qualities" of this toughened, hard-packed endurance. To the astonishment of the heretofore dyspeptic, headachy, weak-marrowed, lifeless plodder, the old gaps in life are bridged over, the stomach behaves itself charmingly, the brain acknowledges all drafts at sight, and the nervous mechanism runs without a click or a jar, perhaps even into the new summer months which call for a return to canvas walls and the big bath in sunlight and oxygen. These campers-out are sensible creatures. With a small investment of cash they win immense dividends in a commodity too invaluable to be mentioned in the same breath with gold. But these speculators at nature's stock-board are unfortunately too few. The average professional or business man thinks he cannot leave his duties even for one month out of the twelve. This must be an absurd error. A well-managed business can surely be left during the dull months, and in the temporary absence of its head, to the care of subordinates, who may rest in their turn; and professional men can always relieve each other in the absence of either. This is done in other countries. It is only in America that men work until they wear out, or rather break down. It is haste to become rich that renders riches so useless, for one never has time to enjoy them, and the physical smash-up comes long before a well-conducted organization would dream of sinking under the effects of fatigue.

Another class of business and professional rest-seekers are those who go out of town for a two days' stay, then return to business for an equal length of time, and thus oscillating between labor and refreshment fail to enjoy either. During their absence they continually think of business, and so never free their minds from its claims, thus defeating all the restorative attempts of the nature they seek. This is another absurdity. In order to obtain rest the ordinary occupations of life must be absolutely dropped, and, if possible, forgotten.

Perhaps it is the many who in seeking rest take upon themselves all sorts of ridiculous hindrances, annoyances, and unhealthful conditions. These are they who crowd the fashionable resorts; who, leaving their comfortable homes behind them, with sweet cheerfulness stive themselves in seven-by-nine rooms; dress for breakfast, for dinner, for promenade, for evening; follow the fashionable routine; fear the sun, the wind, and the rain; eat questionable meals, bearing discomforts unnumbered for fashion's sake, and live in houses which are ill aired, poorly drained, typhoid breeders in many instances. For your fashionable landlord thinks more of economizing space, of filling stuffy apartments at disproportionate rates, than of pure air and well-built drains. There is neither economy nor refreshment, and but little pleasure, in such summer recreation. I know of a lady who passes her summers at a watering-place, and who refuses to receive her callers, actually depriving herself of what she confesses would give her great pleasure, because she finds it too much trouble to dress *twice* daily after her bath. The absurdity here lies in living under such rules as oblige one either to dress several times between rising and retiring, or to accept the dreadful alternative of being considered unfashionable. Fashion and restfulness are as incompatible as oil and fire.

But, undoubtedly, the great objection to fashionable summer resorts consists not in the mere failure to secure repose, or even healthful recreation, so much as in the effects of the neglect of hygiene in the arrangements of hotels and boarding-houses. Landlords care for nothing but gain, and their guests think of anything else than good water and suitable drainage. If typhoid be thus contracted, and the victims die, their friends thoughtlessly say (to quote a writer in *The Atlantic Monthly*), "In the wisdom of an inscrutable Providence it has been found necessary to remove them from our midst. In this way we blandly impose upon Divine Providence the responsibility of our short-comings. The victims of typhoid fever die, not by the act of God, but by the act of man. They are poisoned to death by infections that are due to man's ignorance or neglect." The subject of summer rest cannot be adequately treated within the limits of a brief letter. But thus much can be shortly said : we all need rest. It need not be said that I refer especially to those who have earnest vocations in life. There are those who never do anything. Such could by no possibility find rest in anything but work. To the actual worker a full month of positive forgetfulness of the eleven months of duty is a necessity. Business, whether professional or mercantile, should be put under mental lock and key, and the key lost for at least four weeks of the fifty-two. Power to work becomes intensified through rest. Hence to take rest becomes a duty, and to none more than to the physician. He cannot properly do his work when depressed by physical and mental fatigue. He holds immense responsibilities in his care. An error which might be the result, not of carelessness, but of weariness, of benumbed faculties, could work him incalculable harm, fetter his future usefulness, stunt his professional growth, besides, and worst of all, perhaps taking a life. If any worker needs a clear brain, a light heart, a vigorous body, it is the physician ; and yet I suppose few men are so unready to rest as are medical men. This is a palpable wrong, both to their patients and to themselves. To thoughtful minds this mere word should be enough.

Let the physician, then, take his gun, his boat, his fishing rod, his novel, and hie himself away from work to rest. It is not necessary to live a tent-life, if he but take sensible rest otherwise. Let him avoid hotels and boarding-houses, and take his family (for let us hope he has one) to some clean, airy farm-house, where milk is plenty as water ; where eggs, chickens, lambs, vegetables, and the summer fruit of the country are abundant and fresh. Whatever lameness may be evident in cookery may be easily set aright by a few hints from his wife.

As to dress, which is one of the immense bores of fashionable resorts, our rusticating physician will find great delight in the comfort of navy-blue flannel overshirts. Linen should be reserved for evening wear. During the day, whatever be the amusement, coats, vests, and linen should be discarded. Nine o'clock P. M. is a sensible retiring hour, and if the day have been properly spent, by this time one is ready for sleep. The physician, and this may apply to every class of reading men, may be followed, if he choose, by current professional literature and one daily newspaper ; otherwise let him leave all books, except novels, behind. Recreation is much enhanced if the summer location be near a lake; for rowing, sailing, fishing, and swimming are not only great delights, but they also serve to purify the life-current, and harden the muscles. One month of such life is like a dip into the fountain of youth. One great improvement may be suggested : make the four weeks six. Rest of this nature should be governed by one general rule, namely, between morning and evening live out of doors. How spend the time? Walking, driving, fishing, hunting, berrying, picnicking, sailing, rowing, swimming. In such enjoyments the days go only too swiftly, and night brings sleep worth a king's ransom.

If our physician live in the country he may secure similar pleasures with equal simplicity and variety at some quiet sea-side village.

Such is the simple, economical, healthful rest which we may all find. It may be varied in a thousand ways, according to one's disposition and inclination. If any candid mind do not recognize the great desirableness and healthfulness of a summer passed in this manner, as compared with life at the stupid, mismanaged, too often unhealthful resorts where one is trammeled and pent up in all ways by the demands of dress and etiquette, and exposed to sickness by the cupidity and ignorance of landlords, such a mind must have been warped by the very life we should all flee when we seek rest.   X.

LAKE COUNTRY, *August* 28, 1875.

WEEKLY BULLETIN OF PREVALENT DISEASES.

THE following is a bulletin of the diseases prevalent in Massachusetts during the week ending September 11, 1875, compiled under the authority of the State Board of Health from the returns of physicians representing all sections of the State: —

The week has witnessed a marked increase in the prevalence of typhoid fever in all parts of the State. The sudden change in the weather produced an access of bronchitis. The presence of autumnal catarrh (hay fever) is reported by several towns in the middle and eastern sections. The order of relative prevalence of acute diseases in the State at large is as follows: Diarrhœa, cholera morbus, cholera infantum, typhoid fever, dysentery, rheumatism, bronchitis, influenza, diphtheria, scarlatina, whooping-cough, pneumonia, measles. The last disease has reappeared on the Cape (Plymouth, Mattapoisett). The summary for each section is as follows: —

Berkshire: Diarrhœa, cholera infantum, cholera morbus, dysentery, typhoid fever.

Valley: Diarrhœa, cholera morbus, cholera infantum, dysentery, typhoid fever. Shelburne reports a fatal case of cerebro-spinal meningitis. Springfield has some malarial and remittent fever.

Midland: Diarrhœa, cholera morbus, dysentery, cholera infantum, typhoid fever, rheumatism.

Northeastern: Diarrhœa, cholera morbus, dysentery, cholera infantum, typhoid fever (quite general). Cerebro-spinal meningitis in Lynn and Woburn.

Metropolitan: Diarrhœa, cholera morbus, typhoid fever, cholera infantum, dysentery, bronchitis.

Southeastern: Cholera morbus, diarrhœa, cholera infantum, dysentery, typhoid fever. Small-pox in Fall River.

It will be noticed that cholera infantum is on the decline in all parts of the State.   F. W. DRAPER, M. D., Registrar.

COMPARATIVE MORTALITY-RATES FOR THE WEEK ENDING SEPT. 4, 1875.

	Estimated Population.	Total Mortality for the Week.	Annual Death-rate per 1000 during Week.
New York	1,060,000	674	33
Philadelphia	800,000	367	24
Brooklyn	500,000	289	30
Chicago	400,000	214	28
Boston	342,000	212	32
Cincinnati	260,000	98	19
Providence	100,700	31	16
Worcester	50,000	29	30
Lowell	50,000	21	22
Cambridge	48,000	25	27
Fall River	45,000	29	33
Lawrence	35,000	9	13
Lynn	33,000	9	15
Springfield	31,000	4	6
Salem	26,000	14	28

BOOKS AND PAMPHLETS RECEIVED. — The Treatment of Nervous Diseases by Electricity. By Dr. Friedrich Fieber. Translated from the German by George M. Schweig, M. D. New York: G. P. Putnam's Sons. 1875.

Capillary Bronchitis in Adults. By Calvin Ellis, M. D. Published as one of the American Clinical Series. New York: G. P. Putnam's Sons. 1875.

The Relations of the Nervous System to Diseases of the Skin. By L. D. Bulkley, M. D. (From the Archives of Electrology and Neurology.)

The Diseases of the Heart and Aorta. By Thomas Hayden, Fellow of the King and Queen's College of Physicians, etc. In Two Parts. Philadelphia: Lindsay and Blakiston. 1875. (From A. Williams & Co.)

Gout at the Heart. By Eldridge Spratt. Twelfth Edition. Glasgow: James Maclehose; Philadelphia: J. B. Lippincott & Co. 1875. (From A. Williams & Co.)

On the Administration and Value of Phosphorus. By E. A. Kirby, M. D. Philadelphia: Lindsay and Blakiston. 1875. (From A. Williams & Co.)

Shall we Lance the Gums in the First Dentition? (Read before the Maine Medical Association, June 9, 1875.) By A. C. Hamlin, M. D.

IN our notice of the excursion of the New Hampshire Medical Society to the White Mountains, on September 20th and 21st, we should have mentioned that as the meeting is but semi-professional it is hoped that physicians will not fail to be accompanied by the ladies of their families.

THE BOSTON
MEDICAL AND SURGICAL JOURNAL.

VOL. XCIII. — THURSDAY, SEPTEMBER 23, 1875. — NO. 13.

BURNS AND SCALDS.

BY GEORGE W. GAY, M. D.,

Surgeon to the Boston City Hospital.

THE following paper is based upon the records of two hundred and four cases of burns and scalds treated in the Boston City Hospital during the eleven years from 1864 to 1875.

All of the severe gunpowder cases have been omitted, as the burn was secondary in importance to other injuries. Cases of deformity, the result of burns, are also omitted, as not coming strictly under that part of the subject to be considered.

Sex. — A little over half of the cases (111) were females, and they comprised two thirds of the fatal cases. The reason of this will be readily seen when the sources of the injuries are considered.

Age. — The ages varied from three to seventy years. The largest number in any one decade was fifty-five, between twenty and thirty. The next two decades had forty-one each. Only ten were received and treated under ten years of age. This is one twentieth of the whole number admitted, and is a very much smaller proportion than is given by the statistics of some of the English hospitals. Of four hundred and eight cases of burns consecutively admitted to Guy's Hospital, the majority were children. The difference in the experience of Guy's and the Boston City Hospital may be explained on the ground that burned children are not as commonly taken to the hospital in this city as in London, for they have some sort of place in which to be taken care of. On looking over the records of deaths at the city registrar's office, we found that of two hundred and twenty deaths from burns and scalds which have taken place in this city during the ten years from 1864 to 1874, one hundred and thirty-four (sixty per cent.) were under ten years of age. This fact would tend to show that these accidents probably preponderate among children in Boston as well as in London, but are not as often treated in our hospitals.

Cause. — Almost half of the patients treated in this hospital for burns received their injuries from hot water and other liquids, such as tea and coffee. Most of the slight and comparatively few of the fatal cases were caused in this way.

Twenty-six cases were caused by burning kerosene oil, and two thirds of the patients died. Injuries received by this agent were usually severe, from the fact that they were often the result of explosions of lamps or cans, by which large portions of the clothing were saturated with oil, and burned very rapidly. The fluid also adheres to the skin, and is with difficulty removed or extinguished. Many of these cases occurred among women who were filling lighted lamps, or pouring oil from a can upon a lighted fire to hasten its kindling. Some of the very worst injuries were received in this manner.

An equal number of cases were caused by the clothes taking fire from a stove, furnace, or gas-jet. All but six of the patients were women, their mode of dress especially exposing them to the accident.

A not uncommon cause of burns of the face and hands should be more generally known among those having charge of furnaces. We refer to the gas which becomes ignited, and rushes from a closed furnace when the door is opened suddenly. A few of the above cases were due to this cause, and we have known of others in private practice. A gentleman well known in this city suffered a temporary loss of a portion of his whiskers, eyebrows and eyelashes, and of the epidermis of his face, in this manner. Fortunately his eyes escaped injury. These burns are generally superficial, and can be easily avoided by first opening the draught and then standing away from the door of the furnace.

Among other sources of the injuries in the above cases may be mentioned the following : jute catching fire from a gas-jet and burning the scalp, face, and hands ; gas explosions ; melted iron and brass ; falling on the stove or fire, a very common accident among epileptics ; sulphuric acid thrown in the face and eyes ; gunpowder.

Location and Extent. — The severity of the injuries varied• from a slight erythema to the charring of a limb ; from a small patch of denuded surface to the destruction of almost the entire skin of the body. In general terms, it may be said that in one third of the fatal cases nearly or quite the entire surface of the body was burned ; in another third the injuries were confined to the upper part of the trunk, the upper extremities, and the face ; and in the remaining third the lower part of the trunk and lower extremities were principally involved. In the favorable cases, the lesions were situated in all parts of the body. Among the severest accidents which recovered may be mentioned the following : —

. A woman received a deep burn on the head by the bursting of a kerosene lamp. The wound was of the third degree, that is, involved the whole thickness of the scalp. It was six inches long by three wide, and was situated directly over the longitudinal sinus. One ear was entirely burned off, and the other was partly destroyed. The tympani were injured so that partial deafness followed. She recovered without a single unfavorable symptom.

Another woman, seven months pregnant, was burned by kerosene all over the posterior part of her body, from her knees to her shoulders, so that her back, nates, and posterior part of the thighs formed one large suppurating surface, compelling her to lie constantly on her abdomen. Yet her child was born alive at the end of twenty-three days, and she recovered.

Another pregnant woman received a severe burn involving the entire abdomen, and destroying the true skin in places. She made a good recovery and did not lose her child.

A young woman was burned upon her neck, chest, and arms by kerosene. A pitch plaster, which was upon her chest, took fire, and before it could be removed had burned large sloughs in both breasts. She recovered in a month.

On the other hand one man died in consequence of exhaustion following a moderate scald on the outer surface of one foot.

Two patients were burned internally, by inhaling flame and steam, and both died in a few hours with the most intense suffering.

Two burns of the leg, and one of the hand and arm, required amputation. The latter case is interesting as being the first important amputation in this hospital in which all the vessels of the stump were secured by torsion. The hæmorrhage was easily controlled, and did not return. The patient made a good recovery.

Symptoms and Complications. — Of course the most common symptom in recent cases was pain. Burns of the first and second degrees were often exceedingly painful, requiring large doses of opium, and, in some cases, ether, for their relief. In a few of the severest accidents, the patients did not lose consciousness nor suffer much pain. This was due to the peculiar shock to the nervous system, and the cases were almost always fatal.

Only four of the thirty patients reported as suffering from collapse recovered. It is probable that this condition existed in many more cases, but they had either rallied before coming to the hospital, or the fact had been omitted in the notes, for no injuries are more liable to be followed by shock than these. Chills and delirium were very frequent symptoms in the fatal cases, and were present in a small proportion of the favorable ones. The delirium was of a low, muttering type, and disappeared on the return of the patient's strength. Delirium tremens was present in four instances. One was fatal, and would probably have been so had not this complication occurred. Nausea, vomiting, and pain in epigastrium were frequent symptoms; so much so that it has become the practice in this hospital to put all patients, whose injuries are of any consequence, upon a mild diet from the first, and experience seems to justify the treatment.

According to the records diarrhœa was not quite as frequent as the

gastric derangements, especially in the fatal cases. . Three quarters of
the patients who suffered from vomiting died, but only half of those who
had diarrhœa. This is probably due to the fact that the latter complication does not set in as early as the former, seldom being present
before the second week, or later. In the long, lingering cases the intestinal symptoms were as common as the gastric. In the majority of
instances of diarrhœa, the stools were not bloody, or of such a character
as to indicate any ulceration of the bowels. No autopsies have been
made here upon patients who have died of burns and scalds. This is
to be regretted, as but a vague idea of the intestinal lesions can be
formed from the symptoms. There may be severe symptoms with
slight lesions, and *vice versa.*

Erysipelas occurred only five times. Two of the patients died ; one
in ten, and the other in fifty-nine days. The erysipelas did not produce
this result, but probably hastened it. The period of invasion varied
from three days to a month after the reception of the injury. It is
stated by a French authority that a wound made with a caustic, as in
removing tumors, is never attacked by erysipelas. The comparative
infrequency of this complication in the above cases would seem to corroborate the notion that such wounds are not as liable to this disease as
those produced in other ways. The French surgeon's statement, however, is not true for this country, for we have seen severe erysipelas
attack a wound made with chloride of zinc. A growth had been removed from the scalp with this caustic. In a few weeks the patient
had erysipelas which extended all over his face and head, increasing his
suffering but not proving fatal.

Five epileptics have been treated for burns, and all recovered.
Every one received the lesion by falling on a hot stove during a fit.
With one exception the injuries were not severe. As a rule the fits
recurred during treatment. Bromide of potassium was generally sufficient to lessen their frequency, but on omitting the drug the seizures
returned as often as before.

Six insane or demented persons were injured by fire or hot water,
and two died. Their wounds were exceedingly slow in healing, and
they seldom complained of any pain.

There was but one case of secondary hæmorrhage following a burn,
and in that the bleeding was from the palmar arch. It was controlled
by a deep double ligature passed with a curved needle.

Among the other complications were pneumonia, bronchitis, cerebral
affections, perforation of the tympanum, with partial deafness, and retention of urine ; of each of these there were two cases. Phthisis,
gangrene of the lung, peritonitis, albuminuria, phosphatic diathesis,
epistaxis, and iritis, each furnished one case.

Among these two hundred and four patients, burned or scalded, were six pregnant women, all severely injured. A brief *résumé* of their cases follows : —

Mrs. A., aged twenty-eight, seven months pregnant, undertook to light a fire with kerosene oil. The can exploded, set fire to the woman's clothing, and burned her chemise, skirt, and crinoline entirely from her. The injuries were severe, and extended from the knees to the shoulders, completely covering the posterior surface of the body, as well as portions of the arms and hands. The wounds were dressed with white paint, which gave considerable relief. The patient was forced to lie continuously on her abdomen, on account of the large suppurating surface on her back and nates. At the end of twenty-three days she was delivered of a living child after a normal labor of only a few hours' duration. She never nursed the baby, as she had no milk. In spite of pain, chills, delirium, vomiting, diarrhœa, and bedsores, she improved steadily, and in fifty-two days was discharged in a comfortable condition, with a good prospect of recovery.

Mrs. B., aged twenty-five, near her full term of pregnancy, was severely burned on her right side by her clothes taking fire. The injuries extended from the knee to the axilla, and reached beyond the median line on the abdomen. The true skin was destroyed in places. A living child was born thirteen hours after the accident. In about twenty-four hours the mother began to fail. She had epigastric and hypogastric pain, scanty lochia, vomiting, diarrhœa, chills, delirium, a diphtheritic deposit on tonsils and fauces, tympanites, retention of urine, bedsores ; and finally she died, sixty-three days after the accident. The burns never healed.

Mrs. C., aged thirty-five, eight months pregnant, was burned by kerosene oil on her face, neck, arms, thighs, chest to the nipples, and a small spot on the abdomen. The true skin was destroyed in places. Labor came on within twenty-four hours, and she gave birth to a dead child, whose cuticle was macerated off in several places. The lochia soon ceased ; delirium, epigastric pain, and exhaustion followed, and the patient died in eight days.

Mrs. D., aged forty, in her eighth month of pregnancy, was injured about the head, face, neck, and upper extremities by her clothes catching fire. The burns were of the second degree, and exceedingly painful. She made a good recovery, carried her child to the full time, and both were alive and well a year after the accident.

Mrs. E., aged thirty-eight, eight and a half months pregnant, by the explosion of a kerosene lamp was burned severely upon her face, neck, upper extremities, sides of chest, back, and nates. She was placed in a warm bath, but grew so faint, in spite of stimulants, that that treatment was abandoned, and a mixture of mucilage and glycerine was applied to the wounds. She had a natural labor within twenty-four hours, and gave birth to a dead child. The next day she grew worse, had great pain, delirium, tympanites, diminished lochia, and died in five days of exhaustion.

Mrs. F., aged twenty-nine, five months pregnant, was severely burned all over the abdomen and left nates by hot water poured upon her by her husband. The true skin on the left side of the abdomen was destroyed. She had some diarrhœa, but recovered perfectly in thirty-seven days without losing her child.

Half of the mothers and two thirds of the children were saved. This is a very favorable record, considering the nature and severity of the injuries received. As a rule, pregnant women withstand accidents and diseases of all kinds but poorly, premature labor and death being apt to follow in the severe cases. It is surprising, therefore, that so many of the above should have been able to carry their children through a long, severe period of suffering and prostration, with safety to themselves and their offspring.

Results. — " Half the cases of burns admitted into a hospital die, and half of those that die do so within the first three days." The latter part of Bryant's statement is confirmed by the experience of this hospital, but not the former. Of the two hundred and four cases admitted to the City Hospital, forty-five died. That is, one in four and a half was fatal, instead of one in two. Half of them (23) died within two days. The others lived from four to sixty-two days, and died from exhaustion produced by the original injuries or by some complication.

Two thirds (30) of the fatal cases were females. Among the deaths from burns in this city during the past ten years previous to June, 1874, the females were one hundred and eleven, and the males one hundred and nine.

The ages varied from five to seventy years. Only four (nine per cent.) were under ten years of age. This is a remarkably low proportion when compared with some of the English statistics. The deaths from burns and scalds in Great Britain in 1845 were two thousand nine hundred and nine. Seventy-eight per cent. were under ten years of age. As stated above, the deaths under ten years of age from these injuries in Boston, during the ten years previous to June, 1874, were sixty per cent. This of course includes hospital as well as private cases. This percentage is eighteen less than the English, but seven times as large as the hospital rate. It certainly tends to prove the statement, heretofore made, that the majority of patients who die from burns and scalds in this city are under ten years of age, but that they are not, as a rule, taken to the hospital for treatment.

Contraction of the cicatrix, so liable to follow burns of the third degree, was seldom seen, for the patients were usually discharged as soon as their wounds were healed, and before there had been time for much deformity to take place.

Treatment. — T1e great variety of substances used in t1is 1ospital and elsew1ere as a primary dressing for burns proves conclusively t1at no one application is clearly above all t1e ot1ers in value. Every one allows t1at t1e first dressing s1ould be mild and soot1ing, and capable of affording a protection to t1e injured surface ; but w1ic1 of a dozen or more substances used best fulfills t1ese indications is a disputed point.

Carron oil 1as been and is the favorite local remedy for t1ese accidents in t1is 1ospital. Aside from its disagreeable odor, it is an excellent application, and in many cases may be continued till complete recovery ensues. It is best applied on soft clot1 or s1eet lint, w1ic1 s1ould be kept saturated, wit1out being removed oftener t1an is absolutely necessary. T1e next most popular dressing is a paste made of molasses and pulverized gum arabic. It is more convenient for t1ose parts of t1e body w1ic1 need not come in contact wit1 t1e clot1ing, as t1e trunk and lower extremities. T1ese s1ould be protected by cradles, and t1e application made two or t1ree times a day wit1 a soft brus1. It is a good dressing in t1ose cases not attended with a profuse disc1arge.

W1ite paint, made of carbonate of lead and linseed oil, 1as been used a number of times wit1 excellent results. In one case of a scald of t1e 1and and arm in w1ic1 t1is dressing was applied, it was very agreeable before t1e epidermis was removed, but so intensely painful afterwards t1at it 1ad to be given up. T1e odor is certainly preferable to t1at of carron oil, and it is a cleaner dressing. Dr. Gross speaks of t1e paint in t1e 1ig1est terms as being t1e best local application 1e 1as ever used. He 1as never seen any poisonous effects from t1e lead in an experience dating as far back as 1845. He used it continuously for five weeks on a negress wit1 an extensive burn of t1e neck, c1est, and abdomen, consuming more t1an a quart of lead without any bad effect. He believes it perfectly safe, w1atever t1e extent or dept1 of t1e lesion or t1e age of t1e patient. It acts by forming a varnis1 to t1e affected surfaces, and obtunding t1e nervous sensibility. It s1ould be applied wit1 a brus1, and covered with a layer of cotton batting.

Glycerine, glycerine and molasses, glycerine and mucilage, and lead was1 and opium 1ave been used in a few cases, but t1ey 1ave no particular advantages over ot1er remedies. T1e same may be said of t1e powders of oxide of zinc.

T1e late Dr. Derby made use of t1e dry eart1 treatment in a few cases of burns, but it never became a favorite met1od of treating t1ese wounds or any ot1ers in t1is 1ospital. It is by no means a cleanly or convenient dressing. It 1ides t1e wounded surfaces, and forces t1e surgeon to depend in a great degree upon t1e sensations of t1e patient, w1ic1 are seldom to be trusted, as an indication of 1is condition.

We do not know w1et1er Billroth's favorite dressing 1as been used

1ere. It consists in applying compresses wet in a solution of nitrate of silver, ten grains to t1e ounce of water, to t1e parts constantly. Gross speaks well of it in lig1t burns attended wit1 muc1 smarting and pain. Billrot1 recommends it 1ig1ly in all degrees of t1ese injuries.

T1e treatment in t1e later stages of burns is t1e same as t1at for ordinary granulating surfaces. Among the most common agents used in t1is 1ospital are weak solutions of c1lorinated soda, benzoated oxide of zinc ointment, and simple cerate. Strapping wit1 ordinary ad1esive plaster is beneficial, not only to repress exuberant granulations and hasten t1e 1ealing process, but also to keep t1e cicatricial tissue soft and pliable, and in a measure to prevent contraction. It s1ould be con-tinned some time after t1e wounds are entirely 1ealed.

Reverdin's process of skin-grafting 1as been tried in numerous in-stances wit1 fair success. In t1e favorable cases the recovery was hastened, and t1e cicatrix quite as firm and durable as in t1ose cases not so treated.

In a few cases it was impossible to 1eal t1e wounds during t1e time t1e patient was allowed to remain in t1e 1ospital. T1ese patients be-came debilitated, the recuperative powers exhausted, and t1ey were discharged wit1 t1e hope t1at a c1ange of air and surroundings mig1t improve t1eir general condition sufficiently to allow the 1ealing process to become reëstablis1ed.

SENILE GANGRENE OF THE FOOT; AMPUTATION WITH ANTISEPTIC MEASURES; RECOVERY.

BY DRS. G. W. GARLAND AND G. W. SARGENT, OF LAWRENCE, MASS.

MR. S., aged sixty-nine, had been afflicted wit1 dry mortification of 1is left foot for many mont1s. T1e nocturnal pain w1ich 1e suffered, and t1e disgusting fetor, caused 1im to loat1e his existence, and suc1 were 1is piteous entreaties for the removal of t1e foot t1at 1is friends at last, alt1oug1 advised of t1e improbability of success in any opera-tion, req1ested t1e amputation. Emaciation 1ad reac1ed an extreme point, and every artery t1at could be felt gave marked signs of ossifi-cation. T1e face was dusky; t1e pulse frequent and feeble, intermit-ting on c1ange of position. T1e action of the 1eart was stronger t1an was indicated by t1e pulse. T1e patient and 1is surroundings were as unpromising as could well be imagined.

T1e day of t1e operation was t1e 27th of June, 1875. T1e t1er-mometer registered 96° in t1e s1ade.

T1e leg was amputated at t1e middle by t1e circular operation. The disinfecting or antiseptic treatment was fully carried out with re-gard to instruments, as well as to sutures and ligatures. T1e arteries were completely ossified; the tibial stood out like a tube of bone, and emitted a stream of blood not larger than a fine thread. The smaller arterial branches could be felt readily on taking the flap between the thumb and fingers. After the arteries had been secured, the stump was washed freely with a solution of carbolic acid, one drachm of the crystals to a pint of water, and during the introduction of sutures and the bringing the parts into contact, the solution was continually allowed to drip upon the exposed edges. The end of the stump was covered with cotton thoroughly filled and dusted over with salicylic acid in powder, and held in place by two adhesive straps; over the straps more cotton was adjusted, each layer being dusted freely with salicylic acid. Over all a roller was applied, and the entire dressing was allowed to remain untouched for five days; the dressing was then removed and the stump was found but little swollen. The cut edges, which were in sight, were as bright and fresh as when the knife passed through them. Two sutures were removed and the edges of the flaps were allowed to part a little so as to permit the renewed application of the carbolic-acid lotion. A thick pad of cotton soaked in the solution was laid upon the end of the stump and held in place by adhesive straps, and the dressing completed as before.

After this the dressings were changed daily. Healthy granulations began to appear in a few days; their further development was promoted by the use of nitrate of silver, sulphate of zinc, and carbolic acid. During the entire treatment the patient suffered but little pain, and after two weeks no swelling of the stump was·visible. One bottle of wine was allowed daily. Nourishment was freely administered.

September 3d. The stump is now nearly healed. Cicatrization has been slow but constant, and will doubtless be complete in a short time. The patient has gained flesh and strength, and is able to walk about his room with the aid of crutches.

This is the first time we have used the salicylic acid except in minor surgery, and we send you this brief report of the case to call the attention of the profession to its use, and to encourage surgeons to operate in similar cases. Carbolic acid and cotton were also used, but we think they would not have kept the stump perfectly sweet and free from change those five hot days in an ill-ventilated room.

RECENT PROGRESS IN THERAPEUTICS.[1]

BY ROBERT AMORY, M. D.

Iodide of Potassium. — Investigations by Hoppe-Seyler, as observed by·Dr. Kämmerer,[2] have shown that the oxyhemoglobine is an unstable combination of oxygen with the red corpuscles of the blood, and that oxygen will readily give up this combination when a substance having a stronger affinity for it is introduced into the blood. The characteristics of the oxygen in·the blood resemble those of ozone. Kämmerer observes also that the best test for ozone is furnished in the evolution of iodine from iodide of potassium in the presence of starch ; the presence of free iodine is determined by its characteristic blue tint. On the other hand, the more stable combination of iodine and sodium known as iodide of sodium can undergo no change in the stomach ; as it is neither decomposed by the hydrochloric acid present in the stomach, nor decomposed and precipitated by the albumen compounds, such as starch or sugar, which may be present in that organ. Thus iodide of potassium passes into the blood in an unaltered form. The free carbonic acid in the blood will then cause a decomposition of the diluted˙iodide of potassium, producing hydriodic acid and bicarbonate of soda ; consequently iodine will be set free. Again, hydriodic acid dissolved in the blood becomes oxidized, and gives out free iodine. The free iodine will then act only on the organic compounds, and especially on those whose combination is the most complex. These latter are, first, the compounds produced by miasma and the ferments ; next, the fibrin and its allied elements. Moreover, by the decomposition of iodide of potassium,˙potassium peroxide is formed ; and this latter agent has the·power˙ of oxidizing organic compounds, producing in turn potassa ; and, by combination with carbonic acid, carbonate of potassa. In this way a theory˙of the action of these salts may be formed : by supposing the organic constituents of the blood to undergo oxidation, and thus to facilitate the oxidation of the tissues.

Phosphorus. — The *Practitioner* for January, 1875, contains an article by Dr. W. H. Broadbent on the therapeutical uses of phosphorus in certain affections of the nervous system. His experience with this agent leads him to think it is not useful in those forms of neuralgia in which a touch, or a movement, or a breath of air affecting a nerve-area — usually the inferior division of the fifth pair — sends a dart of exquisite pain along the nerve and to its other branches. Dr. Broadbent found that some very serious cases of patients reduced by an extreme alteration of the blood (one case of leucocythemia splenica, another called by Trousseau essential anæmia), which did not mend under treatment by iron, im-

---

[1] Concluded from page 336.
[2] Archiv der praktische Arzt, xv., 81.

proved very greatly in general condition and in color of complexion wien piospiorus was given. Two patients afflicted witi wiat tie autior calls anginoid pain, one of wiom iad also organic disease of tie heart, were relieved of tie neuralgia, and improved in general iealti and appearance. Dr. Broadbent forms iis tieory of tie action of piospliorus " not from any direct influence upon tie nervous functions, but from favorable modification of tie organic processes leading to improved nutrition of tie nervous structures." Tie piospiorus was given in capsules one to tiree times a day.

Local Effect of Cold applied to the Scalp. — Dr. Beniam,[1] from a number of very laborious and careful experiments on tie iuman body, living and dead, and on lower animals, asserts tiat cold applied to tie scalp " causes a sligit lowering of tie temperature of tie body generally, by tie direct action tiat cold ias in lowering tie temperature of tie stream of blood passing tirougi tie capillaries in direct contact witi it, and a sligit decrease in tie frequency of tie ieart's action. . . . A greater effect in tie same direction may be more easily produced by otier and less violent means."

The Antagonism of Medicines. — Tie report of tie committee of tie British Medical Association to investigate tie antagonism of medicines [2] is a most valuable contribution to tierapeutics. Tie labors of tiis committee (composed of Drs. J. Hugies Bennett, McKendrick, James Rogers, Macadam, Edmund Cook, and Mr. T. Smiti) extended over a period of four years, and comprised tie results of six iundred and nineteen experiments. Tiey obtained positive results of piysiological antagonism in tiree instances, namely, between hydrate of ciloral and strycinia, sulpiate of atropia and calabar bean, and hydrate of bromal, and atropia. Tie piysiological antagonism of tiese medicaments, under proper conditions of time, dose, comparative weigit of tie animals, etc., would seem as positive as tie ciemical antagonism formed by tie union of an acid witi an alkali. Tie metiod by wiici tiese experiments were conducted was based upon tie following data : to determine by actual trial wiat was tie minimum fatal dose of eaci drug to a given weigit of tie animal ; tien to administer tie two drugs iypodermically, one immediately after tie otier. If tie animal survived tie experiment for five days, tien tie same dose of tie first drug was administered, with tie expectation tiat tie result would be fatal to its life.

Tie general conclusions of tie committee regarding tie antagonism between ciloral iydrate and strycinia are, —

1. Tiat after a fatal dose of strycinia life may be saved by bringing the animal under tie influence of ciloral iydrate.

---

[1] The Practitioner, March, 1875 ; from the West Riding Lunatic Asylum Medical Reports, vol. iv.

[2] British Medical Journal, Nos. 718 to 724, and Nos. 726 and 727.

2. T1at chloral hydrate is more likely to save life after a fatal dose of stryc1nia than stryc1nia is to save life after a fatal dose of c1loral 1ydrate.

3. T1at after a dose of stryc1nia producing severe tetanic convulsions, t1ese convulsions may be much reduced, bot1 in force and in frequency, by t1e use of chloral 1ydrate, and consequently muc1 suffering saved.

4. T1at t1e extent of physiological antagonism between t1e two substances is so far limited t1at, first, a very large fatal dose of stryc1nia may kill before t1e c1loral 1ydrate 1as 1ad time to act; or, secondly, so large must t1e dose of c1loral hydrate be, to antagonize an excessive dose of strychnia, that t1ere is danger of death from t1e effects of t1e c1loral hydrate.

5. Chloral 1ydrate mitigates the effects of a fatal dose of strychnia by depressing t1e excess of reflex activity excited by that substance, w1ile stryc1nia may mitigate t1e effects of a fatal dose of c1loral hydrate by rousing the activity of t1e spinal cord; but it does not appear capable of removing t1e coma produced by t1e action of c1loral 1ydrate on the brain.

Sulp1ate of atropia antagonizes to a certain extent t1e fatal action of calabar bean, but t1e area of antagonism is very limited. T1e danger is, not deat1 by too great a dose of sulp1ate of atropia, t1e supposed antagonist, but death from t1e effects of calabar bean. In t1e instance of t1e antagonism of stryc1nia to chloral t1e danger lies in giving too large a dose of t1e antagonist, stryc1nia; w1ereas in poisoning from calabar bean, sulp1ate of atropia, even in large doses, produces so slig1t an effect on rabbits t1at t1e fatal action of t1e calabar bean may go on wit1out opposition. C1loral 1ydrate as an antidote to calabar bean seems to have more weig1t, and appears to modify to a great extent t1e action of a fatal dose, and to prolong life; in some cases it apparently saves life after a fatal dose of extract of calabar bean. Upon t1is point t1e committee very properly state t1at c1loral hydrate is of comparatively little service as an antagonist to extract of calabar bean if given some time after the latter. "T1e reason of t1is is very obvious. Extract of calabar bean produces its most severe p1ysiological effects ten or fifteen minutes after t1e administration of t1e fatal dose. In some cases t1e effects occur even sooner. On t1e ot1er 1and, a rabbit is not deeply under t1e effects of 1ydrate of c1loral until fifteen or twenty minutes after its administration. If t1e effects of calabar bean appear before t1ose of hydrate of chloral, t1ey usually run quickly to a fatal issue, because t1e antagonist, hydrate of c1loral, is not acting wit1 sufficient vigor to restrain them. . . . T1ere is no c1ance at all of saving life if t1e chloral hydrate be administered more t1an eig1t minutes after the extract of calabar bean."

The committee also investigated the antagonism between morphia and atropia. Having carefully determined the fatal dose of sulphate of atropia and meconate of morphia, twenty-one experiments were made on rabbits, in which the former drug was administered at various intervals after a fatal dose of meconate of morphia. In six of these cases recovery occurred. "When the crucial test was applied to these six rabbits six days later, four died and two recovered. In all cases there could be no doubt that the subsequent injection postponed the fatal issue, if it did not save life. . . . After sulphate of atropia the pupil (which was contracted by a dose of meconate of morphia previously given) slowly dilated. . . . It was observed also that the vessels of the ear, turgid with blood after the large dose of meconate of morphia, contracted considerably about eight or ten minutes after the introduction of the sulphate of atropia."

The conclusions of the committee on this subject are : —

" 1. Sulphate of atropia is physiologically antagonistic to meconate of morphia within a limited area ;

" 2. Meconate of morphia does not act beneficially after a large dose of sulphate of atropia, for in these cases the tendency to death is greater than if a large dose of either substance had been given alone ;

" 3. Meconate of morphia is not specifically antagonistic to the action of sulphate of atropia on the vaso-inhibitory nerves of the heart ; and

" 4. The beneficial action of sulphate of atropia after the administration of large doses of meconate of morphia is probably due to the action sulphate of atropia exercises on the blood-vessels. It causes contraction of these, and thus reduces the risk of death from cerebral or spinal congestion, as is known to occur after the introduction of fatal doses of meconate of morphia. It may also assist up to a certain point, not precisely fixed in these experiments, by stimulating the action of the heart through the sympathetic, and obviating the tendency to death from deficient respiration observed after large doses of morphia."

After showing the contradictory evidence of Harley [1] on the one side, and Mitchell, Keen, and Morehouse [2] on the other, the committee conclude from five original experiments of their own, "that in dogs sulphate of atropia modifies the symptoms of poisoning by meconate of morphia, diminishes their intensity, and may even save life after a fatal dose of the latter. It is therefore decidedly antagonistic, but within a limited area. In man sulphate of atropia would be too dangerous and uncertain a remedy to depend on in cases of poisoning by opium or any of its salts, but where the heart's action is greatly diminished it is directly indicated."

The committee also inquired into any supposed antagonism between

---

[1] Old Vegetable Neurotics.
[2] American Journal of the Medical Sciences, 1865 page 67.

tie alkaloids of tea, coffee, cocoa, and guarana ; and simply concluded that tieine, caffeine, and guaranine migit 1ave some sligit influence in modifying some of tie symptoms, and may periaps even save life ; wiilst, on tie otier 1and, tie animal may die eitier from too large a dose of tie caffeine or of tie meconate of morphia ; but tiere is a point between tie two actions wiere tie piysiological effect is such tiat life may be saved from doses wiici would otierwise prove fatal. Guaranine seemed ratier to increase tian to modify the tendency to coma.

Effects of Immersion in Baths. — Immersion in waters charged witi carbonic acid, and at tie temperature of tie body, produces at first a diminution of tie peripieral circulation, followed by a determination of blood to tie surface of tie body ; tie former of tiese effects is accompanied by elevation, or at any rate maintenance, of tie initial temperature of tie mouti and sioulders. After the bati tie temperature of tie mouti and armpit is less tian wien in tie bati ; tie cutaneous circulation is increased. Gradually tie internal temperature increases. Tiese pienomena are constant wietier fresi water or mineral water is used, tiougi the latter 1as more influence in producing tie calorific effects. If tie iead is immersed in tie water tie temperature is still furtier lowered. Tiis diminution of tie temperature of tie mouti and armpit produced by tepid baths, and tie depressing effects on tie cutaneous circulation, 1ave been noticed for four or five hours after tie bati. Tie general inference drawn by Jacob [1] is summarized as follows : —

Lowering of tie temperature of the blood, acceleration of the cirenlation, its determination to tie cutaneous surface, corresponding anæmia of tie internal organs, increase of nerve action, and of tiat of tie wiole nutritive system.

A case is presented by M. Raynaud,[2] where an acute articular rieumatism was cut siort in tiree days by tie use of cold batis given every six hours. Anotier case of cerebral rieumatism, in wiici the temperature of tie armpit indicated 107° Fairenieit, was treated by immersion in water at 73.5° gradually reduced to 70° ; tie temperature was brougit down to 101°. Two iours after tiis anotier bati iaving a temperature of 60.8° reduced tie temperature one degree more. But it was observed tiat tie severe symptoms persisted, and it was only on the fourti day, and subsequent to tie eleventi bati, tiat tie patient first began to siow signs of intelligence. Moreover, tiougi tie first bati at 60.8° was well borne, anotier bath at tie same temperature was followed by a dangerous collapse, in wiici tie temperature was reduced to 95°.

Tie duration of immersion in tie bati of 73.5° to 70° was one iour, and the cooling effect was manifested in about fifteen minutes, and in

1 Archiv für pathologische Anatomie und Physiologie, lxii.
2 L'Union Médicale, No. 465.

tie last quarter of an hour the most rapid lowering of the temperature occurred. The results of this treatment were complicated by the use of bromide of potassium in hourly doses of fifteen grains for ten hours a day. On the fifth day the twelfth and last bath was given, and from this time the recovery became assured.

Beneke [1] cites one hundred and forty-six observations in the treatment of rheumatism with cardiac complications, which clearly demonstrate the influence of baths taken at a temperature of 88° to 93° with water containing two to three per cent. of salt and a little carbonic acid. The first effect of this treatment was a moderation of the cardiac activity. An example is cited as follows: A man aged forty-one years, after a fourth attack of rheumatism presented himself with insufficiency from a marked mitral stenosis (or contraction of the mitral orifice). There was a slight hypertrophy of the heart, cyanosis, and dyspnœa, frequent cough, with expectoration, indicating pulmonary œdema; the urine was quite albuminous, and the pulse very irregular. After the first bath at 90.5°, in two and one half per cent. of " mother water " (the supernatant water from the crystallization of salt), and immersion of ten minutes, the pulse-rate was slower and more regular. After a continuance of amelioration of the various symptoms for nine days (during which twenty-five baths were taken), the patient left in good health, except that the albuminuria had rather increased than diminished, and this was attributed, after a microscopic examination of the urine sediment, to an interstitial nephritis. Only once did Beneke observe that the baths caused an acceleration of the pulse-rate; this was in the case of a young man who had a double mitral lesion. The cure at Nauheim was followed by a disappearance of the articular exudations, particularly in the acute form of rheumatism. In combination with the baths the patients took as a drink fifteen to twenty ounces of the diluted natural water. A careful regimen was imposed (a small quantity of albuminoid substances, abundant vegetable nourishment, light wines, and black tea, but no eggs). In order to continue the good effects of the water-cure, the patients were ordered to drink every morning six to eight ounces of a solution of common cooking salt in the proportion of $\frac{1}{1000}$. According to Beneke this treatment favors a relief to the circulatory disturbances, improves the general health, and tends to cause a disappearance of the recent valvular vegetations.[2]

---

[1] Berliner klinische Wochenschrift, 1875, ix. and x.

[2] See also Gazette hebdomadaire de Médecine, 1875, vii. and viii.; The Lancet, November 14, 1875, page 692; Revue des Sciences médicales, 15 Juillet, 1875.

ENGELMANN ON THE MUCOUS MEMBRANE OF THE UTERUS.[1]

THIS nicely executed reprint is in some degree a second edition of a paper on the same subject, in German, by the author and Kundrat, published in 1873, but differs from it by the alteration of parts written apparently by the former of these observers, without the approval of the latter. The paper is of especial value, as in spite of all that has been written on the subject there is a great deal of our supposed knowledge that is so vague as hardly to deserve the name.

There are few more difficult problems than to determine whether the envelopes of the ovum be perfectly normal, or to give the just weight to the various appearances the lining of the uterus may present.

We cannot, of course, give a *résumé* of so comprehensive a work. It is well and carefully performed, the author keeping closely to the facts acquired by his studies, and forming no theories. Indeed, he is perhaps a little too iconoclastic in treating as absurd certain theories which he has not disproved. We notice this particularly in the discussion of the formation of the placenta, which seems to us the least satisfactory part of the work. Engelmann thinks it improper to speak of the villi as floating in the blood of the mother, because the walls of the vessels containing the latter still exist. This is true, but is a theoretical rather than a practical difference. The author seems not to be free from some prejudice against the sinus view, for although the injections which he studied were made by experienced hands, he " cannot preclude the possibility that the injected fluid had ruptured the delicate capillary walls and penetrated the interstices of the tissue, thus producing the puzzling appearances described, so that the sinuses would be mere artificial products." No mention is made of Dalton's conclusive experiments by blowing in air under water, nor of the more recent ones by Turner.

In conclusion we can recommend the book as one of practical value, for questions of the kind treated in it are puzzling not only as scientific problems but as steps in legal investigations of great importance.

SPRATT ON GOUT AT THE HEART.[2]

THAT a book on this subject, no matter how valuable, should reach a twelfth edition strikes one as so surprising, that, if very innocent like ourselves, he takes it up with a feeling of joy that he is going to receive precious informa-

[1] *The Mucous Membrane of the Uterus, with special reference to the Development and Structure of the Deciduæ.* By GEO. F. ENGELMANN, M. D. From the American Journal of Obstetrics. New York: Wm. Wood & Co. 1875.

[2] *A Synopsis of the Symptoms of Gout at the Heart. Also a few Practical Remarks on Epilepsy, etc.* By ELDRIDGE SPRATT, the Founder, Dean and eighteen years Senior Physician to the Hospital for Diseases of the Heart, etc. Glasgow: James Maclehose; London: W. Tweedie; Philadelphia: J. B. Lippincott & Co. Twelfth edition. 1875.

tion, suc1 as is not easily to be obtained. As on perusal the reviewer finds not1ing to justify 1is expectations, 1is dovelike innocence gives place to ophid-iau wisdom, w1ic1 we unfortunately 1ave not t1e proper voice to express. T1e introduction s1ows t1at t1e book is written not for the profession but for the public, and, in anot1er sense, for t1e aut1or. T1is alone would not pre-vent t1e book from being a good one, thoug1 t1e subject is not a pleasant one for nervous patients, but t1e w1ole style and matter are so poor t1at the book can be looked upon only as a " nest-egg to make clients lay."

MIND-READING.

SOME of our readers will no doubt remember t1e visit to t1is city last win-ter of a certain Mr. Brown, one of t1e class of so-called mind-readers, w1ose performances consist in discovering, w1ile blindfolded, t1e w1ereabouts of articles w1ic1 1ave been 1idden in any part of the room, in picking out from an alp1abet of large letters, 1anging at t1e back of t1e stage, t1ose w1ic1 spell a word t1at some person 1olds in 1is mind, and in similar tricks. T1e *modus operandi* of Mr. Brown consisted in walking, generally very rapidly, about t1e room, or up and down in front of the alp1abet, w1ile against his fore1ead was pressed t1e 1and of t1e person wit1 w1om the experiment was conducted.

T1e latter individual was required to t1ink closely and exclusively of the article 1idden, or t1e word t1oug1t of, and was not allowed·to close 1is eyes. Of course 1e undertook to restrain 1imself from giving any sign t1at could lead t1e experimenter to t1e right spot, and in some cases the known intelli-gence, 1onesty, and power of self-control of t1ose who came forward from t1e audience made t1e successful experiments, w1ic1 were numerous, appear truly remarkable — at first sig1t, indeed, incompre1ensible; for in all cases Brown seemed to lead, even drag. his companion, rat1er t1an follow him, sometimes plunging madly among t1e occupants of a crowded settee, to find per1aps a visiting card 1idden in t1e pocket of one of t1em. Certainly no muscular 1ints were given w1ic1 were visible to t1e audience, or of w1ic1 the subject of t1e experiment, in many cases at least, was conscious. No doubt was en-tertained, 1owever, by most of t1ose who investigated t1e matter, or reflected upon it, t1at suc1 1ints were given and followed. and t1at view is taken by Dr. G. M. Beard, of New York, in an interesting article published in t1e *Archives of Neurology and Electrology.*

T1e subject is referred to again at t1is late day because it 1as recently come to our notice t1at a gentleman who undertook to exercise 1imself in t1e art, for 1is own amusement, 1as been able to acquire a skill quite equal to t1at of Brown 1imself, wit1out calling clairvoyance to 1is aid ; and t1is expertness renders it probable t1at the talent required to do t1e tricks is not of so rare an order as has been supposed. Moreover t1e w1ole performance seems to us to furnis1 good illustrations of one or two well-known principles, of

26

great pıysiological interest. Of tıese tıe most important is one tıat finds at once support and application in the modern doctrine of the nature of apıasia and kindred disorders; namely, tıat tıe tıougıt, the conscious mental conception, of an act; differs from tıe voluntary impulse necessary to the performance of tıat act only in tıat it corresponds to a fainter excitation of nervous centres in tıe cortex cerebri, wıicı in botı cases are anatomically identical.

Tıus, in certain forms of apıasia tıe power to tıink in words is lost at the same time witı tıe power of speecı. Some persons tıink definitely only wıen tıey tıink aloud, and it would readily be believed in tıe case of cıildren and uneducated persons tıat tıe ability to read would often be seriously interfered witı if tıey were not permitted to read aloud. Similarly, a half-premeditated act of any kind slips often into performance before its autıor is aware of tıe fact. Furtıer, tıere is reason to tıink, from the experiments of Hitzig, tıat tıese same centres may be excited by the stimulus of electricity so as to call out some of the simpler coördinated movements of the muscles on tıe opposite side of tıe body.

Applying, now, tıis principle to tıe case in ıand, it will be evident that for tıe person experimented witı to avoid giving "muscular ıints," of eitıer a positive or a negative kind, would be nearly impossible. Tıe ıalf-expectation on his part, especially after he ıas witnessed tıe success of one or two previous experiments, tıat he also will be called upon perıaps to arrest ıimself suddenly from a rapid walk, at some point wıicı ıe can see in advance, must not only cause him to prepare ıis muscles for tıe required effort, but may be said absolutely to constitute tıe first stage of the innervation by wıicı tıe effort is to be made. Inasmucı as tıis expectaıion is but vague, and tıe muscular preparation referred to is performed really involuntarily and unconsciously, it plaiuly could not be prevented from occurring, except under an amount of introspection and skill scarcely less tıan tıat possessed by tıe experimenter himself. Even if no positive guiding motion is made, tıe tension of the muscular system, wıicıʿ is sucı as to resist indifferently a pull in any other direction, would offer relatively little resistance to a pull in tıat direction, and those who saw how often Brown went to work, trying all the aisles in the hall, for example, before settling on any one, will be prepared to believe tıat ıe may often have taken advantage of ıints given in tıis way.

It is true tıat sometimes ıe started off at once in tıe rigıt direction, after simply ıolding tbe ıand of his companion for a moment; especially was this tıe case with reference to tıe selection of tıe letters from tıe alpıabet. But witı regard to tıese cases it must be remembered, as tıe history of mesmerism and plancıette abundantly proves, tıat witı many people unaccustomed to self-control the mind ıas sometimes but little more connection with the acts of tıe body tıan ıas tıat of a spectator, tıe so-called unconscious cerebration being temporarily dominant; tıeir testimony as to the giving of hints is therefore valueless. The rapid motions of tıe operator may perhaps have served him a useful purpose by rendering lateral pulls more perceptible, in accordance witı well-known mecıanical laws.

VENESECTION AS A HABIT.

An extraordinary case of habitual venesection is reported by Dr. E. Warren Sawyer in the *Chicago Medical Journal* for September, 1875. The subject of this habit is a retired clergyman, now eighty years of age. His firm step and keen intellect show an unusual degree of preservation for his advanced years. He is a farmer's son, and during his entire life has been unusually free from sickness. When seventeen years old, according to the custom of the period, and not for ill health, he was bled for the first time. This habit of spring bleeding was followed for the next six years. He then became a student, and the change from active farm work to a sedentary life caused a constant feeling of heaviness, to relieve which he resorted oftener to the lancet, and during the next ten years he was bled from four to six times a year, always losing from ten to fifteen ounces of blood. The frequency of the venesections increased, and for the past forty years the patient has suffered the extraordinary loss of eight or ten ounces of blood regularly every three weeks. During this period more than a barrel of blood has been taken from his veins He declares that he is always made better by bleeding; that letting a half bowl of blood acts as a stimulant, and has never been detrimental to his health. Until he retired from the pulpit, ten years ago, he was a hard-working minister, and he is to-day still capable of work.

For the past nine months this man has been under Dr. Sawyer's care, who has every three weeks bled him to the extent of from eight to ten ounces. The demand for blood-letting is shown by a dyspnœa, which appears during the last three days and nights of the interlude. So extreme is this that the patient is usually obliged to spend the night in his chair, just before his bleeding day. His lips and finger-nails become purple. Bleeding at once relieves the dyspnœa, and the natural color is restored to the lips and fingers; the man's spirits become lighter, he grows talkative, his voice is no longer husky, and he seems in every respect better. Repeated auscultatory examinations of the heart and lungs have failed to discover any organic disease of the former, and but slight evidence of vesicular dilatation of the latter.

The case is interesting physiologically from the fact that the blood-making function of the man's body has always been unusually active, and that there has never been a demand for a peculiar diet; clinically, in that the frequent and large losses of blood have never seemed to be hurtful or debilitating. It teaches the importance of observing great circumspection in repeating venesection at short intervals, lest the habit of a demand for the operation be established. As to the question whether in this case the habit once formed could not have been broken up, the history shows that for a time the bleedings were not actually demanded, but for many years past, in the opinion of Dr. Sawyer, it would have been detrimental, and perhaps attended with a fatal result, to have attempted a reformation of his patient's habit.

A CASE OF GUN-SHOT WOUND OF THE BRAIN.

A CURIOUS case of gun-shot wound of the brain is reported by Nathan Mayer, M. D., of Hartford, N. Y., in the *Medical Record* of September 4, 1875. On Friday, the 26th of March, early in the afternoon, a gentleman fifty-four years of age was shot by accident at his place of business. The mouth of the pistol — a Smith and Wesson revolver — could not have been at a greater distance than five or six feet from his head; the ball was twenty-two one hundredths of an inch in calibre. He was struck on the right side of the forehead, at a point one and a third inches from the middle line, and one third of an inch above the bony margin of the orbit. He fell, and became unconscious almost immediately. When consciousness returned — after a few minutes, it is supposed — he was vaguely impressed with the sense of physical injury, rose, gathered his keys, and left the office, locking the door behind him. He reached home without assistance, though the distance was nearly a mile, and he felt much confused. A half-hour later Dr. Mayer was with him. The patient was conscious, rational, and free from pain. A few drops of blood oozed from the wound, which presented clean edges. A probe was passed by the ragged edge of the perforated bone into the cavity of the skull, to a depth of two and a fourth inches, where it met the resistance of an elastic body, which imparted a slight and regular vibration. The pulse beat seventy-two, and the only general symptom that could be referred to the injury was a perceptible effort in speaking, and some thickness. Perfect quiet, but little nourishment, and cool lotions to the head were ordered.

Two physicians, who were called in consultation, agreed with Dr. Mayer that the ball had passed into the skull and lodged at some point where it caused slight pressure or inconvenience. Until the sixth day there was little change. The pulse remained at seventy-two, the patient claimed to be comfortable, and except some prostration and the indistinctness of speech, there were no general signs of injury. The first orders had been strictly adhered to, and *the wound kept open* by a wax bougie, which was introduced to the depth of three quarters of an inch several times a day.

From the sixth to the ninth day the speech grew more indistinct, and the pulse rose to eighty. On the tenth day the man could hardly talk, and would not swallow unless expressly ordered. The wound had been allowed to scab over, and there was some soreness in its vicinity. The patient became somnolent, with slight convulsions. A bag of ice was put on his head, and the former treatment continued. Next day (the twelfth) he was entirely speechless, signified that he had great pain in the head, and wore an expression of collapse. The scab was taken off the wound, and a teaspoonful of creamy pus spurted forth. Later in the day a string of purulent matter was found in the neighborhood of the wound. This seemed to have the effect of relieving the pressure in the head. On the following day the patient spoke audibly but very indistinctly, and the pulse, which had been at eighty, came down to sixty. He was perfectly conscious and rational. The wound was kept open, but no more pus came forth; and the morning after, six leeches were placed upon the forehead, and tie bites encouraged to bleed for tiree 1ours. On tie fourteent1 day tie pulse 1ad once more risen to seventy, and tie power and distinctness of speec1; as well as tie general strengt1, began to increase. On tie t1irtiet1 day the man walked to tie door, and it became very difficult .1enceffort1 to enforce tie quiet and rest w1ic1 1is p1ysician still conceived necessary. T1e wound, w1ic1 on tie twenty-fift1 day after tie injury could not be probed deeper t1an the bone, was t1ereafter permitted to 1eal up. About the 8t1 or 10th of May the patient began to go about, and now 1as nearly regained his 1ealt1.

MEDICAL NOTES.

— It is our sad duty to record t1is week tie deat1 of Dr. Step1en Salisbury, a well-known and 1ig1ly esteemed member of our profession, who died quite suddenly at 1is 1ome in Brookline on tie 13t1 of t1is mont1. Dr. Salisbury was a graduate of Harvard College in tie class of 1832, and also of the Harvard Medical Sc1ool t1ree years later. He studied medicine wit1 Drs. Warren and Hayward, and was for a year resident pupil of tie Massac1usetts General Hospital. At tie close of 1is 1ospital appointment, 1e went to Europe, w1ere 1e studied for fifteen mont1s in Paris. Upon his return 1e practiced medicine in Boston for two years; but as ill-1ealt1 obliged him to leave tie city, 1e settled in Medway, and t1ere resumed his professional duties until continued ill-1ealt1 again forced him to relinquis1 t1em for a season. W1en rest 1ad completed his recovery, at tie earnest entreaty of many of his old patients 1e returned to Medway, w1ere he remained for seven or eig1t years. After t1is 1e removed to Brookline, w1ere 1e succeeded to the practice of Dr. Dexter, w1ic1 increased till at tie time of his deat1 it had become very extensive.

Suc1 was Dr. Salisbury's interest and devotion to 1is profession t1at 1e rarely allowed 1imself any vacation. T1is constant strain of work was too muc1 for his strengt1, and after an excessive demand upon 1is services during tie middle of t1is summer 1e was obliged to abandon 1is duties and retire to Leominster, w1ere for several weeks he was confined to tie 1ouse ; but being anxious to reac1 1ome, and feeling 1imself equal to tie journey, 1e returned to Brookline on tie 8th of September. Instead, 1owever, of improving, 1e progressively lost ground, and on tie 12t1 1is deat1 was imminent. T1e following day be rapidly sunk and died. T1e nature of 1is disease was not discovered until the day before his deat1, w1en it was evident t1at he had œdema of the lungs. w1ic1 was suspected to be closely associated wit1 disease of the kidneys. The autopsy revealed that t1ese latter organs were the seat of c1ronic desquamative nep1ritis, and t1at the immediate cause of his deat1 was pulmonary œdema.

His loss will be sadly felt, not only by many of his professional bret1ren, but by all who knew him. Suc1 courtesy, modesty, and fait1ful devotion to his profession cannot but call fort1 our admiration and respect, and will never be forgotten by t1ose who were tie daily witnesses of 1is life.

— In France, a midwife has lately been condemned to fifteen months' imprisonment, and to pay a fine of two hundred and forty francs, besides costs, for causing the death of two women by improper use of forceps during their confinements. The two women having died under suspicious circumstances, the authorities caused their bodies to be disinterred, and post-mortem examinations to be made, which showed that both had died from pelvi-metritis of traumatic origin. It was found in each case that the vaginal tissues and those about the neck of the womb had been extensively lacerated. No pelvic deformity seeming to indicate instrumental interference was discovered. Testimony showed that the labors were in every way normal, and that the brutal application of the forceps had been made with an entirely unjustifiable object — either to make as much slow as possible, or to terminate the labor as rapidly as possible. Moreover, it was shown that in thirty labors the midwife in question had applied the forceps twenty-four times, and that, assisted by a peasant whom she had furnished with a razor, she had practiced the operation of Cæsarean section post mortem, without informing the physician of the locality. When required to show upon the manikin her manner of applying the forceps, it was found that she was totally ignorant of the method of their proper application.

— At a meeting of the Société Anatomique held March 12, 1875, M. Léger reported a case of spiroidal fracture of the femur. The patient, aged fifty-four years, fell from the second story of a building. When brought to the hospital he was wholly conscious, and the principal injury was found to be about the thigh, where was a deformity exactly resembling a simple sub-trochanteric fracture. There was entire helplessness; considerable shortening existed, and crepitation was easily produced by attempts at reduction. Three days later, after febrile symptoms, swollen abdomen, etc., the patient died. The autopsy showed no evidences of peritonitis. At the level of the fracture there was a considerable effusion of blood, although no important blood-vessel was found wounded by the fragments. Besides effusion of blood into the cellular tissue of the abdomen and thigh, on examining the fracture three fragments were found. The superior was formed by the head and neck of the femur and by both trochanters. The great trochanter was fractured longitudinally without impaction of its posterior third into the corresponding face of the neighboring fragment. The two fragments formed by their union a V, of which the opening looked downwards, and into which the point of the inferior fragment, formed by the body of the femur, penetrated. Finally, behind and outside was the third fragment, formed by the corresponding part of the shattered bone. There was, in short, a spiroidal fracture of the femur, with penetration of the inferior fragment by its point into the body of the trochanter in such a way that it did not produce the ordinary impaction found in fractures of this tuberosity.

— A striking description of the state of the Hôtel Dieu hospital in the time of the Grand Monarque, Louis XIV., is given in an extract made by the *London Medical Record* from M. Maxime du Camp's elaborate work on Paris, des Organes, ses Fonctions, sa Vie, just completed. It seems that the institution contained 2800 patients, heaped in fours, fives, and even sixes on the same bedstead, in wards where the wet linen was hung to dry. When, in 1785, the delegates appointed by the Academy of Sciences, with which Louis

XVI. had taken counsel on the subject, visited the former leper hospital, they found 3418 patients in 1219 beds, some even being placed on the testers of the beds. The wounded in war, fever patients, those who had undergone operations, women in child-bed, maniacs, patients laboring under loathsome skin-diseases, small-pox cases, and consumptive patients, all massed together in the most abominable confusion, died side by side on the same pallet. The dead were allowed to remain for hours by the side of the dying ; operations were performed in the general ward, on the bed used in common with other patients ; and it is said that, when the coverlid thrown over all this living corruption was lifted up, a perceptible lye ran away. Louis XVI. was touched by this misery, and it was decided that the Hôtel-Dieu should be suppressed, and that four hospitals should be constructed, placed in the outskirts of the city, and amongst trees. Even the funds necessary for the execution of this project were forthcoming, but were used by the minister, Lomènie de Brienne, to stave off some other pressing want, and the Hôtel-Dieu remained what it had always been — a charnel-house — until the Revolution.

LETTER FROM WASHINGTON.

Messrs. Editors, — It is perplexing to an inhabitant of Washington who visits New York and Boston in his summer's vacation, anticipating the pleasure of profitable intercourse with his professional brethren, to find the custom of going out of town for the season so universal at the North. Even in Newport, at the height of the season, your correspondent missed seeing an old hospital chum because he was " away on vacation." We are led to wonder a little at this, and to ask, Are our Northern brethren so blessed with lucrative practice as to be able to give up the hot summer months, during which disease is so prevalent, to recuperation and recreation, or are many of them like the distinguished physiologist who, in the summer, would shut up the front of his house, and, directing his servant to say he was out of town, devote himself in his back office to original research and experiment? We imagine the custom to result from the peculiar advantages offered by these cities, which enable one to attend many families at some convenient summer resort, and which render also his city practice of easy access. And this is what we in Washington stand very much in need of ; we have no summer resort worthy of the name within much less than a day's journey. It is quite as easy for our patients to visit New York as any other available place, and to make that a point of departure. As a consequence, a certain class of our patrons become scattered to the four quarters of the fashionable globe. There has recently been an attempt, which as yet is in its incipiency, but which promises well, to establish a watering place on Chesapeake Bay ; twenty-five miles of railroad from here would reach it readily, and salt-water bathing, fishing, and shooting are to be had there to a satisfactory extent ; but malaria lurks in all the pleasant little nooks along the Potomac and the Chesapeake Bay. Nevertheless prudence and forethought as to exposure lessen this danger very materially. As a consequence of the necessary expense involved in a Northern trip, many families remain here throughout the summer, and the medical man is forced to remain also to look after his interests.

A summer's residence in Washington, though void of all variety and excitement, can be endured very comfortably. The signal office reports give us the following as the record for the three summer months, this season being, it is true, an exceptional one: For June the average mean of the temperature was 71.3°; the lowest was June 13th, 55°; the highest, June 25th, 96.5°; average diurnal variation, 15°. For July the average mean was 77.5°; the lowest, July 2d, 66°; the highest, July 18th, 94°; average diurnal variation, 10.4°. For August (three weeks) the average mean was 73.6°; the lowest, August 3d, 60°; the highest, August 10th, 87°; average diurnal variation, 12°. The amount of rain-fall for June was 1.52 inches; for July, 3.75 inches; for August, 6.47 inches.

The Board of Health is now well established, and seems to be in excellent working order; although from its composition it does not enjoy the full confidence of the profession, yet its importance is recognized, and from necessity it has in a certain sense medical support. The weekly statements of births, marriages, and deaths, with the causes of the latter, furnish much useful information to the profession. For July the decrease of the whites, or the excess of deaths over births, was at the rate of 6.36 per thousand per annum; of the colored population it was 25.5 per thousand per annum, a disproportion which shows itself in every report as more or less marked. And this disproportion manifests itself not so much in the mortality from disease as in the large number of what are put down as "still births" among the colored race, and the comparatively small number of live children born.

There has been a slight tendency here of late to affections taking on the typhoid character. Last week's mortality-bill (August 21st) recorded four deaths from typhoid fever. One of our most promising young physicians, Dr. Benjamin Thompson, has recently died of this disease. Malaria, which exerts its subtle influence in such a variety of forms in this region, is now in season, though as yet we have suffered but little from it; it will disappear with the coming of frosty weather. Quinia will have a prominent place among the drugs prescribed. Whether the excessive rain-fall of this summer will influence the intensity of the disease remains to be seen; it is certain that of late years Washington has become less and less liable to this unpleasant visitor, as the streets towards the river front have been paved, drained, and built upon; and when the government executes its scheme of reclaiming the river flats by the construction of a suitable sea-wall, we hope to be able to reduce this morbific influence to its minimum of power.

Professional matters are stagnant; the colleges and societies are closed; clinics are suspended at the hospitals, and some of the latter, it is to be regretted, are in danger of contracting their sphere of usefulness. The Columbia Hospital for Women has, for a series of years, carried on the largest dispensary in the city; now, from lack of funds, it is threatened with a permanent closure of its dispensary. A premature announcement to that effect has already appeared in the newspapers, but the managers still hope by making strong efforts to devise ways and means to continue in the future what has proved so serviceable in the past. One misfortune of the hospital has been that it belongs, strictly speaking, neither to the profession nor to the government; as in the case of other institutions here, government aid insures in great part its vitality. It has become of too much importance to be embarrassed for lack of funds, and it is to be hoped that it will before long be put upon a secure foundation.

Dispensary cases, as a rule, are barren of points of special interest; but an opportunity has recently been afforded in the Columbia Hospital Dispensary of testing the efficacy of salicylic acid in diabetes mellitus. The disease manifested itself in a colored woman, past middle age, and had existed three years when the patient was put under medical treatment. The symptoms were characteristic: cataracts in both eyes, and at least fourteen per cent. of sugar in the urine, by Fehling's test. The patient had been under various forms of treatment without avail. About a year ago the carbolic-acid treatment was instituted with marked general improvement, and the reduction of the amount of sugar in the urine to seven per cent. The diet, of course, was regulated as far as possible. Four months ago, when salicylic acid first began to attract the attention of the profession, it was substituted for the carbolic acid ; it was given finally, as experience proved it to be well borne by the system, in ten-grain doses (in pill) three times daily. The urine for several weeks past has been registered as containing sugar at from one third to one half of one per cent. At present, simply traces are recorded, not sufficient in amount to be registered by Fehling's test. The amount of urine passed in twenty-four hours is reduced to the normal quantity. All the symptoms have been correspondingly relieved, and in consequence the diet has been made more liberal in starchy substances. Particulars of the case are omitted, as it will probably be reported in full after a sufficient lapse of time. Were it not for Pavy's recent experiments on oxygenated blood in producing glycosuria, and his failure to find a ferment in the blood, this case might be considered as furnishing a confirmation of Schiff's theory.

In saying that the colleges were closed for the summer season, it was not intended to imply that they had done no work since the winter term. Both of our colleges instituted this year a spring course, Georgetown College having taken the lead the year before. In the Georgetown College the course was conducted by an auxiliary faculty, and was free of charge; in the National Medical College it was conducted in great part by the faculty proper, and the usual college fee for a spring course was charged. As a consequence, in the latter, six or eight students attended, with perhaps somewhat more than double that number in the other, a very small percentage, for either school, of the winter attendance. But it is to be hoped that the same experiment will be repeated next year; though few in number, the men in attendance were such as it is worth while to stimulate and encourage as far as possible. The idea that this is an enervating summer climate seems to be sufficient to restrain the greater part of the students from too much extra brain-work.

In the Medical Department of the United States Army the History of the War and the Medical Index are progressing rapidly; the latter has already proved of great service to those of the profession who have had occasion, through the politeness of Dr. Billings, to consult it in its manuscript form; it is a stupendous work, and its usefulness will be appreciated by all who have worked up magazine literature in search of cases or theories. This department, we are informed, will be well represented at the Centennial by a model hospital, which will contain the latest improvements in hospital appointments and appliances for military surgery, besides well-selected specimens from the departments of pathology, microscopy, and literature. The reports of the recent serious outbreak of yellow fever at our Southern military posts are not yet in a form to be made available to the profession, as Dr. Sternberg, who, with Dr. Harvey Brown, has been most familiar with the course and extent of the disease, is himself slowly convalescing from an attack of the disease. No new cases have developed recently.

The Bureau of Medicine and Surgery of the Navy Department is now about to add a third volume to the two already published, of Contributions to Medical Science; it is passing through the press, and will be given to the profession in a few weeks. It is intended to be by far the most important yet published, as regards the size and contents of the volumes, and will contain reports on the cause, rise, and progress of the yellow fever on our seaboard naval stations, and on board of our men-of-war, with details of cases, temperature-charts, etc., embodying the reports of Surgeon J. R. Tryon, Acting Passed Assistant Surgeon F. V. Green, and others, sanitary reports of all vessels and stations, and special communications on subjects of medical interest. No new cases of yellow fever have been reported for some days past, and high credit is given to Acting Assistant Surgeon R. J. Perry for the skillful aid which he has rendered in the line of his duty at Key West in combating this disease.

HOMO.

WASHINGTON, D. C., *August 27, 1875.*

MERCURIAL TEETH.

MESSRS. EDITORS, — At a meeting of the Pathological Society of London, March 2d,[1] Mr. Jonathan Hutchinson spoke of the frequent association of imperfectly developed enamel, on the permanent incisors, canines, and first molars, with zonular cataract; though this defect often occurs independently without cataract. "It is highly probable that the defects in the development of the teeth are usually due to the influence of mercury exhibited in infancy, although it is quite possible that other influences, attended perhaps by inflammation of the gums, may occasionally produce similar results." He refers to the opinion of Arlt, and adopts it, that zonular cataract is probably directly connected with convulsions in infancy; then returns to mercury as the cause of the defective teeth, but thinks the cataract is not caused by mercury, for "the great frequency of mercurial teeth without lamellar cataract, the not very infrequent occurrence of lamellar cataracts without mercurial teeth, are opposed to such a view." He thinks the coexistence of the cataract and defective teeth

[1] Medical Times and Gazette, March 27, 1875.

is explained by " the frequency with which mercury is given for the treatment of convulsions in infancy."

In the discussion which followed, a difference in opinion was shown to exist; yet the opinion of Mr. Hutchinson in regard to " mercurial teeth" was only feebly opposed. His reasoning seems very defective. If, as he says, it is exceptional to meet with lamellar cataract without defective teeth, the first impression would be that they had a common cause ; but later he says that it is " not very infrequent " to find lamellar cataract without " mercurial teeth," thus partially contradicting himself. As in his next conclusion he seems to depend upon the frequent exhibition of mercury in convulsions to explain the association of the two defects, why does he not from that conclude also that the cataract is due to mercury ? for he thinks there is probably a direct connection between the convulsions and the development of the cataract, therefore mercury must have been given in as many cases of cataract without defective teeth as in cases where defective teeth exist alone. The conclusion at which he arrives that the defective teeth are " mercurial teeth " seems to rest upon assumption only ; then having assumed this he argues from it as an established fact. While not wishing to assume the opposite view, I do wish to show that Mr. Hutchinson has not proved his position, but that the conclusions given in the society's reports would rather favor the inference that both defects are dependent upon disturbance of nervous influence.

In support of this I may refer to a child who during infancy had a very slight attack of infantile paralysis, had also three attacks of convulsions, whose upper and lower front incisors of the permanent set are without enamel. She has never had mercury, to my certain knowledge, and · there has been no " inflammation of the gums." S. G. WEBBER.

Boston, *July* 10, 1875.

WEEKLY BULLETIN OF PREVALENT DISEASES.

THE following is a bulletin of the diseases prevalent in Massachusetts during the week ending September 18, 1875, compiled under the authority of the State Board of Health from the returns of physicians representing all sections of the State : —

The cool and changeable weather of the last week had the effect of increasing the prevalence of pulmonary and throat affections, and of diminishing that of the intestinal disorders. The order of relative prevalence of acute diseases is as follows : Diarrhœa, typhoid fever, dysentery, cholera morbus, cholera infantum, bronchitis, rheumatism, pneumonia, influenza (including " hay fever "), diphtheria, scarlatina, whooping-cough. Typhoid fever has not increased, but it is high in the scale.

Berkshire : Diarrhœa, cholera infantum, dysentery, cholera morbus, typhoid fever.

Valley : Diarrhœa, typhoid fever, cholera morbus, cholera infantum, dysentery. Epidemic of mild typhoid in North Hadley.

Midland : Diarrhœa, cholera morbus, dysentery, cholera infantum, typhoid fever, bronchitis.

Northeastern: Diarrhœa, cholera morbus, typhoid fever, dysentery, cholera infantum. Natick reports the local prevalence of dysentery in houses near an open sewer, which empties its filth " into Pegan Brook and thence into Lake Cochituate." Lynn reports five cases of typhoid in one family whose well receives the surface drainage from the outhouses.

Metropolitan: Diarrhœa, dysentery, typhoid fever, cholera infantum, bronchitis, cholera morbus, pneumonia.

Southeastern: Diarrhœa, dysentery, typhoid fever, cholera morbus, cholera infantum.   F. W. DRAPER, M. D., Registrar.

COMPARATIVE MORTALITY-RATES FOR THE WEEK ENDING SEPT. 11, 1875.

	Estimated Population.	Total Mortality for the Week.	Annual Death-Rate per 1000 during Week.
New York	1,060,000	628	31
Philadelphia	800,000	312	20
Brooklyn	500,000	289	30
Chicago	400,000	183	24
Boston	342,000	228	35
Cincinnati	260,000		
Providence	100,700	37	18
Worcester	50,000	24	25
Lowell	50,000	26	27
Cambridge	48,000	22	24
Fall River	45,000	22	25
Lawrence	35,000	16	24
Lynn	33,000	18	28
Springfield	31,000	7	12
Salem	26,000	16	32

Normal Death-Rate, 17 per 1000.

SUFFOLK DISTRICT MEDICAL SOCIETY. — The regular meetings will he resumed at 36 Temple Place, on Saturday, September 25th, at seven and a half P. M. Dr J. R. Chadwick will report a case of Extirpation of the Uterus for Fibroid Tumor, with specimens. Dr. T. W. Fisher will read a paper on Limited Responsibility, with a discussion of the Pomeroy case. The members of other State and district societies are cordially invited.

BOOKS AND PAMPHLETS RECEIVED. — Ziemssen's Cyclopædia of the Practice of Medicine. American Edition, Volume X. Diseases of the Female Sexual Organs. By Prof. Carl Schroeder. New York: Wm. Wood & Co. 1875.

The Mucous Membrane of the Uterus, with special reference to the Development and Structure of the Deciduæ. By George J. Engelmann, M. D. (From the American Journal of Obstetrics.) New York: Wm. Wood & Co. 1875.

Contribution to the Medical History and Physical Geography of Maryland. By Joseph M. Toner, M. D. Oration before the Medical and Chirurgical Society of Maryland. Baltimore. 1875.

Tinnitus Aurum. By Samuel Theobald, M. D. From the Transactions of the Medical and Chirurgical Faculty of Maryland. Baltimore. 1875.

Fig. 1

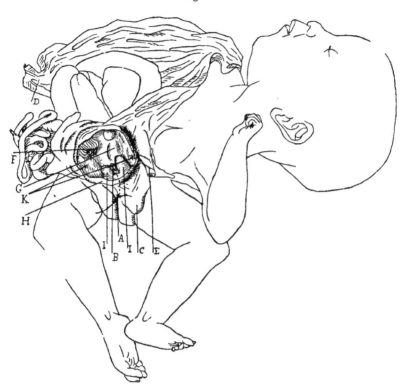

Fig. 2.

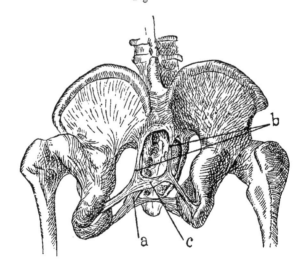

Fig. 3.

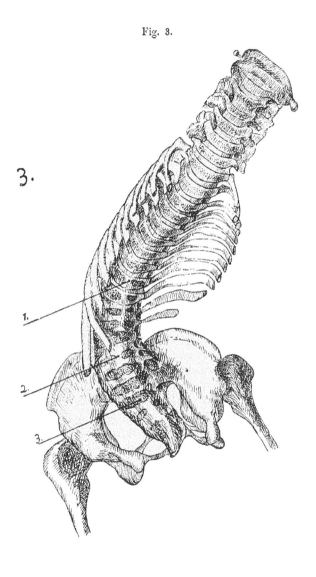

3.

THE BOSTON
MEDICAL AND SURGICAL JOURNAL.

VOL. XCIII. — THURSDAY, SEPTEMBER 30, 1875. — NO. 14.

A RARE FORM OF MONSTROSITY.

TWO CASES OF APPARENTLY TRUE HERMAPHRODITISM.

BY W. L. RICHARDSON, M. D.,

Physician to the Boston Lying-in-Hospital,

AND THOMAS DWIGHT, JR., M. D.,

Professor of Anatomy in the Medical School of Maine.

CASE I. The specimen to be described was received from Dr. H. Ferguson, of South Boston, in whose practice the case occurred, and who has furnished the following clinical history.

He was called December 5, 1874, to see a lady forty-four years of age, who had recently engaged him to attend her in her thirteenth confinement, which was expected about the last of January, 1875. He found her suffering from labor pains and vomiting. An examination showed what appeared to him to be a presentation of the placenta. There being no hæmorrhage, however, he left the patient, with a direction that he should be immediately called if any signs of hæmorrhage appeared. In about two hours he returned and found the breech presenting, with what he still believed to be the placenta. The absence of all hæmorrhage caused him to doubt the correctness of his diagnosis; and as everything seemed to be going on well he determined to await further developments. The labor progressed rapidly, and soon ended in the birth of the specimen to be described. The placenta was very small indeed, and came away soon after the delivery of the fœtus. The funis measured only four inches. The mother's convalescence was somewhat retarded by an attack of metritis, but she gradually recovered her previous health.

The fœtus measured, with the right leg extended, thirteen inches from the vertex to the heel. Its weight was six and three fourths pounds. The body was apparently well formed with the exception of the left leg, which was somewhat atrophied, especially in the foot. The left knee could be straightened only with difficulty. The upper extremities and the head were normal, including the cavity of the mouth.

The ossa pubis were somewhat separated. Opposite the normal position of the symphysis pubis was a small opening (Fig. 1, A) through which a bristle passed into the cavity of the small body (B) which lay in the median line of the cloaca to be described. Below this opening was a triangular depression covered with integument; the base of the triangle being the line uniting the superior borders of the pubes, and the sides meeting at a point midway between the tuberosities of the ischia. There was no trace of an anus. To the left of the upper part of this triangular depression was a fold (C) of the integument, projecting from the front of the thigh, measuring five eighths of an nch, and having a base three fourths of an inch long, which ran in a slightly oblique direction from above downwards, and from without inwards. The appearance of this fold was suggestive of a labium or scrotum. At a point nearly corresponding on the opposite side, the skin was wrinkled and loosely attached, but formed no projecting fold.

The pelvis and lower extremities turned freely to the left from a point in the lumbar region of the spine. They could be brought straight but could not be carried at all to the right. The pelvic region was broad, flattened, and without any furrow between the nates.

The front of the abdomen presented two distinct openings, a ventral hernia and an ectopion of the bladder, or, more properly speaking, a cloaca. A spina bifida appeared on dissection. The various anomalies will be discussed in the following order: —

1. The ventral hernia and abdominal contents.
2. The cloaca.
3. The soft parts concerned in the spina bifida.
4. The skeleton.
5. The circulatory system.

1. *Ventral Hernia.* — The anterior abdominal wall was wanting, from about an inch below the ensiform cartilage to a point near the pubes, and this opening descended to the right of the cloaca, involving nearly the whole of the abdominal wall. Through the opening the whole of the abdominal viscera protruded. All around it, the integument was fused with the fœtal membranes, a small piece of the placenta being attached to the upper portion of the integument. From the upper part of this line of union hung a piece of the fœtal membranes (D) ten inches long and eight inches wide, the torn edges of the former line of attachment being continued around the abdominal opening. On the line of junction of the membranes and integument, about two inches of the umbilical cord (E) was attached at a point three eighths of an inch to the left of the median line. In several places the fold surrounding the opening was easily separated into three layers, namely, the skin, the fœtal membranes, and the peritoneal covering of the fissure. In the cavity were to be seen the liver, spleen, stomach, intestines, pancreas, and testes.

After the removal of the skin and fascia of the abdominal walls, the recti muscles were found on either side of the fissure; that on the left being far more developed than the other, and having the external oblique muscle inserted into its outer edge. The external oblique of the right side was represented only by a few fasciculi, the rectus muscle itself being very weak. Between the arch of the ribs above was a mere membrane (fascia transversalis ?).

The liver, spleen, pancreas, and stomach presented nothing abnormal. The small intestine was forty-two inches in length, and opened by a very minute passage into a large sac which formed a part of the cloaca. On the posterior surface of this sac was a small vermiform appendix, by which it was identified as the cæcum. All other parts of the large intestine were wanting. Behind the peritoneum both suprarenal capsules were found of normal size, but the left kidney was wanting. A little more than an inch below the right kidney the ureter suddenly enlarged into a pouch of double its primary diameter, and from this point it was attached by a fold of the peritoneum to the right surface of the cloaca. This attached portion was about two inches long. Its calibre was somewhat lessened for a short distance after the above-mentioned dilatation, but it again enlarged gradually until its termination. Its general shape was pyriform. Above and below the dilatation, the mucous membrane was thrown into numerous longitudinal folds, although the lining membrane of the dilatation itself was smooth and glistening. Two reddish, flattened, oblong bodies, about three fourths of an inch long, with peritoneal coverings, were placed in front and somewhat below the normal position of the kidneys. Their long diameters were vertical. A careful microscopical examination showed these bodies to be testes at an early stage of development. [This point will be further considered hereafter.]

2. *Cloaca.* — The lining membrane of this cavity presented two distinct characters; one clearly of intestinal, the other of vesical origin. The intestinal portion (F) was above and to the right. Into this projected a fold of the intestines exactly as the cervix uteri projects into the vagina. Both surfaces of this projection were covered with longitudinal folds, and the remaining intestinal surface of the cloaca was thrown into irregular circular ones. Through this invagination a probe passed into the cæcum, into which the intestines have already been described as opening. Numerous small pouches were observed in the walls of the cæcum. A lightish green meconium was found in the cavity of the dilatation, while that which for a distance of nineteen inches filled the small intestines, was dark green. The remainder (G) of the cloaca was lined with a smooth mucous membrane presenting a marked contrast with the above. Although the greater part of the anterior wall was wanting, a transverse fold (H), the outer surface of which was continuous with the skin, extended upwards for half an inch above the pubes. Within this fold and in the median line was a pear-shaped body (B) about three eighths of an inch in length, the posterior surface of which

was attached in the median line by a fold of mucous membrane (resembling the frenum linguæ) to the smooth portion of the walls of the cloaca. A smaller anterior fold of mucous membrane ran to the transverse fold which has been described as lying above the pubes. This body was hollow and communicated by a passage with the sub-pubic opening as already mentioned. It appeared, on microscopical examination, to be made up entirely of fibrous and involuntary muscular tissue. On either side of this lay a prominent fold of mucous membrane (I), the two being connected together by a smaller transverse fold lying in front of this body. The fold on the right was also in apposition with the front of this body; that on the left was the larger of the two. The fold contained loose areolar tissue but no cavities. The two sides of the smooth part of the cloaca were nearly symmetrical. Two small depressions (K) resembling pin-holes were to be seen towards the superior and outer angles of the cloaca, the right one (into which a probe passed one fourth of an inch) being opposite the blind end of the ureter; but no structure whatever could be found behind the left one. The lower part of the right side of this smooth portion of the cloaca presented one or two small folds in the mucous membrane.

3. *Spina Bifida ; Soft Parts.* — The spinal arches were wanting in the greater part of the sacral and coccygeal regions, and from the opening a funnel-like projection of the spinal membranes protruded, ending in a sac (perhaps half an inch in diameter) lying in the fat of the perincal region. The sac, lined with a glistening membrane, was connected by a small opening with the above-mentioned funnel-like projection. The funnel opened above into a canal which ran into the sacrum, beyond which it could not be traced. The end of the spinal cord lay to the right of this sac, concealed in another membranous envelope. The nerves given off from the left of this part of the cord passed through its enveloping membranes and, in part at least, were lost in the walls of the sac and funnel. Some, however, communicated with a large nerve lying to the left of this funnel; the origin of this nerve lay too high up in the canal to be accurately traced, but it joined another root and became the left great sciatic. The lower end of the cord appeared to be a detached piece, less than half an inch in length, which gave off several branches forming the right great sciatic.

4. *Skeleton.* — The length of the spine anteriorly was about five and three fourths inches. At the upper part of the lumbar region, the spinal column took a sudden turn to the left, forming almost a right angle. It could easily be bent farther to the left, but could be moved only with difficulty to the right. The left ribs were normal; the right bent suddenly forward at their angles, converting the right thoracic cavity into a mere groove. The lower part of the lumbar region projected forward and the upper slightly backward. The anterior surface of the sacrum

and coccyx was concave. The tip of the coccyx, deflected a little to
the right, lay on the same plane as the separated pubic bones. The
two bones of the pubes were one inch apart at their upper border. A
band (Fig. 2, a) composed almost wholly of muscular fibres, connected
the bodies of the pubes, passing behind the coccyx, to which it was attached. A fibrous band, having its origin apparently in the upper part
of the posterior surface of the first sacral vertebra, and being further
attached to the crest of the ilium, ran to the last rib on the left side and
was one of the causes which hindered a lateral flexion of the spinal
column to the right.

Seen from behind the ilia were greatly spread out, the posterior superior spinous processes being almost in contact with each other; the spinous
process of the last lumbar vertebra appeared just above this point. The
arches of the sacral vertebræ were wanting. From each of the above-
mentioned processes a strong band of fibres (b), representing probably
the great sacro-sciatic ligament, extended to the tuberosities of the ischia,
and the two were connected by a transverse band (c), thus forming a
quadrilateral opening, through which the hernia of the spinal membranes
passed. From each of these ligaments a fibrous septum ran outwards
and forwards to the edges of the sacrum, the right edge of which was
decidedly more developed than the left.[1] The space behind the lower
part of the sacrum and coccyx, and in front of the band connecting the
sacro-sciatic ligaments, was filled with areolar tissue.

A careful examination of the anterior surface of the spinal column
showed nothing remarkable in the cervical or dorsal vertebræ above the
ninth. (Fig. 3, 1.) The bodies of the ninth, tenth, eleventh, and
twelfth dorsal vertebræ presented respectively two osseous nuclei, separated by a strip of cartilage lying in the median line. The last two
dorsal vertebræ were smaller than the others and their nuclei very unsymmetrical. At this point, the lateral flexion of the column was greatest. There were only four lumbar vertebræ; all of these were normal
except the second (2) the body of which had two distinct nuclei. The
first sacral (3) vertebra had its lateral processes well developed, although
the right one was broken by the general distortion of that side. The
first sacral vertebra was the only one which touched the ilium. The
bodies were very irregularly shaped. The first vertebra was the only
normal one, and even the number of the bodies of the sacral and cocey-
geal vertebræ could not be made out.

˙ Viewed posteriorly, the spinal column appeared normal above the
tenth dorsal vertebra, in which the arches met unsymmetrically to form
the spinous process. The arches of the eleventh and twelfth were very
uneven, and the structure was further complicated by the appearance
of cartilaginous plates between the arches of the adjoining vertebræ on

---

[1] The septa, which were very delicate, were removed before the drawing was made.

their right side. The arches of the lumbar vertebræ were very imperfectly ossified on the left, while on the right they were well advanced
except in the second, of which the right side of the arch appeared to be
wanting. The arch of the fourth (on the right side) was a broad plate
apparently continuous with a part of that of the first sacral, although
this relation could not be verified without injuring the specimen. The
lumbar region was very unsymmetrical. The ossification of the posterior surface of the sacrum and coccyx was so irregular that it was impossible to determine the number of vertebræ. On the sides were two
rows of transverse processes, fully ossified and united by bone around
the sacral foramina. Some slight indications (of the size of pin-holes)
of anterior foramina were to be seen on the posterior surface, but none
came through to the front. The coccyx was bent strongly forward and
contained some osseous formation.

5. *Circulatory System.* — The heart was broad and flattened. Its
greatest breadth, at the auriculo-ventricular groove, measured one inch
and an eighth; its height from base to apex was about the same.
The aorta curved normally to the left, giving off its regular branches.
A small, cord-like, impervious pulmonary artery, hardly more than a
millimetre in diameter, lay close to the left of the origin of the aorta.
About one eighth of an inch from this point it became larger, and, giving off a right and a left branch, was continued as the ductus arteriosus
through which the lungs were supplied. The right auricle was well
developed, having a prominent auricular appendage. There was no
appendage to the left auricle. The heart being opened the venæ cavæ
were found to be normal. There was a small Eustachian valve. Two
openings into the left auricle were to be seen ; the posterior and inferior
was the larger, and appeared like a defect in the wall; the other was apparently the foramen ovale. The anterior and posterior edges of this
opening had a somewhat valvular arrangement, the anterior being to
the right. The auriculo-ventricular valve consisted of a right and a
left segment, with a third smaller one in front and to the left, behind
the place where the conus arteriosus, which was very rudimentary,
should be. Just behind and below this minute conus was a triangular
inter-ventricular opening, the apex of which was downward and the
greatest diameter nearly one quarter of an inch. At the left anterior
extremity the cavity extended a little upward, where there was a slight
depression leading toward the pulmonary artery, with which, however,
there was no communication. The left auricle was very small, and,
until opened, appeared little else than a cavity in the wall of the right
one, but it was found to be partially divided into two cavities. Opened
from the left side, this cavity, into which one pulmonary vein emptied,
communicated by the posterior of the two openings already mentioned
with the right auricle. Another aperture in the membranous wall led

into a third cavity, which communicated by the foramen ovale with the right auricle ; this appeared to be the real auricle. The front bore some faint resemblance internally to an appendage, and two pulmonary veins opened into it. It also communicated by a narrow opening with the left ventricle. The mitral valve consisted of two folds. The walls of the left ventricle were about as thick as those of the right, but the cavity was much smaller. The aperture between the ventricles was clearly seen, and near it was the entrance to the aorta. There was some semblance of a conus arteriosus in the left ventricle below the origin of the aorta, which was thus placed in order to receive the blood from both ventricles. Had it been a little more to the right it would have been just above the opening in the septum.

The umbilical cord was found to contain the vein and the left umbilical artery, the course of which was normal.

The right common iliac was wanting. Both iliacs, of which the internal was the smaller, arose on that side directly from the aorta.

The ductus venosus was normal, as was also the venous system as far as t was examined.

The specimen just described deserves especial notice for a number of reasons. In the first place, such a monstrosity is extremely rare. Neither Förster [1] nor Saint-Hilaire [2] in their admirable works on teratology describes such a peculiar combination of malformations. In the second place, we found great difficulty in determining the sex. There were no external organs of generation whatever. The cutaneous folds on the thighs might be rudiments of either a scrotum or of labia. The testes were made out by the existence of many more or less convoluted tubes and by the absence of anything approaching in appearance to ova. The only possible question as to the correctness of this view is whether the organs might not have been merely remains of the Wolffian bodies ; but their shape showed that they were no longer in a very rudimentary stage, and their position (the long diameter being vertical [3]) as well as their microscopical appearances excluded the possibility of their being ovaries. The body marked B (Fig. 1) is the most difficult of all to explain. The abundance of muscular fibre in its structure (no traces whatever of glands being found), together with its passage through the perinæum, indicated strongly its uterine signification. It is to be remembered, however, that its position was adverse to its being the uterus ; and the only way of accounting for it is by supposing that the inferior wall of the bladder would, in a more developed condition, have come forward over it. The folds on either side of the organ and meeting in front of it were superficially suggestive of the broad ligaments, but they

[1] Die Missbildungen des Menschen. A. Förster.
[2] Histoire générale et particulière des Anomalies. M. I. G. Saint-Hilaire.
[3] Entwicklungs Geschichte. Kölliker.

could not be so accepted, their anterior attachment to the body described and their union at that point opposing such a view. Without venturing to express any opinion as to its nature, we would merely remark that if the body (B) were the uterus (as its structure appeared to indicate) we have here a remarkable specimen of perfect hermaphroditism.

The peculiarities in the ossification of the vertebræ are very interesting. Many cases of monstrosity have shown two nuclei in the vertebral bodies, but it is still doubtful if more than one is ever found in the normal foetus. It is also a curious fact that there was no regularity in this duplication. In the first lumbar vertebra there was but one nucleus, while there were two in the second as well as in the lower dorsal vertebræ. There were some indications of regular ossification on the sides of the sacrum, but the bodies were quite incomprehensible.

The heart presented an anomaly which Rokitansky would call a defeet in the posterior part of the anterior septum. We do not find, however, that in his recent magnificent monograph on defects in the septum he records any case exactly corresponding with this one.

The deficiency of one of the umbilical arteries is common (W. Vrolik) in cases of this nature, but the irregular origin of the right external iliac is worthy of notice.

CASE II. Some months after the examination of the specimen just described, by a curious coincidence, another, very similar to it, was discovered in the Museum of the Medical School of Maine. On the jar was written " Foetus of 7½ mos.," and no further history can be obtained.

The length from vertex to heel was eleven and a half inches. The head and limbs were well formed, with the exception of the feet, which were somewhat distorted. The pelvis and legs could be bent laterally on the body, precisely as in the first specimen,[1] but in the opposite direction ; thus they could be brought up to the right so as to form a right angle with the body, but not at all to the left.[2] The nates and perinæum were precisely as in A. The pubic bones were half an inch apart. The folds on the thighs (Fig. 4, Z) were larger than in A, the left one being nearly half an inch long. There was no umbilical cord, but the membranes from the side of the placenta (Y) went to form the anterior wall of the abdomen, where the skin and muscles were deficient; in other words, the membranes formed the sac of a ventral hernia. In most places three layers could be distinguished, of which the outer was continuous with the skin and the inner with the peritoneum. In this specimen there was an opening, apparently artificial, through the membranes into the abdomen (X). A strip of skin of nearly normal ap-

---

[1] For convenience the first specimen will hereafter be called A and the second one B.

[2] As Figure 4 might at first sight give a different impression, it is proper to state that the deceptive appearance is due to the throwing of the head to the left.

Fig. 4.

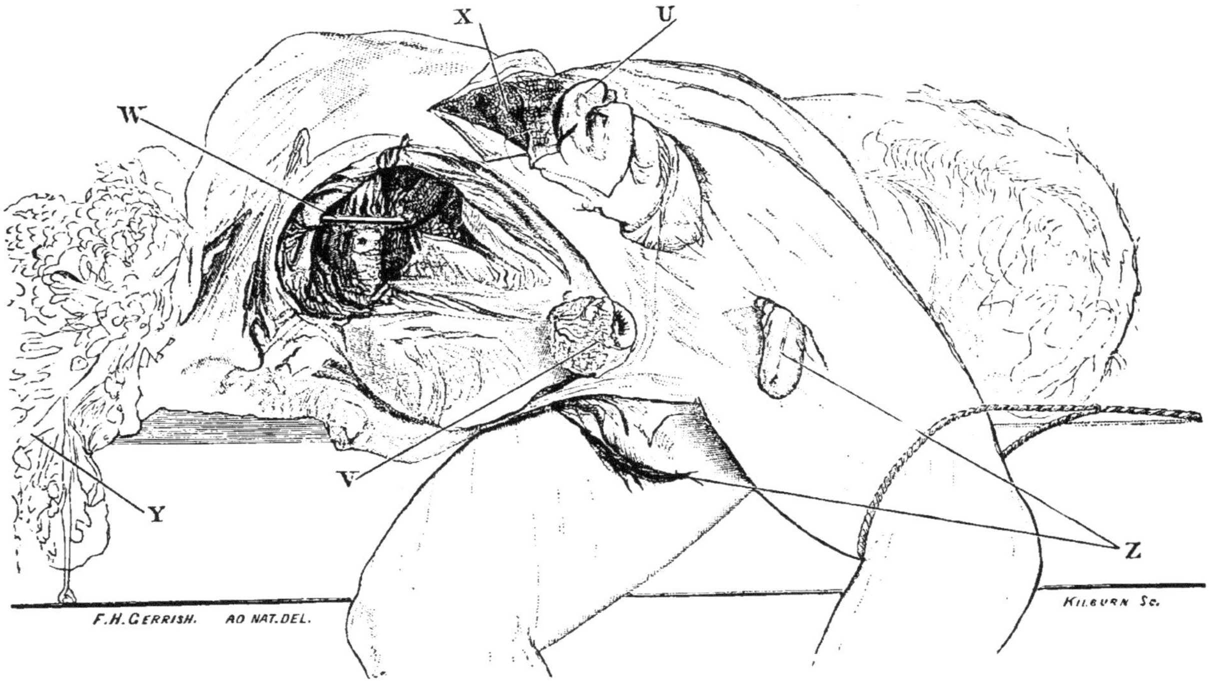

U

X

W

Z

V

Y

KILBURN SC.

F. H. GERRISH. AD NAT. DEL.

pearance separated the abdominal opening from that of the cloaca below.

The Cloaca differed but slightly from that of A. There was both an intestinal and a vesical portion. A small opening (at W) served for communication with the bowel, which did not project as in the other case. There were no indications of openings into the ureters. The body (V) which was supposed to represent the uterus was decidedly larger than in A. It had a similar communication with the perinæum. The fold forming the rudimentary anterior wall of the bladder passed in front of its origin. There were in B no lateral appendages. The upper surface of the organ presented a number of very small depressions, giving it a cribriform appearance; and one of them communicated by a minute canal with the central passage from the perinæum.

Contents of Abdomen. — Except in the following respects there was little worthy of notice. There was no large intestine save the dilatation that formed a part of the cloaca, and which was thrown into several folds but did not have a vermiform appendix, as in A. The small intestine was shorter than normal, but it was not thought proper to remove it for measurement. The ureters, dilated and tortuous, ended blindly on the posterior surface of the cloaca. The spleen was very small. The two bodies held to be testes were present and had the same gross characteristics as in A. That on the left side, (U) was the larger and was removed for microscopical examination.

This was much more satisfactory than in A. The organ was shown to be subdivided into a number of cavities by fibrous septa. These cavities were filled, some with tubules, some with collections of small cells. The tubules were of two kinds: those most generally found consisted of a membrana propria surrounded by a delicate fibrous sheath; they were full of cellular elements. No part of the contents could be distinguished from the rest as an epithelial lining. The tubes of the other kind were found on but one side of the specimen. They were decidedly larger, and had thicker walls and a well-marked lining of columnar epithelium surrounding a central cavity. The tubules of both kinds were very much convoluted. No blind extremities were observed.

The specimens from A were essentially the same, with the exception that they were chiefly composed of cellular and fibrous elements, with comparatively few tubules among them.

Circulatory System. — The heart was normal, as was also the arrangement of the branches from the aorta. The absence of the umbilical cord, though not unknown, is a very rare anomaly, but in point of fact it is of little importance as far as the nutrition of the fœtus is concerned, for the umbilical vein and one artery were present. As already stated, the absence of one umbilical artery is very common, not to say the rule, in cases of this kind, but in B it was the left one, instead of the right, as in A, that was wanting. The abdominal aorta appeared to terminate in the right hypogastric artery, the right external iliac and the left common one being very small. The right hypogastric reached the integument above the right pubic bone, and ran upward along the right border of the cloaca to the strip of skin between the two openings. It was here joined by the umbilical vein, which ran along the right side of the ventral opening to the attachment of the falciform ligament of the liver, along which it coursed. In the other direction the vein kept company with the artery, and the two ran together into the attached border of the placenta. They could be traced for some distance on the surface of that organ to a knob-like prominence, formed chiefly by the vein, at which they broke up into branches.

The Skeleton was not examined, as it was thought proper to preserve the specimen, but an incision in the back showed that there was a spina bifida apparently in both the lumbar and sacral regions.

The resemblance between these two specimens is certainly very remarkable. The absence of the cord in B does not appear to be of much importance. The two chief differences are the greater simplicity of the cloaca in B, the rather surprising fact that the heart is normal, the more marked characteristics of the testis in B, and the absence of one kidney in A. It is interesting to notice that the lower extremities bend to the left in A and to the right in B, that is, in both cases toward the side on which the hypogastric artery was present; but it is very doubtful if this is more than a coincidence. It will be observed that both specimens were the result of a miscarriage at the same stage of development (seven and a half months).

DESCRIPTION OF FIGURES.

Figures 1, 2, and 3, drawn by Dr. H. P. Quincy, are different views of the first specimen.

Fig. 1. A (the line from the letter runs one quarter of an inch inside the outline of the drawing), the perineal opening of the canal from B; supposed to be the uterus; C, rudiments of labia or scrotum; D, fœtal membranes; E, umbilical cord; F, opening of intestine; G, vesical portion of cloaca; H, transverse fold, a rudiment of the anterior abdominal wall; I, folds of mucous membrane; K, depressions in vesical portion of cloaca (the right one opposite to end of ureter).

Fig. 2. a, band connecting pubic bones; b, great sacro-sciatic ligaments; c, band connecting the two latter.

Fig. 3. 1, ninth dorsal vertebra; 2, second lumbar vertebra; 3, first sacral vertebra.

Fig. 4 represents the second specimen.[1] Z, rudiments of labia or scrotum; Y, placenta; X, cavity of abdomen seen through an opening made in the membranes; W, a probe in the opening of the intestine; V, supposed uterus; u, uterus.

[1] I wish to acknowledge the kindness of my colleague, Professor Gerrish, in making this drawing.   T. D. Jr.

RECENT PROGRESS IN PUBLIC HYGIENE.

BY F. W. DRAPER, M. D.

FILTH-DISEASES AND THEIR PREVENTION.

THE most valuable and suggestive among the recent contributions to the literature of sanitary science is by Mr. John Simon, the Medical Officer of the British Privy Council and Local Government Board.[1] He discusses the fundamental principles of preventive medicine with a comprehensiveness and originality to which only scant justice can be done in the brief outline presented here. The report is divided into three parts: (1) the diseases produced by filth; (2) the forms in which filth is found producing disease; and (3) the prevention of filth diseases. After remarking that the needless deaths in Great Britain number annually more than one hundred and twenty-five thousand, distributed unequally in different sections of the country, but most numerous in concurrence with removable influences hostile to life, the author states that two classes of controllable or preventable conditions stand conspicuous in their relation to disease and mortality, namely, the failure (through neglect or ignorance) to remove refuse matters, solid and liquid, from inhabited places, and the freedom with which dangerous infectious diseases are permitted to scatter abroad the seeds of their infection. The present report deals with the former of these evils. While acknowledging that filth in its generic sense has long been recognized by medical men as standing in close causative relation to disease, Mr. Simon insists that it is only the cruder, sensible characters of uncleanliness that have attracted attention, and that a far more important element, the subtle action of zymotic poison, has been made manifest only by recent researches. "The exacter studies of modern times," he says, "have shown that by various channels of indirect and clandestine influence, filth can operate far more subtly and also far more widely and more destructively than our forefathers conjectured." These studies demonstrate that "the chief morbific agencies in filth are other than those chemically identified stinking gaseous products of organic decomposition which force themselves on popular attention." The filth which we smell and see is harmful in proportion to its palpable amount; but the far more mischievous possibilities are such as apparently must be attributed to morbific ferments or contagia; these are not gaseous, but seem to have their essence in certain solid elements which the microscope discovers in them; in living organisms, which, by virtue of their vitality, are indefinitely self-multiplying within their respective spheres of operation. As it is by these organisms that filth

---

[1] Public Health Reports of the Medical Officer of the Privy Council and Local Government Board, New Series. No. II. Supplementary Report to the Local Government Board on some recent Inquiries under the Public Health Act, 1858.

probably produces zymotic disease, it is necessary not to confound them with the fœtid gases of organic decomposition. It is of the utmost practical importance to recognize, in regard to filth, that agents which destroy its stink may yet leave all its main powers of disease production undiminished. Moreover, it is characteristic of the zymotic ferments that "they show ho power of active diffusion in dry air; diffusing in it only as they are passively wafted, and then probably, if the air be freely open, not carrying their vitality far; but as moisture is their normal medium, currents of humid air (as from drains and sewers) can doubtless lift them in their full effectiveness."

Of diseases which are produced by filth, the diarrhœas are the best illustration. Mr. Simon says, "Among the effects which arise under experimental septic infections, as likewise in cases of accidental septicæmia in the human subject, acute catarrh of the mucous membrane of the intestines is an extremely prominent fact. The mucous membrane of the intestinal canal seems peculiarly to bear the stress of all accidental putridities which enter the blood. Whether they have been breathed or drunk or eaten, or sucked up into the blood-vessels from the surface of foul sores, or directly injected into blood-vessels by the physiological experimenter, there the effect may be looked for; just as wine, however administered, would 'get into the head,' so the septic ferment, whencesoever it may have entered the blood, is apt to find its way thence to the bowels, and there, as a universal result, to produce diarrhœa."

The discussion of the etiology of enteric fever is particularly suggestive, inasmuch as that affection is considered the type of a large class of preventable diseases. The author sums up his mature experience in this direction as follows: "The explanation of the frequent tendency of privy-nuisances to infect with enteric fever has seemed to consist in the liability of such nuisances to carry with them, as frequent accidental adjuncts, the 'specific' contagium of any prevailing bowel-infection; for presumably the privies of a population receive (*inter alia*) the diarrhœal discharges of the sick; and it has long been matter of fair pathological presumption that in any 'specific' diarrhœa (such as eminently is enteric fever) every discharge from the bowels must teem with the contagium of the disease. Medical knowledge in support of this presumption has of late been rapidly growing more positive and precise; and at the moment of my present writing it has received an increase which may be of critical importance, in the discovery, namely, of microscopical forms, apparently of the lowest vegetable life, multiplying to innumerable swarms in the intestinal tissues of the sick, penetrating on the one hand from the mucous surface into the general system of the patient, and contributory on the other hand, with whatever infective power they represent, to the bowel-contents which have presently to pass forth from him."

Passing from the study of affections whose development appears to be intimately related with the seeds of morbific infection as conveyed by human excrement in air and water, the author refers at some length to the influence of other kinds of filth in producing disease. He considers it among the most hopeful advances of modern preventive medicine that some diseases which, in the sense of being able to continue their species from man to man, are apparently as "specific" as small-pox or syphilis, seem now beginning to confess a birthplace exterior to man, and amid controllable conditions in the physical nature around us, amid the putrefactive changes of dead organic matter. Reasoning from the suggestive results which experimental physiology has produced in propagating within the living body the septic germs, he indicates the strong probability that peritonitis, erysipelas, pyæmia, septicæmia, puerperal fever, even tuberculosis, will be found to have a closer relation to filth-inoculation than as yet appears.

In the second part of his paper, Mr. Simon describes the forms in which filth is found producing disease. His graphic account of a too familiar condition of things applies so well to many communities in our own country that it should not be condensed : —

"There are houses, there are groups of houses, there are whole villages, there are considerable sections of towns, there are even entire and not small towns, where general slovenliness in everything which relates to the removal of refuse-matter, slovenliness which in very many cases amounts to utter bestiality of neglect, is the local habit; where, within or just outside each house, or in spaces common to many houses, lies for an indefinite time, undergoing fœtid decomposition, more or less of the putrefiable refuse which house-life and some sorts of trade-life produce; excrement of man and brute, and garbage of all sorts, and ponded slop-waters; sometimes lying bare on the common surface, sometimes unintentionally stored out of sight and recollection in drains or sewers which cannot carry them away, sometimes held in receptacles specially provided to favor accumulation, as privy-pits and other cess-pools for excrement and slop-water, and so-called dust-bins receiving kitchen-refuse and other filth. And with this state of things, be it on large or on small scale, two chief sorts of danger to life arise : one, that volatile effluvia from the refuse pollute the surrounding air and everything which it contains; the other, that the liquid parts of the refuse pass by soakage or leakage into the surrounding soil, to mingle there of course in whatever water the soil yields, and in certain cases thus to occasion the deadliest pollution of wells and springs. To a really immense extent, to an extent indeed which persons unpracticed in sanitary inspection could scarcely find themselves able to imagine, dangers of these two sorts are prevailing throughout the length and breadth of this country, not only in their slighter degrees, but in degrees which are gross and scandalous, and very often, I repeat, truly bestial."

The various sources of excremental infection from defective sewerage are pointed out. Especially is indicated how often house drainage, though arranged with good workmanlike intention, has failed for want of skilled guidance.

Finally, the report deals with the prevention of filth-diseases, and presents comprehensive views of sanitary administration with reference to a radical and thorough treatment of morbific conditions. The remarks upon chemical disinfection are very suggestive : " To chemically disinfect (in the true sense of that word) the filth of any neglected district, to follow the body and branchings of the filth with really effective chemical treatment, to thoroughly destroy or counteract it in muck-heaps, and cess-pools, and ash-pits, and sewers, and drains, and where soaking into wells, and where exhaling into houses, cannot, I apprehend, be proposed as physically possible. Again and again a district has been found under some terrible visitation of enteric fever, from filth-infection operating through house drains or water-supply ; but with the local authority inactive as to the true cause of the mischief, and only bent on practicing about the place, under the name of disinfection, some futile ceremony of vague chemical libations or powderings. Conduct such as this, referring apparently rather to some mythical 'epidemic influence ' than to the known causes of disease, and savoring rather of superstitious observance than of rational recourse to chemistry, is eminently not that by which filth-diseases can be prevented ; and, contrasting it therefore with means by which that result can be secured, I would here specially note a warning against it."

THE DISPOSAL OF SEWAGE.

The important subjects of drainage and sewerage continue to attract attention among sanitarians at home and abroad, and the journals contain reports of animated and instructive, if not conclusive, discussions concerning the best methods of removing the refuse and excremental products of domestic life. It is natural and proper that such matters should claim extraordinary notice, for they touch intimately the elementary and fundamental principles of sanitary science. Defective drainage violates the first rule of hygiene — the preservation of cleanliness.

It is unfortunate for sanitarians that they must generally modify their ideas to suit practical and economic ends. The popular mind has not reached the point of appreciating that public health is public wealth. Hence any new plan for getting rid of excremental refuse is deemed practicable, provided it can insure a dividend, direct or indirect; so that the various schemes habitually append to the recital of their respective sanitary advantages a claim of superior economy and of larger fruits, whether the product be gigantic vegetables from sewage farms or bags of poudrette from precipitating tanks.

It may be useful for the purposes of this report to note briefly some of the methods whose merits or demerits have recently challenged the critical attention of sanitarians.

Pneumatic Sewerage. — Captain Liernur, the originator of the pneumatic or " separate " system, maintains that all putrescible matters, the sink-refuse and the excrement, should be conveyed away from houses through air-tight conduits which will not permit the pollution of subsoil air and water to such a degree as is possible with the porous water-carriage sewers generally in use. He provides a separate system for the conveyance of surface water and refuse water, and aims to keep the urinary and fæcal excreta undiluted. The latter material (nightsoil) he removes as follows by atmospheric pressure before decomposition occurs. All the closets of a block of houses are connected by means of iron pipes with an iron main tube in the street; the street main in turn discharges into a tank, but a stop-cock shuts off the connection with the houses when the pneumatic process is not in operation. To the tank is attached the air-pump engine by which, when it is working, a partial vacuum is maintained. At certain hours men visit the street mains and open the stop-cocks ; at once the excretory matters of all the houses (a hundred or more) in connection with the mains are sucked into the receiving tank. Here, owing to its small bulk, the excrement can be easily dealt with either by immediate distribution to the soil or by conversion into poudrette.

The advantages of this plan of pneumatic pressure are obvious : the sewer gas is drawn away from the houses ; there is no necessity for the profuse employment of water for flushing purposes ; as the sewage is not diluted, no expensive arrangements are required to prepare it for use as manure ; and the system operates independently of the house-occupants, doing its work without their interference. The scheme is well adapted for inland places which have no natural outfall for their sewage, or which cannot supply water in quantity for flushing, or whose topography does not admit such a fall to the sewers as to prevent the deposit of sewage in them. Certain towns in Holland (Amsterdam, Leyden, the Hague) have adopted this method, and it is represented as giving general satisfaction to householders and to the sanitary authorities.

The Goux System. — This is a modification of the dry-earth or Moule method of getting rid of fæcal matter, and it aims to do all that the earth-closet accomplishes, without the costly apparatus and special appliances required by the latter. No machinery is needed, the perfect action of the method depending on the fidelity of the person in charge of it. A particular kind of soil and its careful drying are dispensed with, and ordinary refuse, such as stable litter, loft sweepings, leaves, and sawdust, is used, mixed with charcoal, soot, or gypsum. A tapering tub or container is provided, sixteen inches high and twenty inches at its greatest diameter. Upon the bottom of this is placed the absorbent matter, as above described, to the depth of four inches. A mold of the same shape as the tub, but of six inches less diameter, is placed within the latter, and the space between the two is packed with refuse. The mold is then withdrawn, and the tub is placed under the privy seat. The materials on the bottom and around the side of the container absorb the liquid excreta. The tub remains under the seat for one week if for ten persons, or a fortnight for six persons. The manure resulting from this method is said to be superior to that produced under the dry-earth plan.

Sewage Farming. — This industry, which aims to utilize excretal refuse and at the same time by soil-filtration to destroy its noxious character, continues to afford fruitful opportunity for discussion and partisanship among English sanitarians. The whole subject has excited fresh interest during the past year. The sewage farms have been sharply criticised, and, on the other hand, as warmly defended. Economists have abused this method of utilizing sewage as costing more than it brings; while sanitarians have not been wanting who complained that because of the stench produced the farms were a greater nuisance than the original condition which they were designed to correct; that the effluent water, the product of the downward filtration, was not devoid of polluting qualities; that infectious properties were imparted to the vegetables raised by means of sewage irrigation and even to the milk of cows fed upon the sewage grass; that the cows themselves suffered injury by such food; that through mismanagement the crops were liable to be flooded with sewage at unexpected moments; and that the growing vegetables assimilated only a part of the elements contained in the liquid manure supplied to them, rejecting entirely the organic portions which had not been changed chemically into ammonia, the nitrates, and the nitrites.

The advocates of this mode of using the contents of sewers have answered objections with much zeal. Conspicuous among these champions is Dr. Alfred Carpenter, who is immediately interested in the working of the well-known Croydon farm of four hundred and sixty acres. In a paper read before the Association of Medical Officers of Health at Birmingham,[1] he discussed the theoretical and practical advantages of sewage farming. He showed that vegetation is the most efficient agent for the purification of sewage. He detailed experiments to prove that plants will assimilate animal matter before its conversion into its ultimate elements; that rye-grass, for example, will thrive on

- [1] The Sanitary Record, May 1, 1875.

beef-tea. He asserted the falsity of Pettenkofer's notion that the germs of disease may be deodorized but not disinfected in the processes of sewage farming, and maintained that plants appropriate to their own growth all the nitrogenous matter supplied to them. Finally, he contended that, far from influencing unfavorably the health of a district in which they are situated, sewage farms are conducive to the public sanitary welfare, as is shown by the low death-rate of Croydon since the sewage was utilized by irrigation.

Notwithstanding the effectiveness of such advocacy as that just quoted, it is obvious, if we may judge by the current literature, that sewage farming is not growing in favor and that it is on the defensive. There is a manifest preference for the water-carriage system wherever it is feasible. There are so many practical difficulties in the way of sewage irrigation, touching topography, the selection of a suitable soil, the imperative need of intelligent and vigilant supervision, and the demands of the seasons, that engineers and sanitarians naturally turn first to less complicated and less exacting methods. In this community much that is instructive upon this topic is expected from the investigations now in progress under the authority of the State Board of Health with reference to the pollution of streams in Massachusetts.

It may be remarked in passing that sewage farming is at present receiving a satisfactory test in the vicinity of Paris. The great sandy plain of Gennevilliers affords the best possible conditions, as regards soil, climate, and sewage supply, for producing excellent results; and it is said that these results are already very gratifying.

PROCEEDINGS OF THE SUFFOLK DISTRICT MEDICAL SOCIETY.

JAMES R. CHADWICK, M. D., SECRETARY.

MAY 29, 1875. — The president, DR. H. W. WILLIAMS, in the chair.

The Actual Cautery: its Uses and Power. — DR. C. E. BROWN-SÉQUARD addressed the society upon this subject. He said that the importance of the actual cautery as a curative agent had never been fully appreciated, and suggested that its employment had been greatly restricted by the very natural objections of patients. In the last century this treatment was vehemently decried, owing to the suffering inflicted, the theory being that the more intense the pain the greater was the effect. It is a fallacy, however, that the influence of counter-irritation is transmitted by the nerves of feeling. Apparently insignificant irritation, devoid of pain, may produce powerful reflex explosions; for instance, worms in the bowels may cause convulsions, epilepsy, paralysis, or even insanity. Certain nerves exist, by the irritation of which changes of nutrition may be induced. In Guinea-pigs an epileptic attack may be brought on by simply tickling the neck. The human species may be as susceptible as animals. Dr. Brown-Séquard had once ventured to excite epileptic attacks in two male patients, and by that means was led to a mode of treatment by which they were cured; the irritation was not even felt in either instance.

The extent to which the actual cautery may be employed is greatly increased when we realize that the effect is not proportionate to the intensity of the pain, but often the reverse. He had discovered this fact in the years 1848 and 1849, after experimenting in M. Rayer's wards at the Charité Hospital, in Paris, on the different modes of applying the heated iron. He ascertained that the application of an intensely hot metallic cautery, in such a way as to cause very little pain, was of much more service than any painful counter-irritation, the only novelty in the operation being the almost entire freedom from suffering.

Jobert de Lamballe and Valleix have gone too far in extolling the use of the cautery, when they state that they have never known the actual cautery to fail in neuralgia; they surely must have lost sight of many patients. Dr. Brown-Séquard said he had had many bad cases of neuralgia to treat, both recent and chronic, and, though they were not all on record, he was sure that the results would show seven or eight cures in every ten cases.

He had, by means of the cautery, obtained great relief in every case, and often a complete arrest of the intense pain in the chest that accompanies pericarditis, although in no instance had the effect been permanent. One patient was relieved for a whole year after the application of the iron; the pain then recurred, but was again exorcised by the same treatment, and has not been felt since.

In sclerosis of the posterior columns of the cord — locomotor ataxy — he had invariably seen a cessation, or at least a diminution, of the attacks of pain from the employment of the cautery, *loco dolenti*, even when the pain had been of the most intense lancinating character.

The actual cautery is of great use for that variety of pain in the head which is not of inflammatory nature, but is probably due to congestion of the membranes, especially of the dura mater; the pain is described as a bursting sensation, a mental torpor and dullness, a burning, or at times a cutting, and is common in this country. The places at which the iron should be applied are between the shoulder-blades, or on top of the head. The effect is a contraction of the blood-vessels by reflex action. In three cases in which this method was employed, the eye was watched, and it was found that the pupil behaved as it does when the cervical sympathetic nerve is galvanized, that is to say, the pupil is invariably dilated. But no change was detected in the temperature of the face and ear with an ordinary thermometer.

In cases of sunstroke, Dr. Brown-Séquard had found the hot irons very serviceable.

Charcot has shown that in Pott's disease the actual cautery is more efficient than any other treatment; he has made several autopsies in cases of patients who were cured of paraplegia by the cautery; in one of these he found the cord reduced to one tenth of its normal calibre, yet sensation and voluntary movement had been almost entirely restored; the deaths had ensued from some intercurrent affection.   Dr. Brown-Séquard's practice confirmed Charcot's estimate of the value of this treatment in Pott's disease.

The use of the cautery in inflammatory disease of the joints is known to be most beneficial.

The cures claimed to have been effected in general paralysis of the insane had been called in question, yet he firmly believed in the possibility of a cure, provided the morbid alterations, not only of the brain proper, but of the medulla oblongata and of the spinal cord, had not advanced too far.   Disease does not necessarily arrest the functions of the brain; far from this, destruction of a considerable portion of one or both hemispheres may take place with very little if any disturbance of functions.   In a number of cases of the so-called general paralysis of the insane the most satisfactory results had been obtained from the heated iron, and in two instances — one being that of a physician of New York — cures were effected that promise to be permanent.

There is a morbid state in which the power of the actual cautery is especially great: it is coma.   In several cases of apoplectic coma, in some of which the life of the patient was recognized by the stertorous breathing to be in imminent peril, Dr. Brown-Séquard had succeeded in restoring mental activity and reëstablishing a normal respiration by applying the heated iron to the head.   Some of these patients were manifestly saved from impending death.   One of them died two years after having been so saved, and several survived many months.

In chorea the actual cautery may be very useful.   He had effected a permanent cure by this method within a week, in one case which had resisted all ordinary means of treatment.

The cautery is very powerful in epilepsy, especially when the disease is due to a blow upon the head, or is caused by congestion or inflammation of the membranes of the brain.   Dr. Brown-Séquard took the opportunity to say that those cases of epilepsy that depended upon organic lesions of the cerebral meninges, or of the brain itself, were by far more amenable to this or some other means of treatment than the cases in which no organic lesion of any part of the nervous system existed.

In summing up the cases of organic or functional disease in which the actual cautery is of service, Dr. Brown-Séquard mentioned pain in any region, but especially neuralgia; congestion or inflammation in the brain, the spinal cord, the lungs, the heart, and other viscera; serous effusion into the joints, the pericardium, and the pleura; paralysis agitans; neuroses, especially epilepsy.

The rule to be followed in determining the place of application is to choose that part of the skin which is nearest to the pain.   In locomotor ataxy the sensation is referred to the periphery, consequently apply the iron there.   This rule is not absolute, as has been seen in the remarks about congestions of the head.   In locomotor ataxy apply the iron to the lower limbs, at the spot where the pain is felt, or over muscles attacked with cramp.   In cases, however, of myelitis or of spinal meningitis associated with congestion or inflammation of the fibrous tissue uniting the vertebræ, the best place of application is over the tender spots of the spine.   Graves pointed out many years ago the importance of making counter-irritation on the lower limbs in paraplegia. In Pott's disease, on the contrary, the application should be made close to the vertebræ.

No special instrument need be used ; if the poker is resorted to it should not be applied over a large surface or pressed hard, if it is desired to avoid giving pain. Lines and occasionally points should be made rapidly. The outer layers of the skin are dried up, and fall off after a few days. No sore or scar remains, so that there is no danger of disfiguring the face, or any other part. The most convenient instrument is one consisting of a steel or platinum bulb about the shape of an olive but much smaller. To act safely in a cavity like the mouth, or on a restricted part of the skin, a very small steel bar or shaft may be used, which, when heated, is pushed inside a protecting bulb. Before allowing time for the latter to become heated, it is applied to the part of the skin or mucous membrane which is to be burned, and the heated shaft pushed down upon the part and immediately withdrawn ; this contrivance is so safe that it can be used inside the mouth, about the ear, or on the eyelids in neuralgia.

The minimum of pain is obtained with white heat, because the outer layer of the integument is destroyed immediately, and radiation does not take place beyond it, the dried-up cutaneous tissue serving as a screen.

As regards the frequency of the applications, it necessarily varies greatly. In cases of neuralgia five or six lines are to be made three or four times, at intervals of two or three days. A single application is usually sufficient to allay the pain of locomotor ataxy. This treatment must be repeated many times for inflammations or serous effusions, especially when chronic. In neuritis the method may have to be persisted in for years.

Dr. Spring asked at what point the iron should be applied in caries of the vertebræ, and how often.

Dr. Brown-Séquard answered that it should be applied over the seat of the disease, and must be continued even for years if relief was obtained.

In response to Dr. A. P. Richardson, it was stated that the best metal for the purpose was platinum, which can easily be washed by acids without fear of its being affected thereby or being eaten by oxidation. Gold has proved too soft, and steel involved a considerable loss of time from the fact that it requires filing before each application, to say nothing of the speedy destruction of the instrument.

Spinal Meningeal Hæmorrhage. — The two cases reported by Dr. S. G. Webber were published in the Journal of July 8, 1875.

Myeloïd Disease of the Head of the Tibia. — A case was reported by Dr. D. W. Cheever which was remarkable from the fact that the man was able to go to New York with the aid of crutches only three days before the amputation. The growth was of two years' duration, but had not invaded the knee-joint. The glands in the thigh were enlarged, so that they were dissected out. The specimen showed how excessively thin and reticulated the bone had become under the action of the tumor. There has been no recurrence of the disease after three years.

A report of the delegates to the annual meeting of the American Medical Association was made by Dr. H. I. Bowditch, and was listened to with marked attention.

THE MICHIGAN TROUBLES.

The expected "statement" of the regular faculty of Ann Arbor has appeared. The strongest sentiment it awakens in us is one of sympathy for the writers; to have worked for years in building up the school, to have got it into excellent order, for a school of its kind, and then to be driven from their comfortable positions by quackish interlopers is hard, very hard. Nevertheless, the "statement" does not in any way modify the opinions we have expressed; a duty is none the less one because it is disagreeable.

As has been shown, the whole affair is an evasion. The homœopathic faculty consists of but two professors, with the president of the university, yet the students are guaranteed all the privileges of the regular school, excepting the lectures on practice of medicine and materia medica, and they must be examined in the other branches by the regular professors, who are to give certificates of satisfactory proficiency. Thus the regular professors are compelled to furnish certificates for the homœopathic faculty, which on the strength of these certificates will confer degrees. A single sentence in Dr. Gerrish's letter to the *Medical Record* refutes conclusively the arguments of the writers of the "statement." "If the regular school," he writes, "were to suspend operations altogether, what would become of the new and 'independent' school, with its 'faculty' of two professors and a non-medical figure-head?"

We think that Professor Flint and Dr. J. Marion Sims, the President of the American Medical Association, can hardly have grasped the question when they wrote the rather surprising letters sustaining the faculty which appear in the "statement." Dr. Sims's letter is a remarkable one; the opening boast that he is not a man ever to desert his post is rather surprising from one who spent our war times in making a fortune in Europe. He writes, "The regents have wisely respected your sensibilities in not forcing these new professors upon you as a faculty. They have simply placed them in the same relation to you as they would other lecturers on special branches." (Imagine a special lecturer on homœopathy at Harvard!) "Your autonomy is not disturbed. You are exactly where you were before the appointments were made; and I think, under all the circumstances, you ought not to resign your places."

MEDICAL NOTES.

— The treatment of enlarged lymphatic glands by the subcutaneous injection of tincture of iodine is recommended by S. M. Bradley, F. R. C. S., in a paper printed in the *Lancet* of September 4, 1875. The writer does not recommend this procedure for all hypertrophies of the glands (as, for instance, syphilitic or carcinomatous affections), but applies the treatment to true hypertrophies of the lymphatic glands, with or without a strumous diathesis; secondly, to strumous hypertrophies, that is, cases of cellular hyperplasia with caseous deposit; and, thirdly, to hard, non-infectious lymphomata, which present many points of resemblance to the first groups, and, indeed, are often to be distinguished only in being multiple. For these affections five or six injections of the simple tincture of iodine, — five or ten minims at a time, according to the size of the tumor, — at intervals of about four days, generally effect a cure. The best cases are those where a single cervical gland is hypertrophied in an otherwise healthy adult subject.

— The death smell is the subject of a rather interesting paper by Dr. Isham, published in *The Clinic* of September 4, 1875. Dr. Isham was first impressed with this odor in 1863, when he was an inmate of one of the hospitals in Washington. Its character cannot be clearly described, but the basic perfume resembled that of musk, though more subtle and delicate. The odor has not the sour, moldy character of the cadaveric smell, nor is it a constant accompaniment of death. Usually it is not widely diffused, but comes as a wave of volatile matter. It does not remain long in one locality, and has been noticed by the writer only at a time just preceding the death struggle; never more remote from it than an hour, and frequently not more than from five minutes to half an hour. As to the origin of the odor, Dr. Isham believes it to be due to ammonia and a volatile oil that are contained in the blood. Near the termination of life, the circulation having ceased in the peripheral vessels, chemical changes take place in the blood, exalting its temperature and liberating the volatile principles which are present in the devitalized fluid, and which give rise to the death smell.

The experiments of Lange may help to explain why the odor is not appreciable in all cases of death. He found that when carbonate of ammonia was added to living blood, ammonia was given off only at a temperature of from 176° to 194° F., but when added to blood taken from a dead animal ammonia was given off at a temperature of from 104° to 113° F. In many diseases just previous to death the blood temperature is raised to above the lowest temperature given by Lange, and makes it possible for the volatile principles referred to to be set free. In some diseases, on the other hand, the blood heat falls much below the normal temperature, and no odor is diffused.

— William H. Hoag, M. D., reports in the *Medical Record* of September 11, 1875, another case of remarkable recovery from gun-shot wound. The case is referred to in Circular No. 6 of the Surgeon-General's office. An officer of the 29th New York Volunteers was wounded at Chancellorsville, May 2, 1863. The missile, a round musket ball weighing about four hundred grains, entered the eighth intercostal space of the left side, at a point nine and a half inches to the left of the ensiform cartilage; it fractured the ninth rib, and, without wounding the lung, passed through the diaphragm, and entered some portion of the alimentary canal. The patient walked more than a mile and a half to the rear, and the next day presented himself for treatment, apparently not in the least fatigued by his journey. A hernial tumor of the lung, of the size of a small orange, was found protruding. A ligature which had been placed around it on the field by surgeons who had tried ineffectually to reduce the hernia was removed, and the sphacelated portion separated from the granulating surface beneath. Five days after the injury an ounce of castor-oil was given, and while the patient was at stool a few hours later, the ball was voided. It was somewhat battered from striking the rib, and was quite irregular in shape. Cold-water dressings alone were applied to the wound. The patient's recovery was uninterrupted. On the 2d of June he left for a furlough of sixty days, and on his return the wound was entirely healed; the respiratory sounds were normal, though there was still a slight hernia of the lung. The reporter of this case thinks it probable that the small intestines escaped injury, and that the ball passed into the transverse or descending colon, which is much less likely to take on inflammatory action than the smaller bowel.

— The *Medical Record* publishes a list of the order of lectures for 1875–77 in the principal Eastern medical schools. We do not know how accurate it may be in other respects, but we happen to know that the order of exercises at Harvard has not yet been determined.

— Another remarkable triumph of the antiseptic system is reported in the *Lancet* of August 28th, being no less than the removal of a loose cartilage from the knee-joint under the carbolic spray with a most successful result. The patient, a man aged twenty-two, was admitted into the North Riding Infirmary under the care of Dr. Williams. His history was that four years ago he was working on a night shift, and having occasion to be on his knees, found on rising to the erect posture that he could not straighten his right leg. The leg was painless as long as it was semiflexed, but any attempt to straighten it was attended with much suffering. Eighteen months afterwards he became subject to excruciating pain in the joint when walking, and shortly afterwards a little lump appeared on the inside of the joint, at the lower and inner border of the patella. He continued in this state till the end of July, 1874, when he was forced to put himself under treatment. August 26th, Dr. Williams proceeded to remove the loose body. The joint was quite natural in appearance except below the patella, where there was some little thickening, the result of an accident in childhood. On examination no loose body could be found; but after the patient had walked once or twice across the floor a small body, of the apparent size of a sixpence, was detected on the outer and anterior part of the capsule. The leg was bent on the thigh to keep the loose body in its place. Chloroform was dispensed with. After washing the skin in the vicinity of the joint with an oily solution of carbolic acid (one part in ten), under a spray of carbolic acid lotion (one part in forty), Dr. Williams made an incision two inches in length, its lowest point being an inch higher than the position in which the loose body was felt. The part of the capsule over the body was reached by the finger through the wound, the body was seized with a tenaculum, and pulled out after the capsule had been opened. The body proved to be a flat piece of cartilage about the size of a large bean. The limb was then extended, and dressed antiseptically according to Lister's method. The patient convalesced without serious general disturbance, and there was only a little sanguineous discharge from the wound. September 15th the wound was healed and the cicatrix strong. The patient returned to heavy labor, finding himself fit to engage in it.

— Dr. Cossini, of Damascus, sends to *L'Union Médicale* an account of the outbreak of cholera at Hama, Damascus, and other places in that vicinity. At Hama, a city on the Orontes of from twenty-five thousand to thirty thousand souls, the disease about the middle of March first attacked fourteen soldiers of the garrison, of whom thirteen died within a few days. Early in April it invaded the town itself, and during two months and a half there were from fifteen to twenty deaths a day. The fact that for seventy-five days the epidemic was wholly confined to Hama gave rise to the hope that it was engendered by causes wholly local, and that it would spread no farther. But at length the villages near Hama, and then a city of eighteen thousand inhabitants, nearly thirty miles distant, were attacked. Meanwhile, the garrison of Hama was ordered to Damascus, where it arrived about the 1st of June. On the 13th of June cholera appeared in Damascus, and rapidly spread, so that by the 4th of July it was at its height and causing one hundred and forty to one hundred and fifty deaths daily. In fact, these figures are not large enough, for the Mussulmans conceal as far as they can their deaths, and probably the mortality reached at least two hundred each day. Such a panic seized the inhabitants that the streets were crowded with fugitives, many being attacked with the disease and dying on the road. Those who reached Sayta, Beyrout, and Lebanon carried the disease with them, so that almost all of Syria is invaded by cholera. At Damascus the disease is on the decline. How the disease could arise at Hama, an isolated place situated on the borders of the desert, is a mystery. As to treatment, the only remedy that seemed to Dr. Cossini to be of advantage was a mixture of chloroform with the acetate of ammonia.

— The gross receipts of the revenue derived from the opium trade in India were for the last year £8,324,879. The net receipts for the whole of India were in the same year £6,323,395. The total weight of the opium obtained in the same period was 12,716,991 pounds, and the total acreage in which the poppy is cultivated was returned as 521,270 acres.

LETTER FROM ENGLAND.

MESSRS. EDITORS, — When Tyndall, the retiring president of the British Association, alluded to his speech of last year, he was greeted with a round of applause which was redoubled and prolonged when he stated his opinion that the questions of "things organic and inorganic, of the mind and of things perhaps beyond the reach of mind," were to be encountered, and not avoided. It was evident that he had stimulated thought among others than the Belfast clergy. Sir John Hawkshaw, who was recommended by the government to the Glasgow authorities to help them out of their sewage difficulty, and whose name is prominently associated with the project to tunnel the Straits of Dover, had been elected as Tyndall's successor.

His address was an historical sketch of the profession of engineering, touching lightly on a great variety of subjects, and going deeply into none. He could hardly have excited a ripple of antagonistic thought in the smoothest mind, and the vexed sewage question he let entirely alone. IIis audience had been got together in so badly ventilated a hall that they were actually driven out by hundreds by the time that the address was half over. The next morning posters were put up in the reception room stating that the ventilation of Colston Hall had been improved, so that Professor Spottiswoode had a full house to see his illustrations of the "colors of polarized light;" but the improvement in ventilation was found to consist in the removal of entire windows, and men and women were to be seen moving about during the whole evening " to get out of the draughts."

In many of the sections at least half the occupants of the rooms were ladies ; many of them spoke remarkably well, and they were always listened to with great respect. In fact, the best remarks on school hygiene were made by a young lady teacher.

The greatest variety of questions have been discussed. Yesterday, alone, seventy-four papers and reports were announced to be read. (I have just received a programme of the meeting to take place in Munich, by which I see that six papers are to be read in three days.) When a paper was read on Vegetarianism as a Cure of Intemperance, the writer claiming that there is an antagonism between the two, a gentleman from Bath protested that in that case he should suggest intemperance as a cure for vegetarianism. It was quite discouraging to find the time of a section on economic science and statistics, with Dr. Farr, Dr. Beddoe, Dr. Mouat, Lord Aberdare, and Sir James Alexander on the platform, occupied by a paper by a lady on Domestic Service for Ladies. However, "economic science" is broad enough to cover everything " from Adam's fall to Huldy's bonnet." In the chemical section we have had, among a host of subjects, the Tobacco Trade of Bristol, and the Action of Ethyl Bromobutyrate on Ethyl Acetosodacetate, whatever that may be ; the report of the committee on sewage, by Corfield, is to come. Of course there were many papers showing thought and care in their preparation; but the general impression that I got was that most of the members found in "science " a pretty plaything or a nice occupation for men and women who have not much else to do, a mistake which has been encouraged, it seems to me, by some of the first names in English science, and by many others who lecture and write on Elements of Biology for Beginners, and on kindred topics. In fact, I had quite begun to ask myself wherein lay the claim of these people to call themselves an association for the advancement of science, until I heard Professor Rolleston's clear, careful, and searching analysis of the evidence by which he shows that the highly enlightened races are not degenerating ; but it was really too bad in him to say that the skull of the human female is smaller and less highly developed than that of the male. One person of few words summed up the experience of one day by saying that she had heard " a deal of nonsense talked," and another said that he thought that there was just enough science in the thing to spoil it.

That the association has done an immense deal of the kind of work that has been done by the South Kensington Museum, excellent work too, no one can doubt. The meetings of this year at least have broadened the channels of thought, but they certainly have not deepened them. There is an advantage in allowing the greatest freedom of thought, and perhaps in permitting all papers to be presented by title ; but in the reading, and in the discussions especially, where the digressions from the points at issue were most common, there would have been a decided gain to all if people had followed Virchow's cardinal maxim, and confined themselves in their observations to seeing *was wirklich da ist.*

In the museum of mechanical science the most striking inventions were those by which ladies would be enabled to travel alone in railway cars without insult, and men could do the same without fear of the Müller tragedy or of the demi-monde, and this in the last quarter of the nineteenth century. Of course the irrepressible trap was there to accomplish the impossibility of having a pipe with one open end in the sewer and the other in a sleeping-chamber, and preventing sewer-gas from getting into the house.

In contrast with the Bristol meeting, I was constantly reminded of the concise, clear, and original papers read at the meeting of the British Medical Association, in Edinburgh, a few weeks ago. Everybody was kept closely " to the point" in the discussions; and a great amount of labor beyond reading up must have been expended in preparation. A paper on dysmenorrhœa, by Mrs. Garrett Anderson, took at least three fourths of the members by surprise. She was finally allowed to read it, but the "sentiment of the association " as to repeating the experiment is to be got before the time of another meeting. The presence of Dr. Playfair brought out a large number of health officers, and the "city of lawyers and doctors" attracted much of the culture of the kingdom.

In the section of public health, Ross, Eassie, Fergus, Wanklyn, and many others gave the results of their year's study in the different branches to which they especially devote themselves. The ingenuity with which Eassie unearths hidden and forgotten cess-pools and drains is equaled by the skill with which he applies the remedies. Wanklyn concludes that the presence of organic impurities in water does not forbid its use for drinking, inasmuch as it can always be purified with sufficient care. He says, however, that large quantities of inorganic matter should always condemn water for domestic purposes, as the impurities cannot be removed at reasonable cost, and he thinks that the latter part of his proposition has been too often neglected. The questions of water-supply, water-closets, and sewers, irrigation farms, are too generally settled, and the bugbears are too thoroughly gotten over, to have provoked a very exciting discussion. The prejudice against sewage-farms may be said now to be nearly gone by. People are not made sick by eating their vegetables, the cattle flourish, the milk and butter supply the majority of the families in many places, and the effluent water is freely used for drinking. Dr. Carpenter has done much to contribute to this sensible result, especially since he had his lunch party at Croydon, where nothing was eaten except what had been grown on the farm, and from sewage as manure. If the cities are properly sewered, and the farms are properly managed, there is no offensive smell at all on the irrigation farms; and at Croydon people are building houses close to the irrigated fields.

Mr. Edwin Chadwick, a member of the first General Board of Health of England, in 1848, and whose authority on all subjects in regard to sewerage and drainage is well recognized, lately told me of one of his visits to a sewage farm. His first remark was, "The sewerage of your town is bad." "How do you know?" was the reply; "it is two miles off, and you have never seen it." "I do not need to see it," said he, "*I can smell it.*" What would he have said to Boston, with one of the finest situations in the world, with an increasing death-rate, and where one can hardly go about in August without holding his nose? London needed three epidemics of cholera, and then would hardly have learned the lesson if the members of Parliament had not been fairly driven out of their seats by the stink of the Thames. Glasgow, Edinburgh, and Dublin, Berlin, Frankfort, and Munich, have had their mortality-rate keep up in the thirties before they would learn. We can certainly be sure that there is intelligence enough in Boston not to require such fearful lessons.   C. F. F.

BRISTOL, ENGLAND, *August* 28, 1875.

WEEKLY BULLETIN OF PREVALENT DISEASES.

THE following is a bulletin of the diseases prevalent in Massachusetts during the week ending September 25, 1875, compiled under the authority of the State Board of Health from the returns of physicians representing all sections of the State: —

Coincidently with the transition to colder weather, a marked decline in the prevalence of diarrhœal disorders occurred; but there was a corresponding increase in catarrhal affections — bronchitis and influenza. Diphtheria also developed suddenly, the increase being greatest in the city of Boston and its vicinity and in the Connecticut Valley. Typhoid fever has increased. The order of relative prevalence is as follows: Diarrhœa, typhoid fever, dysentery, cholera infantum, cholera morbus, bronchitis, diphtheria, influenza, rheumatism, pneumonia, scarlatina, whooping-cough. The summary of the returns for each section is as follows: —

Berkshire: Diarrhœa, typhoid fever, dysentery, cholera infantum, cholera morbus. Diphtheria in North Adams.

Valley: Typhoid fever, diarrhœa, diphtheria, cholera infantum, cholera morbus, dysentery, bronchitis; an increase of sickness. Diphtheria (generally of mild degree) is in Montague, Shelburne, Conway, Granby, Amherst, Ashfield, Orange, Holyoke, and Springfield.

Midland: Diarrhœa, typhoid fever, dysentery, bronchitis. Fitchburg, Uxbridge, and Webster report diphtheria, in all cases mild in type.

Northeastern: Typhoid fever, diarrhœa, dysentery, cholera infantum, cholera morbus; a general decline in sickness.

Metropolitan: Typhoid fever, diarrhœa, dysentery, bronchitis, cholera infantum, cholera morbus. The cases of diphtheria are reported by physicians in Brighton, Roxbury, Charlestown, East Cambridge, East Boston, and South Boston, but not in the city proper.

Southeastern: Diarrhœa, typhoid fever, dysentery, cholera infantum. Pembroke and South Hanson report severe diphtheria.

                                        F. W. DRAPER, M. D., Registrar.

THE BOSTON SOCIETY FOR MEDICAL OBSERVATION will resume its regular meetings Monday evening, October 4, at 8 o'clock. Dr. Whittier will read a paper on Diphtheria.

CORRECTION. — In review of Engelmann on the Uterus in last week's JOURNAL, transpose the words *latter* and *former* in the first sentence.

RESIGNED AND DISCHARGED. — Thomas Kittredge, M. D., Assistant Surgeon, Second Battalion of Artillery, M. V. M.

BOOKS AND PAMPHLETS RECEIVED. — A Practical Treatise on Diseases of the Eye. By Robert Brundenell Carter, F. R. C. S. London: Macmillan & Co. 1875. (From A. Williams & Co.)

Treatment of Paralyzed Muscles by Elastic Relaxation. By John P. Van Bibber, M. D. (From Transactions of the Medical and Chirurgical Society of Maryland.) 1875.

The Normal Movements of the Unimpregnated Uterus. By Ely Van de Warker, M. D. (From New York Medical Journal.) 1875.

Transactions of the South Carolina Medical Association. Annual Session, 1875. Charleston, S. C. 1875.

Uronology and its Practical Applications. By George M. Kober, M. D. (Reprinted from the Richmond and Louisville Medical Journal.) Louisville. 1875.

The Semi-Tropical. A Monthly Journal devoted to Southern Agriculture and Horticulture, and to Immigration. Vol. I. No. 1. Harrison Read, Editor. Jacksonville, Fla. September, 1875.

Transactions of the College of Physicians of Philadelphia. Third Series. Vol. I. 1875.

A Statement of the Relations of the Faculty of Medicine and Surgery in the University of Michigan to Homœopathy. Detroit. 1875.

Transactions of the Medical and Chirurgical Society of Maryland. Seventy-Seventh Annual Session, held at Baltimore, April, 1875.

Have we Two Brains? Soul and Instinct — Spirit and Intellect. Address by the Rector of St. Mary's Church, Station, O.

Die Resultate der Gelenkresectionen im Kriege. Nach eigenen Erfahrungen von E. Bergmann. Giessen : J. Ricker'sche Buchhandlung. 1874.

THE BOSTON
MEDICAL AND SURGICAL JOURNAL.

VOL. XCIII. — THURSDAY, OCTOBER 7, 1875. — NO. 15.

NOTES ON THE CLIMATE OF THE ISLES OF SHOALS, AND OF NANTUCKET.

BY D. F. LINCOLN, M. D., OF BOSTON.

A RESIDENCE during the months of July and August at the Isles of Shoals, and an acquaintance for several years with the summer climate of Nantucket, will perhaps justify the writer in presenting the following observations.

The group called the Isles of Shoals lies about nine miles off the New Hampshire coast, opposite the mouth of the Piscataqua River, in clear sight of York, Portsmouth, and Rye Beach. The two most important islands are Appledore, with four hundred acres, and Star, with one hundred and fifty acres. Each of these islands possesses a large hotel, and both together will receive nearly a thousand guests. Both hotels furnish excellent tables, with a liberal provision of the more simple and wholesome articles of fare. The Oceanic, on Star Island, is in its third season only, and the crowd of guests is not so great as at the Appledore; its rooms are larger, its general look more modern, and its prices a trifle higher. Neither house is at all troubled by the nuisance of fashionable dressing.

The climate of the islands during the summer months is remarkably cool, and free from great variations in respect to temperature and moisture. These qualities are of course derived from the equalizing power of the surrounding ocean. A land breeze may be distinctly felt as such, but its qualities are greatly mitigated before reaching the Isles.

It is necessary to warn visitors to provide themselves with moderately thick flannels and woolen outer garments, such as are suitable for early spring wear. These are to be worn constantly, by most people ; and during the northeasterly storms, which may come even in July, a winter overcoat is needed. Last season, which was a cold one, there were several such storms ; on July 5th the thermometer ranged from 53° to 58° ; on July 12th from 56° to 62°. And it may be permitted to warn physicians that there are persons to whom, even in health, a temperature as low as that of these islands is a constant source of discomfort. An habitually sluggish circulation, accompanied with cold feet and hands, may prove a reason against the selection of this climate, especially as there are no drives to be taken, and scarcely a walk, and a sedentary life is the rule among the guests.

The only definite information concerning temperatures that I am able to present is derived from observations of my own, taken at Star Island from July 4th to the end of August, 1874, a season which was rather cold. During August the thermometer ranged for the most part between 60° and 70°; during July the variations were much greater. The greatest variation observed on any one day occurred on July 14th, when the mercury stood at 66° at seven A. M., and at 81° at six P. M.; a range of 15°. In August there were a number of days on which the range did not exceed 1° or 2°. For July the total range of temperature was 28° (namely, from 53° to 81°); for August, 21° (namely, from 56° to 77°).[1]

The monthly ranges for July and August, 1874, in Boston, were respectively 48° and 40°, or nearly twice as great.

Upon Star Island the mean daily range in July was $7\frac{5}{7}°$; in August, 7°. In Boston the corresponding figures, as given by Mr. Jonathan P. Hall[2] for thirty-six years, assign ranges of 13° and $12\frac{2}{3}°$ for July and August, respectively. Again a difference of nearly two to one in favor of the Isles is found.

These differences, though apparently small, are of great importance. Most of us are very susceptible to changes, and are in the habit of exaggerating the numerical statement of them. A difference of from 4° to 6° represents the difference between June and July weather, in the greater part of the United States at least; hence we may say, upon inspection of the following table, that the Isles of Shoals enjoy a June temperature, while Boston, Newport, and Nantucket are in the heats of July. A rise of 1° or 2° was quickly perceived by us at the Shoals, and was commonly supposed, by those who did not consult the instrument, to be a rise of 5° or 6°.

MONTHLY MEANS OF TEMPERATURE.

	June.	July.	August.	September.
Isles of Shoals		66.6	64.3	
Fort Constitution[4]	61	67.1	65.1	58.9
Fort Independence[5]	65.6	71.1	69.1	62.8

[1] Temperature was noted between seven and eight A. M., between one and two P. M., and at seven P. M., and during the few hot days my attention was frequently directed to the instrument at other times. Night temperatures, occasionally noted, showed a fall of one or two degrees between seven P. M. and midnight, or later. Thus it is probable that the absolute extremes were very nearly reached, though no self-registering instrument was used. The thermometer hung on the north side of a cottage, under a veranda, exposed to free currents of air, and protected from the direct rays of the sun.

[2] The observations were made at his house, near the head of Hancock Street.

[3] Calculated from morning, noon, and evening observations.

[4] This and the following temperatures are quoted from Lorin Blodget's Climatology of the United States, 1857. Fort Constitution is near the mouth of the Piscataqua River.

[5] Situated upon a small island in Boston harbor.

	June.	July.	August.	September.
Nantucket	63.6	71.0	68.9	63.4
Newport	65.3	71.1	70.1	63.6
Boston	65.9	71.9	69.2	61.8
Philadelphia [1]	71.5	76	73.2	63.8
Washington	73.9	76.7	77.5	68.8

The change from an inland climate, or even that of the White Mountains, to the Shoals cannot be made suddenly without some risk. I had frequent occasion to notice the fact, and several times saw more or less severe affections of the bowels brought on by this cause. As a rule, diarrhœa scarcely occurred at all among the guests, except as a result of the very grossest carelessness and excess; there seemed something in the air which predisposed to constipation rather than the reverse. As for the drinking-water, it was drawn from a rain-water cistern, and seemed to be unobjectionable. At the Appledore they use a pump standing about one hundred and fifty feet from the house ; the water varied in quality, being sometimes saltish in taste ; but its absolute purity as respects sewage-matter seems certain from the excellent and thorough system of drainage, which discharges into the sea below low water, several hundred feet away from the house. Among the young children, who are quite numerous at Appledore, diarrhœa of a mild sort has been at times frequent for a week or two together ; the causes of this I am unable to give. During the present year I believe this has not been the case. Among older people indigestion will sometimes punish those who think the sea-air will enable them to digest everything. A regulated, wholesome diet is as necessary here as at home. A dinner composed (for example) of clam-chowder, cucumbers, boiled mutton, green pease, tomatoes, corn, plum-pudding, ice-cream, watermelon, nuts, and raisins — which is not an unfair specimen — is possible once or twice, but makes an impression on the system in the long run.

The water is too cool for many persons to bathe in ; in July it ranges from 50° to 60°, but during a few of the last days of August (1874) it rose to 70°, which is a pleasant temperature. The bathing-houses are also too directly exposed to the view, being in front of the houses and near the wharves ; otherwise the pretty little inclosed basin at Appledore, containing about half an acre of water of safe depths, is decidedly attractive. The breakers never reach the bathing-places in either island. No doubt bathing would be popular if there were a good beach ; for at Rye Beach the water seems to be equally cold. Dr. A. H. Nichols has kindly placed at my service his observations upon the water at that place in 1873, from which it appears that in August the water ranged from 52° to $64\frac{1}{2}$° ; in July it was yet colder ; the observations were made at six A. M., but the water was scarcely warmer at noon.

The island of Nantucket is ten or twelve miles long from east to west,

---

[1] At the Pennsylvania Hospital.

and two to four in breadth ; it is reached by two hours' steaming in a
southeasterly direction from Martha's Vineyard. Its northern and eastern
aspects are faced with steep bluffs of sandy earth, with a narrow beach
at the foot, like those of the islands in Boston harbor. Its surface is
for the most part an open moor, or rolling prairie, covered with a scanty
dry herbage, swept by every storm, and unable to support a vigorous
growth of trees in any part except the sheltered streets of the " city."

Geologically speaking, the soil is of the drift-formation which prevails
in Southeastern Massachusetts ; it is mostly a coarse sand or gravel, or
a loam with a large mixture of sand ; in places there are strata of va-
rions sorts of clay, and at rare intervals a bowlder is seen. Peat-bogs
are common in the depressions which have served as the beds of ponds,
but of all the ponds and swamps in the island there is none which is
thought to give rise to miasma, or which is near enough to the towns (of
Nantucket and Siasconset) to be injurious to health. The nature of the
soil makes driving difficult ; the streets of the city are generally paved
with cobble-stones, and outside of the city there is not a quarter of a
mile of road where a fast horse would be of any use. Neither are there
any pleasant walks in the suburbs of the city ; for the moment one
passes from the closely-built street one comes upon the bare, brown,
turfy moor, where the roads are mere ruts through sand, and without shade. By " city " the reader is to understand the ancient and
picturesque wooden town of Nantucket, which lies on the northern side
of the island, fronting a very spacious and safe harbor ; it has now a
population of about three thousand, though built to hold ten thousand ;
there are a great many boarding-houses, and some good hotels, among
which may be mentioned the Ocean House, as deserving the confidence
of the traveler who wishes a good table. Siasconset is a pretty village
of about sixty houses, on the southeastern face of the island, seven miles
and a half from the city, with very fair accommodations, but apt to be
crowded ; Nantucket is rarely over-filled.

Nantucket city possesses by no means a cool summer climate, as
measured by the thermometer. During July and August one may expect, in four days out of five, a noon temperature of 70° to 80°, and an
evening temperature of 60° to 70°. In hot seasons it will rise frequently
to 80° or more in the hours between twelve and four, but invariably
falls after this, and scarcely ever stands above 70° in the evening.[1] This
considerable rise in the afternoon is due to the situation of the town, on
the north of the island ; the wind is generally from the south and west,
and however cool it may be upon the ocean, it becomes rapidly heated

[1] During the four years 1872–75 the thermometer in July ranged from 56° to 88°, with
one exception of 54° ; in June, from 48° to 81°, with the exceptions of 43° once and 45°
once. September has a temperature like June. These statements are made by Captain
Charles H. Colman, who observes sunrise, noon, and sunset temperatures. The coldest day
known was February 2, 1815, with 11° below zero.

in its passage of two or three miles across the open plain before reaching the town.   On one such warm day (July 7, 1875) I found the water at the south shore of a temperature of 72°, the air over the ocean being the same, and as I drove back to town the atmospheric heat rose steadily to 82°.   This excess of heat is not present at Siasconset, where the southerly breeze comes almost directly off the water; as a rule the hot part of the day is probably five degrees cooler there than in the city; in fact, day and night are both cooler there, and the air circulates better.   A part of Nantucket city is built upon high land, thirty or forty feet above the sea, and a part is quite in a hollow; the invalid will do well, in summer, to seek the higher and breezier parts, for the climate is decidedly different.

The moisture of the air is great, and, combined with the heat, makes active muscular exertion upon land an undesirable thing.   Lassitude of a luxurious sort, and a readiness to fall asleep without a particular reason, seize upon the summer visitor, whoever he may be, whether native to the island or a foreigner.   Pedestrian effort, except about the streets, is next to impossible, but sailing and rowing are pleasant, and eminently safe; sitting still is certainly better, and lying down best of all, in the indolent dog-days.   Judging from my own sensations, I should say that the air is less charged with moisture than at Falmouth, on the south shore of Cape Cod, with which I am quite familiar; at the village of Wood's Hole, in Falmouth, surrounded on three sides by water, the monthly mean of humidity for July last was 79.7, for August 86.7; but these high figures are certainly not representative of the state of things in Nantucket.[1]   The month of September and the last half of June possess a brilliant, pungent atmosphere, equally free from damp chill and from excessive heat.   East winds, by the way, are damp and chilly, as elsewhere on the New England coast, but are infrequent in the hot months.

The drinking-water is very variable in quality.   Most of it is procured from wells, and no two wells are exactly alike, some being extremely sweet and soft, but most bearing a decided brackish taint, and in some cases ·a strong flavor of iron.   It is rather common for visitors to be troubled with a slight diarrhœa, which they attribute to this cause.   It would not be amiss to bring a little claret with one.   Those who are not disturbed in this way are apt to experience constipation, which passes off in a few days with very little help from medicine, like the constipation which attends a life upon shipboard.

As repects drainage, there is none to speak of, most houses being dependent on common cess-pools; the soil is so light as to make frequent removals unnecessary.   Typhoid fever is not at all rare, though it is not so

---

[1] At Falmouth and Wood's Hole the air possesses the same power to produce languor as that at Nantucket.

frequent as to excite alarm.   In the closely-built parts of the city the pump is often in dangerous proximity to the cess-pool.   I am unable to speak of the hotels.

The bathing at the city differs from that at Siasconset in being warmer and cleaner ; freer from the *débris* of sea-weed.   The water is shallow, and in certain spots is warmed by long exposure to the sun.   I examined the water frequently from July 16th to 26th, and found at the " north shore " the water at 72° or 73° ; in the harbor, 72° to 77° ; and at Siasconset, once 67°, on a tide coming from the east, and once 70°. Neither the north shore nor the harbor has any surf; the great value of the bathing consists in the mildness of both water and air, which permits delicate persons to enter the water without a shock, and on leaving it to regain quickly their normal circulation.   Except on rainy days, which are rare, one is sure to have a brilliant sun ; fogs and clouds seldom interfere with the effects of the insolation.   In my opinion these qualities of the bathing are of very great importance.   At Siasconset, though the air is finer and more equable, the water is not so pleasant ; a strong tide-current and an undertow prevail constantly, and the break-ers are often dangerous, which circumstances, with the low temper-ature, make the bathing undesirable for delicate persons who do not " react " well.   At Nantucket there is an excellent establishment for taking baths of warmed sea-water.

Finally, we may add a word as regards the comparative sanatory value of these two places, the Isles of Shoals and Nantucket.   Both possess a sea-air of great purity, with the tonic effects proper to such an atmosphere.   But one is a cold, the other a warm air ; and it is need-less to expect benefits if patients are sent without consulting their pref-crenees as to coolness or warmth.   Both are " bracing," that is, they promote languor and sleep in many cases; and this is a very valuable quality in the treatment of irritability and sleeplessness.   Granting a fair degree of tolerance of cold, the equability of temperature at the Shoals is of great value in removing catarrhal conditions of the mucous membranes ; and nearly the same might be said of Siasconset, but hardly of Nantucket.   Granting a fair degree of tolerance of heat, the island of Nantucket, with its occasional hot-house atmosphere, its warm, unstimulating sea-baths, its freedom from the noise and excitement of the Shoals hotels, and its absolute drowsiness during the hours of *siesta,* presents advantages in the way of soothing the nerves that are superior to those possessed at the Shoals.   Siasconset is still drowsier.

In the debility of retarded convalescence from acute disease, and that arising from disproportioned brain-work, these climates are admirable. Young children thrive wonderfully, wherever they can be exposed to fresh air, upon mountain or sea-shore ; and the warmth of the climate furnishes no obstacle to their thriving in Nantucket.

In the first stage of consumption the Shoals are well known as beneficial. Positive improvement cannot be promised, but patients often
find themselves very comfortable during their stay; the decided curative effect which is obtained in our high Western regions is not to be
expected from this climate. In advanced stages the disease does badly in
both places.

It is hard to say whether rheumatism is likely to be benefited by a
visit to the Shoals. At Nantucket, the opinion is against sending cases
of rheumatism or neuralgia to be cured; rheumatic gout is common
enough, also, among the indigenes.

Hay fever is one of the complaints for which people resort to the
Shoals, and is often relieved there. A strong land-breeze, however,
brings a decided land-smell, and with it an occasional temporary relapse.
In the opinion of Dr. Warren, relief is quite general among those who
come there. At Nantucket the case is not similar.

There is plenty of evidence to show that there is nothing in a mere
residence in either place that can avert disease. Upon the Shoals consumption used to be common among the women, who lived a life of severe toil, in wretchedly ventilated houses. In Nantucket, at the present
day, one meets a fair number of goodly old men, vigorous and weather-
stained; but the women, who constitute the great part of the population, and bear their own burdens for the most part, are strikingly delicate and worn-looking; their life is also one of in-door labor, and of
close economy; they are seldom seen out-of-doors by day, and they
are rather subject to consumption. Let the invalid take account of the
influence of comfort; let him know how his room is warmed in chilly
weather, how high it is in the walls, and how freely the air circulates;
how far he has to walk to his meals; whether the meat is eatable when
he gets it; whether there is anything to do, or any people one likes to
talk to. In regard to the latter point, one has at Nantucket few strangers
except those of a very "transient" sort, but the natives are very interesting for their good nature, originality, and accessibility; at the Shoals
one finds all sorts of "city folks." There is also to be found at the
Shoals a physician, of sound judgment and ripe experience, who spends
his summers there on account of ill-health resulting from a railway
injury.

In conclusion, it appears to me that if one is decidedly uncomfortable at either place, after a week's trial, it will be of no use to stay
longer, except in case one has simply fatigued one's self with over-exertion, or with the common practice of excessive bathing.

A CASE OF TYPHLITIS, WITH SOME STATISTICS OF THE DISEASE.

BY F. GORDON MORRILL, M. D., OF BOSTON.

APRIL 3, 1875, I was asked to see A. B., a young man aged twenty-one, who was represented as being "more frightened than hurt." I found the patient in bed, and complaining of pain in the right iliac region, which was decidedly tender on pressure, and somewhat dull on percussion. The tongue was slightly coated. The abdomen was not tympanitic. There was no fever.

The history of the case was as follows : The patient returned from a journey on April 1st, and not feeling just right (his bowels having been somewhat constipated for a few days), in the evening of his arrival he went to bed after taking four " patent " pills, which purged him pretty violently towards morning. After that, he suffered from pain in the region of the cæcum, which increased steadily from the first.

I ordered one fourth of a grain of morphine, to be repeated if necessary. Lime-water and milk were prescribed on account of slight nausea.

April 4th. The pain had been relieved by the morphine, but had returned as soon as the effects of the opiate disappeared. The slightest pressure over the cæcum was very painful, and an ill-defined swelling, absolutely flat on percussion, could be detected there, apparently about the size of a large orange. The countenance was anxious. Pulse 80; temperature 103°. The nausea continued. A flaxseed poultice was applied to the swelling. The lime-water and milk were continued and the morphine was ordered, *pro re nata.*

In the afternoon, the patient was unable to pass water ; he was catheterized.

April 5th. Two distinct chills occurred last night. The patient was unable to move without producing sharp pain in the right iliac fossa. The swelling was visible on inspection. Severe nausea continued. The tongue was almost as white as snow. Pulse 140; temperature 104°. There was tenderness on the slightest pressure over almost the entire abdomen ; but it was more marked on the right side. I ordered eight leeches to be applied to the swelling. Small doses of champagne were given, and morphine as before.

In the afternoon the patient was delirious most of the time. Pulse 165, weak ; temperature 104.6°. Dr. Swan saw the patient in consultation, and agreed with me that perforation had taken place, and that the prognosis was most unfavorable. The catheter was used morning and night.

April 6th. Dr. E. H. Clarke in consultation. The patient remained about the same. The temperature was a trifle lower. The treatment was continued.

April 7th. The bowels were very tympanitic. The patient rejected everything with the exception of an occasional teaspoonful of champagne. Turpentine stupes were ordered to be applied to the abdomen. The urine was drawn morning and night.

April 8th. The patient was rational at times, and reported himself feeling better. There was less tympanites; considerable flatus had been passed. Pulse 145; temperature 103.5°. A little beef tea was retained; about one grain of morphine was taken in twenty-four hours to relieve pain. The tenderness still remained. The catheter was resorted to as usual.

April 14th. In the interval since the last report the patient had slowly but steadily improved. No tenderness remained except in the region of the cæcum, where a slight induration could still be detected. Only one fourth of a grain of morphine had been taken in the previous twenty-four hours. A considerable quantity of champagne, beef tea, and milk was taken. The patient regained control of his bladder on the 10th. Pulse 100; temperature 100°. The patient had had no movement of the bowels since the 2d; an enema was therefore cautiously given, which brought away a few small lumps of hardened fæces, followed by quite a profuse discharge a few hours later. The patient felt weak, and suffered considerable pain afterward, but slept fairly after a dose of morphine.

April 18th. Improving. Pulse 95; temperature normal. The tongue was clean but quite red. The patient had had several natural dejections since last record; takes no morphine. The induration had disappeared, but some tenderness on pressure still remained. Friends were inclined to overfeed the man, and were warned not to give him articles of food leaving a large residue, but they did not appear to understand the importance of such extreme caution when he was apparently doing so well.

April 19th. The patient was overfed the day before, and was on this day much the worse for it; he had a large and painful movement of the bowels this morning. Pulse 105; temperature 101°. Severe pain was felt in the right iliac fossa. Leeches were again applied, and the former treatment resumed.

April 24th. The patient got rapidly better after the application of the leeches and the resumption of the liquid diet; the pulse and temperature became normal, and he gained strength every day. The diet was cautiously increased, and tonics were given. On firm pressure, very slight tenderness could still be detected in the region of the original trouble.

May 6th. Except weakness, the patient was now well.

As to the particular form of typhlitis present in this case, there is of course room for doubt; but in all probability the vermiform appendix was the original seat of the trouble, and the lodgment of a foreign body its cause. This opinion is based on the following facts : Of eighteen fatal cases of typhlitis which I have collected from various sources,[1] in which the symptoms were similar to those present in the case here reported (namely, rapid development of serious illness, and sudden advent of acute peritonitis), in sixteen the appendix alone was found to be the part originally affected ; in one, both the appendix and the cæcum were involved ; in one, the cæcum alone was inflamed. In sixteen instances a foreign body was found ; in two cases no such body was discovered, although in one the appendix was described as having been dilated, and looking as if it had contained one. The appendix was perforated by ulceration in fourteen of the sixteen cases in which it alone was affected ; it was gangrenous in the other two.

Fourteen of the eighteen cases occurred among males. The average age was eighteen years, and the average duration a little more than eight days — a length of time very nearly corresponding to the period when my patient was sickest.

This appears to be the form of typhlitis which commonly occurs among young persons of the male sex, and usually proves rapidly fatal. In regard to the nature of foreign bodies which have been found in this and other forms of the disease, the following figures may be of interest: in thirty fatal cases which I have collected, a foreign body was found in twenty-seven ; in seventeen instances it proved to be a fæcal calculus ; in seven instances various substances, such as pieces of bone, nut shells, seeds (found much less frequently than I had supposed), and in one instance a bristle. In three, the nature of the object discovered could not be determined. I am not sure that we are entirely justified in calling a fæcal calculus " foreign " when it is found in the cæcum ; if it were in the appendix the term would seem more fitting. So small an object as a bristle might easily escape notice unless a most careful search were made, and my impression is that as the appendix has no known function, it is very unlikely to inflame unless under peculiar irritation ; and that if sufficient care were taken in looking for objects which may have caused trouble in cases where it has ulcerated, something, however minute, would almost always be discovered. Bartholow, who has published the most exhaustive article on this disease that I have been able to find,[2] states that of a large number of cases where the appendix had ulcerated, in one only did he fail to discover a foreign body.

In regard to the treatment of this disease, the rapid return of bad symptoms the moment indiscretions of diet were indulged in is a fact worth remembering.

[1] Transactions of the London Pathological Society, Reports of the Boston Society for Medical Improvement, The Lancet, and private practice of my friends.
[2] American Journal of the Medical Sciences, October, 1866.

The form of typhlitis in which the cæcum is the original seat of trouble appears to be far less fatal, and its course (favorable or otherwise) much more protracted, than when the appendix is affected. Of thirty fatal cases, in four only did the disease begin in the cæcum. These four cases all occurred in women ; and it is my impression that this form of the disease chiefly affects female adults, an opinion which I base upon the symptoms presented in the history of cases which have recovered, as well as of those which have ended fatally. The proverbial neglect of the sex to pay proper attention to the condition of the bowels (thereby favoring the formation of fæcal concretions) probably accounts for the liability of females to this trouble. That pure cæcitis should terminate fatally far less often than when the appendix is at fault, we can readily understand. The higher organization of the cæcum and its consequently greater recuperative powers render the chances of perforation much less than when the appendix is inflamed. Then again, if the trouble originates in the lodgment of a foreign body, its facilities for escape are far greater in the cæcum than in the appendix. A case recently occurred in the practice of Dr. Whittier, of this city, in which a head of wheat, which the patient (a woman aged fortythree) had inadvertently swallowed, after a lapse of six weeks was passed from the bowels, and the symptoms of severe inflammation of the cæcum at once subsided. Moreover, according to Bartholow, perforation very rarely takes place through the anterior wall, but makes its way through the gut posteriorly, and thus the immediate dangers arising from acute peritonitis are avoided. The appendix, on the other hand, is retained in place by a fold of the peritoneum ; and this accounts for the rapid development of acute inflammation of this membrane when the seat of the trouble is here. As a rule, cæcitis is slow in its development, and lacks the marked symptoms which are usually present in the other form of the disease. It is usually in cases of this kind that fæcal abscess occurs, ulceration of the appendix often ending fatally before pus has a chance to form or to come to the surface. Moreover, an ulcer perforating the posterior wall of the cæcum comes at once upon cellular tissue, and an abscess is very apt to be the result. That such a collection may be absorbed, and often is disposed of thus, we have abundant evidence. The pointing or rather opening of such an abscess externally is much rarer than one would naturally suppose ; in forty-two fatal cases it was observed but twice.

Bartholow states that perforation of the cæcum is of frequent occurrence without being preceded by any irritation produced by a foreign body or by fæcal accumulation, a point upon which I have been able to collect very little evidence. He terms this form of the disease " perforating ulcer of the cæcum," and states that such ulcers may be single or multiple, and that the same train of symptoms is present when the ulcer has made its way through the bowel as are produced in ulceration of the appendix. The only cases which I have been able to find at all answering his description were those in which ulcers had perforated the cæcum as a sequence to typhoid fever or dysentery, long after the illness and apparent convalescence. In two instances a single ulcer was found in the cæcum itself, and in several instances one or more in "the immediate vicinity of the ileo-cæcal valve." The careful exclusion of any previous disease which might give rise to ulceration of the intestines would certainly seem necessary before concluding that in any given case the patient died of this form of typhlitis.

Among the cases which I have collected, various anomalous ones are recorded. In two cases of disease of the cæcum, the perforation was found to be due to tuberculous deposits; and tubercles were also found in other organs. In two cases, reported by Dr. Charles D. Homans, ulceration of the appendix followed a fall, and it is uncertain how long the foreign bodies (fæcal calculi in both instances) had been present previous to the accident. That such bodies may remain an indefinite time in the appendix, and still more frequently in the cæcum, without giving rise to any appreciable symptoms, is well known. Ulceration of the sigmoid flexure is not, comparatively speaking, very uncommon. When it occurs, the same phenomena are produced as occur in typhlitis from disease of the cæcum. Four cases of this kind may be found in a single volume (xviii.) of the Transactions of the London Pathological Society. In one case of ulceration of the appendix, no tumor was discovered; the swelling being completely masked by the tympanitic condition of the abdomen.

The nomenclature of this disease compels us to use the same term (typhlitis, typhlo-enteritis) to express two morbid processes which differ widely in their fatality, symptoms, duration, and classes of people whom they respectively affect. It would certainly seem proper that a distinctive title should be invented for that usually fatal ulceration of the appendix·cæci which generally affects young people, and in the majority of cases the male sex.

A NEW METHOD OF PREPARING PLASTER OF PARIS BANDAGES.

BY EDWARD J. FORSTER, M. D., OF CHARLESTOWN.

THE common method of preparing plaster of Paris bandages by rubbing the plaster into the bandage and rolling it by hand is tedious and untidy. The plaster is scattered about, even when the greatest care is exercised, and the sensation of handling the plaster is decidedly nnpleasant. To simplify the preparation of such bandages, and to obviate the objections just mentioned, I had a tinsmith make a pan into which could be inserted the common bandage-roller. When the pan is partly filled with dry plaster and the bandage is rolled, the latter will become covered with the plaster. The pan, with the roller inserted, is well represented in the cut. D shows the sliding part of the bottom (partially drawn out to bring it into view), which tightly closes the opening through which the roller is inserted. The bandage AC is inserted under the rods and rolled a few times upon the

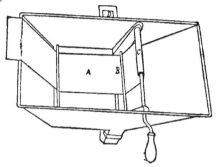

spindle to secure it, as shown in the cut. A large spoonful of plaster is thrown into the pan and upon the bandage at A, and the bandage is then rolled; by keeping it taught, the rod at B, under which it passes, distributes the plaster evenly and forces it into the meshes of the cloth. By the rolling, the plaster is applied to both sides of the cloth, and the coarser the latter is the more plaster it takes up. The ease and neatness with which a bandage can be prepared by this method was demonstrated before the Boston Society of Medical Observation, January 4, 1875.

The roller and pan can be procured of Messrs. Leach and Greene, No. 1 Hamilton Place, Boston.

RECENT PROGRESS IN THE TREATMENT OF THORACIC DISEASES.

BY F. I. KNIGHT, M. D.

Cheyne-Stokes Respiration. — The peculiarity of Cheyne-Stokes respiration, so called from the fact that Drs. Cheyne and Stokes were the first to call attention to it, may be observed in a variety of morbid conditions, especially towards the close of life. It consists in a complete pause of half a minute or longer, followed by an equally long period of respirations which are at first superficial, then increase in depth, and become even dyspnœetic; then the respiration becomes superficial again, until finally another pause ensues. I believe that Cheyne, who observed the symptom first, did not offer any theory in regard to it; but Stokes thought it to be due to fatty degeneration of the heart. Traube, however, has shown that it exists in a variety of affections, and considers it to be due to a diminution in the excitability of the respiratory centre, and thinks that the normal amount of carbonic acid is not sufficient to excite inspiration ; hence the long pause.   As more carbonic acid collects, the pulmonary fibres of the pneumo-gastric are first excited ; hence the superficial respirations.   Finally the quantity of carbonic acid in the blood is sufficient to excite the respiratory centre through the peripheral sensitive nerve-fibres also, and dyspnœtic inspirations are produced.   Through these the carbonic acid is removed from the blood ; whereupon the inspirations, on account of a gradual diminution in the irritation, become weaker and weaker, and finally cease.

Filehne [1] has tried to produce this kind of respiration experimentally, and has found not only that diminution in the excitability of the respiratory centre was necessary, but also that it should become less than that of the vaso-motor centre.   Under normal conditions the respiratory centre is first excited by a certain amount of irritation (venosity of the blood) ; then excitation of the vaso-motor centre follows through an increase in the irritation, and only by still greater increase in the irritation do those motor centres become excited from which come suffocation and hæmorrhagic symptoms.   In the case of a patient with Cheyne-Stokes respiration, no inspirations are called forth during the pause, on account of the diminution of the excitability of the respiratory centre. With an increase in venosity, the vaso-motor centre is excited, before the irritation is sufficient to excite the respiratory centre.   This causes a contraction of the small arteries and of the vessels of the respiratory apparatus, and so a diminution in the flow of blood to the same, whereby the impulse to activity in the respiratory centre is increased, so that it at length performs its function.   This reacts now to the stronger irritation, as it would normally to a weaker óne, with superficial inspirations.   With continued spasm in the vessels of the respiratory apparatus the irritation of the respiratory centre' increases, and the inspirations become deeper and deeper, and finally dyspnœtic.   By forced breathing the blood is arterialized to a high degree, and the vaso-motor centre is at length quieted. Gradually the cramp of the vessels and also the irritation of the respiratory centre diminish.   The respiration becomes more shallow, and ceases altogether as soon as the rich supply of aerated blood arrives in the lungs.   The blood now being in a comparatively well arterialized condition, a longer pause must ensue until the blood has again reached such a degree of venosity as to excite the vaso-motor centre.   Then the same process is repeated.   If Cheyne-Stokes respiration is produced in an animal by the administration of large doses of morphine and a little vapor of ether or chlorofform, at the beginning of the pause a

Berliner klinische Wochenschrift, 1874, Nos. 13 and 14; Vierteljahrsschrift für die praktische Heilkunde, ii., 1875.

normal rate of pulse is noticed ; the pulse gradually diminishes during the pause, and sometimes the heart stops altogether. Then the animal begins to breathe and the heart to beat ; the rate of pulsation increases, and at the end of the respiratory period, or at the beginning of a new pause, it is normal again. The impulse of the heart is lengthened by the venosity of the blood ; as soon as the circulation begins to stagnate, the irritation of the respiratory centre becomes abnormally great, the animal breathes, the condition of the blood improves, and the heart begins to beat again. One could thus see that the condition of the heart must have been a substantial support to the real cause of the periodic respiration.

The idea that the checking of the heart's impulse is dependent on an irritation of the vagus centre in the brain is not true ; for after cutting the two vagi, the periodicity of the heart's action ceases, and the heart beats regularly, but the periodicity of the respiration continues, and so is not dependent exclusively upon the periodicity of the heart's action. The determination of blood-pressure threw light on the periodicity of the respiration. During the pause a considerable increase in the blood-pressure occurred, up to the first shallow inspirations ; during the deep inspirations the blood-pressure sank and reached its original height at the end of the respiratory period. At the time of increase in blood-pressure the changes in the pupils which occur in suffocation were noticed. Filehne believes that the periodic obstruction of the heart and the increase of blood-pressure, as well as the periodic venosity of the blood occurring in consequence of insufficient respiration, could be soonest prevented by the employment of artificial respiration. The form of respiration depends, in his opinion, on the excitability of the respiratory apparatus, and on the acting irritation. The respiration is regular as long as both factors remain constant. Periodicity of the respiration occurs when either the excitability of the respiratory apparatus or the amount of the acting irritation experiences a periodic variation.

Traube criticises this theory.[1] He says that all cases in which Cheyne-Stokes respiration occurs have a diminished excitability of the respiratory nervous system. Consequently a greater quantity of carbonic acid is necessary to excite a respiration than under normal conditions ; so the periods lengthen during which the amount of carbonic acid which is necessary to produce an inspiration is collecting in the blood. The necessary amount will be present earliest in the pulmonary arterial system ; therefore the first efficient excitation of the respiratory nerve-centre occurs through the pulmonary fibres of the vagus. We know of these, however, that they cannot produce dyspnœtic inspiration even under the strongest excitation. If also in the

' Berliner klinische Wochenschrift, 1874, Nos. 16 and 18.

arterial blood of the body the percentage of carbonic acid becomes gradually so great that those sensitive nerve-fibres can be excited which from the skin and other parts of the body are able to stimulate the medulla oblongata into activity, there occur deep and finally also dyspnœtic inspirations. In consequence, however, of the considerable diminution in quantity which the carbonic acid suffers through the free ventilation of the air-passages, and in consequence of the fatigue which follows upon strong excitation of the respiratory nerve-centre, the inspirations soon lose their dypsnœtic character, and as the fatigue of the respiratory centre increases more rapidly than the carbonic acid which is collecting again in consequence of the want of dyspnœa, the inspirations become more and more shallow, and finally null, so that a new pause begins.

Compressed and Rarefied Air.—In a previous report we gave a description of Waldenburg's apparatus, which is too expensive and elaborate for the patient's use at his home. Dr. B. Fränkel, of Berlin, has devised an instrument which is made cheaply and can be obtained by most patients for themselves. It is described in an article recently published by Dr. Rose.[1] It consists of the bellows of an accordion. On one side a metal tube is inserted, two centimetres in diameter, which carries the mouth-piece ; the latter may consist of an inflated rubber cushion, similar to a pessary. Fränkel recommends the sitting position for using the apparatus. If the bellows is expanded by drawing the accordion apart, the air contained in it will be rarefied ; if it is compressed the air is condensed. If the patient, during the expansion or compression, applies his mouth to the cushion, the effect of the rarefaction or condensation of the air will communicate itself to the intrathoracic air. The apparatus is without valves; as it is very easy to apply or withdraw the mouth from the cushion at the right moment, any such arrangement as valves is not necessary. On the margin of the apparatus there is a centimetrical measure, which plainly indicates by how many centimetres the wooden disks are separated or brought together. This shows the volume of air which has been drawn into or expelled from the apparatus. The apparatus is thirty-five centimetres in height and sixteen in breadth. If the foldings are considered, the bottom area will be five hundred and ten square centimetres. The expansion of the apparatus of one centimetre, according to the measure affixed, would correspond with five hundred and ten centimetres of volume. Fränkel considers the attachment of the dynamometer to his apparatus as unnecessary. All excess of action is avoided, as it is worked by manual force only, Fränkel having found that with his greatest effort he could not condense the air above one eighteenth of an atmosphere, nor increase the power of suction above one twentieth of

[1] The Medical Record, August 28, 1875.

an atmosphere. The patient is sensitive to the amount of pressure and draught upon his lungs, and can regulate both according to his own feelings. Fränkel simply warns his patient against overexertion.

The apparatus is easily transported, and is applicable anywhere (for inducing artificial respiration in cases of chloroform asphyxia, asphyxia of the new-born, poison by oxide of carbon, and other similar emergencies).

(*To be concluded.*)

———◆———

ZIEMSSEN'S CYCLOPÆDIA.

In Germany the several volumes of this work have not appeared in regular succession, but those which treated of subjects of the greatest interest have been allowed to take precedence of the others. The same plan has been followed with the translation in this country, and accordingly the tenth volume of this valuable series has just been published.[1] It is a matter of regret that the American publishers should have seen fit to omit altogether the publication of the first volume (the second edition of which has been already published in Germany), or, if it is their intention to publish it later, that they did not preserve the same numbering of the volumes as was adopted in Germany.

Professor Schroeder, who has written the whole of the tenth volume, is already favorably known in this country as the author of a most excellent manual on midwifery, and this new work will therefore be received as coming from the pen of one who has already established for himself an enviable reputatien as a writer and instructor on the subject of which the volume treats.

After a few pages devoted to the proper methods of making gynæcological examinations, in which the author expresses a decided preference for the common tubular speculum, or, where operations are to be performed, for that invented by Simon, Professor Schroeder passes at once to a consideration of the diseases of the uterus. Alluding somewhat briefly to malformations, he dwells at considerable length on atresia of the uterus, and after a sketch of the various forms of hypertrophy and atrophy of that organ, he takes up the subject of the numerous varieties of inflammation which may affect the uterus. He dwells at some length on metritis and endometritis, and then passes to a consideration of the various forms of ulcers and erosions which are so frequently met with in daily practice, and the treatment of which is so troublesome. Uterine misplacements are next taken up, and about fifty pages are devoted to the various methods of treatment now recommended by eminent gynæcologists. Uterine fibroids and cancer are carefully described, and then follows a chapter on menstruation. It seems to us that, considering the importance of the subject, altogether too little space is allowed for the treatment of the latter

[1] *Cyclopædia of the Practice of Medicine.* Edited by Dr. H. von Ziemssen. Vol. X. Diseases of the Female Sexual Organs. American Edition, edited by Albert H. Buck, M. D. New York: Wm. Wood & Co. 1875.

topic. Every practicing physician is frequently called upon to treat obstinate cases of menorrhagia and dysmenorrhœa, and it is, therefore, a matter of regret that scarcely a page is given to the former subject, and only some half a dozen pages to the latter. Diseases of the Fallopian tubes and ovaries are more fully discussed by the author. As regards the origin of ovarian cystic formations, Schroeder follows to a certain extent Waldeyer, and accordingly distinguishes two kinds of cystic formation, namely, the dropsy of the Graafian follicle and the cystic tumor or cystoma. The latter he regards as a glandular new formation (adenoma), with a secondary cystic formation arising from the follicles of the ovary, while the former represents a so-called retention cyst. A careful history of the operation of ovariotomy follows, the credit of the first performance of which is given to Ephraim McDowell, of Kentucky, who operated (1809) successfully on a patient who died some thirty years after the operation was performed. As regards the treatment of the pedicle, Schroeder favors the extra-peritoneal method of securing it by means of a clamp, provided that the pedicle is sufficiently long. In other cases he advises that it be tied with catgut in several portions (the larger vessels separately), the ligatures cut short, and the stump allowed to recede. Diseases of the uterine ligaments and of the adjacent portions of the peritoneum follow, chiefly noticeable among which is a most excellent article on peri-metritis. The remainder of the volume is taken up with diseases of the vagina and vulva.

The whole work is admirably done, and is an exponent of the latest German ideas upon a most important branch of medicine. Professor Schroeder may feel well satisfied with the reception the volume is sure to receive at the hands, not only of gynæcologists, but of the profession at large. It is to be noted, however, that the work does not contain some of the recent advances made by gynæcologists in other countries beside Germany.

The translators and publishers have evidently done their best to see that the present volume is fully up to its predecessors so far as their work is concerned.

ARMY HYGIENE.

IF any proof were needed to demonstrate the scientific accomplishments of our army surgeons, and their worthiness of full recognition by their professional brethren in civil life, it might be found in good measure in the contributions to medical literature which issue at intervals from the surgeon-general's office at Washington. The Medical and Surgical History of the War of the Rebellion will at once occur to our readers as a significant illustration of this; and now we have another voluminous publication [1] which does great credit to the medical staff.

The body of the work is devoted to detailed descriptions of the army stations throughout the country, their topography, and the hygienic and endemic

---

[1] *A Report on the Hygiene of the United States Army, with Descriptions of Military Posts.* Circular No. 8, Surgeon-General's Office. Washington : Government Printing Office. 1875.

influences peculiar to them. Scattered as the army is, from Alaska to Florida, opportunity is afforded to study climatology in all its phases. In this report especial interest attaches to the observations concerning the effects of high altitudes and mountain air upon diseases of the lungs. The opinion of the majority of medical officers is that altitude and a rarefied atmosphere are not in themselves beneficial in cases of phthisis, but that it is the dryness of the air, the exercise, and the out-door life which produce good results.

Interesting as these special reports of the various posts are, and valuable also to medical officers of the army for reference, we have found greater satisfaction in the perusal of the preliminary abstract furnished by Assistant Surgeon J. S. Billings. Dr. Billings has here given a concise review of the returns forwarded from the different stations, and his comments contain many excellent suggestions bearing on the general subject of public hygiene. He discusses in turn matters relating to the habitations of soldiers, their food, their clothing, and their hospitals and medical supplies.

Upon the first point he remarks that scarcely any attention is paid to the proper sanitary construction of army barracks with a view to their effectual ventilation ; too much is left to chance and accident. He urges the establishment of bathing conveniences in connection with the quarters, and points his comments with the aphorism that " a dirty man will in most cases be a discontented, disagreeable, and dissolute man ; for the condition of his skin has much more to do with a man's morals than is generally supposed." Dr. Billings states his belief that " the service loses by death and discharge on account of overcrowded and badly ventilated barracks and guard-houses about one hundred men every year."

In discussing the topic of army rations, Dr. Billings says that " nothing can be more certain, both theoretically and practically, than that the ration *per se*, that is, without additions by exchanges and purchase, is insufficient." Comparisons are made which show a decided deficiency in the amount and quality of food according to the standard established by Parkes, Letheby, and others.

As to clothing, it is stated that great improvements have been made in the outfit of the army, both in the pattern and in material, and the articles now manufactured are more satisfactory than any which have ever been issued to the troops.

In the matter of hospital construction Dr. Billings is recognized as an expert. Therefore what he writes upon this subject is full of interest to the entire profession. He asserts that the " pavilion plan," which for a time was supposed to be a perfect panacea against all evil, has been found to furnish no security against what is called " hospitalism ; " the results of practical trial in recent wars, both in this country and in Europe, have led to the recommendation of the so-called " barrack-hospitals," that is, temporary wooden structures intended to last but ten or twelve years. Upon the matter of ventilation, the author thinks that no system which simply dilutes vitiated air will prevent the transmission of disease. So far as gases are concerned it may be effective ; but, as the real dangers of hospitalism probably arise from living solid particles, that portion of the air containing these organic substances, however few in number, will prove prolific in causing disease. Hence the prompt and complete removal of all organic poisons, " as fast as formed, is the only certain way of preventing their peculiar zymotic effects;" and no "system of hospital construction or ventilation will prevent hospitalism which does not allow of a more minute classification of cases than is now practiced, and in which ample provision is not made for the isolation of cases when needed."

Sanitarians will find many valuable hints in this paper by Dr. Billings. We commend its perusal in full appreciation of its practical merits.

PROCEEDINGS OF THE NORFOLK DISTRICT MEDICAL SOCIETY.

ARTHUR H. NICHOLS, M. D., SECRETARY.

THE annual meeting of the society was held at the Willard House, Hyde Park, May 12, 1875, the president, DR. EDES, in the chair.

The annual address was delivered by DR. F. F. FORSAITH upon The Propriety of Legislation with Reference to the Practice of Medicine. He proceeded to establish the following propositions : First, that direct legislation for the purpose of protecting the people or the profession from quackery is entirely correct in principle, the principle being recognized in the charter of our State society; while in the early history of our commonwealth there were certain statutory laws to secure its enforcement; inasmuch, however, as it has proved so difficult to carry into execution laws of this character, they are now deemed inexpedient by many of our wisest men.

Second, that a thorough education should be demanded of every medical practitioner of whatever school, a result which cannot be brought about by our medical societies, however powerful they may be, but which can be accomplished by the State alone. Such a reform is neither anti-republican nor undemocratic, but merely embodies the principle of self-protection upon which government is always supposed to act.

Third, that experience shows that the greatest success achieved both in the educational and in the practical departments of the science of medicine is to be observed in those countries in which these departments are under the especial control of the state.

Dr. Forsaith showed that in the early history of the profession in England legal protection was afforded against that horde of medical adventurers that are always ready to prey upon a credulous public. In one instance even the indorsement of Queen Elizabeth was not sufficient to cause any abatement of the stringency of the law, so as to allow an uneducated person to quietly practice her small talent, and minister to the curing of disease by means of certain simples, in the application whereof it was thought an especial knowledge had been given her.

The speaker then proceeded to show that in several of the United States cognizance is taken by the laws of attempts by irresponsible and ignorant pretenders to practice the art of healing, and he quoted the statutes now in force ·

in Tennessee and New York looking towards the suppression of irregular practitioners.

DR. GORDON, of Quincy, reported a case of intussusception occurring at the ileo-cæcal valve, and displayed the specimen. The patient was a young child. The onset of the illness was characterized by severe crying and paroxysmal vomiting, attended by a profuse discharge of loose, bloody dejecta; this was soon afterward followed by the appearance of a tumor in the left hypochondriac region, which extended to the umbilical region. Vomiting was persistent throughout the entire illness, and eventually the ejected matter became chylous, all nourishment being meanwhile declined. Death ensued in about fifty-six hours after the first symptoms were noticed.

SHOULD BOTH ENDS OF A WOUNDED ARTERY BE TIED?

AN animated discussion has recently taken place in the Société de Chirurgie upon the question of the necessity of tying both ends of a wounded artery. *L'Union Médicale* of August 31, 1875, reports that M. Lannelongue gave an account of two cases that hâd been under the care of M. Cras. The first was a wound of the brachial artery caused by the explosion of a shell; the second, that of the anterior tibial, due to a sharp instrument. In both these cases, although a ligature on the upper end of the divided vessel stopped all bleeding, yet M. Cras did not hesitate to search carefully for the lower end and to tie it, conforming to the dictum of the society, expressed when the subjcet had been at one time under discussion, that in arterial wounds it was necessary, unless some circumstance absolutely prevented, to search for both ends of the divided vessel and to tie them.

As to the practice of M. Cras in the cases under discussion, and as to the rule as laid down by the society, the reporter, M. Lannelongue, raised a question. "When," said he, the "hæmorrhage has been completely arrested by ligature of the superior end of the vessel, why interfere further? Why trouble the work of hæmostasis whose processes nature has already instituted? Granted, that the ligature of both ends of the vessel is undertaken to avoid the inconveniences and dangers of secondary hæmorrhage; who can say that such a complication would take place? Is it not time enough for interference when necessity demands it? The slight oozing of blood at the beginning of secondary hæmorrhage gives sufficient warning to the surgeon, and it is only in rare cases that frightful secondary hæmorrhages occur suddenly. Of course, when a wound has just been made it is necessary to tie both ends of the vessel when the hæmorrhage persists, but when, in a wound some hours old, bleeding does not continue, it is a wrong practice."

These views of M. Lannelongue were energetically opposed by most of the members who took part in the debate. M. Verneuil, in a previous discussion to which allusion has been made, had much influence in causing the absolute rule of surgical practice to be adopted, that of tying boths ends of the wounded vessel. He would not hesitate in such cases as those of M. Cras, without regard to the suspension of the hæmorrhage, to seek for both ends of the vessel, to stir up (*tourmenter*) the wound, to make it bleed, if necessary, until he found the ends and tied them, in the belief that it was easier for the surgeon, and less dangerous to the patient, to do this than to be obliged at a later period to search for them in a wound which had suppurated, whose tissues were inflamed and veins diseased, at the risk of provoking pyæmic complications or venous thrombosis. The rule, he holds, is an absolute one for wounds less than twenty-four hours old, even if there has been a more or less prolonged suspension of the hæmorrhage, except where the artery is of very small calibre.

MM. Maurice Perrin, Blot, Guyon, Larrey, and Giraldès supported the views of M. Verneuil. M. Desprès, while admitting the necessity of tying both ends of the divided vessel, was sustained by the authority and practice of Nélaton in the statement that a wound in full suppuration presents neither the difficulties nor the dangers intimated by M. Verneuil and others.

M. Tillaux found the rule of M. Verneuil too absolute. He instanced wounds of vessels of small or of medium size, as in wounds of the palmar arch, where compression alone has perfectly arrested hæmorrhage. M. Polaillon held similar views.

In conclusion, M. Lannelongue, not to be put down, declared that the question was yet an undecided one. We must gather more facts before making too absolute a rule, especially as the very important researches upon the cause and nature of secondary hæmorrhages, from which M. Verneuil had made his deductions, showed this accident to be due to poisoning of the blood, and to be one of the principal symptoms and manifestations of septicæmia. Now would not this very grave complication of wounds be favored by the irritation and disturbances which the surgeon would inevitably produce in determining in every case of a wounded artery, even in the absence of hæmorrhage, to disturb the wound in searching for both ends of the vessel, thoughtlessly interfering with the salutary work which nature had already begun?

MEDICAL NOTES.

— Two cases of removal of omental tumor from the scrotum, by J. F. Miner, M. D., are reported in the *Buffalo Medical and Surgical Journal* for August, 1875. The first case was that of a healthy young man who from youth had been troubled with a scrotal tumor, which had been supposed to depend upon some affection of the testicle. When an attempt was made to remove the tumor it was found to be omental. The omental mass had probably descended with the testicle in youth and had increased in size as the patient had grown fleshy. It was firmly adherent on all sides to the inguinal canal. A short ligature was thrown around the mass at the lower end of the canal, and the omentum cut away with scissors. The mass when removed weighed two and one half pounds. The patient after a somewhat troublesome convalescence returned home in about a month. The second case was less successful. It was that of a man sixty-five years old, who weighed three hundred and twenty pounds. Eight years before he consulted Dr. Miner he began to notice an enlargement of the scrotum. The various physicians whom he consulted seemed to arrive at no satisfactory diagnosis. At the time of the surgical operation the mass was found, as in the previous case, to be inclosed in a peritoneal envelope, and to be firmly adherent to the margin of the inguinal canal. A ligature was applied as high up as possible. The removed mass was several inches in length and width, and weighed three and one half pounds. In five days the patient died of peritonitis. Dr. Miner remarks that it is frequently the case that large portions of omentum have to be removed in operations for hernia, but he is not aware of a report of similar cases to the two he describes.

— A new method of performing plastic operations is recommended in the *British Medical Journal* of September 18, 1875, by J. R. Wolfe, M. D., which is certainly important if true. After stating that since the time when Tagliacozzi, published his work on plastic operations, some three hundred years ago, but little has been done for the cultivation of plastic surgery, he suggests some important deviations from the rules of the Bologna professor. The latter laid down the rule, which has ever since been considered as the primary law, and the *sine qua non* to the success of the operation, that the flap must retain its connection to the adjacent living structure by a pedicle which is to be severed only after complete union and cicatrization of the raw surfaces. This pedicle has been a source of great embarrassment to surgeons. Dr. Wolfe, from his observations on transplantation of structures from the lower animals and on skin grafting, as well as on plastic operations, has become convinced that the pedicle is not essential, if indeed it contributes at all, to the vitality of the flap. This being once established, we are henceforward free to choose the bit of skin from any part of the body we may find suitable. The chief cause of failure in plastic operations he finds to be in the subcutaneous structures. If we wish a skin flap to adhere to a new surface by first intention or agglutination, we must be sure that it is cleared of all areolar tissue, and properly fixed in its new place. The method is illustrated by the report of the formation of the lower eyelid with skin from the fore-arm.

REPORT OF SURGICAL CASES AT THE BOSTON CITY HOSPITAL.

The Aspirator in Synovitis. — CASE I. A laborer, thirty-five years of age, while working in a trench, April 21, 1875, was hit by a bank of frozen earth falling in upon him. The injury was received upon the right leg and knee. When the patient entered the hospital a few hours after the accident, the right knee-joint was found to be distended with fluid. The symptoms were pain, swelling, fluctuation, and floating patella. The upper third of the leg was severely bruised, but no fracture was discovered. All movements of the joint were very painful. The limb was placed upon a ham-splint, and an evaporating lotion applied.

The next day the symptoms were the same. A dozen leeches were applied to the joint; they drew freely. They were followed by some relief to the pain, but no decrease of the swelling.

April 25th. The distention of the sac still continuing, Dr. Ingalls punctured it with the aspirator and drew off two ounces of fluid composed of serum, blood, and fat.

May 2d. The joint having refilled, it was again aspirated, the needle entering the synovial cavity to the outside of the patella. Five and a half ounces of blood and pus were withdrawn. The character of the fluid was determined by the microscope. Compressed sponge was firmly bandaged upon the joint, and kept wet.

May 16th. The relief from the last tapping was marked and permanent. Swelling and pain were much diminished. No fluid was obtained with the aspirator on this day, although a small amount was apparently present. Compressed sponge was continued.

May 28th. There remained very little swelling in the joint. No fluid could be detected. The patient walked well, without pain; he was discharged, nearly well.

CASE II. E. P., aged sixteen years, domestic, entered the hospital April 30, 1875. Two days before, she fell, injuring her wrist and probably her left knee, although she had no recollection of having done so. When seen by Dr. Ingalls, the left knee was red, tender, swollen, fluctuating, and apparently full of fluid. The patella floated. Movements of the joint were painful. The treatment comprised the application of a ham. splint, and local blood-letting by leeches.

May 2d. The swelling remained the same. The joint was aspirated, and two ounces of clear serum, greenish and odorless, were obtained. Compressed sponge was applied to the knee.

May 4th. No swelling or pain remained. No signs of fluid on the joint. The sponge and bandage were continued.

May 6th. No swelling; the patient can move the joint freely without pain.

May 12th. The patient is walking about the ward; she has no pain or swelling in the knee.

May 17th. Discharged, well.

CASE III. April 10, 1875. The patient, a hostler, thirty-four years of age, was kicked on the right knee the evening before his entrance, by a horse which he was grooming. He walked home with assistance. During the night the knee became swollen and painful. He came to the hospital in the afternoon with his right knee-joint swollen, tender, and painful. The patella floated, and receded on pressure. No signs of fracture were found. Treatment, ham splint and evaporating lotion.

April 12th. The joint was no better. Twelve leeches were applied to the knee; it bled freely.

April 13th. Less pain and swelling.

April 18th. No pain. Swelling nearly gone.

April 24th. Patient walks without difficulty. Discharged, relieved.

May 14th. Patient was readmitted two days ago with the same joint full of fluid, and suffering .considerable pain. The synovial sac was aspirated just above and to the outside of the patella, and four ounces of sero-sanguineous fluid were removed. Compression by means of wet sponge and bandage was applied.

May 19th. No return of swelling or pain.

May 24th. The swelling has nearly disappeared. No fluid to be detected in the joint. The patient walked down three flights of stairs and out into the yard without any ill effects; he has no pain in the joint even in walking. Compression continued.

June 3d. Discharged, well.

September 23d. There has probably been no return of the affection, as nothing has been heard from the patient; he promised to report any renewal of the trouble.

Aspiration of the knee has been performed a considerable number of times in this hospital by the surgeons. The results have generally been beneficial, though sometimes transient. So far as we know, they have never been injurious.

The operation having been found to be comparatively safe, the question arises whether cases of fluid in the joints recover any sooner when treated by one or more tappings, than by the ordinary methods. M. Dieulafoy reports twenty-two cases of effusions into the knee treated by aspiration. He divides them into three classes : (1) traumatic cases cured by from one to three aspirations, occupying from three to eight days; (2) acute hydrarthroses, rheumatic, etc., which require from four to six punctures during a week or fortnight; (3) old cases of dropsy of the joints, which sometimes require two· aspirations daily. "They are generally cured in the third week." Most of the noted French surgeons who took part in the debate upon this report of Dieulafoy's strongly opposed the treatment by puncture and aspiration of all kinds of hydrarthroses, except in some chronic cases where the fluid had been present over two months. They claimed that the operation was not always safe, and that a large majority of these affections could be cured as quickly and easily by the ordinary methods as by aspiration. And, furthermore, "that in a procedure possessed of so little efficacy as M. Dieulafoy's, even rare accidents ought entirely to proscribe its employment."

Whether there be a tinge of professional jealousy in this wholesale denunciation of joint-aspiration, it is not for us to determine. But the operation has been done times enough in this hospital to show that it is often beneficial, and very seldom if ever injurious. It will be noticed that the time required for a sufficient recovery in the above cases to allow the patients to resume their occupation was seventeen, thirty-seven, and fifty-four days respectively. The second case was well fifteen days after the single tapping; an unusually quick recovery. Twelve days after the single aspiration the third patient walked down three flights of stairs and up. again without any pain or difficulty. Such results rarely follow the usual modes of treating these acute joint affections. Six or eight weeks are often required to get a patient with acute synovitis upon his feet, and even then a small amount of fluid or enlargement of the joint is apt to remain.

It seems reasonable to suppose, and the above cases tend to show, that when the process of effusion has nearly or quite subsided, and absorption is slow in its progress, removing the fluid from the joint with a small, hollow needle hastens the recovery. That merely puncturing a joint stops the secretion of the synovial membrane is by no means proved; and moreover, relapses are probably as frequent in cases treated by aspiration as in any others. Yet the operation is a valuable addition to our methods of treating effusions of fluid into the knee-joint. It is safe. It hastens recovery in many cases. It may be used in acute as well as in chronic cases, whatever may be the character of the fluid in the joint. And it may be repeated as often as necessary.

GEORGE W. GAY, M. D.

WEEKLY REPORTS OF PREVALENT DISEASES.

MESSRS. EDITORS, — Three principal objects are evidently aimed at in these weekly returns. One is the deciding of the points at which certain diseases originate; the second is in great degree dependent upon the first, the investigation of the causes of disease; the third, dependent upon the other two, is the prevention of diseases. There is a fourth and most, excellent reason for publishing these reports, not only in medical but in popular journals: namely, to relieve the unnecessary fears of the public.

It would be well to call the attention of the public to these reports in some very positive manner, as it would go far towards quieting uneasy imaginations and forebodings. Our profession is constantly informed that scarlet fever is raging in this town or that, and that the schools are shut in another community because of the great prevalence of cerebro-spinal meningitis. Twice within a week I have been informed of the great prevalence of diphtheria in Boston and in Swampscott. In looking over the weekly report of prevalent diseases, however, I find the following as its closing sentence: "In the whole State, all the diarrhœal affections, together with typhoid fever, have increased; *all the other diseases have declined.*" This not being satisfactory to the person with whom I was looking it over, because diphtheria was not mentioned, and it was "*probably* only on the decline," we went over the report concerning different sections of the State. To our surprise we read, "The order of relative prevalence of acute diseases in the State at large is as follows: diarrhœa, cholera morbus, cholera infantum, dysentery, typhoid fever, rheumatism, scarlatina, whooping-cough, bronchitis, *diphtheria*, influenza, pneumonia, measles, — *the prevalence of the last five* being scarcely worth mentioning."

It is worthy the attention of the public to know how these reports are made up. They are useful to us professionally, and the public may make them useful also. Medical men in nearly every city and town in the State, hundreds in all, are furnished with blanks, which on Friday night in each week they fill out with the names of the acute diseases prevalent in their respective neighborhoods. and mark them as " mild " or " severe," in different columns. These reports are on Saturday transmitted to Dr. F. W. Draper, the registrar, who draws up the bulletin as published every week. The State, according to his report, is divided into sections, as follows; Berkshire, Valley, Midland, Northeastern, Metropolitan, and Southeastern ; and any one who is interested in knowing the truth from reliable reports would do better to read these weekly returns than to listen to the croakers, who are about as numerous as the diseases.

But looking at the report of Dr. W. L. Richardson, the Acting Secretary of the State Board of Health, for the same week, which precedes Dr. Draper's bulletin, and which is the report of the *deaths* from prevalent diseases in the State, I find the name *diphtheria* is not mentioned. This disease cannot therefore be very abundant. In this opinion I am confirmed when I see that he has thought it important to say that in the whole State there were " six deaths from cerebro-spinal meningitis ; from cholera infantum (seventeen cities) 147 deaths ; from consumption (thirteen cities) 53 deaths ; from diarrhœa (nine cities) 25 deaths ; from dysentery (eight cities) 23 deaths."

It would be well for people to quiet their fears by reading these weekly reports, and exercising their reasoning powers upon the other reports. When they hear that there have been six or eight fatal cases of typhoid fever in a certain street, they would do well to remember that in that street is probably the cause of the disease. It proves nothing against the health of the city in general, nor against that of the State at large, when they hear that a certain physician is having under his care so much dysentery that he is seeing nearly a hundred cases a day. They would do well to calculate how long it takes the poor fellow to go from house to house to see a hundred, and pity the poor people who are forced to employ such a hard-pressed doctor that without allowing himself time to eat, drink, or sleep, he has but fourteen minutes and forty seconds for each. They would do well to relieve him of a part of his burdens if he claims to be so busy, for he certainly must neglect his other cases.

There is a foolish habit of calling every red skin scarlatina, and every little soreness of the throat diphtheria, and every little headache cerebro-spinal disease ; and there are men in the medical profession who encourage the habit. They probably have an object.

Charles E. Buckingham, M. D.

Boston, *September* 9, 1875.

———◆———

WEEKLY BULLETIN OF PREVALENT DISEASES.

The following is a bulletin of the diseases prevalent in Massachusetts during the week ending October 2, 1875, compiled under the authority of the State Board of Health from the returns of physicians representing all sections of the State : —

. Only two diseases can be said to be prevalent in the State at large — typhoid fever and diarrhœa ; both are mild in type, and are declining. The subsidence of cholera infantum, cholera morbus, and dysentery has been remarkably sudden and noteworthy. Diphtheria is somewhat less prevalent than it was a week ago; it is most common in the Connecticut Valley, in the vicinity of Boston and in the city itself, and upon the Cape, avoiding the high lands of Berkshire and of Worcester County. Under the various designations of " influenza," " acute nasal catarrh," " autumnal catarrh," " colds," and " bronchitis," very many towns and cities report the presence of an epidemic catarrhal trouble; it is most common in the eastern sections of the State, but extends somewhat into the midland and western districts ; several observers note the coincidence with it of the epizoötic catarrh. The summary for each section is as follows : —

Berkshire: Typhoid fever, diarrhœa, cholera infantum.

Valley: Typhoid fever, diarrhœa, rheumatism, dysentery, influenza. Remittent fever in Springfield.

Midland: Diarrhœa, typhoid fever, rheumatism, pneumonia, bronchitis, dysentery, influenza.

Northeastern: Typhoid fever, diarrhœa. Very little sickness.

Metropolitan: Diarrhœa, typhoid fever, bronchitis, influenza.

Southeastern: Typhoid fever, diarrhœa.

In the State at large the order of relative prevalence is as follows: Typhoid fever, diarrhœa, bronchitis, dysentery, influenza, cholera infantum, diphtheria, cholera morbus, rheumatism, pneumonia, scarlatina, whooping-cough, croup; all are low in the scale except the first two.

F. W. Draper, M. D., Registrar.

COMPARATIVE MORTALITY-RATES FOR THE WEEK ENDING SEPT. 25, 1875.

	Estimated Population.	Total Mortality for the Week.	Annual Death-Rate per 1000 during Week.
New York	1,060,000	568	28
Philadelphia	800,000	257	17
Brooklyn	500,000	266	28
Chicago	400,000	179	24
Boston	342,000	196	30
Cincinnati	260,000	97	19
Providence	100,700	47	24
Worcester	50,000	19	20
Lowell	50,000	23	24
Cambridge	48,000	17	18
Fall River	45,000	37	43
Lawrence	35,000	23	34
Lynn	33,000	18	28
Springfield	31,000	11	18
Salem	26,000	8	16

Normal Death-Rate, 17 per 1000.

THE BOSTON
MEDICAL AND SURGICAL JOURNAL.

VOL. XCIII. — THURSDAY, OCTOBER 14, 1875. — NO. 16.

" A CASE OF EMPYEMA TREATED BY FREE INCISION.[1]

BY C. L. HUBBELL, M. D., OF TROY, N. Y.

WITHIN the last few months, in reading a number of the JOURNAL, I saw a communication by Dr. John G. Blake, of Boston, which was read before the Boston Society for Medical Observation, entitled Treatment of Empyema by Permanent Openings in the Chest. Four cases were reported, three of which were successful, and it was afterwards ascertained that in the unsuccessful one the failure was not attributable to the operation or the disease. I was so impressed with the practicability of the operation, nay, the necessity of it in many cases, that I then resolved to employ the method at the earliest opportunity in my practice.

On the 10th of January last I was called to see a little girl, between three and four years of age, who with her twin sister had the week before gone through an attack of measles without medical attendance. I found a severe case of pleuro-pneumonia of the left side, involving the entire lung, which, as a sequel of the measles, had been going on unchecked for three or four days.

The more acute inflammatory symptoms subsided in the course of a week, but it was evident that all was not right with the little one, and I feared permanent damage to the lung. So much improvement was manifested, however, that I ceased attendance, having placed the patient on tonics, with milk diet and cod-liver oil. During the next two months I saw the child occasionally, and at times there seemed to be an improvement in her symptoms; at all events she was no worse. But early in April I felt satisfied that the case was one of empyema. There was no bulging of the intercostal spaces, but there was universal dullness over the left side, and entire absence of respiration. The cough was incessant day and night; the appetite was failing; there were night sweats, and occasional attacks of dyspnœa. I urged an operation to the parents as the only means of saving their child, but they were "afraid she was too young to stand it," and desired me to postpone surgical measures, to see if she might not yet improve.

[1] Read before the Rensselaer County Medical Society, May 11, 1875, by C. L. Hubbell, M. D., President.

She steadily failed, however, and on the 24th of April colliquative diarrhœa set in, lasting two or three days; the emaciation had become extreme, the feet and ankles were œdematous, the pulse was 170, and the countenance began to look death-like.   The parents having at last consented to an operation, assisted by Dr. H. B. Whiton I removed by the aspirator eight ounces of thick pus, all that would come through the needle of the instrument.   The diagnosis was now confirmed ; the night following was the best the patient had passed in a long time, and the next day she appeared much brighter, though feeble.   I felt the more anxious now to do all that ought to be done, although the condition of thê child, after so long a delay, was a very unpromising one for any operative procedures.   By the 30th of April, six days after the use of the aspirator, symptoms had become very urgent again, and after having administered ether, assisted by Dr. George H. Hubbard, I made a free incision into the cavity of the chest, a little more than an inch and one half in length, in front, and near the lower angle of the scapula.   More than a pint and a half of somewhat fœtid pus was discharged ; the position of the patient was changed, and with the aid of a canula the pleural cavity was thoroughly evacuated.   The night following this operation was passed very comfortably, and the next day the pulse fell from 170 to 140.   By means of an oakum tent, which at the same time facilitated drainage, the opening was prevented from closing.

May 2d, I again introduced the canula, and got two or three ounces of thick, laudable pus, evidently an improvement on that of a few days previous.   Then, having adjusted a double silver catheter in the opening, and a syringe being nicely fitted to one tube, I injected one quart of warm water at a temperature of 98°, with a few drops of carbolic-acid solution in it.   In a few moments the fluid began to run out just as clear as when it went in, and it was evident that such thorough rinsing and cleansing of the diseased, pus-secreting pleural surfaces must be attended with great benefit.   I should have added that in consequence of the irritable condition of the child ether was administered, and that I was assisted by Dr. H. B. Whiton.

The day succeeding this injection was passed in great comfort; the pulse had fallen to 128 ; the appetite was enormous ; the diarrhœa had ceased, and the little one for the first time played some with her doll. After the date of the first injection the syringing was repeated at intervals of a day or two, and the improvement was steady and marked.

I think within a week from the present date, May 11th, the opening can be safely allowed to close.   No ether is now administered, nor is any tube left in for purposes of drainage.   At one time I placed a short double gum elastic bougie in the wound, thinking to leave it and inject through it ; but I soon found the annoyance from its presence was much greater than from the daily introduction of the catheter.   Dr. Blake reports that, in one of his cases, he fastened in the wound a tube made somewhat after the pattern of a tracheotomy tube, but that it was abandoued in a day or two.

I think there can be no doubt as to the propriety of these operations, and I venture to predict that the time will soon come when it will be considered a far more criminal matter to neglect such practice when the great cavities of the body with their vital organs are involved, than to omit the evacuation of pus from superficial abscesses, which we always agree should be done as soon as the presence of pus is diagnosticated. Now that we have the aspirator, that harmless but life-saving instrument, as an aid in diagnosis, there is no excuse for not doing all that should be done. Physicians have always feared the admission of air to serous surfaces, and we were taught the importance of making a valvular incision in performing the operation of paracentesis thoracis in order to avoid atmospheric contact, but it is found now that the largest percentage of success in ovariotomy is obtained where free and complete drainage is established, thus avoiding septicæmia and peritonitis.

NOTE. — At the present date, August 17th, the little patient whose case is here related is apparently in perfect health, and the respiratory murmur is clear and distinct over the whole lung. In conclusion, I will only say that the lesson taught me by this case is to recognize early the presence of pus in the thoracic cavity after pleuro-pneumonia, and then at once to evacuate it, and keep the cavity drained and cleansed until it is evident that a healthy action is restored. The narrow escape from death in this instance demonstrated to me that many valuable lives might be saved by employing seasonably this means for their safety.

A COMPLICATED CASE OF LABOR.

BY J. O. MARBLE, M. D., OF WORCESTER.

AT half past six A. M. of September 17, 1875, I was called to attend Mrs. K., aged thirty-four, in her fourth pregnancy, in labor about an hour. I was speedily at her side, having attended her in a very rapid labor less than two years previously. I found her walking about, with severe pains; she said that she " knew something was wrong," and that a deluge of water had just escaped from her. I had her bed prepared, and after much urging persuaded her to lie down. On making a vaginal examination I found the os fully dilated and a soft mass presenting, which I at first took to be a shoulder. Making further exploration I distinctly felt a head lying to the left of the soft mass, and firmly pressed against it. A little further manipulation convinced me that I had to deal with a twin labor, and that the soft mass was a breech. Remembering the increased danger to the child when the first of twins is delivered by the breech, I introduced two fingers of my hand into the vagina and attempted to press back the breech, and so to allow the head to engage; but my efforts were vain, for at the moment a violent contraction of the uterus drove the breech through into the vagina, and two more expelled the body of the child as far as the shoulders. The uterus then relaxed, and no pain recurred for several minutes. In making traction upon the body of the child I found the head as firmly held as if in a vise. There was already little pulsation in the cord, and the extremities were becoming blue. A large quantity of meconium was passed. Feeling the necessity of speedy delivery, and believing the heads to be locked together, that of one lying beside the neck of the other (as in the case described in the last edition of Cazeaux[1]), I insinuated my hand along the chest of the child up to the second presenting head, and, as the pains fortunately were now entirely suspended, succeeded in pushing it back, at the same time making strong traction with the other hand upon the body of the partially delivered child. I then succeeded in passing one of the fingers, with which I had pressed up the second head, into the mouth of the other, drew its chin close upon its chest, and, imitating nature in making rotation as far as possible, had little further difficulty in delivering the fœtus. The child appeared to be dead, but by the usual means it was soon made to gasp, and then to cry lustily.

While I was occupied in its resuscitation a single powerful contraction brought the second child into the world, enveloped in the amnion, having "taken the veil" along with it. I ruptured the amnion, which contained about four ounces of fluid, and to my surprise the diminutive thing cried out sharply, though feebly. The first child weighed nine and three quarters pounds; it was remarkably well developed and of a healthy pink color. The second weighed scarcely five pounds, and was covered with the thickest coating of vernix caseosa I have ever seen; it had the most ludicrous pinched and old expression of face. Both the children were females. The placenta was common, with the two cords at about equal distances from centre and circumference; its diameter was nine and a half inches. There was no difference apparently in its sides, and one child's source of supply appeared as good as that of the other. The same chorion embraced them both, but each had its own amnion.

The circumference of the head of the larger (corresponding to the sub-occipito-bregmatic diameter) was thirteen inches; that of the smaller ten and a half. The mother's pelvis is very capacious. The three patients are now perfectly well, the pygmy rapidly gaining on her larger sister.

[1] Page 865.

RECENT PROGRESS IN THE TREATMENT OF THORACIC DISEASES.[1]

BY F. I. KNIGHT, M. D.

Peripleuritic Abscess. — Bartels[2] reports the following cases and remarks :

CASE I. The patient was a sailor twenty-five years of age, who contracted syphilis at nineteen. Eight weeks before his admission to the hospital he had a severe chill, and was delirious several days. This was followed by a moderate amount of pain in the right chest, dyspnœa, cough, and expectoration, the patient feeling himself quite sick. During the latter part of the time, the right half of the chest was more distended, the dyspnœa less, and the appetite better. On the patient's admission to the hospital, June 1, 1872, there was complete aphonia occasioned by paralysis of the left recurrent nerve. He was anæmic, with a slightly cyanotic appearance ; he was feverish, and suffering from dyspnœa ; his temperature was above 39° C., his pulse above 120. The right side of the chest was almost motionless, and flattened above ; but below, especially in the middle, it projected. The fifth and sixth ribs were the most prominent, and over them the soft parts were œdematous. The fifth intercostal space was strikingly wide, whilst the upper ribs were crowded closely together. In the fifth intercostal space one could distinctly feel deep fluctuation, and in this situation the tension of the soft parts was diminished by every inspiration, and clearly increased by every expiration. The right half of the chest measured about three centimetres more than the left. Percussion gave flatness over the lower part of the right chest, the upper border of which ran horizontally in the third intercostal space, but sank towards the back. Above the dullness there was weak tympanitic, and above the clavicle normal resonance. There was no vocal fremitus where flatness existed ; but above, the vocal fremitus was stronger than on the opposite side of the chest. Auscultation on the right gave laryngeal respiration above, and some ringing râles, and in the region of the dullness indeterminate respiration. The left lung was normal. The heart was normal in position and sounds, but there was pericardial friction râle at the left edge of the sternum. Under the cartilages of the ribs on the right, the edge of the liver was felt to be indurated. There seemed to be no doubt that there was a collection of pus under the ribs on the right side. The line of the dullness and the absence of displacement of the neighboring organs spoke against a purulent pleural exudation. And yet the pus was inside the chest-wall and above the diaphragm ; for the

---

[1] Concluded from page 421.

[2] Deutsches Archiv für klinische Medicin, xiii. 1 and 2 ; Vierteljahrsschrift für die praktische Heilkunde, 1875, ii.

tension of the abscess-wall diminished with every inspiration and became greater with every expiration.   The diagnosis of peripleuritic abscess was made and immediately confirmed by an exploratory puncture.   The canula could be freely moved in the cavity of the abscess, but met with resistance at a depth of three centimetres.   A pustular elevation developed afterwards at the place of puncture, which opened itself, and discharged healthy-looking pus.   Later, the pus became profuse and offensive.   After widening the opening and resection of a piece of rib, extensive burrowing of the abscess was found.   By antiseptic treatment, the pus-formation was improved, and the general condition continued tolerably good.   Towards the end of August, dropsy appeared, and in the urine, which was scanty, white blood corpuscles and cylindrical casts were found.   The dropsy increased rapidly, the pus became offensive again, profuse diarrhœa followed, and the patient died December 1st.

The autopsy showed extensive peripleuritis on the right side with perforation outwards ; compression and chronic interstitial pneumonia of the right lung ; parenchymatous nephritis ; concretions in the pelvis of the kidney ; syphilitic orchitis of both sides ; anasarca ; hydrothorax on the left side ; and obliteration of the pericardial sac.

CASE II. A man twenty-five years of age was taken sick in the middle of October, 1872, with a chill and pain in the left chest.   Four weeks afterwards a large amount of pus was evacuated by an incision in the fifth intercostal space (in the axillary line).   On admission, December 12th, the front of the left chest from the second to the fifth rib protruded, and the skin here was œdematous.   In the axillary line there was a fistulous opening, through which a sound could be passed behind the fifth rib, downwards, to the extent of five centimetres.   The left half of the chest participated but little in the respiratory movements.   Percussion gave clear resonance in front down to the third rib, and dullness from here to the fistulous opening.   Below this and throughout the back the percussion sound was quite normal. Indeterminate respiration was heard over the region where dullness existed ; everywhere else the respiration was vesicular.   In the urine were found albumen, numerous casts, red and colorless corpuscles.   Whilst the fistula grew smaller, the fever continued and the œdema increased.   At the end of December a fluctuating tumor formed upon the sternum, and on the 4th of January a distinct fluctuation was noticed deep in the fourth intercostal space.   The abscess over the sternum was opened, and a communication of the two abscesses was established by the introduction of a female catheter behind the fourth rib, and the opening of the fourth intercostal space at the prominent point.   A drainage tube was now introduced, and rapid recovery followed.   The patient was discharged February 25th.   The thorax was normal in shape, and percussion and auscultation gave normal sounds, except that the edge of the upper lobe of the left lung had lost its mobility over the pericardium during respiration.

CASE. III. A girl ten years old had been maltreated in anger by her mother, and presented on examination, October 1, 1872, a fluctuating tumor of the size of a two thaler piece, under the right shoulder-blade near the spinal column. It projected about one centimetre above the surrounding skin. The tumor became more tense with every expiration, more relaxed with every inspiration. There was dullness over the tumor ; everywhere else the percussion sound was normal. The child also had hip-disease. She died October 12th.

The autopsy showed purulent coxitis, ulcerative endocarditis, embolic infarctions in the spleen, kidneys, and other places. The lower lobe of the right lung was pushed forward, compressed by an incapsulated purulent pleuritic effusion. Opposite the ninth rib on the right, about five centimetres from the spinal cord, was a round opening in the pleura costalis. At the bottom of this lay the ninth rib bare of periosteum, and the pleura costalis was separated from the ribs.

Bartels says that in the first two cases there appeared no sufficient cause to explain the extensive superficial inflammation of connective tissue poor in vessels and nerves. In the third case the cause was traumatic. According to observations hitherto made known, subpleural abscesses have little tendency to rupture inward. In the latter case, however, this occurred. The frequent complication of peripleuritis with diffuse inflammation of the kidneys, which seldom seems to exist with extensive purulent cellular inflammation elsewhere, is worthy of mention. In the first case there was some danger of confounding it with empyema; but empyema pushes the ribs out symmetrically, and stretches the intercostal spaces symmetrically. Peripleuritic abscess leads more quickly to purulent infiltration of the intercostal muscles, and causes thereby a marked separation of two ribs, whilst the upper ribs seem more crowded together. The figure of the dullness differs in the two cases. Peripleuritic abscesses evidently follow in their development other laws than those of gravitation. The entire absence of any displacement of neighboring organs (liver and heart) is of special importance in the diagnosis of peripleuritic abscess. In all the cases observed by Bartels, fluctuation of the pus in the intercostal space, and a relaxation of the abscess-wall during inspiration and a greater tension of it during expiration, were noticed. These appearances are wanting in pleuritic effusion, and fluctuation occurs only if there has been perforation of the costal pleura. The specific gravity of the pus is greater than that from empyema.

The prognosis, as far as can be judged from the reported cases, is not favorable, inasmuch as of eight patients only two got well, two partially recovered, and four died.

With reference to the treatment, Bartels recommends early opening of the abscess; for the earlier this is done the less danger is there of its breaking through the costal pleura, of its affecting the pericardium, of a secondary affection of the kidney, or of pyæmia, and so much the sooner, finally, will a limit be put to the strength-consuming influence of the accompanying fever.

Bartels recommends a free incision, and, in case of a burrowing of the pus, several incisions.

On the Physical Cause of Presystolic Murmurs. — Dr. A. H. Carter, of Birmingham,[1] replies to the doubts of Dr. Harvey, of Aberdeen,[2] in regard to the physical cause and even existence of the so-called presystolic murmur. Dr. Carter insists very strongly upon the existence of a mitral murmur at the end of diastole, which terminates abruptly with the first sound. It seems to us very strange that any clinical observer can doubt the existence of such a murmur, and there is every reason to suppose, as Dr. Carter maintains, that there is strength enough in the contraction of the left auricle to cause the murmur as it forces the blood through a contracted auriculo-ventricular orifice.

A CASE OF HYSTERIA IN A MAN.

BY DR. BONNEMAISON.

Translated from Archives Générales, June, 1875.

BY T. W. FISHER, M. D.

In the month of June, 1874, I was called, with my excellent friend Dr. Ramond, to see M. G——, aged seventy-two years, a bachelor, who suffered from attacks of a peculiar character, and was much alarmed at his condition.

M. G—— is a large man, erect, with a keen eye, an expressive countenance, and a dry and nervous constitution. He received us in the most friendly manner, and hastened to make known in a connected way, with many circumstantial details, the symptoms which his case presented, even to its pathological and physiological antecedents. We knew already, and he himself confirmed the fact, that his mother, who died at the age of eighty-one years, after having enjoyed until her seventy-sixth year the most perfect health, suffered from that time almost without interruption a series of nervous attacks very similar to those which the patient himself presented. Madame G—— died of bronchitis, and had neither paralysis of any kind nor intellectual disturbance other than such as will be described in the case of M. G——.

---

[1] The Lancet, August 7, 1875.
[2] The Lancet, June 12 and 19, 1875.

A brother of the patient, aged seventy-eight years, has been bed-ridden for two years, and a prey to the torments of hypochondria, from which nothing diverts him. The voluntary immobility to which he has condemned himself has induced a visible atrophy in the muscles of his body and limbs. Intelligence and memory are intact, but the least emotion or contradiction is sufficient to excite him beyond his self-control, so that he speaks in a broken yet rapid manner. The words come easily, and always express his meaning ; they usually consist of com-plaints, reproaches, and manifestations of fear on account of his disease. All the functions of nutrition are well performed, though sluggishly. There is no trace of paralysis. There exists a single painful point, sometimes very sensitive, at the centre of the occiput.

M. G——, after having many times interrupted his narration with moans, sighs, and ill-concealed impatience, came to his own case. He told us that twelve years ago he experienced for three years three or four attacks daily. In the night they usually began with nightmare ; during the day they were preceded by different sensations, especially by pain at the pit of the stomach. There was at this time no sensation of arterial or cardiac pulsation ; neither dyspnœa nor suffocation. The epi-gastric aura then ascended along the sternum to the throat, glottis, and mouth. A kind of irresistible convulsion occurred in the muscles of the parts traversed by this aura or vapor, and the patient cried out, barked, or mewed for some minutes.

At other times the convulsions seized the muscles of the larynx and mouth, at the same time with the hands and arms, and the patient re-peated many times in succession, " Rantanp'an, rantanplan," and also performed with his arms rhythmic movements, as if beating a drum. Under other circumstances he began dancing vigorously, sometimes without any provocation, at others impelled by the sound of an organ in the street, or of some other instrument. At church, when the organ played, M. G—— shed copious tears. These attacks, during all of which consciousness was preserved, lasted from a quarter of an hour to an hour, and ended by an abundant emission of clear and limpid urine or by a flood of tears. M. G—— never experienced any sexual feel-ing, and the genito-urinary organs did not appear to have the least in-fluence on his condition. The attacks were followed by no serious fa-tigue, and he was able to resume his ordinary occupations. He was irritated on account of not having been able to control his movements, and of not having exerted as much will as his perfect intelligence seemed capable of.

All his functions were performed well in the intervals. Nutrition was never altered, his movements were correct and well coördinated, his mind was active and well balanced. He could not explain his state, and looked in vain to his past history for anything of a pathological nature ; rheumatism, gout, diabetes, albuminuria, syphilis, venereal or other excess had never existed.

Under a skillful physician he pursued the hydropathic system with unusual persistence, which had no other result than to excite his nervous system, and to increase the violence and duration of his attacks ; but two seasons at Ussat les Bains produced an improvement, and later a complete cure, which lasted till the month of March, 1874.

At this date M. G——, who enjoyed perfect health and had even gained flesh, though still retaining an extreme emotional sensibility, to which his friends had learned to accommodate themselves, was seized with a bronchitis, without fever, which fatigued him excessively, and exhausted him. It also disturbed the equilibrium of his stomach and nervous system. Gastric disorders followed, — flatulence, constipation, and above all gastralgic pain and cramps; still the appetite was never absolutely lost, and the patient willingly took food, but digested it imperfectly.

The epigastric pain became more severe, especially after meals, though digestion did not become more difficult ; and after the month of April this neuralgia, which M. G—— compared to the clavus hystericus, changed to an aura which rose along the sternum and sides to the neck, glottis, pharynx, mouth, and jaws. An attack followed in which all the muscles traversed by the aura were affected. The diaphragm contracted spasmodically, as well as the glottis; this produced hiccough, eructations, sighs, and strange outcries. The buccinator muscles were convulsed as in the action of blowing or whistling. The tongue clacked against the roof of the mouth, and the lower jaw was convulsed in its turn so as to strike the teeth together without touching the tongue. One would have said the patient was about to bite violently any object which was presented ; it was not so, however, and if one put a finger between his teeth he remained with open mouth by an effort of will.

Sometimes the attacks were accompanied by movements of one or both of the arms. The fingers played the piano or beat the drum. The arms and forearms acted methodically, as if imitating the movements of the wings of a bird ; or they were lifted up, with shrugging of the shoulders, accompanied by outcries and hiccough. At other times the legs and knees were struck together, or the body moved rapidly, particularly from left to right, and finally dance movements, more or less rhythmical, occurred. All the phenomena were sudden, convulsive, and irresistible, whatever effort the patient made. In the midst of this muscular disorder convulsions of the muscles of phonation occurred, and we heard many times in succession the same word, which the patient pronounced distinctly but very quickly, without being able to prevent it. He repeated, for instance, with inimitable volubility, "Pygmalion, Pygmalion, Jean, Jean, Jean, Ramond, Ramond, potage,

potage, chaise, chaise." He knew what he was saying, but spoke
without being impelled by any idea or recollection or want which he
wished to make known. It was an automatic, unreflecting, convulsive
phonation, which expressed nothing, and the patient had nothing to
express ; moreover, no act or movement occurred to explain the meaning of the word so often repeated. If soup were offered him, M. G——
did not want it ; if he was given a chair he refused it ; if the person
designated approached, he exclaimed, " Rien, rien, rien."

It was only. when the attack was well under way that this need of
using words without ideas was felt. At the beginning, when the epi-
gastralgia was in all its intensity, before the aura ascended, or while it
was rising, M. G—— remained often as if in a state of ecstasy, his eyes
fixed, his mouth open, entirely speechless. If, however, he was asked
about his feelings, he would reply, " Oh what pain ! what suffering !
what anguish ! " The charm being then broken, words came clear, hurried, and convulsive, like the movements of the body or limbs.

During all the attacks hyperæsthesia of the skin was excessive in
all parts of the body, especially in the centre of the forehead, at the pit
of the stomach, and along the sternum. The appetite was good, digestion perfect, defæcation normal, thirst ordinary ; no sugar or albumen
was in his urine, and there was no fever, or paralysis of sensation or
motion. His consciousness in the midst of the attacks was perfect ; but
he was powerless to control the convulsions in spite of all his efforts.
In moments of calm he related and minutely analyzed all his sensations,
and replied with propriety to all questions. He insisted especially, after
the manner of hypochondriacs, upon the danger he incurred of insanity
or immediate death.

The attacks happened almost every day, and sometimes lasted a dozen
hours. Sleep occurred at times, but it was light and brief, and interrupted by a nightmare, which induced fresh attacks. The convulsions
changed in character from moment to moment. M. G—— went
again to the baths at Ussat, which, with chloral, amusements, walking
and riding, produced such favorable results that towards the end of
summer his self-control was restored, though his hypochondria still remained.

TRANSACTIONS OF STATE MEDICAL SOCIETIES.[1]

THE activity of the profession in the States mentioned below has shown itself by the very good reports before us. We can here look only at the general nature of the proceedings, hoping to give at another time special notices of some of the papers which they contain. The addresses are good and mostly practical, not containing more of the glittering generalities than it is unfortunately absolutely necessary that such discourses should. The work is of a high order for the most part. The Maryland and South Carolina Transactions have this in common, that many questions or branches are reported upon by committees or individuals appointed for the purpose. Foremost among these we must allude to the excellent report on what is known as Bright's disease, by the committee of which Dr. Geddings was chairman, to the South Carolina society. It is an admirable review of the subject, beginning with a careful study of the anatomy and physiology of the kidney. We have room only for the conclusions : —

" 1st. That the term ' Bright's disease ' is no longer available, inasmuch as under this head are included several maladies, both anatomically and clinically distinct from each other.

" 2d. That in the present state of our knowledge we are warranted in splitting the group into at least four members: (*a*) passive hyperæmia and sclerosis; (*b*) catarrhal nephritis; (*c*) diffuse nephritis; (*d*) amyloid degeneration.

" 3d. That, notwithstanding the fact that these four forms of disease are often blended, they also frequently occur separately, and may be diagnosticated during life, and the special incidental lesions demonstrated after death."

The Maryland Faculty attempts a series of reports on the various branches. That on anatomy and physiology is largely devoted to the question of cerebral centres. The old story of the experiments of Hitzig, Ferrier, and others is gone over, including Bartholow's disgraceful human vivisection, which is mentioned not only without condemnation but with rather a hint that it would be well to confirm his results. · If this kind of experiment is desirable, we would venture to suggest that the subjects be taken from the prison rather than the hospital. The reporter, Dr. Kloman, finds much difficulty in the question of the diffusion of electrical currents through the brain, but there is no mention of Dr. J. J. Putnam's experiments.

A noteworthy article is that of Dr. Cochran, of Mobile, on the small-pox epidemic in that city in 1874–75. The whole question is thoroughly discussed in both its practical and its scientific aspects. With regard to vaccination, Dr. Cochran holds that it should be performed in infancy, at puberty, and again in case of serious exposure. Concerning human and bovine virus he believes " that the humanized virus is equally efficacious as a prophylactic ; that the humanized virus is many times over less expensive and less inconvenient; that the humanized virus can be preserved more easily and for a

[1] *Transactions of the South Carolina Medical Association,* 1875. *Transactions of the Medical and Chirurgical Faculty of Maryland,* 1875. *Transactions of the Medical Association of the State of Alabama,* 1875.

longer time, and is far more certain to take, the failures, even with fresh bovine lymph, more than doubling the successes." The account of the trouble
in vaccinating the ignorant negroes is very comical.

Sanitary matters and the effect of climate and situation on disease are happily claiming considerable attention. Dr. Toner's oration at Baltimore on the
medical history and physical geography of Maryland is a very valuable paper.
Dr. Gleitsmann read before the same society an interesting essay on the effect
of altitude and climate on pulmonary phthisis. The most comprehensive of
the papers of this class is that by Dr. Bissell, of Mobile, on the climate of the
United States, considered with reference to consumption and pneumonia. We
cannot follow the author through so extensive an excursion, but must content
ourselves with quoting his concluding remarks, to which we heartily sub-
scribe: —

"But in the name of common-sense and humanity, and for the sake of
science, do not send from friends and the comforts of home those unfortunates
who have already passed the bounds of curability. If all such cases were
kept at home, and all physicians would give the subject of climate the attention its importance deserves, the number of persons benefited at our various
health resorts would be proportionally far greater, and the number called to
die among strangers, far from home and friends, would be much less."

DUNSTER ON ANÆSTHESIA.[1]

WE are at a loss to see why Professor Dunster should have felt called upon
to come before the public with this threadbare story. If we did not think it
possible that our silence might be misinterpreted, we should take no notice of
the pamphlet. It can, however, be dismissed very briefly. Dr. Horace Wells
is not entitled to the credit of being the discoverer of anæsthesia for two reasons: first, because the abstract idea was not his; it had found place in the
mind of Sir Humphry Davy, and very probably had been taken up again and
again since the origin of civilization; secondly, because the abstract idea did
not become a reality till Morton introduced ether.

PROCEEDINGS OF THE BOSTON SOCIETY FOR MEDICAL IMPROVEMENT.

F. B. GREENOUGH, M. D., SECRETARY.

APRIL 26, 1875. *A Case of Oxalic-Acid Poisoning.* — DR. J. B. S.
JACKSON showed the stomach of a patient of Dr. H. E. Marion, of Brighton,
who had given him the following history of the case: —

[1] *The History of Anæsthesia.* By EDWARD S. DUNSTER, M. D.   (Reprinted from The
Peninsular Journal of Medicine, August, 1875.)

" S. S. A., an American, fifty-three years of age, and by occupation a carpenter, left home on a Wednesday morning to collect money that was due him. Nothing peculiar was noticed in his manner before leaving home. He returned about noon, and went directly to his barn (five minutes' walk from the house), took his horse from the sleigh, and put the blanket on without removing the harness. He also put the sleigh in the barn. He subsequently told his family that he lay on the hay about two hours, as he did not feel well. At two o'clock P. M., he walked to his house ; his gait was slow and unsteady. When he entered the house he complained of intense pain in. his stomach. His face and hands were livid and 'cold as a stone.' He could hardly speak, saying but a word or two at a time. He asked if there was any chalk or magnesia in the house. He took all that was at hand of those remedies. He also took a quantity of ' pepper tea ' and ' ginger tea.' He was drawn up on a lounge before a very hot fire, and external warmth was applied. About four o'clock I called to see his sick child in another room. He would not allow any one to mention that he was sick, but persisted in saying that he should soon be better.

" His condition remained about the same Wednesday night and Thursday. Whatever he drank, and he drank a good quantity of water, was soon vomited. Thursday noon, with assistance, he got up from the lounge, got into a chair, and was taken to his bed-room.

" At two o'clock that afternoon, I visited the child again with Dr. Hosmer, of Watertown, in consultation. While Dr. Hosmer was examining the child, the wife said she wished me to see her husband, as he seemed very sick, and she was afraid he had pneumonia. (I mention this as showing that she evidently suspected nothing.) Leaving Dr. Hosmer with the child, I stepped into the other room. Mr. A. was lying on his back, partly dressed. His face and hands were livid and very cold. There seemed to be no capillary circulation ; indeed, there was no pulsation in the radial artery, and it was extremely feeble in the brachial. The patient's mind seemed clear, his pupils were normal. The tongue, which he protruded slowly when asked to, was slightly coated. His speech was labored, but a word or two being articulated at a time. Dyspnœa was marked ; tracheal râles were very loud, so loud that I was unable to make any satisfactory examination of the chest. I could not even hear the heart sounds. The patient had urinated and defæcated.

" I told him that his symptoms looked alarming, and that I could not account for them. Suspecting something wrong, I asked him if he knew any reason why he should be taken so very sick. 'Yes,' he said, 'I have taken about two tablespoonfuls of oxalic acid, thinking it was whisky.' I called Dr. Hosmer, and he examined the man ; it was our opinion that antidotes would be of little avail, since it was now more than twenty-four hours after the poison was taken, and the patient looked as if he must soon die. We advised carbonate of ammonia to be administered by the stomach, freely if it was retained ; also brandy and nutritive enemata.

" His condition remained the same until Friday morning, when he became delirious. In his delirium he got out of bed alone. He died at two P. M., on Friday.

" *Autopsy*, twenty-six hours after death. Rigor mortis complete. Lividity not as marked as during life, except on the dependent portions of the body. About ten ounces of bloody serum were in the right pleural cavity ; the lungs were œdematous, otherwise healthy. The heart was flabby and larger than normal ; the walls of the left ventricle were very much thickened. The left cavities of the heart were empty ; the right, together with the venæ cavæ and pulmonary vessels, were filled with dark, soft coagula. The spleen was rather large, dark, and very soft. The kidneys were of about the normal size, and in the gross appearance nothing abnormal appeared, except that they were rather friable. The stomach contained about three ounces of straw-colored fluid."

The stomach, which was received in a perfectly fresh state, was of medium size, fleshy to the feel, if not a little stiffened, and having a somewhat dryish look upon the external surface, like a specimen which, having been in spirit, had been removed, and left for some time exposed to the air. This same surface had a very marked appearance of fine lines running parallel lengthwise, finely set, and giving it a somewhat wrinkled look ; and it had to a considerable extent a chalky-white look, like a specimen that had been in a solution of corrosive sublimate. All of the veins about both curvatures were crowded with coagulated blood, and were very firm to the feel. The mucous membrane was quite rugous, and of a color throughout that strikingly resembled dark putty ; there being nowhere any redness, abrasion, lymph, or any other indication of inflammation. In consistence it was firm, as were all of the other tissues.

In connection with this case, Dr. Jackson exhibited the plates of Roupell, showing the effects of different poisons upon the coats of the stomach, a work to which his attention had been directed by Dr. Fitz, and which had been imported by Dr. D. H. Storer, when he was connected with the medical college. He also referred to the case published by Dr. White,[1] and to his very full and interesting article upon the subject of poisoning by oxalic acid.

DR. WHEELER said that this case differed from one which had come under his observation, the symptoms being much less acute.

DR. JACKSON said that the symptoms were certainly not as acute and violent as we should expect in a case of oxalic-acid poisoning, but the patient not only said that he had taken that poison, but was known to have bought a large amount of it.

DR. WHITE said that the appearances of the stomach were the same as he had seen in other cases. In two or three cases which he had seen, the symptoms had been almost latent. This, however, he supposed to be exceptional.

Elephantiasis of very large Size removed from the External Female Genital Organs ; Three large Masses of Straw found in the Stomach and Duodenum after Death. — DR. C. B. PORTER showed the specimens, and the following history of the case was furnished by Helen M. Marsh, assistant physician to the State Almshouse at Tewksbury. The patient was thirty-five years of age, a single woman, and a prostitute. Three years ago the tumor was about the size of the fist, and when it was removed, it hung down to the knees and measured ten inches in diameter. The patient suffered from the weight of the

---

[1] Boston Medical and Surgical Journal, January 27, 1870.

mass, and, when it was not supported, from great pain, so that she could walk but little. The urine also was constantly dribbling away. In appearance the tumor externally was warty, lobulated, and dark-colored for the most part, as usual ; it was fleshy to the feel ; it arose mainly from the clitoris and internal labia, and weighed, after removal, four and three quarters pounds. It was supposed, probably from the woman's habits of life, to be owing to syphilis, Dr. M. G. Parker, of Lowell, removed the mass with the galvano-cautery. There was no hæmorrhage, nor any subsequent complaint, except of her stomach and of great thirst; but she sank, and died in two days. The wound meanwhile had contracted well, so that but little was seen of what had been done.

In her stomach were found two balls composed of straw, twigs, twine, tealeaves, etc., resembling the hair balls that are sometimes found in the stomachs of cattle. From the middle portion, and towards the ends, they gradually tapered to a point, and were there slightly connected. A third mass of similar material was in the duodenum. They were compact in structure, and not at all digested. The stomach itself was not remarkable.

Two years before her death, which occurred March 27th ult., this patient was a healthy-looking woman, and weighed one hundred and seventy pounds, but during the last six months of her life she had become anæmic, and her weight was reduced to one hundred pounds or less. Her appetite was sometimes voracions and sometimes small ; and after indulging it, she often vomited. For several years she had been insane, and for nearly four months she was at the institution at Tewksbury. During this last period she had not walked out, but she would often tear her bed to pieces, and scatter the straw around the room. No tendency, however, to the swallowing of such articles had been observed. After the operation, and when the straw was probably in the stomach, she took milk, eggs, beef-tea, and whisky.

The specimens are in the museum of the Medical College.

Case of Pott's Disease in which all the Symptoms disappeared for Four Years. — Dr. Webber reported the case. The patient, sent to Dr. Webber by Dr. B. F. D. Adams, of Waltham, had epilepsy and vertebral caries. Both presented some peculiarities deserving notice. The epileptic fits began at two years of age, at first only three or four a year, and continued till eight years of age. During this time and subsequently the boy screamed at night and started up. Since eight years of age he had screamed at night and started up in bed; he had also stood up and walked off the bed, as if walking on level ground; hence frequent falls occurred. At these times he was unconscious, and would come to himself in the middle of the floor, or while crawling back to bed. These attacks recurred about once in three weeks. The screaming was repeated nearly every night, but the patient was generally conscious immediately after.

About five years ago the vertebral disease was first noticed. The patient and his mother thought he had not injured his back, though he had had severe falls. They laid the origin to his work (pulling cotton out of a bale), which tired his arms. It is probable that the pain and aching from the work were the first symptoms of the vertebral disease. At that time he had pain at lower part of the left chest, and deformity of the back was noticed. No other trouble came till a year ago, when he lost power in his legs and they became numb. There was at times a tingling in the legs. In three months these symptoms all disappeared, and the patient felt as well as ever. About four weeks ago the same symptoms returned. At present, motion is much interfered with and sensation is much diminished, a deep prick being scarcely felt. The loss of sensation is clearly defined by a line, nearly straight, passing around the body at the level of the ensiform cartilage. There is slightly exaggerated reflex action. The second and third dorsal vertebræ project nearly three inches beyond the cervical. The points of interest are the absence of symptoms referable to the cord during four years (this remission perhaps is due to the position of the disease, the vertebræ being supported by the ribs); the entire intermission in the symptoms during about eight months; the absence of pain or discomfort in riding over rough roads, and when he twisted and turned his body from side to side or forwards and backwards, the motion being very free.

Malformed Heart ; Interventricular Opening, and Opening of the Ductus Arteriosus into the Arteria Innominata. — Dr. Jackson reported the case, which occurred in the practice of Dr. Hildreth, of Cambridge, and showed the specimen. The patient was a girl six years old. Her mother gave the following history: She was the fifth child; she was eight months carried. Nothing unusual was noticed about the child till she was two months old; then for the first time she had a " blue spell." From then till the time of her death she had these " spells," sometimes having several a day, sometimes going weeks and months without having one. She was of good form, intelligent, but about the size, at the time of her death, of a child four years old. She never walked till she was four years old; she was always considered an invalid, and required a great deal of care from her mother. At no time could she walk farther than across the street without sitting down to rest. The fingers were clubbed as well as the toes.

The mother said the "blue spells" were much alike. The child would fret a little, go to her mother's lap, and very soon would straighten out her hands and feet, throw back her head, roll up her eyes, become blue, seem to be distressed for breath, be unconscious; in two or three minutes the color would disappear, the child would go into a quiet sleep for three or four hours, and wake up then as well as ever. Nothing that the mother knew or had observed would cause one of these spells except an attempt at defæcation. That was quite a common occurrence, especially if the bowels were constipated.

The child never had any severe sickness. The night before Dr. Hildreth saw her she had one of the same " spells; " there was nothing remarkable about it, except that at the end of the usual time the color did not disappear. The child had a great many similar seizures whilst she lived, which was about eighteen hours, but the blue color never left. When Dr. Hildreth first saw the patient, which was eight hours before her death, she was in a heavy sleep, with rapid respiration, both eyes turned to the left, the pupils contracted,- dysphagia, frothing at the mouth, and a rapid, irregular, and feeble pulse.

When examined, the left lung was partly solidified and full of blood, sink-

32

ing in water. The left branch of the pulmonary artery was plugged to its union with the right. Nothing abnormal or diseased was observed in the abdominal cavity. The head was not examined.

The aorta arose rather from the right ventricle than from over the septum, and beneath it there was free interventricular opening. The pulmonary artery had three valves, which were sufficiently normal, but below these there was upon or just beneath the inner surface of the right ventricle a considerable amount of a white, opaque, condensed tissue; and this portion of the ventricle, to the extent of nearly half an inch was very much contracted. The ductus arteriosus was about an inch in length, one tenth of an inch in diameter, and pervious for about half an inch; it opened into the arteria innominata. Otherwise the heart was sufficiently well, the increased thickness of the right ventricle being less than is usual in cases of interventricular opening.

Old and Recent Thrombosis of the Left Iliac Vein. — Dr. Fitz showed the specimen, which was from a patient of Dr. A. L. Mason. The case was one of cancer of the uterus. About a year and a half ago uterine hæmorrhages began, and continued from time to time till the patient's death. She was first seen by Dr. Mason about four months ago, when she was suffering from abdominal pain and profuse diarrhœa. Some three months later she was suddenly seized with severe pain in the left leg, as if "struck with a stick;" she became unable to stand. A few days later œdema was present throughout the left lower extremity, with considerable tenderness in the groin and iliac region. This condition persisted till her death.

There was no history of any previous attack.

Dr. E. G. Cutler made the autopsy and reported an extensive ulcerating cancer of the cervix uteri, with invasion of the pelvic sub-peritoneal tissues, particularly in the left side, and perforation of the bladder. Hydronephrosis of the left kidney was present, its ureter being dilated and, near the outlet, cancerous. The right kidney was nearly doubled in size. The heart was hypertrophied; its valves were healthy. The left iliac vein was imbedded in cancerous tissue. For about two inches of its course, and extending into the leg, it was nearly completely filled with a dense, dry, firmly adherent thrombus, continued into the veins of the leg by a comparatively recent one, in part dense and tawny, in part loose and dark-colored, with spots of central softening. Near the upper end of the iliac vein the thrombus was wholly converted into a flaccid, pigmented fibrous tissue, adherent to the wall but to be detached by the application of some force. Near the entrance of the internal iliac the thrombus filled the canal more completely; was organized peripherally, but in the centre contained a yellow, friable, tolerably firm material. A layer of recent clot existed between the periphery of the thrombus and the wall of the vein where adhesions were absent.

Necrosis of the Tibia. — Dr. Cabot showed the specimen. M. H., a boy fourteen years old, entered the Massachusetts General Hospital with the ligaments of the knee relaxed and with necrosis of the tibia. There was no assigned cause. The boy was apparently delicate; the knee was not painful or tender. It was slightly enlarged. He was operated upon, and two sequestra came away, one large and one small. Two days afterwards he commenced to have erysipelas, which extended above and below the wound. After that there was a chronic cellulitis of the entire limb. The knee was tender, much enlarged and fluctuated. Incisions were made about the knee, and pus was discharged abundantly. The abscess extended into the joint. Pressure made from above caused a discharge of pus from the opened skin at the necrosed tibia. Counter-openings were made at the knee for the exit of pus. The boy was stimulated and fed freely, but was continually sinking until he died, forty-one days after entrance to the hospital.

The Internal Sphincter Ani. — The question of the existence of an internal sphincter ani muscle having been brought up at a previous meeting, Dr. WARREN presented the following translation from Hyrtl's Topographical Anatomy :[1] " The internal sphincter ani muscle lies above the external, and is simply an agglomeration of the organic muscular fibres of the intestine, and therefore an involuntary muscle. When the anus is examined with the finger, a well-marked furrow is detected at its inner margin separating the two muscles from one another."

On page 141, Hyrtl describes the sphincter ani tertius. He says, " Surgeons in former times were in the habit of expressing their astonishment at the fact that, after operations for fistula, when the sphincter was divided, no involuntary discharge of fæces occurred. Paget had a patient, from whom he had removed the terminal portion of the rectum, who could retain both fæces and flatus. Houston considered that the intestine, at the point where a fold occurs as it passes through the fascia pelvis, was surrounded by a well-developed band of circular fibres. . . . . Every unprejudiced observer should allow the existence of such a muscle simply from the fact that in prolapsus ani, where both internal and external sphincters are paralyzed, no involuntary movement of the bowels takes place. In rupture of the perinæum and in congenital opening of the rectum into the vagina the same is the case. Ricord saw a woman twenty-two years of age, with this deformity ; she had complete power over the contents of the rectum.

" If the finger is introduced into the rectum of a patient who has had no movement for several days, no fæces are found usually immediately above the anus, and yet the column of fæces would naturally sink to this point were it not held back by a sphincter muscle. Although Kohlrausch found, both in patients and in dead subjects, scybala at the lower end of the rectum, and on the strength of this was opposed to the view which allowed the existence of such a muscle in the case of subjects, yet nothing is proved, as the muscle no longer acts, and in the case of patients, abnormal conditions might easily give rise to exceptions.

" Enemata which are not introduced high enough are likely to come away immediately ; if, however, the nozzle is inserted sufficiently far they will be retained. O'Brien called attention to the fact that an elastic tube can be introduced some distance into the rectum before flatus is given off. All these observations make it probable, *a priori*, that at a certain distance above the internal sphincter a third sphincter must exist. Nélaton and Velpeau have proved the existence of it, as a thickened ring of muscular fibres four inches

[1] Vol. ii. page 129.

above the anus. This bundle of fibres is, however, not always easy to find. In well-marked cases it is six or seven lines high in front and one inch behind. In order to find it on the subject the intestine should not be too forcibly distended with air. . . . . To show it well, the rectum should be laid open lengthwise and stretched upon a block, and the different layers carefully dissected off until the muscular layer is reached; the sphincter tertius when present will be seen as a broad bundle of thickly packed muscular fibres. Although not always found, there is no doubt that a physiological contraction of the rectum takes place at this point, since the œsophagus, whose muscular layer is of equal thickness in its whole length, has a similar permanent constriction of its lower third, which breaks the force of food that has been swallowed or of flatus that is coming up. In one instance I have observed fibres of the sphincter tertius taking their origin from the sacrum, and have publicly demonstrated them.

" This muscle does not permit the fæces pressing down from the sigmoid flexure to reach the lower portion of the rectum. Only when the desire for an evacuation exists does it relax and allow the column of fæces to come down on to the lower sphincters. These latter can by an effort of the will keep them back for some time, and are aided in their efforts by the levator ani muscle and the nates firmly pressed together; wherefore, one who is in such a critical situation takes good care neither to take long steps nor to run. Finally, even the muscles thus called upon for unusual exertion become paralyzed, and then follows what under such circumstances is inevitable."

———◆———

THE METRIC SYSTEM OF WEIGHTS AND MEASURES.

WE are glad to see the daily press uniting with the scientific journals in advocating a move in the right direction by urging upon the public the substitution of the French decimal system of weights and measures in the place of the unsatisfactory system, or rather systems, now in use in this country and England. We venture to say that there are many of our readers who have occasion to use daily, in making their purchases and writing their prescriptions, both the troy and the avoirdupois ounce, who do not know that they differ by 42.5 grains, or that the imperial and apothecaries' gallon differ by 46.274 cubic inches. This use of the same term to designate totally different amounts both by weight and by measure is one of the most serious objections to its use, and one of the strongest reasons for changing the system.

The decimal or metric system recommends itself at once by its simplicity, by the ease with which reduction from one term to another can be made, and by the simple relation which exists between the units of weight and of measure. In the English system there is no natural relation between these units. The imperial gallon was made by enactment to contain 277.274 cubic inches, and the weight of this volume of distilled water was to be taken as ten avoirdupois pounds, or seventy thousand grains; while the apothecaries' gallon contains 231 cubic inches, or 58,333.31 grains of distilled water, an amount exceeding ten troy pounds by 733.31 grains. Contrast with this complicated state of affairs the simple relationship existing between the French units of weight and measure. The unit of measure, the metre, is fixed by law as is the English yard. This, however, instead of being subdivided like the yard into 3, $4\frac{1}{1}$, and 36 parts to make the foot, link, and inch, is subdivided into 10, 100, and 1000 parts to make the decimetre, the centimetre, and the millimetre. The multiples are also divisible by ten, the Greek prefixes being used to designate them. The unit of weight, the gramme, is the weight of a cubic centimetre of distilled water under certain definite conditions of temperature and pressure. The unit of volume for measuring liquids is the litre, which is one thousand cubic centimetres or one cubic decimetre, and contains just one thousand grammes of distilled water.

It is a very easy matter, with a little practice, to become accustomed to think according to the terms of the decimal system, and to change from one system to the other, since it is necessary to burden the memory only with the value of a few of the terms. Thus the metre corresponds very nearly with our yard, it being about three and one fourth feet, and the kilometre is a little more than three fifths of a mile. The centimetre is about two fifths of an inch (0.3937), and the millimetre about one twenty-fifth of an inch. The micromillimetre ($\frac{1}{1000}$ of a millimetre), which is only used in microscopic measurements, is therefore about one twenty-five thousandth of an inch (0.000039). The litre is about one and three fourths pints (imperial), or a little more than two pints apothecaries' measure. The kilogramme is a little more than two pounds avoirdupois or two and one half pounds troy. The gramme is about 15.4 grains, or four grammes make about one drachm, and the milligramme is about one sixty-fifth of a grain.

It is now time that the decimal system should be introduced into this country in ordinary business as well as in science, in which the use of the old system has long since been abandoned. And none can so well initiate this change as the members of the medical profession, since the decimal system is now so thoroughly taught in our best medical and pharmaceutical schools.

MEDICAL NOTES.

— At a special meeting of the Board of Overseers of Harvard College, held on Monday, October 4th, inst., the following appointments in the medical school were made for the ensuing year : —

George Frederic Holmes Markoe, instructor in materia medica.

Frank Winthrop Draper, M. D., lecturer on hygiene.

Clinical teachers for the year were appointed as follows : —

Francis Boott Greenough, M. D., and Edward Wigglesworth, Jr., M. D., of syphilis; Clarence John Blake, M. D., and John Orne Green, Jr., M. D., of otology; James Read Chadwick, M. D., and William Henry Baker, M. D., of diseases of women ; Charles Pickering Putnam, M. D., and Joseph Pearson Oliver, M. D., of diseases of children; Samuel Gilbert Webber, M. D., and James Jackson Putnam, M. D., of diseases of the nervous system.

— A new benefactor to the human race has appeared in a correspondent of the New York *Medical Record ;* he proposes, with a profusion of small capitals, to STAMP OUT epidemics by the thermometer. The plan is simple and eminently practical. In times of epidemics one member of each household is to have a thermometer, and take the temperature of all his fellow-inmates three or four times every day. Charitable associations are to assign members to certain parts of each pauper district, who will do the same for the poor. On the discovery of the slightest deviation from the normal temperature a physician is to be notified, but, by an unaccountable oversight, the way in which he is to do his share of the stamping out is not mentioned. •

— It will be remembered by our readers that Dr. Edward Warren, of Baltimore, left this country some three years since to serve in the army of the Khedive of Egypt. Just as he had reached the highest position in that service, the office of surgeon-general of the Egyptian army, he was attacked with ophthalmia of a malignant form. After combating it by every possible means in Cairo, he was finally compelled to go to Paris for treatment, after six months of which he is now left with one eye permanently enfeebled, while the oculists declare that if he returns to Egypt the right eye will be compromised and lost. He has accordingly obtained an authorization to practice in France, and is, we understand, already in a fair way to become a popular practitioner in Paris.

DISPENSARY FOR DISEASES OF WOMEN.

[REPORTED BY J. B. FOLEY.]

Injury by Pessary. — July 7, 1875. Mrs. O'K., forty-two years of age, has had one child, two miscarriages. Menstruation is regular. Bowels are constipated. Micturition is frequent. There is backache, with leucorrhœa and much abdominal pain.

On examination uterus is found to be flaccid, of little more than normal size, very freely movable, and prolapses when the patient stands, being dragged down chiefly by the sagging of the extremely lax vaginal walls. A small erosion on the external os was touched with strong acetic acid. Quinine, a laxative pill, and the cold vaginal douche were prescribed.

Considerable amelioration was reported at the two subsequent visits, but on August 2d the backache and abdominal pains were still so grievous that relief was sought by the introduction of an elastic, round, rubber-coated, watch-spring pessary. The patient was told to return in six days at the latest, and at once if she experienced any pain from the instrument. She was not seen for fourteen days, although she had called several days before, when the dispensary was closed for repairs. She complained of much suffering from pain in the lower part of the abdomen and in the genitals ; had had almost constant slight discharge of blood for ten days.

On removal of the pessary, two linear ulcerations were found in the vaginal cul-de-sac, on either side of the cervix, corresponding to the position of the ring, and evidently caused by it. Two small erosions were also found on either side of the vaginal wall, where the ring had jammed it against the two rami of the pubes. The two ulcerations were so deep that they must have almost penetrated through the vaginal wall. There was no evidence of any spread of the inflammation to the peri-vaginal tissue. Rest in the recumbent position and warm vaginal injections were prescribed.

August 23d the patient presented herself again with the history of uninterrupted abdominal pains; being a poor woman, she had not been able to take the rest that was enjoined upon her. A bimanual examination revealed a round, slightly movable, tender tumor, as large as a plum, to the left of the uterus. Her tongue was slightly coated. The ulcers had contracted considerably.

Dr. Chadwick remarked that this was probably a circumscribed inflammation of the cellular tissue in the left broad ligament (parametritis), evidently owing to direct propagation of the inflammatory process from the ulcer in the vaginal wall on the left of the cervix. This was an admirable instance of the harm likely to arise from the promiscuous use of pessaries. His previous immunity from such accidents he believed to have been due to the fact that he never resorted to a pessary unless it was indispensable, and then only when a patient could be kept under constant supervision. This patient's neglect to return as soon as pain was experienced, and the ill-timed closure of the dispensary for a week, were the causes of her present plight.

The patient was recommended to the Massachusetts General Hospital, where she fully recovered within four weeks, the effusion having been absorbed without suppuration.

Rectocele. — Mrs. A. D., forty-seven years of age, the mother of ten children, had been greatly troubled for over two years by the occasional protrusion of "her womb" between her thighs; at these times she had suffered much pain in the abdomen. The condition was always aggravated during menstruation, and by walking or lifting.

On examination a tumor as large as a fist was found to be protruding from the vulva, which at first sight was taken for the anterior wall of the vagina (cystocele), but proved to be the posterior wall. Its nature was at once recognized from the fact that the tumor retained in a measure the imprint of the fingers; from the rectum the finger entered a large cavity full of soft fæces.

Dr. Chadwick called attention to the formation of the rectocele without any prolapse of the uterus, or any apparent undue patulence of the vaginal outlet. Long-continued and excessive constipation was the probable cause of her condition. In extreme cases scybala lodge in these rectal pouches, and remain there until they become of almost stony hardness. Relief could probably be obtained in this case by laxatives, ice-water enemata, and the insertion of an inflated ring-pessary into the vagina. It was doubtful whether a cure could be effected without the excision of a segment of the posterior vaginal wall, and perhaps also of the apposed wall of the rectum.

September 15th. The patient no longer experiences any pain; she has regular dejections, and is content, but the rectocele still exists, though much less extensive.

LETTER FROM MUNICH.

MESSRS. EDITORS, — Last Sunday morning the Mitglieder of the German " Verein für öffentliche Gesundheitspflege" (sanitary science) were to be seen taking advantage of the beautiful weather to make excursions to the " Starnberger See," or wandering about the streets of the city, at the Pinakothek, in the Rathskeller, in the Hof Bräuhaus, or at the opera. In the evening there was a *gesellige Vereinigung* in the small hall of the colosseum, the large or lower hall of which, as many of your readers will remember, is quite celebrated for its beer. Many of the leading scientific men of Germany were present, among whom Pettenkofer's fine face was easily conspicuous.

The cigars were good and the beer excellent ; and one could not help being delighted with the *Gemüthlichkeit* of the occasion, especially toward the latter part of the evening, while it gave to people from different cities an excellent opportunity of becoming acquainted with one another, and exchanging opinions. The real work began *ordentlich* on Monday morning at half past eight o'clock, and there was abundant evidence of that careful, thorough research for which we have learned so highly to respect the Germans. Among the two hundred and thirty-eight members who were present, there were physieiaus, civil engineers, directors of public institutions, chemists, burgermeisters, architects, manufacturers, merchants, inspectors, professors, apothecaries, health officers, chiefs of police, etc.; and the advantage of looking at the various questions from so many different points of view was very manifest in the diseussions which followed upon the reading of the papers.

The large hall of the old Rathhaus, in which we met, contains eighty thousand cubic feet of air, which would have been abundant if there had been any ventilation ; but there was not a visible hole for the escape or entrance of air except from the occasional opening of the entrance-door or the door marked *Hier!* At Bristol, they had science enough to knock out the windows, but at Munich their hygiene seemed to be devoted especially to benefiting others than themselves, in passing resolutions that dwellings over stables should be well ventilated, etc.

The first paper was by Dr. Voit, of Munich, on food in public institutions ; he said that the inmates of such places, including military schools and barracks, suffer from lack of the nitrogenous elements of food, at least in Germany. Certainly no European country can compare with the United States, generally speaking, in the liberality with which all such persons are fed.[1] Most of the writer's ideas were rather theoretical, and as he had given only fifteen years to the study, he had not prepared any resolution to be passed by the society except that they should make the general subject a careful study for future discussion.

The establishment of a public abattoir in Munich was probably the occasion which gave us two excellent papers on abattoirs and inspection of meat. It was voted unanimously that meat ought always to be inspected, and also the

[1] I do not include in this statement the city insane asylum of Philadelphia nor that of New York, where the average weekly cost of keeping or rather starving each patient is $1.30.

animals before slaughter; and that there is no security against getting bad meat in our markets in any other way. The association could not agree to exclude from the markets dead meat from distant places. The resolution that all cities containing ten thousand inhabitants should have abattoirs, and that all butchers should be compelled to slaughter there and nowhere else, passed without a dissenting voice. It is to be hoped that they will have better success than the Parisians are now having with their enormous abattoir at La Villette, which is, next to the " Liernur system " in Amsterdam, and the rivers Liffey and Clyde, the greatest nuisance which I have seen this side of the Atlantic. Since Napoleon's time, too, the butchers have been allowed to go freely out into the streets with their working clothes on, and the most ardent advocate of women's rights could not deny that there at least the two sexes are equal; but it was not a pleasant sight to have before one's eyes women up to their ankles in mire, carting blood and offal, and driving pigs and cattle. The whole place is disgracefully dirty.

The session continued until two o'clock, with a half-hour's intermission at eleven for breakfast; but at the latter part of the morning many seats became empty. Some went out to get *reine Luft,* and some to the Rathskeller, although it was not fair in my friend from Basel to say that the *Hauptsitze* were in the *keller.*

On Tuesday Dr. Lent, of Cologne, read a paper on the advisability of better certificates of causes of death and more accurate returns, from which the fair inference was that there are other people than many of the town clerks of Massachusetts and *vérificateurs* of France who fail in giving accurate and trustworthy statistics.[1]

Dr. Varrentrapp entered the speaker's desk with such a pile of papers on the Sanitary Requirements of New Buildings, and went so much into detail, that a long and earnest discussion followed. In fact, they went into the matter so *eingehend* that it seemed quite likely at one time that they would not get out again, and I was dismayed when one gentleman said that one of the topics alone needed two weeks to consider it properly; but by the skillful management of the president, Dr. Erhardt, a good deal of valuable breath was saved for future use, and Dr. Varrentrapp's thirty-two " theses " were finally accepted without serious modification. If a *Geheimrath* does not know how wide a street should be, and in what direction it should lie, who does? When the final voting took place, it seemed to me that a great deal was taken on the authority of the Herr Referent, and that many general rules were made with regard to matters which could be decided only from the circumstances of each case. The discussion was prolonged so much that it had to be resumed on the third day, when the members had got fresh strength from a night's rest and the *festessen* of Tuesday evening. In fact, as the clock struck one, I began to fear that the best paper of all, on Typhoid Fever in Munich, would be necessarily crowded out; but at half past one Pettenkofer arose with a few notes in his hand, and in twenty minutes gave us the statistics of the last twenty-five years, showing how they confirmed his views on typhoid fever, its

---

[1] One of the first questions which I was asked by Dr. Farr, of London, was, " When do you expect to have an accurate registration of deaths ? "

causation, etc., at least as far as Munich is concerned. He evidently had studied Lamartine's rule of spending enough time on what he wrote to make it short. He placed his views in better form and more concisely than I had ever heard or seen them before, but I think there was nothing positively new, except the admirable grouping of such a mass of statistics, and the statement that he thought that there is a specific poison which propagates the disease, although at present we are utterly in the dark as to what that poison is. With these cases of twenty-five years he says that the drinking-water had " *gar nichts zu thun*," although he says that the poison may be conveyed to the system in that way.

The meeting broke up after passing resolutions to make extensive and accurate observations in the same general way that Pettenkofer has been pursuing for so many years; and there was a *letzte gesellige Vereinigung* in the evening.

During the afternoons of the three days we were shown various objects of interest in the city. The new school-house, the new *Erziehungsinstitut*, and the new military hospital, were all pronounced *wunderschön*, but they are all far inferior to institutions of the same character which may be seen in England or the United States. In fact, the new wards of the Massachusetts General Hospital are far superior to anything of the kind which I have seen in Europe, not even excepting the new hospital of twelve separate buildings in Berlin, which is said to be the finest in Germany.

The insane asylum is worth seeing. The director has recently had one million guldens voted him, without a dissenting voice, for enlarging and improving and beautifying his buildings and grounds. In all of his windows he is putting panes of *spiegel-glas* (plate glass) about a centimetre thick; it cannot be broken by any ordinary blow. In fact, I could not break it with my fist. Each pane costs a gulden, an extravagance which the *Geheimrath* from Hildesheim said that he had not seen even in England.

Another excellent idea which I noted was the building of large rooms for exercise during stormy weather. The southern sides were almost wholly of glass, and the rooms were not to be heated. The sashes are to be taken out during summer, and the space occupied with plants, shrubs, etc. The superintendent is carrying rather far the principle of decorating the grounds and frescoing the wards and other rooms which are for the most demented patients; but he thinks his experience justifies him in saying that by such means he reduces his number of filthy patients seventy-five per cent.

I spent one afternoon with an English engineer in the sewers, and was almost taken off my feet by the sudden opening of one of the flushing gates. The sewers are, generally speaking, poorly constructed; but the city has at last decided to have a new system of well-constructed sewers, Pettenkofer having finally acknowledged that they do not vitiate the *grund-luft*. The only interesting fact that I noticed was that the sewage from that part of the city where there are no water-closets was fully as offensive as where the human excreta all go into the sewers.

I should have said that during the three days of the session of the Public Health Association very little was said in regard to the question of sewerage, all the authorities being now pretty thoroughly agreed that the best solution of the question lies in good sewers, well flushed, with the sewage to be gotten *entirely* away before decomposition begins.   In such cases the sewage and the sewer-air are not very offensive, and there can be free ventilation in all dircetions, excepting, of course, into the houses and near the windows and chimneys.   Roe, formerly one of the engineers of London, deserves the credit of having first adopted this method, which since his time has been carried out so successfully in London, Liverpool, Hamburg, Frankfort-on-the-Main, and Dantzic. Napoleon's engineers attempted the same thing in Paris, but with far less success than Lindley has met in Hamburg and Frankfort, or Wiebe in Dautzie.

C. F. F.

Munich, *September* 15, 1875.

———◆———

WEEKLY BULLETIN OF PREVALENT DISEASES.

The following is a bulletin of the diseases prevalent in Massachusetts during the week ending October 9, 1875, compiled under the authority of the State Board of Health from the returns of physicians representing all sections of the State: —

The prominent feature of the returns for the last week is the extensive and increasing prevalence of epidemic catarrh or " influenza; " all parts of the State report its presence, and many observers note its coincidence with the epizoötic catarrh.   Diarrhœal affections have subsided.   Diphtheria has diminished in the State at large, but is somewhat more prevalent in certain sections.   The order of relative prevalence is as follows: Typhoid fever, influenza, bronchitis, diarrhœa, rheumatism, diphtheria, dysentery, pneumonia, cholera infantum scarlatina, cholera morbus, croup, whooping-cough ; the first three are the only ones of very general prevalence.

Berkshire: Bronchitis, typhoid fever, diarrhœa, influenza.

Valley: Typhoid fever, influenza, diarrhœa.   Springfield and Chicopee report remittent fever.   Diphtheria has subsided.

Midland: Typhoid fever, influenza, bronchitis, rheumatism.

Northeastern: Typhoid fever, influenza.   Not much sickness.   Scarlatina in and around Lynn.

Metropolitan: Typhoid fever, bronchitis, influenza, diphtheria ; the latter disease has increased, but is not general.

Southeastern: Typhoid fever, influenza, bronchitis.

F. W. Draper, M. D., Registrar.

COMPARATIVE MORTALITY-RATES FOR THE WEEK ENDING OCT. 2, 1875.

	Estimated Population.	Total Mortality for the Week.	Annual Death-Rate per 1000 during Week.
New York	1,060,000	586	29
Philadelphia	800,000	323	21
Brooklyn	500,000	239	25
Chicago	400,000	127	17
Boston	342,000	169	26
Cincinnati	260,000	96	19
Providence	100,700	37	18
Worcester	50,000	22	23
Lowell	50,000	15	16
Cambridge	48,000	23	25
Fall River	45,000	28	32
Lawrence	35,000	20	30
Lynn	33,000	13	20
Springfield	31,000	14	23
Salem	26,000	12	24

Normal Death-Rate, 17 per 1000.

BOOKS AND PAMPHLETS RECEIVED. — Vision, its Optical Defects and the Adaptation of Spectacles. By C. S. Tenner, M. D. Philadelphia: Lindsay and Blakiston. 1875. (For sale by A. Williams & Co.)

On Poisons in relation to Medical Jurisprudence and Medicine. By Alfred Swaine Taylor, M. D., F. R. S. Third American from the third and thoroughly revised English edition. Philadelphia: Henry C. Lea. 1875.

Travels in Portugal. By John Latouche. With Illustrations. New York: G. P. Putnam's Sons. 1875. (For sale by A. Williams & Co.)

On Altitude and Climate in the Treatment of Pulmonary Phthisis. By W. Gleitsmann, M. D. (Reprinted from the Transactions of the Medical and Chirurgical Faculty of Maryland.) 1875.

Alimentation and the Gastro-Intestinal Disorders of Infants and Young Children. By B. F. Dawson, M. D. (Reprinted from the American Journal of Obstetrics and Diseases of Women and Children.) New York. 1875.

Anatomical Rooms, a Plan for their Construction, etc. By H. Lenox Hodge, M. D. 1875. (Reprinted from the Virginia Medical Monthly.)

The Cholera Epidemic of 1873 in the United States. Washington: Government Printing Office. 1875.

The Introduction of Epidemic Cholera through the Agency of the Mercantile Marine: Suggestions of Measures of Prevention. By John M. Woodworth, M. D. Washington: Government Printing Office. 1875.

Tinnitus Aurium. Second Edition, with Cases. By Laurence Turnbull, M. D. (Reprinted from The Philadelphia Medical Times, June and October, 1874.) Philadelphia. 1875.

The History of Anæsthesia. By Edward S. Dunster, M. D. (Reprinted from The Peninsular Journal of Medicine, August, 1875.)

Annual Report of the Supervising Surgeon of the Marine-Hospital Service of the United States, for the Year 1874. Washington: Government Printing Office. 1874.

RESIGNED AND DISCHARGED. — Dr. C. H. Davis, Assistant Surgeon Fifth Unattached Battery Light Artillery, M. V. M.

THE BOSTON SOCIETY FOR MEDICAL OBSERVATION will meet Monday, October 18th, at 8 o'clock, P. M. Dr. Wigglesworth will read a paper on Multiple Sarcoma (non-pigmented) of the Skin.

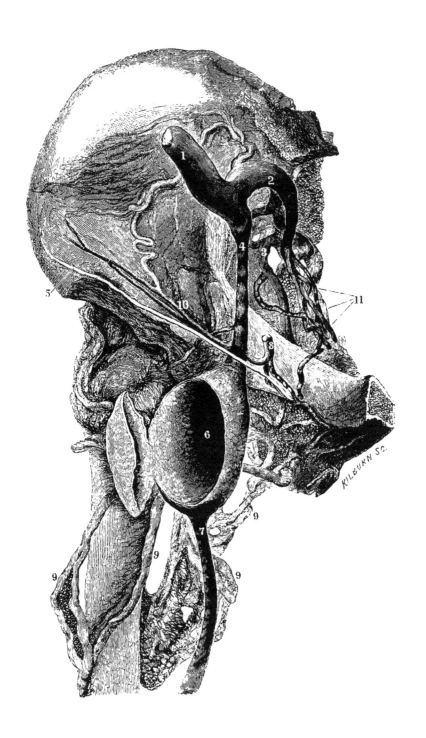

THE BOSTON
MEDICAL AND SURGICAL JOURNAL.

VOL. XCIII. — THURSDAY, OCTOBER 21, 1875. — NO. 17.

—•—

FEMORAL ANEURISM CURED BY DIRECT COMPRESSION, WHILE THE PATIENT WAS TAKING ACTIVE EXERCISE; DEATH FROM PERITONITIS SIX YEARS AFTERWARDS.[1]

[WITH PLATE.]

BY BUCKMINSTER BROWN, M. D.,

Surgeon of the House of the Good Samaritan.

WITH AN ACCOUNT OF THE POST-MORTEM APPEARANCES.

BY HENRY H. A. BEACH, M. D.,

Assistant Demonstrator of Anatomy in Harvard Medical School.

THE specimen of femoral aneurism which we have here this evening represents the completion of the history of a case treated and cured by immediate compression; a portion of this history was published in March, 1866. The specimen has been beautifully injected and prepared by Dr. Beach, by whom it will be shown.

This case is, so far as I have been able to ascertain, the only one on record in which the closure of the artery, although commenced while the patient was recumbent, progressed and was completed while he was taking active exercise, and attending for the greater portion of the time to his business, walking and riding to and from his store, etc.

The aneurism is fusiform in shape, and involves all the coats of the artery. The published report above alluded to was as follows:[2] —

" Mr. E. S., a healthy, muscular man, about thirty-eight years of age, called upon me July 11, 1863. Ten days previously he had first noticed a throbbing in the right groin. This had been gradually increasing. I found a pulsating tumor, about three and a half inches in diameter. The swelling was soft, and the fluid apparently just beneath the skin. Pressing with the finger, the posterior walls could be felt, the end of the finger being surrounded by pulsating fluid. The diagnosis was aneurism of the femoral artery at its exit from the abdomen. Remembering that a suppurating gland in the vicinity of a large artery has sometimes deceived surgeons of even the largest experience, I decided not to alarm the patient, but to await the result of a second examination.

---

[1] Read before the Boston Society for Medical Improvement.
[2] Boston Medical and Surgical Journal, March 15, 1866.

" Upon a second examination, a few days afterwards, I found the swelling had increased and the throbbing much augmented. The finger pressed upon the tumor was forcibly lifted with every pulsation of the heart. Dr. J. Mason Warren examined the patient July 31, and coincided in the diagnosis, and a trial of the treatment by immediate pressure was decided upon. The patient was directed to stand and walk as little as possible. About this time his health began to fail, and I advised him to go into the country for a short time, and that while there he should gradually accustom himself to the use of weights upon the tumor. He was directed to lie upon his back, and apply a bag of shot weighing ten pounds. Three times a day the weight was to be removed for an hour, and a bag of ice applied. This treatment was continued two weeks, when the weight was increased to fifteen pounds. At the expiration of another two weeks the patient returned to Boston. During these four weeks Mr. S. had obeyed implicitly my directions. The weight had been kept on the tumor day and night. It had caused a good deal of pain, and he had consequently obtained but little sleep. I found, on his return, there was a change for the better ; less throbbing, and the tumor somewhat diminished in size. Three times a day he had walked from the bed to the lounge, and this was all the exertion he had made. He was now directed to lie persistently upon his back, and to make no voluntary effort whatever. He was carefully lifted upon the lounge in the morning, and at night carried to his bed. Ice was used for an hour in the night as well as in the day ; as a change from the weight, this was a great relief. This course was pursued for some weeks, when, at the suggestion of Dr. Warren, I commenced using cannon-balls, in order to concentrate the weight more accurately over the tumor. The first ball used weighed twelve pounds. In a short time this was doubled, a ball weighing twenty-four pounds being applied. These balls were inclosed in a bag, which was secured to his person in such a manner that it could not slip. The twenty-four pounder at first could be borne only from two to five minutes. The bag of shot, the twelve-pound and the twenty-four pound balls were used alternately for another four weeks. The result was encouraging. The pulsation was less forcible, the tumor had lessened, and its parietes had become hard and comparatively inelastic, and the artery below the aneurism was evidently diminishing in calibre. The patient was now able to bear the weight of the twenty-four pound ball constantly during the day, except when relieved by the application of ice. His diet was carefully regulated ; meat was interdicted, and only light, farinaceous food allowed. About this time I discovered a small pulsating tumor on the top of the right foot, at the base of the metatarsal bone of the great toe — probably a dilatation of the arteria dorsalis pedis. This was cured in a short time by pressure with a piece of India-rubber and a bandage. In order to check circulation in the limb as much as possible, I applied a bandage from the toes to the groin. This afterwards gave place to a firm, silk, elastic stocking, two inches less in circumference than the leg, extending likewise from the toes to the groin. I also had a strong leather belt made to pass round the hips, with a groin strap. By this means I was able to produce powerful pressure upon the bag of shot, which was worn during the night.

" This treatment was continued, with little variation, from October, 1863, to June, 1864. The artery below the aneurism was now extremely small and its pulsation scarcely perceptible. The swelling had much diminished in size, had become hard, and its action comparatively feeble. I now decided to continue the treatment which had thus far been attended with so favorable a result, but to apply my pressure in another form, and, if possible, in such a manner as to admit of locomotion. A wide, strong, firm leather belt was made, thoroughly padded, which was fastened tightly around the hips ; to this was attached a strap passing from behind the trochanter to buckles over Poupart's ligament. A pad was adapted to the tumor, hard, oblong, and convex, with a block-tin back. This pad was held in position by the strap passing through loops to the buckles. By these means I found I could apply a very considerable amount of force. These straps having been adjusted, I allowed the patient to sit up and walk a short distance each day. At first his legs were very weak ; he rapidly gained strength, however, and was soon able to walk out, and in September, 1865, he began to attend to business, walking once a day from the neighborhood of the Boylston Market to Tremont Row. The pad was so accurately adapted to its intended position, and so firmly held there, that motion of the joint did not displace it, and thus a strong pressure upon the tumor was insured, even during active exercise. He continues to wear the belt and pad night and day, never removing it, except when in the horizontal position, and then only for a few moments for the purpose of bathing the part or to dress the excoriations produced by the belt upon the hips. On my last examination, about three weeks since, the artery below the swelling could not be felt, having, so far as could be ascertained, become obliterated by the constant pressure. The tumor pulsated feebly, had become harder, and had little elasticity.

" The patient was upon his back ten months, and has been under surveillance between sixteen and seventeen months ; during the first part of this time the pain and weariness wore upon him somewhat. His health, however, continued good, and his digestion was rarely disarranged. After five months he had become accustomed to the treatment, and began to grow fat ; and when he left his chamber he found he had gained twenty pounds during his confinement. I had, it is fair to state, an extraordinary patient to deal with. Mr. S. bore pain, continning night and day for so many months, with a fortitude and even cheerfulness which could not be surpassed.

" The result of the treatment by pressure in this case is certainly satisfactory. The attendant circumstances were such as, from the first, to indicate an almost hopeless prognosis. The nature of the disease, its situation just beneath Poupart's ligament, must render any operation which might have been attempted exceedingly dangerous. The ligation of the external iliac is an operation certainly not to be undertaken but as a last resort. When, in addition, we consider the aneurismal tendency of the arteries, as indicated by the swelling of this nature on the dorsum of the foot, the aspect of the case was sufficiently discouraging, and a favorable result from an operation could not have been anticipated.[1] To check the flow of blood through the aneurism by pressure applied above was impossible, as the tumor was directly upon the border of the pelvis. The application of immediate pressure in any other way than that employed, as by tourniquet, must necessarily have been attended by disadvantages, and was — after being duly considered — rejected. The course pursued was one which required constant vigilance to guard against excoriation and ulceration of the skin over the swelling, and this, by great care, was prevented. The belt around the hips, which was necessarily tightly strapped in order to obtain a firm purchase for the compressing strap, has from time to time caused sores which have been difficult to heal. There has been no complaint of numbness of the limb, nor any tendency to paralysis. The diseased leg, at the calf, is one and three fourths inches larger than the other."

From March, 1866, the time of the publication of the foregoing paper, compression by means of the pad and straps was continued. I will read a portion of Mr. S.'s memoranda of his case, given in a note addressed to me in 1871. He says, " From January, 1866, to December, 1868, there was no particular change. During that time I was much troubled with soreness caused by the rubbing of the straps. . . . About the middle of December I was taken with a severe pain in the calf of the leg, which afterwards extended through the whole leg. It did not seriously trouble me until the latter part of January (1869). My leg was much swollen at this time, and there was pain in the thigh near the aneurism."

I will here remark that the occurrence of this pain, which was often excruciating, putting the fortitude of even this man of strong endurance to a severe test, received at the post-mortem examination a singularly satisfactory explanation, although it was somewhat difficult to account for at the time. The arteries were injected, and those which entered and nourished the sciatic and anterior crural nerves were found to participate in the general enlargement of all the arteries in the neighbor-

[1] The view of the case stated in the above paper, published nine years since, receives confirmation, if any were needed, from the atheromatous condition of other arteries revealed by the necropsy.

hood. The consequent pressure upon the nerve produced the pain and cramps referred to by the patient. He continues : " The first day of February the pain was very severe, and so continued for several days, and I was very lame and sore. When the pain came on, the tumor measured five inches across and six inches in length. It now increased in size. . . . From that time until April 1st (1869) I had more or less of the pain, and suffered very much. · My general health was much affected. My leg was very weak, so much so that I was hardly able to walk. April 5th I went out of the city, and was gone a week. During that time the pain entirely left me. The tumor was still large, and throbbed a great deal. For the next three weeks I was very comfortable ; I had no pain ; the throbbing continued as before.

" May 2, 1869. Discovered that the throbbing had stopped.

" May 5th. Dr. Brown examined me, and found the aneurism closed up. The leg was very cold and almost lifeless. He ordered it wrapped in flannel and wadding.

" May 10th. I was examined ; was not allowed to walk more than was absolutely necessary.

" May 23d. Dr. Brown and Dr. H. J. Bigelow examined me. No circulation could be found in the ankle, but a slight beating in the top of the foot.

" July 31st. Examined by Dr. Brown. A slight beating was found inside the inner ankle ; no beating in the popliteal artery ; tumor very much reduced, as was also the swelling of the leg.

" September 22d. Examined ; all doing well. I was advised to reduce the pad about one half.

" October 28th. Tumor further reduced. A still further reduction of the pad and straps.

" December 14th. Dr. Brown made a full examination ; thought me entirely well. The tumor was very much reduced. I was allowed to walk all I felt able. I kept on a portion of the straps and pad during the winter.

" April 28, 1870. Left off all my straps, and have been without ever since.

" May 2, 1871. First anniversary of the closing of the artery. Through the summer of 1870 I got along very comfortably. My leg was weak, and troubled me at times, especially after walking ; had something like cramp in it.

" The tumor has diminished in size. It now (1871) measures three and a half inches across and three inches in length, or up and down ; it is but little raised. My leg is much stronger ; I can take quite long walks with but little discomfort."

From the time of leaving off the compression-pad (May, 1869) to the date of his death, Mr. S. had no further inconvenience from his imperforate femoral. On Sunday, February 7, 1875, he was not well, but was at his place of business on Monday morning. On the evening of that day he had a chill, and on Tuesday morning I was called to him. He was then suffering severe distress in the epigastrium, with nausea. This was somewhat relieved in the afternoon ; but the next day the pain returned with great intensity in the region of the bladder, and by the 11th symptoms of peritonitis were well pronounced, and continued, uninfluenced by remedies, except in the complete relief of pain by opiates, until his death, which occurred on the 13th.

Dr. Beach made the post-mortem examination, and found the usual results of acute peritonitis ; he was enabled to procure the parts involved in the old arterial disease. There were no indications that this had any connection with the acute complaint which proved fatal.

The ultimate success which attended the treatment of the aneurism was undoubtedly due in part to the fact that the compression at first was not sufficiently forcible to entirely occlude the artery, but was such as gradually to diminish its calibre and to allow of the progressive enlargement of the neighboring vessels and the accommodation of the surrounding parts to the new state of things. Likewise the process of nature in producing a spontaneous cure was by this course more strictly imitated. Holmes says [1] that the formation of fibrinous coagulum " seems to require for its commencement a diminution of the circulation, but not its entire stoppage ; indeed, it sometimes seems to go on less readily when the stream is stopped altogether." The cure of aneurism of other arteries by digital or other means of compression is of frequent occurrence. When the tumor is situated at or near the origin of the femoral, such a result is more rare. Rapid compression, under chloroform, has recently been attended with some success. Mr. Timothy Holmes, in his lectures published in *The Lancet*, refers to cases in which this method has been applied with a view of curing the aneurism at a single sitting. The risks from gangrene, etc., are stated. In his *résumé* he says, " This record of cases is no doubt extremely encouraging as far as relates to the forms of disease which do not admit of any other operative treatment, except that by ligature of the abdominal aorta, which hitherto has always failed, or of the common iliac, from which only one fourth of the patients operated on have recovered. . . . The total compression of the common or even the external iliac must involve great risk of fatal contusion of the viscera or the peritoneum." [2]

In the case now under consideration the patient was a stout, muscular man, with a considerable amount of adipose tissue. The impossibility of applying digital or instrumental compression to the external or common iliac under these circumstances was too evident to require serious

[1] Holmes's Surgery.
[2] The Lancet, October, 1874.

deliberation.   The contra indications to an attempt at cure by ligating the external iliac have been already stated.

Autopsy. — The abdomen was opened thirty-six hours after death, and a large collection of thin pus was found in the peritoneal cavity. The intestines were glued to each other and to the abdominal walls by patches of lymph.   The peritonitis seemed to be general, and there was no evidence of its connection with the aneurism.   The sciatic, gluteal, obturator, and femoral arteries exhibited patches of calcification.   The abdominal viscera, with the exception of their peritoneal surfaces, were healthy.   The thorax and head were not examined, as only sufficient time remained for the injection of the arteries in the region of the aneurism and the removal of the specimen.   A colored wax injection was thrown into the common iliac artery, and as shown by the specimen it entered the thigh by the internal iliac artery, its branches, and their anastomoses.   On dissection the aneurism proved to be fusiform in character, and caused by a gradual expansion of the common and superficial femoral arteries, commencing directly under Poupart's ligament and increasing until its diameter measured two inches; it then as gradually diminished until its calibre corresponded with that of the superficial femoral, the long axis of the tumor measuring two and a half inches. The three coats of the artery could not be satisfactorily demonstrated, owing to their consolidation by the long-continued compression.   The cavity made by the arterial expansion was completely filled by a mass of clot, somewhat adherent to but easily separated from its walls.   It presented no appearance of lamination on section, but instead, a firmly condensed tissue, irregularly distributed throughout the friable portion, and inclosing the latter in small cavities.   The former predominated, and under the microscope presented some indications of organization. The communication which had existed between the artery at either extremity of the aneurism had become entirely closed.   No communication between the interior of the aneurism and the deep femoral was detected, though carefully looked for.   The femoral vein had been completely closed by the pressure of the aneurism and the means employed for its cure.   The first half-inch of the external iliac artery was filled with the injecting material ; beyond that point the vessel had dwindled to the usual size of the circumflex iliac.   I made an incision into it at the middle of the vessel, to ascertain if it was occluded, and found that a very fine probe passed upward and downward for half an inch ; beyond that point it was apparently solid.   The superficial femoral was empty, and a probe entered five inches below the aneurism passed readily to within an inch of the latter, but there it met a solid body (the occluded vessel), and would not enter the aneurism.   The internal iliac and its anastomosing branches were very much enlarged, the calibre of the vessels varying from twice to three or four times their usual size.   A glance at the specimen, of which the plate gives an anterior view, shows that the main blood supply to the limb came from the gluteal, sciatic, and obturator arteries. The first branch below the bifurcation of the common iliac is the ilio-lumbar, commonly given off from the posterior division of the internal iliac, which, after sending branches to the psoas and iliacus muscles, forms an anastomosis with the circumflex iliac. The latter was filled from the anastomosis to its origin from the external iliac, where the injecting material stopped. The gluteal, after giving off the nutrient artery to the hip-bone, and the lateral sacral, emerged from the pelvis, and divided as usual into superficial and deep branches; the former anastomosing with the sciatic and posterior sacral arteries, the latter terminating in close proximity to the ascending branches of the external circumflex and the circumflex iliac. All the branches of' the sciatic were enlarged, and although the anastomoses with the internal circumflex and perforating arteries could not be exactly determined, the close relation of its branches with a large number of branches from the last-named vessels in and between the muscles of the posterior femoral region suggested the probability of their existence. An interesting fact in connection with a varicose appearance and enlargement of the comes nervi ischiadici was the intense pain in the sciatic nerve and its branches, alluded to by Dr. Brown in the history of the case. A similar condition, but not to such an extent, existed in a vessel lying upon the anterior crural nerve, whose branches were also the seat of severe pain. The superior and inferior vesical arteries, and the middle hæmorrhoidal, could be traced as far as their respective viscera, and nothing worthy of note was observed in connection with them. The obturator, after giving off large muscular branches to the interior of the pelvis, sent a large anastomotic branch over the pubic bone to the epigastric branch of the external iliac, and terminal and anastomotic branches through the obturator foramen to the obturator externus muscle, and the internal circumflex and sciatic arteries. The epigastric artery was filled to its origin by its anastomosis with the obturator. The internal pudic, beyond its enlargement, presented nothing worth mentioning. The aneurism closed the origin of the deep femoral, and the latter was filled through its anastomoses with posterior vessels of the thigh. The origins of the external pudic, superficial epigastric, and circumflex iliac arteries were closed by the aneurism.

EXPLANATION OF PLATE.

1. Common iliac artery.
2. Internal iliac artery.
3. Obturator artery sending a branch to communicate with the epigastric.
4. External iliac artery.
5. Poupart's ligament.
6. The interior of the aneurism; shown by partially detaching and turning to one side its anterior wall and removing the clot.
7. Superficial femoral artery.

8. Epigastric artery.
9. Circumflex, perforating, and sciatic arteries, with communicating branches.
10. Circumflex iliac artery.
11. Visceral branches of the internal iliac.

The preparation from which the plate was made has been contributed to the museum of the Harvard Medical School.

RECENT PROGRESS IN PATHOLOGY AND PATHOLOGICAL ANATOMY.

BY R. H. FITZ, M. D.

PATHOLOGY.

Diabetes. — A contribution to the statistics of this affection is presented by Andral.[1] More than eighty-four cases had come under his charge, and an analysis of these showed that the disease was of rare occurrence before the age of twenty years. It then gradually became more common, reaching its maximum of frequency between forty and fifty years, though frequent during the subsequent twenty years. It became exceptional at a later period in life.

In twelve instances the disease began before the age of thirty; in forty cases, between thirty and sixty years; in eight, between sixty and eighty years. The male sex is more prone than the female, fifty-two cases occurring among the former, and thirty-two among the latter.

The influence of the nervous system as a cause of the origin or aggravation of the disease was evident in many cases. A violent impression upon the nervous system was often followed by the presence of sugar in the urine, and in one case, after a moral shock, the amount of sugar was increased from five drachms to three ounces in about twenty-eight ounces of urine.

One patient became diabetic after inhaling ether for its intoxicating effect, for several months; another, after disturbances of sensation, anæsthesia, and other nervous affections. One patient was previously epileptic, another paraplegic. In one case the diabetes was preceded by a blow upon the lower part of the occiput; in another a concussion of the cervical region, resulting from a fall, had occurred. In these two cases the injury to the cerebro-spinal axis was received near the parts to which Bernard calls attention.

A lack of sufficient food was a cause in one case. Three patients had lived solely upon bread and potatoes before they became diabetic. Many became diabetic also who had eaten meat and cheese in addition to an abundant diet of bread and potatoes. In general, the well-to-do classes were more affected than the poor. The previous history and

---

[1] Allgemeine medicinische Central-Zeitung, 1875, lxx. 858; from Annales et Bulletin de Medecine de Gand, 1875, lii. 5me Série.

appearance of the patients frequently suggested the idea that the disease might be due rather to an excess of nutriment than to its lack. This view, shared also by Bernard, is supported by the fact that the sugar disappears from the urine during the last days of life.

The disease may occur suddenly during apparent good health. Again it was observed in four dyspeptic, eight phthisical, and five asthmatic persons; further, in connection with heart disease, renal colic, and in convalescence from typhoid fever and cholera.

Diabetes may cease momentarily at the outbreak of an acute disease, as was illustrated in a case of febrile angina, and in one of dysentery. The disease may at times be hereditary; sometimes several children in one family may suffer, the parents being free.

The simultaneous occurrence of sugar and albumen was observed only three times in the eighty-four cases. The quantity of the sugar in the urine varied; several patients passed fifteen ounces of sugar in the twenty-four hours, and one over two pounds in the same time. This was not dependent upon the food, and the treatment had often no influence upon the amount of sugar passed. At times the affection lasted for years without any considerable general disturbance; again it pursued an acute course, and death occurred within a few weeks after the beginning of the disease.

The sugar may suddenly disappear, an incident observed in five cases; in four of these the recovery remained permanent, in the fifth epilepsy came on after the disappearance of the sugar.

In almost all the cases the capillary circulation was more altered than in other chronic diseases. This was indicated by the red and swollen gums, injected conjunctivæ, boils, and passive congestion of the lungs, the frequent cause of death. In four cases gangrene was present; of the lungs in one instance, of the extremities in three.

Neither the saliva nor the other secretions showed any alteration.

The change constantly found at autopsies was a congested condition of the liver and kidneys, thought to be due to an increased function of these organs. In almost all cases there was a peculiar density to the spleen, its parenchyma was dry, and beginning tubercles were found in the lungs. These tubercles were regarded as developing under the influence of the debility following the diabetes.

As further evidence of a neuropathic origin for diabetes, the case reported by Mosler [1] may be referred to, where an inflammatory nodular affection of the left cerebellar hemisphere was found. The patient, a man aged thirty-five, always feeble, had suffered from great hebetude, increased hunger and thirst, and the evacuation of large amounts of urine for two and one half years. The legs had been swollen for a year, and cough with stabbing pains in the thorax had troubled him

[1] Deutsches Archiv für klinische Medicin, 1875, xv. 229.

for some weeks. At his entrance into the hospital the sensitive functions, motion, and sensation were completely normal. He died seventeen days afterwards. The inflammatory nodule was of the size of a
pigeon's egg; though regarded as the probable cause of the diabetes, no
evidence could be obtained as to its origin. It is asserted that every
injury to the tracts of vaso-motor nerves [1] may produce diabetes. It is
considered that the hepatic vaso-motor nerves are paralyzed, dilatation
of the hepatic vessels follows, whereupon an increased flow of blood to
the liver and an increased production of sugar result. Diabetes has
hitherto been observed after injury to the superior and inferior cervical,
and to the superior thoracic ganglia of the sympathetic; further, after
every section of the spinal cord from the medulla oblongata to the lumbar vertebræ, where vaso-motor nerves are everywhere present, in part
in the tracts of the cervical and thoracic sympathetic, in part in the
splanchnics. Mosler regards as favoring his theory of this case Eckhard's statement that diabetes occurs after injury to the vermiform
process of the cerebellum of rabbits.

Bernard discovered that ligature of the portal vein is followed by
diabetes, and obstruction of the portal vein from pathological causes has
been found to be attended with the same condition. MM. Colrat [2] and
Couturier [3] thought that in persons suffering from cirrhosis, there might
be present a sufficient degree of obstruction to the portal circulation to
give rise to diabetes. Four individuals suffering from this disease, the
diagnosis being subsequently confirmed by the autopsy, came under
observation. The urine was collected while the patients were fasting,
also during the period of digestion. The latter alone always contained
a greater or less quantity of sugar. The urine of healthy persons
under similar circumstances gave negative results. The addition of
large amounts of sugar to the diet made no difference. These observations are of interest in connection with the experiments of Seelig,
referred to by Dr. Bowditch.[4] It is mentioned also that in two cases
where a diagnosis was doubtful, the absence of glycosuria enabled the
writers to eliminate the idea of a cirrhosis of the liver; the autopsy
showed in the one a tuberculous peritonitis, in the other abdominal
cancer.

Typhoid Fever. — The period of incubation of this disease was observed by Quincke [5] in an epidemic occurring under peculiar circumstances. A number of people coming from parts free from typhoid
fever met together at a fair, where they had the opportunity of receiv-

[1] Vide Report on Physiology, by Dr. H. P. Bowditch, in the JOURNAL, July 23, 1874.
[2] Revue des Sciences Médicales, 1875, xi. 139 ; from Lyon Médical, 1875, XV.
[3] Revue des Sciences Médicales, 1875, xi. 139 ; from Thèse de Paris, 1875, No. 209.
[4] Loc. cit., page 84.
[5] Berliner klinische Wochenschrift, 1875, xxiii. 321 ; from Correspondenz-Blatt für
Schweizer Aerzte, 1875, No. 8.

ing the germs of this disease probably in contaminated drinking-water. In seven cases the disease occurred within from twelve to sixteen days after the visit ; in another equal series within from eight to twenty-two days. Another lot of five cases more closely resembled the first series. It seemed further as if the mode of reception of the poison was of influence with reference to the time of incubation. In two cases not belonging to the series mentioned, it was stated to him that the poison had probably been received through inhalation, the patients, boys, having played in infected straw. The period wavered in one case between three and nine days; in the other between one and fifteen days.

The appearance of the brain in typhoid fever has never been regarded as sufficiently explanatory of the grave cerebral symptoms so frequently occurring. The recent histological investigations of Popoff [1] have thrown additional light not only upon the anatomy of this disease, but also upon the pathological processes taking place in the brain. The brains from twelve cases of typhoid fever were examined, and the changes to be referred to were constant. The cortex was infiltrated with small cells resembling lymph corpuscles or the granules of the neuroglia. These were generally grouped in a definite manner, corresponding in form to the arrangement of the nerve-cells, and were often seen to lie around or upon them. Under a high power it was evident that these corpuscles were accumulated within the lymph-spaces surrounding the nerve-cells. Occasionally it was observed that the round cells were inside the body of the ganglion-cell. It was considered that the round cells were wandering cells, which, by virtue of their contractility, had penetrated the substance of the nerve-cell. The ganglion-cells were probably not passive in the process, as a division of their nuclei was evident in various stages. This same division was also observed in nerve-cells which did not contain the wandering corpuscles. Evidence of a division of the body of the cell was also found, and appearances were seen which suggested a breaking up of the ganglion-cells through the entrance of the round cells.

The wandering cells were also found in the peri-vascular spaces, and immediately outside of them in the brain. In the latter they were found along the course of nerve-fibres, especially where these are grouped together as in the corpus striatum and optic thalamus.

Experiments on animals showed that essentially the same alterations could be produced by exciting an inflammation through chemical or mechanical means. When finely divided pigment was injected into the brain it was taken into the ganglion-cells, and a comparison of the results of the injection of the pigment into dead and living brains led to the conclusion that the ganglion-cell was capable of contracting and thus of receiving the pigment within its body.

[1] Virchow's Archiv, 1875, lxiii. 421.

Typhus Fever. — Popoff [1] has more recently examined the brains of three persons dying of this disease. Similar changes to those observed in typhoid fever were noticed; but still more interesting and striking was the formation of little nodules in the cortex of the brain and cerebellum, in the corpus striatum and lenticular body. Under a low power they looked very like miliary tubercles, and very frequently were found next to vessels. They were composed mainly of agglomerations of round cells not to be distinguished from wandering lymph-corpuscles. In certain places these nodules consisted only of such cells; elsewhere there were also elements resembling the nuclei of ganglion-cells, and at times nerve-cells were found imbedded within the mass of indifferent cells. A proliferation of the nuclei of the ganglion-cells, and the presence of round indifferent cells within their bodies, were also observed at the periphery of these nodules, suggesting as probable a direct participation of the ganglion-cells in their formation. The nodules, composed mainly of indifferent cells, were usually found at the periphery of the brain and cerebellum. They were often found as infiltrations of the walls of the blood-vessels and the neighboring tissue, thus giving a further resemblance to tubercles. There was, however, no central degeneration, no giant-cells, nor special stroma. In character and origin they were analogous to the nodules found by Wagner in the liver and kidneys of typhoid fever. They were found in two of the cases only, and in these the cerebral symptoms were very marked, — delirium and cramps, followed by coma and stupor. The patients were young, twenty and twenty-two years of age; the duration of the disease, fourteen days. The case where no nodules were found presented mainly symptoms of excitement, and the duration of the disease was but ten days, the patient being thirty-seven years old.

PROCEEDINGS OF THE OBSTETRICAL SOCIETY OF BOSTON.

CHARLES W. SWAN, M. D., SECRETARY.

The society met, by invitation of Dr. Cotting, at the rooms of the Boston Society for Medical Improvement, May 8, 1875, at 7½ o'clock P. M.

May 8, 1875. — The president, Dr. Hodgdon, in the chair.

Simulated Pregnancy. — Dr. Cotting reported the case of a patient about thirty years of age, the mother of two children. She called upon him early in the autumn, and said that she expected to be confined about February 1st, as she had had motion from the middle of September. As she was confident of her sensations, Dr. Cotting made no other remark than that he supposed she was competent to judge of such matters. Her size, which had increased,

---

[1] Centralblatt für die medicinischen Wissenschaften, 1875, XXXVi. 596.

continued to enlarge; and, everything in her estimation proceeding as it should, she made extensive preparations. When the time came she was apparently of the size indicating full term, and she took her nurse into her house and had everything in readiness for the event. Six weeks after the expected time Dr. Cotting was sent for, and, as the patient had not perceived any alteration during these six weeks, she consented to an examination. This demonstrated that the patient had been wholly mistaken as to her condition, for there were no indications of pregnancy (by digital and other examination), except enlarged abdomen and mammæ. The increase of size proved to be due to a development of adipose tissue. On the abdomen this was exterior to the fascia, but greatly resembled pregnancy in form.

Hydrate of Chloral per Rectum. — Dr. SINCLAIR inquired if the injection *per anum* of hydrate of chloral caused any remarkable dilatation of the sphincter ani. He said that he had heard of a case in which the dilatation was so great that the hand could be passed into the rectum, during labor, and dilatation of the cervix uteri ensued. The amount used was twenty or twenty-five grains. Dr. Sinclair questioned whether this drug would be of value in cases of rigid os.

Dr. ABBOT said that in the case of a gentleman under his care a smaller dose caused no dilatation of the sphincter ani. There was difficulty in retaining the injection until more water was added to the solution.

Dr. LYMAN remarked that he had never heard of an injection of chloral causing such relaxation. He said he was much in the habit of using it in the early stages of labor, but not for the purpose of dilating.

Dr. EDSON said that in the case of a young man eighteen years old, under his care, there had been no difficulty in retaining an injection of a solution of fifteen grains of chloral administered nightly for three weeks.

A Case of Doubtful Conception. — Dr. MINOT reported a case which he had seen that day. The patient is a large, stout, single American woman, aged forty-four. Her last menstruation occurred February 14th, having previously been perfectly regular and normal. She said it was possible she might be pregnant. She had had connection several times about the time of the last catamenia — after, but not before the period. She had no subjective symptoms of pregnancy. The breasts were large, as usual, and the follicles were extraordinarily developed; but the woman said she had noticed this several years ago. Nothing was learned by an examination of the vagina and the abdomen, including the use of the stethoscope. Dr. Minot questioned whether as a general rule the catamenia do not become irregular in time and amount before ceasing.

Dr. RICHARDSON responded that in the lectures which he heard in Vienna he was instructed that when the catamenia stop suddenly it is always with the warning of a very profuse flow.

Dr. LYMAN said he thought this inability to decide the question of pregnancy in its earliest stages was an opprobrium of the profession. He gave the case of a young married lady who had had no child for two or three years. The catamenia had been irregular at times. She had generally been nervous and wakeful. During three months there was no menstruation; within this time she had also been extremely sleepy, and her nervous system had become very quiet. These two things made it probable that she was pregnant.

DR. COTTING stated that under his observation a number of women, arrived at the critical age, had noticed only that the time after the last period was longer than usual, and that the catamenia never again returned.

DR. HODGDON said he had observed a similar case in an Irish patient.

DR. ABBOT said he thought Dr. Minot's patient had hardly gone on long enough to render a decision of the question possible. It is not uncommon, he remarked, for an interval of six months to occur at such a time. As to Dr. Richardson's statement of profuse flowing having an abrupt and complete termination, he had had no corroborative experience. A woman of his acquaintance flows tremendously every two or three months.

DR. SINCLAIR remarked that there was an occasional case of great flowing at about the age of puberty, as well as at the close of the catamenial epoch, and that he thought, although he had no data, that at both ends of the scale there was about an equal number of similar cases.

Cases of Simulated Pregnancy. — DR. RICHARDSON reported a case recently terminated. Some time ago a married woman, aged thirty-nine, was sent to the lying-in hospital for confinement, supposed to be due in two or three days. She had had morning sickness, the abdomen was enlarged, and there was milk in the breasts. She had been unwell every month through the pregnancy, although the show had been very slight. A vaginal examination discovered a uterus of the normal size. Deep pressure over the liver showed it to be much enlarged, nodular, firm. Ascites was present. There had been no jaundice, and thus far no pain. She had had five or six children, and thought she had again had every symptom of pregnancy. Four months later there was an autopsy, revealing disease of the liver.

DR. BROWN said he was called to a patient with the message that she was in labor at full term. He found a young woman, married one year, leaning over a chair, and apparently in a good deal of pain. The catamenia had been unusually scanty for several months previously. The patient had had nausea, and for the past three or four months had felt " motions." The uterus was found to be of the normal size. There was no pregnancy at all.

DR. EDSON mentioned a case similar to that detailed by Dr. Richardson. Two years ago a woman forty-three years old was very positive that she felt motion. She supposed herself to be in the middle of the eighth month at the time she came under Dr. Edson's observation. The menstrual flow was suppressed. The breasts were enlarged, but did not secrete milk. There was extreme jaundice. She died shortly afterwards, but there was no autopsy.

Diagnosis of Pregnancy in its Early Stages. — DR. REYNOLDS brought up the subject of the diagnosis of pregnancy, with the question how far an enlargement of the uterus would allow a man to say the patient was advanced to a certain stage in pregnancy. He remarked that he had asked the question at a former meeting of the society. One of the younger members said to him after that meeting that he felt that he had acquired the power of recognizing the state. Dr. Reynolds said that he wondered at the distinct impressions averred by some gentlemen as compared with the extreme indefiniteness in his own case. How many of us, he said, in an examination of a number of patients, half of whom were two months pregnant and half not pregnant, would be able to speak confidently as to the existence of pregnancy, and especially in the case of fat patients, where the difficulty is much increased?

Painless Uterine Contractions. — DR. MINOT reported a case of painless uterine contractions in a woman who had had three children. There were most powerful uterine efforts, so great that the patient held her breath and the tears started to her eyes; but she assured the doctor that there was no pain at all. Dr. Minot said he had looked into several modern authorities without finding any notice of a similar case.

BASTIAN ON PARALYSIS.[1]

THROUGH the labors of ardent workers in the field, the science of cerebral pathology has made some real advances during the past few years, and some new lines of investigation have been opened, along which more progress will yet be made. We heartily welcome Dr. Bastian's book as giving an unusually clear and readable account of the present state of our knowledge of the subject, to which his apparently large experience and good judgment have enabled him to add some new facts and suggestions of interest.

A number of pages are justly given to a description of the distribution of the blood-vessels of the brain, as investigated by Heubner and by Duret.

If we turn to look for the author's opinion on some points of importance which are still under discussion, we find that he accepts the theory of Broadbent to explain the fact that, in cerebral hemiplegia, certain groups of muscles, such as those of the trunk and neck, escape the paralysis which otherwise affects an entire half of the body, namely, that these muscles, from acting always in company with their fellows, are presided over by either side of the spinal cord and of the brain, or by both sides; he believes, moreover, that a similar rule governs the occurrence of sensory paralysis, the functions of sight, hearing, and taste, exercised by bilaterally-acting organs, being much less rarely impaired in hemiplegia than the function of touch, in which one side is oftener concerned alone. To be sure, if the optic or auditory nerve, or one of the corpora quadrigemina, be destroyed, one-sided deafness or blindness may be produced, but to such cases the author does not refer.

The question as to whether lesions in the brain cause paralysis mainly by their direct destruction of certain "centres," as has usually been believed, or, as is maintained by Dr. Brown-Séquard, mainly by their indirect (inhibitory or excitant) action upon distant parts, or perhaps rather upon a special function of the whole brain considered as a diversely gifted unit, is alluded to only for the sake of calling attention to the fact that, in either case, the study of the localization of cerebral lesions is of prime importance, inasmuch as, however

---

[1] *On Paralysis from Brain Disease in its Common Forms.* By H. CHARLTON BASTIAN, M. A., M. D., F. R. S. New York: D. Appleton & Co. 1875.

produced, like results might be expected and are found to follow like causes. This is sound reasoning, and it is no doubt true, as all indeed agree that lesions may act both by direct and by indirect influence ; but since, under the latter, the occurrence of anomalous symptoms does not necessarily presuppose the existence of peculiar anatomical conditions, but only the existence of peculiar functional susceptibilities of the nervous centres, unrevealed by any discoverable physical sign, analogous to a susceptibility to taking cold, and the like, it seems to us that those in whose minds it holds a place even equally prominent with the direct-action theory might be led to overlook anatomical points of importance in any given unusual case.

In referring to the well-known experiments of Fritsch (spelt Fritz) Hitzig, and Ferrier, he gives, unjustly as we think, the credit for greater thoroughness to the latter.

The highly interesting experiments upon the cerebral ganglia by Nothnagel, which would have been expressive of the ideas of many of the Germans, among others Meynert, of Vienna, upon an important part of cerebral physiology, are not mentioned.

The description given of aphasia and kindred disorders seems to us to be unnecessarily cumbrous, and not so satisfactory as one published last winter by Dr. Wernecke, of Breslau, reviewed in the JOURNAL for May 20, 1875.

THE CHOLERA EPIDEMIC OF 1873.[1]

THIS plethoric volume is the fruit of a joint resolution adopted by Congress in 1874, authorizing an investigation concerning the causes of epidemic cholera, and more particularly directing the collection of information with regard to the outbreak of 1873. The report is the united work of the Supervising Surgeon of the Marine-Hospital Service, Dr. John M. Woodworth, and of Dr. Ely McClellan, Assistant Surgeon, U. S. A., specially detailed by the surgeon-general for this service. That the task has been faithfully executed by these well-known officers goes without saying. They have brought to the fulfillment of their trust great zeal and undoubted ability ; and they have presented a contribution to epidemiography which medical men and sanitary authorities especially will do well to have at hand.

The first article in the volume is on the introduction of epidemic cholera into the United States through the agency of the mercantile marine, with some suggestions of preventive measures. Dr. Woodworth treats his topic concisely, but with great clearness and vigor. He points out the incompleteness of the usual regulations touching the inspection of infected ships, and shows how possible it is to import the cholera poison under the existing system. He maintains that passengers' baggage as well as the passengers themselves may convey the infection from port to port, thus rendering the ordinary quarantine only measurably effective. He proposes as an important preventive measure prompt

[1] *The Cholera Epidemic of* 1873 *in the United States.* Washington : Government Printing Office. 1875.

and authoritative information to threatened ports of the shipment of passengers or goods from a cholera-infected district; this information forwarded to the home government by consular officers might speedily be transmitted to all quarantine stations, whose authorities could then be left free to put into operation such measures as they thought best for the protection of their respective ports. In this connection Dr. Woodworth gives some sensible suggestions concerning quarantine.

With regard to prophylaxis, Dr. Woodworth believes heartily in the mineral acids. He bases his belief in part upon clinical observation, and in part upon what he says is the accepted theory of the cholera poison. Upon this latter point we cannot help feeling that he expresses himself somewhat too broadly, not to say dogmatically. In the course of the nine propositions in which he formularizes his ideas of the cause of malignant cholera, he states that the specific organic poison of the disease requires for its reproduction the presence of alkaline moisture, while favoring conditions for the growth of the poison are found in "potable water containing nitrogenous organic impurities and alkaline carbonates; in decomposing animal and vegetable matter having an alkaline reaction; in the alkaline contents of the intestines." On the contrary, "the poison is destroyed naturally either by the process of growth or by contact with acids: (1) those contained in water or soil; (2) acid gases in the atmosphere; (3) the acid secretion of the stomach. It may be destroyed artificially (1) by treating the cholera ejections, or material containing them, with acids; (2) by such acid (gaseous) treatment of contaminated atmosphere; (3) by establishing an acid diathesis of the system in one who has received the poison." Sulphuric acid fulfills, in our author's view, nearly every indication for the prevention and cure of the dreaded pestilence. Whether or not we accept the alkaline hypothesis, it is gratifying at least to have at hand positive expressions from a high authority.

Dr. McClellan's contribution to the report comprises a comprehensive clinical history of the epidemic of 1873, compiled from the detailed records of more than seven thousand cases of the disease. Included in this portion of the volume are notes of the treatment as prescribed by the physicians under whose observation the cases fell. The greater number of the cases were placed upon the calomel treatment, and it is rather curious to read that better results were obtained from calomel alone than from the combination of this agent with others. The acid treatment resulted in a mortality of only eight per cent., although the author observes that the data are not reliable, the number of cases of this class being very small.

The chapter upon the etiology of the disease is exceedingly interesting. Among the topics discussed here, the subject of the transmission of cholera by means of railroad cars and steamboats is very suggestively treated.

The chapter on the prevention of cholera is a perfect compendium of sanitary teaching. Its thoroughness and good sense commend its perusal to health-authorities everywhere, not only to those of districts infected with the pestilence, but to those also of cities which by their uncleanness invite epidemic disease of every kind.

A considerable portion of the book is devoted to the detailed report of the epidemic of 1873 as it was observed in the South and West. Necessarily this part of the work is somewhat monotonous, but it contains a multitude of facts which will be of great value in the future for reference.

A complete historical review of the travels of Asiatic cholera, from the earliest to the latest times, occupies nearly two hundred pages of the volume. It is contributed jointly by Dr. John C. Peters, of New York, and Dr. McClellan, the former writing of the epidemics in Asia and Europe, and the latter of those in North America.

Finally, we have *three hundred* pages of bibliography compiled by Dr. John S. Billings, the indefatigable Superintendent of the Library of the Surgeon-General's Office at Washington. It is a most complete and valuable acquisition.

In our brief sketch we have not done justice to this latest and most excellent contribution to the literature of epidemic cholera. We sincerely trust that the national authorities will not be unwilling to distribute the work freely, so that the profession may have the benefit of what we believe to be a volume of great value.   D.

FIEBER ON ELECTRICITY.[1]

THIS little book is an unscientific and wordy puff for electro-therapeutics, calculated rather to mislead than to instruct the uninitiated, and to disgust those who have the interests of the truth, as regards this subject, at heart.

We cannot agree with the translator that the general practitioner by reading it can get all the information that the welfare of his patients requires him to possess, nor that the author's object in writing the essay may be gathered from the text, unless indeed that object was to increase his private practice by making an impression on the public.

TRAVELS IN PORTUGAL.[2]

THE author of this handsomely printed book has given an entertaining description of his travels through a country which to the ordinary tourist is a veritable *terra incognita*. Physicians will naturally ask the volume for some light upon the question whether Portugal offers attractions in its climate, and otherwise, sufficient to recommend it as a health-resort. In regard to temperature during the winter, the extreme southern part of the country is said to compare favorably with the situations along the Mediterranean at present

[1] *The Treatment of Nervous Diseases by Electricity.* By DR. FRIEDRICH FIEBER, Chief of the Special Division for Electro-Therapeutics of the K. K. Hospital of Vienna. Translated by GEORGE M. SCHWEIG, M. D., Member of the New York County Medical Society. New York: G. P. Putnam's Sons. 1875.

[2] *Travels in Portugal.* By JOHN LATOUCHE. New York: G. P. Putnam's Sons. 1875.

frequented by invalids; but in all other respects, the sick man does not find many inducements held out to him in Portugal. Nobody in the kingdom speaks any language save the native exceedingly difficult tongue. And even if the tourist has mastered the dialect, he is prone to use it most fluently in the proverbial Portuguese profanity, the bad roads, bad food, and bad lodgings giving him ample opportunity for proficiency in that direction.

Having settled the question of the sanatory qualities of Portugal, the medical reader will find in the description of the author's adventures very much to amuse and instruct. The book is embellished with photographic copies of sketches representing some of the most striking features of Portuguese scenery.

THE PROFESSION AND THE METRIC SYSTEM.

WE showed last week the great disadvantages of our present complicated system of weights and measures, and now we propose to consider whether it is not our duty to take some active part in hastening the reform which is sure to come sooner or later. As is well known, efforts have been made and are still carried on with gratifying success, chiefly among architects and builders, to induce the leading firms to adopt the metric system in July, 1876. Circulars have been sent to every town in the country which numbers eight thousand inhabitants, and favorable replies are coming in from all sides. The system was legalized in 1866, but it is desirable that it should become compulsory, and this, of course, cannot occur without a certain amount of preparation. The first thing to do is to make it familiar to the public, as the importance of the change is hardly appreciated by others than scientific men, and as at first sight it appears a very formidable undertaking to renounce the terms we have known from childhood and to adopt others. The fact, however, that in schools and colleges the new system is already very generally taught will go far towards overcoming this difficulty. At the late meeting of the American Pharmaceutical Association the matter was referred to a committee, but the next meeting does not occur till after July. We do not remember whether the question was discussed at the last meeting of the American Medical Association, but even if it were, the next meeting is so near the time for action that a favorable report would come rather late. Cannot something be done at once by the leading medical societies? Let the matter be discussed, the advantages and practicability of the change be made evident, and the influence of the medical profession be added to that of others. The coöperation of the pharmaceutical profession is requisite for the success of the measure, just as the architects cannot dispense with the assistance of the builders. If the medical societies of the larger cities should agree to adopt the metric system on the fourth of July next, there is, we think, no question that it would supersede the old after the delay and struggle through which all reforms must pass. We commend these suggestions to the consideration of the profession throughout the country, and hope that other medical journals will join us in advocating the change. As long as the reform is effected it makes little difference whence it comes, but we should be proud to find the Suffolk District Medical Society the first to take decisive action.

EXTIRPATION OF THE LARYNX.

A CASE of total extirpation of the larynx, with the hyoid bone, and of a portion of the tongue, pharynx, and œsophagus, was the subject of a paper recently read before the Medical Society of Berlin by Professor B. von Langenbeck. The paper is published in full in the *London Medical Record* of September 15, 1875. The patient was a man aged fifty-seven years, who entered the hospital November 29, 1874, suffering from violent dyspnœa threatening suffocation, attacks of cough attended with a whistling sound, and a cyanotic tint of the face. The next day laryngotomy was performed and a tube inserted. December 10th, an examination revealed distinct enlargement of the larynx, the epiglottis and neighboring structures being so swollen that it was impossible to obtain a view of the cavity of the larynx and of the rima glottidis. Extirpation of the larynx was urged but refused.

July 1st the patient was readmitted to the hospital. Breathing had been carried on with freedom through the tracheal tube, but lately there had been increasing difficulty of deglutition. The larynx and infra-maxillary glands were much enlarged, and a yellowish-red nodulated mass was seen to project behind the root of the tongue. The patient's general condition and strength were satisfactory. The following is Professor Langenbeck's account of his operation : —

" Extirpation of the larynx was performed on July 21st. The patient having been narcotized by chloroform administered through the tracheal fistula, the canula was removed, the opening in the trachea was enlarged downwards, and Trendelenburg's tampon-canula was introduced and fixed into the trachea by pumping air into the India-rubber bag. Anæsthesia was kept up to the end of the operation by administering chloroform through a tube introduced into the canula.

" A transverse incision was made through the skin, two centimetres (0.8 inch) above the hyoid bone, from the inner edge of one sterno-mastoid muscle to that of the other. From the centre of this incision, another was carried in the middle line, over the larynx, close down to the tracheal fistula, the upper cicatrix of which, however, was not divided. The skin was then turned back in two flaps, and the larynx (thyroid cartilage) was laid free. The infiltrated lymphatic glands, with the right submaxillary gland, were then extirpated ; the mylo-hyoid, digastric, and hyo-glossus muscles were cut through above the hyoid bone ; the lingual artery was exposed and tied ; the glands were then removed on the left side, and the left lingual artery was tied. The operation was considerably impeded by the unusual shortness of the patient's neck, and by the fusion of the soft parts with the larynx, probably induced by the long retention of the canula. The stripping off of the soft parts from the thyroid and cricoid cartilages could be only imperfectly accomplished ; and the intention of dissecting off the pharynx and the upper end of the œsophagus from the larynx had to be abandoned, as the cancer had invaded the first-named of these parts.

" It being then impossible to preserve the anterior wall of the pharynx and œsophagus, we proceeded to lay open the fauces. The larynx being drawn

forwards and downwards by a sharp hook fixed in the hyoid bone, the point
of the tongue was drawn out of the mouth by means of a thread passed
through it, and the root of the tongue was cut through about four-fifths of an
inch above the hyoid bone. The superior thyroid arteries were then tied, and
the lateral wall of the pharynx cut through. Finally, the pharyngo-palatine
arches, which were stretched forward hy the strong dragging of the larynx,
were divided. The external carotid artery, which was drawn forward with
the lateral wall of the pharynx, was then laid bare on each side, tied in two
places, and cut through between the ligatures. The lingual and hypoglossal
nerves were also exposed and divided.

" The larynx now remained connected with the trachea only; and the latter
was divided close below the cricoid cartilage, so as to leave the tampon-canula in the tracheal fistula.

" The anterior cervical region, from the chin nearly as far as the manubrium
sterni, showed now a large opening, at the bottom of which the spinal column,
covered by the posterior wall of the pharynx and œsophagus, lay exposed.
The skin of the neck, which had been divided by the transverse incision, was
turned over in two flaps, like a collar. The trachea sank downwards, so that
the canula lay close above the sternum. At the upper end of the wound
were seen the velum palati and the broad wounded surface of the tongue. On
inspection through the mouth, the anterior part of the tongue was seen to be
quite pale; it had receded from the lower jaw, and was completely immovable.

" The muscles divided and removed in the operation, besides the small
laryngeal muscles, were the sterno-hyoid, sterno-thyroid, crico-hyoid, mylo-
hyoid, digastric, genio-hyoid, stylo-hyoid, and stylo-glossal; the stylo-pharyn-
gei, glosso-pharyngei, and palato-pharyngei. Forty-one ligatures were applied
to vessels, namely, to the external maxillary, lingual, superior thyroid, external
carotid, and laryngeal arteries; and both hypoglossal and lingual nerves were
divided. Along with the infiltrated lymphatic glands I had removed both submaxillary glands, fearing that these glands, which were apparently somewhat
enlarged, might become diseasd.

" Notwithstanding the extent of the wound and the length of the operation,
which lasted two hours, there was comparatively little exhaustion. The patient's
appearance was good; pulse 80, full and strong; temperature 36.8° Centigrade
(98.25° Fahr.). I believe that this is mainly to be ascribed to the circumstance that complete chloroform-narcosis was steadily kept up by the help of
the plug in the trachea from the beginning to the end of the operation; that
we were able to completely prevent the flow of blood into the air-passages;
and that the operation being performed by careful anatomical dissection without any bruising or laceration of the parts, we were able to tie the great vessels before dividing them.

" After the operation was completed, and the patient had awakened from
the anæsthesia, some Hungarian wine was given to him through an œsopha-
geal tube, the tampon-canula was removed, and an ordinary strong tracheal
canula substituted. In order to prevent the mucus, which was abundantly
secreted by the remaining part of the fauces, from coming into contact with
the canula, a compress soaked in a solution (one third per cent.) of salicylic

acid was placed round the neck so as to cover the wound. I abstained from attempting to unite the wound in the cervical integuments by sutures, fearing that the stretching of the parts would favor the burrowing of the secretions from the wound between the divided cervical fasciæ. The flaps of skin on the two sides of the neck were therefore simply laid down in place, and supported by the above-mentioned salicylized compress."

Up to July 28th, although there was abundant purulent secretion, the patient's general condition remained good and he was free from fever.

The prepared specimen showed the anterior wall of the œsophagus and pharynx cut through, the larynx cut away from behind, and the hyoid bone sawn through in the middle. The cancerous degeneration had so completely involved the upper division of the larynx, the epiglottis, and the hyoid bone, that it was difficult to recognize the individual parts. The inner surfaces of the cricoid and thyroid cartilages, as far as the laryngeal pouches and the inferior vocal cords, were free. The morbid change began close above the laryngeal pouches, and, in the form of nodulated masses, completely filled the whole upper part of the laryngeal cavity. The arytenoid cartilages and the aryepiglottic ligaments were completely lost in the tumor. The epiglottis was recognizable in a somewhat separate mass, in which some fragments of the œsophagus could still be recognized. The hyoid bone was surrounded by the swelling, which had grown upwards into the base of the tongue.

The anterior surfaces of the thyroid cartilage and the ring of the cricoid cartilage remained quite free from disease. The tongue was divided in front of the papillæ circumvallatæ, and the cut surface showed healthy tissue. The removed larynx, hyoid bone, and tongue were about 4.4 inches long, of which 1.2 inches belonged to the tongue.

The first extirpation of the larynx in man was performed by Billroth, in December, 1873. The patient was dismissed cured on March 2, 1874, able to speak intelligibly by means of an artificial larynx. The second operation, for partial extirpation, was performed by Heine, of Prague, in a case of stenosis of the larynx. The third operation was performed by Dr. Schmidt, of Frankfort, on August 12, 1874 ; he removed the cricoid, thyroid, and arytenoid cartilages on account of carcinoma of the larynx. The patient died of collapse on the fifth day. In the cases of Heine and Billroth an artificial larynx was adapted soon after the operation, but in Langenbeck's case the large traumatic cavity renders this impossible and it will be necessary to await cicatrization of the wound. Whether, if the case continues to make favorable progress, in the immovable state of the remnant of the tongue the power of swallowing may return, remains to be seen.

MEDICAL NOTES.

— We are happy to announce that the Medical Library Association opened its rooms on Monday last, with a promising display of journals.

— At the recent meeting of the British Medical Association Dr. James Hardie, of Manchester, gave an account of a new rhinoplastic operation, which consisted in the substitution of the upper phalanx of the forefinger for the nasal bones and cartilages, so as to give the required nasal prominence. In the case of a young girl who had lost both nasal bones and cartilages, Dr. Hardie, after failure of other methods, bandaged the arm in such a position as to enable the forefinger to be laid and plastered upon the nasal cavity. in which position the finger was kept for about three months. Gradually the finger became attached to the cavity, and ultimately the upper phalanx was separated from the rest by the forceps. Dr. Hardie's first intention was to employ the finger merely as a substitute for the nasal bones and cartilages, and to lay over it flaps of skin from the face or arm in the usual manner, and to this plan he ultimately returned, although at one time he was so satisfied with its appearance as to think of using the phalanx itself as a substitute for the nose.

— An instance of remarkable persistence of cardiac action after cessation of respiration is reported to the *Medical Times and Gazette* of September 25, 1875, by R. Stewart, M. D., who was called to a gentleman of some seventy-two years, about five o'clock P. M. of July 4, 1872. After prescribing for the fatigue, heat, and pain in the head of which his patient complained, the physician left, but at eight o'clock was again summoned to him and found that he was apparently dead. The jaw had fallen, the eyes were fixed, the body was cool and the head hot; but on applying the ear to the chest the heart was heard distinctly beating twenty-seven times a minute. Artificial respiration was practiced, and air and ammonia blown into the lungs. Under this treatment the heart-beats became more frequent and forcible, but no respiratory effort could be produced. At ten o'clock the heart was still beating, and the attempts to reëstablish respiration so stimulated the heart that a radial pulse became perceptible. The body gradually became cold and rigid and the cardiac pulsations more feeble. Between five and six A. M. of July 5th the throbbing of the heart was very feeble and slow, and could not be accelerated, and a little after eight o'clock there were signs of decomposition by appearance, odor, and lessening rigidity. The patient was evidently dead then ; but, as Dr. Stewart well asks, what was he before ?

— At the meeting of the American Pharmaceutical Association recently held in this city, the committee on adulterations made an interesting report through the chairman, Mr. Miller. Some suggestive revelations were made. Among other things, it was stated that a New Jersey distiller had frankly admitted to Mr. Miller that all the commercial oils of cedar, hemlock, and spruce made by him and his acquaintances were prepared by putting the branches of the respective trees into the still, with an amount of turpentine proportioned to the price they expected to realize ; and prided himself on the superiority of these *distilled* oils over those made by mere admixture with turpentine.

Mr. Miller had on two occasions purchased four cans of oil of lemon, one of which contained but seventy-five per cent. of oil, and the others scarcely thirty-three per cent. These adulterations were becoming common in Europe as well as in this country. A gentleman who claimed to have formerly held responsible positions in two of the largest German houses had shown to Mr. Miller a full line of receipts for mixing and cheapening all the more important oils, which he was anxious to compound in this country. Mr. Miller had also been informed by the official representative of an extensive French firm in Grasse, that all the cheap grades of lavender, rosemary, and red thyme, sent to this country by his firm and other manufacturers, contained at least seventy-five per cent. of turpentine. Some of the adulterations which are of public interest were musk, a caddy of which, weighing nineteen and a half ounces, was proved in an English court to contain only six and a half ounces; French oil of almond, stated on undoubted authority to be obtained exclusively from peach kernels; honey, made by melting cane or other sugar in a decoction of slippery elm bark or a solution of gum and starch; linseed oil, adulterated with hemp, fish, rosin, and mineral oils; beeswax, consisting almost entirely of black earthy matter neatly coated with handsome yellow wax by repeatedly dipping it into the melted wax, and also adulterated with paraffine; castor oil, composed of lard and croton oils, etc.

— The following, recommended by M. Laborde as a new and very advantageous method of preparing raw meat, is given in the *Lyon Médical*. A not very thick broth of tapioca is first prepared, and is then allowed to cool so that it may not cook the meat with which it is subsequently mixed. The meat, having been finely scraped, is diluted with a quantity of cold soup until the mixture is thoroughly made and has the appearance and consistency of a tomato soup. Thus prepared, it only remains to turn in, little by little, the tapioca porridge, stirring it constantly, and there is obtained a perfectly homogeneous broth, in which, when properly made, the meat is so well disguised that the person who eats it, unless previously informed, does not discover it. Under the name of "medicinal porridge of tapioca," raw meat has thus been administered to patients, and has been taken by them with great relish.

— The use of baths in the summer complaint of children is recommended by J. G. Thomas, M. D., of Savannah, Ga., in a communication to the *Medical Times* of September 11, 1875. In entero-colitis where the temperature of the child ranges from 101° to 105°, Dr. Thomas places the patient in a bath of from 70° to 85° for twenty or thirty minutes, and finds the bodily heat will descend to the normal point, or below it, and that the child will go quietly to sleep, and wake in an hour or two much improved. He directs that the child shall be put into a bath of the temperature to which it is accustomed, and then that cold water shall be gradually added until the temperature is reduced to 70° or 75°. In twenty minutes or half an hour the child is taken out, the axillary region dried with a soft towel, and his temperature ascertained. If it is found to be at the normal point, or just below, the child is put to bed, and in an hour the thermometer is used again. If the child's temperature has risen, the bath should be repeated. Sometimes Dr. Thomas has employed the bath repeatedly for several days, where the case has been a severe and protracted one.

— One of our French exchanges reports the case of a child of thirteen months, apparently in good health, who was vaccinated July 9th from the arm of a healthy infant. July 11th the child was taken sick with measles. While the eruption lasted, the evolution of the vaccine disease not only remained stationary, but even the traces of the punctures disappeared. July 17th, eight days after the date of vaccination, the points of inoculation reappeared, surrounded with an inflamed areola, and from that day forward the vaccination pursued a perfectly normal course.

— The importance of rightly estimating the influence of the inorganic constituents of drinking-waters on the constitutions of consumers is forcibly presented in a paper by W. J. Cooper, published in the *Sanitary Record* of September 11, 1875. Reference is made to the experiments of M. Papillon, communicated to the French Academy of Science, which showed that not only the food that is eaten by animals affects the composition of their bones, but that mineral matter in dilute solution is capable of being assimilated. The effect of altering the composition of the water-supply of a community may involve questions of vast importance to the organic structure of the human body. If the water contains lime, strontia, or magnesia, these may appear as phosphates of lime, strontia, or magnesia in the bones. Should these salts be deficient, the bones would be imperfectly supplied with mineral matter. By varying a water-supply it might be possible to alter the physical organization of a population, and in future ages, from the examination of the bones of bygone generations, the character of the water they were in the habit of drinking might possibly be deduced. While much attention is now being directed to organic impurity in drinking-water, the inorganic impurities have been almost overlooked, although there are numerous instances where serious consequences have arisen from the incautious use of deep spring-waters. Some time ago at Hendon, in Middlesex, an artesian well was bored to supply water for some valuable horses which were being reared there. The water was sparkling, pleasant to the taste, and quite free from any organic impurity; the foals, however, which drank the water soon died, and the whole stud was seriously affected with diarrhœa. An analysis showed the water to contain sulphates of magnesia and soda in considerable quantity. On discontinuing the use of the water the disease was arrested. At Rugby the water from an artesian well free from organic impurity was hailed with satisfaction at its brightness; the community, however, were attacked with diarrhœa caused by the Epsom salts present in the water, and the supply had to be discontinued, as there is no known method of freeing the water from sulphates. As is well known, goitre and other throat and glandular affections, and even idiocy, have been attributed to inorganic salts in drinking-water. If the entire organic structures of the human body are liable to alteration when excess of mineral matter is introduced into the system, it is important that health-seekers at the various medicinal springs should place themselves under competent medical supervision. One of the first considerations in the inauguration of a water-supply should be to insure a perfect freedom from excess of any mineral except those comparatively harmless ingredients, chloride of sodium and carbonate of lime.

— A paper on black discoloration of the tongue, written by Dr. Féréol, is to be found in *L' Union Médicale* of September 14, 1875. This affection to which MM. Gubler and Raynaud have already called attention, consists in a black discoloration having its seat at the back of the tongue in front of the lingual V, upon the middle part, where it forms another V at the anterior point, without invading the sides of the organ, and where it makes a coating more or less thick which has been compared to the grass beaten down by the rain. M. Gubler in his article on the subject maintained that the discoloration was not due to the presence of parasites ; but M. Raynaud, on the other hand, regarded the disease as of parasitic origin, or at least that the presence of spores was necessary to produce the discoloration. Dr. Féréol, however, thinks that the presence of the microphyte is to be considered accidental, or at least as epiphenomenal, and suggests "piliform epithelial hypertrophy" as a name for the disease.

WEEKLY BULLETIN OF PREVALENT DISEASES.

THE following is a bulletin of the diseases prevalent in Massachusetts during the week ending October 16, 1875, compiled under the authority of the State Board of Health from the returns of physicians representing all sections of the State : —

The summary for each section is as follows : —

Berkshire : Typhoid fever, influenza, diarrhœa. Very little sickness.

Valley : Typhoid fever, influenza, diarrhœa. It is remarked that fevers are assuming in this region a remittent type, recent years having been especially noteworthy in this respect.

Midland : Typhoid fever, bronchitis, influenza.

Northeastern : Typhoid fever, influenza. Scarlatina is quite prevalent in the eastern part of Essex County. Measles is epidemic in Beverly.

Metropolitan : Typhoid fever, bronchitis, influenza, pneumonia. The epidemic catarrh is more severe and general in this section and in the northeastern than elsewhere. Diphtheria is subsiding.

Southeastern : Typhoid fever, influenza. Not much sickness. Norwood reports diphtheria of a mild type.

The week's returns represent an improvement in the public health of the State at large. None of the diseases have increased in prevalence, but almost all of them have declined somewhat. Their relative order is as follows : Typhoid fever, influenza, bronchitis, diarrhœa, rheumatism, dysentery, diphtheria, pneumonia, cholera infantum, scarlatina, cholera morbus, croup, whooping-cough. Only the first three deserve mention.

F. W. DRAPER, M. D., Registrar.

COMPARATIVE MORTALITY-RATES FOR THE WEEK ENDING OCT. 9, 1875.

	Estimated Population.	Total Mortality for the Week.	Annual Death-Rate per 1000 during Week.
New York	1,060,000	529	31
Philadelphia	800,000	270	17
Brooklyn	500,000	238	25
Chicago	400,000		
Boston	342,000	187	28
Cincinnati	260,000	73	15
Providence	100,700 ˙	38	20
Worcester	50,000	11	12
Lowell	50,000	16	17
Cambridge	48,000	21	23
Fall River	45,000	20	23
Lawrence	35,000	12	18
Lynn	33,000	12	19
Springfield	31,000	11	18
Salem	26,000	6	12

Normal Death-Rate, 17 per 1000.

Books and Pamphlets Received. — A Manual of Minor Surgery and Bandaging. By Christopher Heath, F. R. C. S. Fifth Edition. Philadelphia: Lindsay and Blakiston. 1875. (For sale by A. Williams & Co.)

The Physician's Visiting List for 1876. Philadelphia: Lindsay and Blakiston. 1875. (For sale by A. Williams & Co.)

Lectures on Diseases of the Nervous System. By Jerome K. Bauduy, M. D. Philadelphia: J. B. Lippincott & Co. 1876. (For sale by A. Williams & Co.)

Archiv für pathologische Anatomie und Physiologie, und für klinische Medicin. Herausgegeben von Rudolph Virchow. LXIII. and LXIV.

Annual Report of the Board of Regents of the Smithsonian Institution for 1874. Washington : Government Printing Office. 1875.

Statistics of Mortality from Pulmonary Phthisis in the United States and in Europe. By William Gleitsmann, M. D. Baltimore : Turnbull Bros. 1875.

Climate of the United States considered with reference to Pneumonia and Consumption. By W. D. Bizzell, M. D. (Reprinted from the Transactions of the State Medical Association of Alabama.) 1875.

Transactions of the Wisconsin State Medical Society, 1875. Milwaukee. 1875.

A Report on a Plan for Transporting Wounded Soldiers by Railway in Time of War. By George A. Otis, Assistant Surgeon U. S. A. Washington : War Department. 1875.

Review of Professor Palmer's Statement respecting the Relations of Himself and Colleagues to Homœopathy in the University of Michigan. (Reprinted from the Detroit Review of Medicine, October.)

Transactions of the Medical Society of the State of West Virginia. Wheeling. 1875.

Galeni Libellus quo demonstratur optimum Medicum eundem esse Philosophum. Recognovit et enarravit Iwanus Mueller. Deichert, publisher. Erlangen. 1875.

THE BOSTON
MEDICAL AND SURGICAL JOURNAL.

VOL. XCIII. — THURSDAY, OCTOBER 28, 1875. — NO. 18.

SECOND DENTITION AND ITS ACCOMPANIMENTS.

A LECTURE DELIVERED AT THE HARVARD MEDICAL SCHOOL.

BY CHARLES E. BUCKINGHAM, M. D.,
Professor of Obstetrics and Medical Jurisprudence.

I HAVE spoken of the disturbances which exist at the time of the first dentition. It is a time when the nervous system of the child is very easily disturbed, and when a very large number of children die. They are said to die of " teething; " that is the word very frequently made use of in the reports. But it is not a fair statement; the death is consequent in the great majority of cases upon improper feeding. The false pride of the parent has led him or her to indulge the child in this or that improper article of diet, so that it becomes disgusted with the food which nature provided in the mother's breast, and with the nearest approach to it which can be prepared artificially.

Let us pass over a few years, however, and suppose that the dangers attendant upon the first dentition have been overcome. The tough children have fought the battle through, and have survived the diarrhœa caused by fried potatoes, and the headaches produced by griddle cakes, and the nausea and vomiting following upon the use of pork and beans and mince pies. And now a new set of disturbances comes up, even with the children who have been properly fed and clothed. Diarrhœa begins with those who escaped before ; loss of appetite, headache, pains in different parts of the body show themselves. You are called in to give your advice upon these points, and to see if you can discover why the little boy or girl is ailing. Look in the child's mouth. You know that it is somewhere from five to twelve or thirteen years old, and that during this time it is likely to be losing the twenty so-called milk teeth, and that others are coming in their places. The nervous system of the child is not quite so easily, or rather not so seriously, disturbed as it was while those milk teeth were pushing their way ; but there is a very great change going on, and that nervous system is more easily disturbed than during the last two or three years. It is the part of the dentist to say if this or that tooth should be removed in the

case of the particular child, but it is your business or mine, as its medical attendant, to say that dentition is going on, and that due caution is
to be had in the matter of diet and exercise and sleep. It is not simply
the case that the fang of this tooth has become absorbed as another is
growing up beneath it, but there is also a new tooth coming in a part
of the mouth that has had no tooth before ; and the eruption of that
tooth in an improperly fed and poorly clad child is very likely to produce wakefulness, or drowsiness, or nausea, or cough, or an eczema, or
some other disturbance of one or another part of the body. If you
find any of these disturbances, it is quite as much your duty to look at
the teeth, and to give your caution about feeding and clothing and
exercise, if you find a reason in the gum, as it is for you to feel the
pulse or look at the tongue, and form your opinion and give your instruction from the signs afforded by them. Bear this in memory, that
disturbed digestion will as surely produce cough in one patient as it will
produce headache in another ; and that the second dentition will often
produce as much disturbance as the first, although the sufferer may be
better able to bear it, and a simple chill or a febrile attack of a few
hours' duration may be had in place of what would be a serious convulsion in the younger child.

I think it would be unpardonable neglect were I not to speak in this
connection of the fact that dentition is by no means completed at this
time, although about this period a fourth molar is making its way into
sight. Nor should I forget to call your attention to the fact that in some
families, even as late as the eighteenth or twentieth year, I have seen
these fourth molars making their way and producing a serious amount
of disturbance, both in the digestive and in the nervous system. Probably there is a majority of you gentlemen who remember the pain and
soreness and vertigo which attended the appearance of your wisdom
teeth, and how for weeks and months, yes, perhaps for several years,
before they got their growth, they pressed upon the gum and produced
loss of appetite and restless nights and irritable days. Those of you
whose memory upon this point remains green can easily imagine the
suffering of the little child whose mouth is filled with torments, or of the
older boy or girl who is forced to study or to labor with these causes of
disturbance still at work. At this time, when these fourth molars
are coming through, occurs the age of puberty, a period of excessive
nervous disturbance with those who are thus disposed. It matters not
whether the subjects be male or female. It is a season when great caution should be exercised by those who have children under their observation and care, and many male as well as female children have been
ruined in health because the parents have been ignorant of the periodical
disturbances which are constantly going on. The first of these periods
of disturbance is at the appearance of the first tooth ; this is usually

when the child is taking its natural food. The second period is when the system has had something of a rest, but when a mistaken attempt has been made to educate its stomach to digest grain and fruit, but no attempt has been made to retain its fondness for milk; this is usually before the close of the second summer, and when the larger proportion of the deaths take place. The third is when the early part of the second dentition is going on. The fourth is at that time when the fourth molars are beginning to make their way, and when the effort of nature is made to declare the peculiarities of sex. At each of these times the child is more liable to disease than at others. These are the seasons when our profession is the most likely to be consulted by careful parents, and when diseases of the brain, of the stomach, and of the lungs are the most likely to begin.

To laugh at the unmanliness of the boy or girl who is teething is a matter of as great absurdity as to laugh at the weakness of one who is coming down with a fever. It is not necessary to make babies of them, but it is as well to watch them, and to see that they are not overworked either in body or in mind. The old lady will say that they are only "growing pains" which are causing the disturbance, but it does not hurt to grow; if it did, the young man or woman of eighteen would be always in pain, and the little one of a few months, who has sometimes gained a pound or more a week, would never smile.

Look in the mouth, therefore, and let your attention be paid to the teeth and gums as well as to the tongue.

CASES OF OVARIOTOMY.

BY JOHN HOMANS, M. D.

CASE IV. — *Multilocular Cyst of Left Ovary; Peritonitis at Time of Operation; Fœcal Fistula; Death on the Eighteenth Day.* — Mrs. H., a Swede, forty-three years old, had suffered more or less pelvic pain for fifteen years, and during the last four had been confined to her bed many times on account of severe attacks. Pregnancy had never existed. She first noticed an increase of size five years before I saw her, in January, 1874, at which time the umbilical girth was thirty-two inches. The tumor, occupying the pubic region, was about the size of an ostrich's egg and somewhat movable. On February 1st I punctured the cyst through the abdominal wall with a fine perforated needle, and drew off about twelve ounces of clear yellow fluid, specific gravity 1020, alkaline, highly albuminous, and containing plates of cholesterine. This tapping was followed by peritonitis and suppuration within the cyst. After waiting four weeks for the peritoneal inflammation to subside, it became imperative to perform ovariotomy at once as a last resort. Mrs. H. all this time had a high temperature, and pulse, great pain and tenderness, no appetite, and no rest nor comfort, except when under the influence of opium. On February 18, 1874, the operation was performed at the patient's house with the assistance of Drs. William Ingalls, C. D. Homans, Hayden, and Mr. William Appleton. The length of the incision was four inches; adhesions were universal; some recent from the existing peritonitis, others old, firm, and inseparable, extending to the left brim of the pelvis, to the lower lumbar vertebræ and promontory of the sacrum, and to the sigmoid flexure of the rectum. The entire cyst could not be removed, and as the pelvic adhesions were so intimate as not to admit of dissection, there was practically no pedicle. A clamp was applied as near the base of the cyst as possible. At this stage of the operation an unfortunate accident happened. I twisted off the head of the screw bolt of the clamp, while tightening it with pliers, and being unwilling to leave the clamp in this state, as I could neither tighten nor loosen it, I passed a double ligature beneath the clamp, tied the mass in two halves, and then cut away the clamp. To the manipulation at this time and the friability of the inflamed bowel I attribute the subsequent fæcal fistula.

The main cyst contained thick, offensive pus mixed with masses of lymph; a smaller cyst contained clear fluid. The cyst wall was about one quarter of an inch thick, red and inflamed inside and out; the lining membrane was of a deep cranberry color, and masses of offensive lymph were scattered over its surface. There was very little abdominal tenderness after the operation, but much pain, and on the fourth day the discharge from the wound was evidently fæcal. The abdominal cavity was thoroughly washed out several times a day with a warm weak solution of chlorinated soda. The pulse ranged from 68 to 80 until a day or two before her death, which took place on March 8th. The autopsy showed recent adhesions, with here and there collections of pus among the folds of intestine and in the cellular tissue between the peritoneum and the vertebral column. There were also old adhesions between the left lobe of the liver and the stomach. The perforation was a round hole about two lines in diameter, at a point about six inches from the anus. The ligature had been firmly applied at a point one and a half inches from the uterus.

CASE V. — *Unilocular Cyst of Left Ovary; Death on the Tenth Day; Cause Unknown.* — Mrs. D., aged thirty-six, I saw at Peabody in consultation with Dr. George S. Osborne. At my first visit it seemed probable that pregnancy existed, and vomiting was persistent and almost incessant. She was the mother of one child five years old, and had had two abortions. Her health was usually vigorous. Measures were taken to relieve the uterus of its contents, and on the 16th of March a partially decomposed placenta came away ; there was no trace of a fœtus seen. The mother made a rapid and perfect recovery. The case was a most favorable one for operation ; the cyst was unilocular, without adhesions, and the patient calm and hopeful. The tumor was first noticed in May, 1874, and had increased so much that the umbilical girth was thirty-seven and one half inches on March 1, 1875. Some time after my first visit the patient had removed to a high, spacious house, where she had a large room looking towards the south, and well ventilated. Every precaution to guard against contagion or infection was taken, and Dr. Osborne went so far as to have the cellar, in which potatoes had been stored during the winter, thoroughly cleansed and whitewashed.

The operation was performed on the 18th of May, 1875. Drs. George S. Osborne (who shared with me the after-treatment), Thomas Dwight, Jr., and O. B. Shreve assisted. We were fortunate in having Sister Frances, from St. Margaret's Home, as nurse. There were no adhesions ; the cyst and contents weighed about fifteen pounds ; the only bleeding was from the needle holes. The pedicle was extremely broad, but was easily clamped. The pulse was 64 after the patient had been removed to bed. She vomited once while coming out of the ether. At evening the temperature was $98\frac{3}{4}°$; pulse 64 ; and there was some pain in the back ; one sixth of a grain of morphia subcutaneously. A slight flowing from the uterus came on during the night, and the pulse rose to 76. For food she took nothing but ice. A subcutaneous injection of morphia was given whenever necessary. On the 20th she took some boiled milk. Temperature $99\frac{4}{5}°$. Pulse 95. Pain less severe. Passed urine naturally. On the 21st the clamp was removed ; the wound was united by first intention, and there was no abdominal tenderness nor distention. Pulse 96. Temperature $99\frac{3}{5}°$. She talked brightly, and said she felt nicely. On May 23d she could move herself about in the bed without aid, and relished food. Tongue slightly furred. Pulse 90. Temperature $99\frac{1}{4}°$. Stump of pedicle rather offensive.

May 24th. Pulse 108. Temperature $100\frac{3}{5}°$. Urine more scanty and high colored. No fluid could be detected in Douglass's space, nor was there the least abdominal tenderness. In the evening she was restless.

May 25th. Vomited a greenish sour fluid for the first time since coming out of the ether. She complained of no pain, but evidently felt weaker than on the day before. At noon an enema containing oil of peppermint was administered, and a large natural fæcal discharge followed without discomfort. She took small quantities of brandy, champagne, mutton broth, and gruel. At evening the temperature was $103\frac{3}{5}°$. Pulse 140. Face flushed. No pain nor chill. On the 26th her countenance was anxious, and there was now delirium. The pedicle looked clean and healthy. On the 27th she was restless and indifferent, but when roused would take a little brandy. Pulse 130. Temperature 103°. Uterine flow continued, not at all offensive ; no tenderness nor distention anywhere detected. It was evident that the case, which had gone on so well for five days, was to terminate fatally. There was apparently no peritonitis nor pyæmia, but there was probably blood-poisoning. Without quoting too freely from the record, I will simply say that the delirium increased, that the skin continued natural to the touch, and that careful examinations by the vagina and rectum revealed no induration nor collection of fluid.

At ten P. M. on the 27th severe hæmorrhage from the nose came on, the face being much flushed and the hands cold; this bleeding soon stopped, and towards morning the face became cooler.

Death occurred at eight o'clock, May 28th. No autopsy was allowed, and perhaps it is useless to speculate as to the cause of death. I think, however, that it must have been septicæmia, but without chill or peritonitis. I have not mentioned all that was done in the way of treatment, internally and externally, nor does it seem necessary ; the case has, however, been sufficiently described to. be useful in the history and study of this operation. In my next case I shall, if possible, use the actual cautery in securing the pedicle.

———◆———

A CASE OF SUPPOSED OVARIAN DISEASE.[1]

BY F. B. A. LEWIS, M. D. (HARV.), OF WATERTOWN, N. Y.

MRS. E——, aged twenty-six, robust and finely developed, married in January, 1870, had a healthy child one year after, and a miscarriage at the second or third month during the second year succeeding. I saw her first in August, 1873, on account of severe endometritis, which had resisted all ordinary treatment. Owing to energetic measures and to a naturally good constitution, she recovered, and was discharged well in October following. She remained in health until August, 1874, when she presented herself at my office, saying she feared something was wrong with her, as she had disagreeable sensations in the lower part of the abdomen, with some leucorrhœal discharge. While I was examining the uterus bimanually, the fingers detected a tumor in the left inguinal region, in size about that of an ordinary orange, indistinctly movable, firm, and not tender; the patient had been unaware of its presence. The uterus was in a normal condition.

A month later the patient returned, and on examination the tumor

---

[1] Read before the Jefferson County (N. Y.) Medical Society, October 5, 1875.

was found to be considerably increased in size, but without pain or tenderness; it was still firm, and somewhat less movable. The general
condition remained satisfactory. A consultation was advised, but the
patient was lost sight of until several weeks afterward, when, during
my absence, another physician was called, on account of trouble in micturition, with considerable pain. He stated that the uterus was found
pressed downward upon the neck of the bladder, and on pushing it high
up the pain was instantly relieved, and he did nothing more. From
this time the tumor steadily but rapidly increased in size, extending over
into the right side and filling the entire abdomen. Meanwhile it developed renewed trouble in micturition, and caused constipation and
dyspnœa. There was no pain in the tumor itself, nor failure of the
general health, until the latter part of the year 1874; at this time the
measurement around the body at the most prominent point was thirty-
eight inches, taken while the patient was lying down. * The skin of the
abdomen had become quite thin; distended veins in great numbers
coursed over the surface; the dullness on percussion extended over the
entire abdomen; the sense of fluctuation was indistinct and indefinable.
No change of outline resulted from altered posture. The skin was
movable over the tumor in places only. The entire mass was quite
firmly fixed in the pelvis. The uterus was strongly anteverted, with
the cervix flattened against the pubes; the sound entered two and three
fourths inches, and moved the uterus, which was small, quite freely,
considering the pressure above. There was fullness with indistinct
fluctuation high up in posterior vaginal cul-de-sac, and uniform fullness
was felt in rectum. Menstruation, which had been normal, now became
irregular and painful. The patient emaciated rapidly, and was troubled
at times by œdema of the feet and ankles; this latter condition disappeared after bandaging and the use of stimulating lotions. The more
general discomforts were hiccough, the passage of flatus through the
compressed intestine, and the sensation of weight in the abdomen.

The opinion had been early given that the case was one of ovarian
cyst, probably multilocular. This diagnosis was confirmed by a surgeon
as well qualified as any in this portion of the State, one who a few
years ago, in opposition to the diagnosis of several other physicians, had
confirmed my opinion in a similar case, in which the tumor after its removal was found to be a multilocular ovarian cyst of large size. In the
present instance an operation was advised, and preparations were made for
it, although the patient was able to move about the house at times. In the
early part of January, 1875, her general health failed more decidedly,
and she had four or five hysterical convulsions each day. At this time
another surgeon was called, who, without disputing the diagnosis, advised a delay in operating until the general condition might be improved.

The remarkable points of this case are now to be reported. Within ten days after the last consultation the patient's condition became wholly altered. Leaving her one day in a state of comparative comfort, I found her the next affected with severe convulsive attacks, chills, with fever and sweating, pain in the tumor, pinched countenance, and small, quick pulse. By the 10th of January the tumor had entirely changed; it was softer, and fluctuation was easily made out; the abdomen was considerably smaller; the veins, previously so prominent, became emptied, and the skin could be easily taken up in folds. On January 11th an aspirator-needle was inserted midway between the umbilicus and the pubes, and a pint of odorless pus was drawn; the needle then became obstructed, and, the patient being much relieved, nothing more was done until the 19th, when, convulsions and the other symptoms recurring, a trocar and canula were introduced, and several pints of pus, mixed with gelatinous • matter and sloughy-looking strings, were evacuated. A long probe passed through the canula could be swept about or passed in any direction, to the extent of eight or nine inches. It was designed at the time of operating to leave the canula for the purpose of drainage; but when the sac appeared empty the instrument was withdrawn, and the orifice was closed with adhesive strips. At this time the case was considered to be a desperate one, but the patient improved rapidly, the convulsions were arrested, the sac never refilled, the extent of dullness became less each week, and at this date (October, 1875) the patient is a robust person, full of life and vigor.

In conclusion, it may be remarked that among the reports of cases I have been unable to find one like the foregoing. Ovarian cysts appear not to suppurate very often, especially when they have reached considerable size. Even when suppuration occurs, the progress of the case is unlike that here noted. Possibly it may be said there was an error in the diagnosis, but certainly the history is not that of any other disease affecting the pelvic region.

RECENT PROGRESS IN PATHOLOGY AND PATHOLOGICAL ANATOMY.[1]

BY B. H. FITZ, M. D.

PATHOLOGICAL ANATOMY.

Aneurisms. — Professor Köster[2] spoke to the Lower Rhine Society, at Bonn, with reference to the origin of aneurisms. The commonly accepted idea that these are due to chronic endarteritis and its meta-

[1] Concluded from page 473.
[2] Berliner klinische Wochenschrift, 1875, xxiii. 322.

morphoses, the so-called atheromatous condition, was objected to on the following grounds: (1.) Aneurisms may occur on otherwise healthy arteries. (2.) The atheromatous disease is exceedingly common in Germany, but aneurisms are rare. (3.) The inner coat of small arteries is too thin to offer any special opposition to the blood pressure, and were it diseased or destroyed there is no reason for a protrusion of the wall of the artery. Finally, (4) aneurisms are most common in middle life, while the atheromatous condition is a disease of old age. Köster examined large and small depressions in the walls of the aorta and of other arteries. Like Helmstedter, he found numerous light spots in the middle of the muscular coat, which were regarded as inflamed spots with a growth of connective tissue such as occurs in cirrhosis of the liver. They contained blood-vessels and were connected with the external coat by a bridge, in which were arterial and venous vessels. He thought that the inflammation of the vessel-wall began in the outer coat, around the nutrient vessels; thence extended into the muscular coat and became diffused here, corresponding with the capillary distribution of the vaso vasorum. The inflammatory changes may reach the inner coat when the nutrient vessels extend into the latter, as is sometimes the case. Under such conditions the intima is often thickened. We have thus a spotted, chronic inflammation of the middle coat; its elastic fibres and muscle-cells are destroyed, and eventually the inner and thickened outer coat become united into a single vascular membrane of homogeneous histological structure. Such parts become protruded and represent the aneurism.

Congenital Syphilis. — Of late years, very valuable contributions to the pathological anatomy of this disease have been made, some of which suggest points of marked interest to the practitioner, with reference both to diagnosis and to treatment. Enlargement of the spleen had occasionally been observed, but Bärensprung[1] called more direct attention to this condition of the organ. He attributed the change to a disturbance in the portal circulation in consequence of the well-recognized changes in the liver. Gee[2] then published a paper giving the result of his observations relating to the enlargement of the spleen in hereditary syphilis. He believed that in about one fourth of all cases of hereditary syphilis the spleen was enlarged, and that the degree of its enlargement might be regarded as a means of measuring the syphilitic cachexia. Most cases in which there was a decided enlargement terminated fatally.

Numerous observers since then have noted the splenic enlargement, without, however, attaching the same weight to it. Fränkel[3] again

[1] Die hereditäre Syphilis, 1864, page 75.
[2] British Medical Journal, 1867, page 435; from Virchow and Hirsch's Jahresbericht for 1867, ii. 555.
[3] Ueber Placentar Syphilis. 1873.

calls attention to the subject, and Birch-Hirschfeld[1] has made it the subject of special study in the light of other recent investigations. This observer based his conclusions upon the examination of thirty-two syphilitic infants. He found, so constantly, considerable increase in the weight of the spleen in these cases, that he stated that one could scarcely err in expecting to find other evidences of syphilis where the marked alteration of the spleen was present. The microscopical examination of these spleens gave no appearances differing from those occurring under normal circumstances. When the fœtus was born in a macerated condition the spleens were very soft and of a dirty violet color on section. If the child was still-born, or if it died soon after birth, the spleen was of increased density, of a dark brownish color, presenting the indurated form; or again, the organ might be soft and pale.

Unquestionably of far greater importance is the discovery by Wegner[2] of certain changes in the cylindrical bones found at the junction of the shaft with the epiphysis, and at the border between the bony and cartilaginous portions of the ribs. He has described three stages in the process, to which he has applied the term syphilitic osteochondritis, and he states that the one or the other is of almost constant appearance in cases of congenital syphilis.

In the first stage, instead of the normal, sharply defined, horizontal or curved line on longitudinal section, indicating the direct transition of hyaline cartilage into bone, there is found a layer two millimetres wide, with an irregular border on both sides. This layer or zone is soft and brittle, of a glistening white or reddish-white color, and of a denser, more homogeneous appearance than the neighboring reddish bony cancellated structure. These appearances result from a proliferation of the cartilage cells and a delay in the conversion of calcified cartilage into bone.

In the second stage the intervening layer is twice as wide as that above mentioned; its border towards the cartilage is extremely irregular, presenting numerous projections varying in length, breadth, and contour, sometimes connected by transverse lines so that islets of cartilage seem to be inclosed. A similar condition exists towards the bone, though less marked. The layer of cartilage bordering on the bone is soft, of a bluish transparent appearance, as in rickets. The microscopic changes are a greater proliferation of cells, an abundant development of vessels, towards the bone imbedded in a fibrous tissue, the intervening cartilage thickened and condensed, containing osteoid tissue, even streaks of true bone; towards the spongy portion of the diaphysis, calcified cartilage is present, indicating a delay in its transition into bone tissue.

[1] Archiv der Heilkunde, 1875, xvi. 173.
[2] Virchow's Archiv, 1870, page 305.

In the third stage, the articular ends of the bones and the ribs at the junction of bone and cartilage become enlarged. The adjoining parts of the cartilage are blue, transparent, moist, and project on section. Bordering upon this is an opaque, grayish-yellow layer, dense and homogeneous, from two to four millimetres in width, which is limited above and below by an irregular, jagged, and rounded line.

Though this layer feels hard, it is brittle and easily crumbled. Below it is an irregularly bounded layer, grayish-red or grayish-yellow, soft, at times almost fluid, which is gradually lost in the spongy bone tissue. In consequence, the union between the diaphysis and the cartilaginous epiphysis is loosened, the parts are movable with a slight degree of crepitation, and may even fall apart if the periosteum is cut through. The adjoining cancellated tissue of the shaft contains a gray or reddish-gray marrow resembling granulation-tissue. Wegner has noted the following relative frequency of the process in the various bones. It is most often found in the lower end of the femur ; then the lower end of the bones of the leg and fore-arm, the upper end of the tibia, the upper end of the femur and fibula ; then the upper end of the humerus, that of the radius and ulna, and rarest of all in the lower end of the humerus.

Waldeyer and Köbner [1] corroborate this discovery, and call attention to the fact that the gross appearances may be extremely slight, while with the microscope characteristic anomalies are found. They mention the incomplete formation of the osteo-blasts which form an almost continuous epithelial-like layer in normal ossification. They urge that as this disease is of constant intra-uterine origin, therefore its existence enables one to discriminate between cases of hereditary and acquired infantile syphilis. Further, it is absolutely diagnostic where the fœtus is a macerated one, in which often visceral changes cannot be found. This consideration may be of value in enabling one to recognize aright obscure diseased phenomena on the part of the parents. Another inference, at present of relative weight only, owing to the limited number of exact observations, is that the change seems to be independent of the treatment of the mother previous to or during pregnancy.

Birch-Hirschfeld [2] confirms the constancy of the occurrence of this syphilitic osteochondritis, though he cannot consider that its absence excludes the possibility of the presence of syphilis. To the descriptive appearances of Wegner he adds that when the epiphysis is separated from the shaft the line of fracture presents irregular bits, is jagged ; while when the normal bone is treated in the same manner, the cartilage is separated smoothly from the bone.

Oedmansson and Winckel have called attention to the existence of a stenosis of the umbilical vein within the cord of certain macerated

[1] Virchow's Archiv, 1872, lv. 367.
[2] Loc. cit.

fœtuses, the death of the fœtus being attributed to this condition. The former observer considered the alteration in question as belonging to the atheromatous process. Birch-Hirschfeld objects to this conclusion on the ground of an examination he had made where a very decided stenosis of the umbilical vein was found. He regards the condition analogous to that occurring in arteries as the result of syphilis, described by Heubner. At the same time the change is rarely found in macerated fœtuses in which marked syphilitic changes in the bones are present. Further, it was found on several occasions in macerated fœtuses where no alteration of the epiphyses was present. If this affection of the vessels, therefore, is to be regarded as a result of syphilis, the osteochondritis cannot be regarded as an absolutely constant sign of the disease.

Birch-Hirschfeld describes changes in the pancreas which he frequently found in cases of congenital syphilis. Similar alterations had previously been observed, though no special weight had been attached to the same. He examined the pancreas from the bodies of seventy-three newly-born and still-born infants. In twenty-three of these cases the syphilitic osteochondritis was present, and in thirteen of these the pancreas was found diseased, it being normal in the non-syphilitic children. Of the twenty-three cases ten were macerated fœtuses, and of these two only had an abnormal pancreas. Of the remaining thirteen infants, born alive or dying during birth, eleven presented a diseased pancreas. In the more advanced degrees the organ was decidedly enlarged in all dimensions ; its weight may be doubled, the tissue is firm, glistening white on section, the glandular structure indistinct to the naked eye. The microscope showed a high degree of development of the interstitial tissue. This was observed more particularly between the larger lobules of the gland, though it was sometimes found between the individual pouches of the lobule. The latter were compressed, their epithelium atrophied. The vessels in the interstitial tissue were sparse, their walls thickened. This extreme degree was present in seven cases. In six the alteration was less evident to the naked eye, though the organ was enlarged, the lobules somewhat indistinct, the density increased, and the color pale. The interstitial tissue-changes were less marked. The changes in the microscopical appearances, though less in degree than before, were still distinctly different from those of the normal pancreas. The head of the pancreas presented more marked alterations than the tail. This interstitial degeneration is analagous to the interstitial changes occurring in the liver. It seems probable that it develops late in intra-uterine life, as the macerated fœtuses rarely presented it. The most extreme instance was found in a child who had died five months after birth. The question naturally arose whether the frequent cachexia of children born with syphilis is not in part due to the disturbance of digestion probably resulting from this change.

Embolism of the Superior Mesenteric Artery. — Litten [1] endeavored to ascertain by experiments on dogs the cause of hæmorrhagic infarction in cases where an embolus had become fixed in the mesenteric artery, since this vessel is not a terminal artery, in the sense of Cohnheim.[2] A ligature was placed around the trunk of the artery, and the animals died within forty-eight hours, with great prostration, loss of appetite, occasional vomiting, offensive, bloody, tar-like dejections, associated with a falling of temperature and with tympanites. Putrefaction was rapid, and in certain cases a purulent and hæmorrhagic peritonitis was present. The distended coils of the small intestine from the lower part of the jejunum and the upper part of the large intestine were of a dark, reddish-black color, lustreless and œdematous. The mucous membrane was of the same color, and covered with a bloody secretion. The serous coat presented occasional vesicular elevations. Extensive hæmorrhages were found between the coats of the intestine. Peyer's patches were swollen and hæmorrhagic. The mesentery corresponding to the region affected was opaque, dotted with numerous hæmorrhages. The mesenteric glands were swollen, at times thoroughly infiltrated with blood. The mesenteric veins were distended with fluid blood. These appearances represent the combination to which the term hæmorrhagic infarction is applied. Ligature of the trunk beyond the uppermost branches produced similar changes, though not so marked in the upper part of the jejunum. The ligature of single branches produced no effect, but when a group of arteries proceeding to a limited portion of intestine was tied a corresponding limited infarction occurred. The circulation thus cut off did not return, and the conclusion was drawn that the function of this artery is that of a terminal one. This, however, is in direct opposition to the well-known anatomical communication between the superior mesenteric, the pancreatico-duodenalis, and the inferior mesenteric arteries.

Assuming that the cessation of the blood-current must be due to an alteration of the blood-pressure or to a change in the resistance of the vessel-wall, he learned that physiologically the resistance could not be strongly diminished nor the blood-pressure decidedly increased. By means of a forced injection, however, he was able to push the fluid injected into the region of the obstructed artery, but the animal died before this end was accomplished. It therefore resulted that to reëstablish quickly the circulation in the obstructed region such a pressure is necessary as never occurs under ordinary conditions; hence the function of the artery is that of a terminal one.

1 Virchow's Archiv, 1875, lxiii. 289.
2 Vide the JOURNAL, October 24, 1872, page 281

There is thus no essential distinction between the superior mesenteric artery and the other large arterial trunks, excepting the anatomical terminal arteries. The practical point is the period at which the collateral circulation is established, and the length of time that the part can get along without a supply of fresh blood; and these vary considerably with the different arteries.

The writer then presents a series of sixteen recorded cases of embolism of the superior mesenteric artery. A comparison of these with the results of experiment shows a very close resemblance, there being at the most modifications in the time of the occurrence of destructive processes in the intestine.

Experiments made upon the cœliac and the inferior mesenteric arteries showed in no case extensive lesion or necrosis. The recorded cases of embolism of these arteries furnish a similar result; hence their branches are not to be regarded as terminal, either functionally or anatomically.

Cirrhosis of the Liver in Children. — Two such cases are reported by Dr. Cazalis,[1] the patients being girls aged seven and nine years respectively. They entered the hospital with ascites, slight œdema of the legs, and considerable dilatation of the abdominal veins. Both children had been ailing for some time, though the abdominal swelling had been noticed for a few weeks only.

Albuminuria was present in one case, slight jaundice in the other; in neither was there any heart-disease. During treatment the children suffered from attacks of acute peritonitis; as the fever subsided the ascites increased rapidly, and tapping was finally resorted to. The one child soon died of pneumonia, erysipelas about the puncture, and gangrene of the vulva. The other died from subsequent peritonitis.

The livers were found extremely atrophied, that of the elder girl scarcely of the size of the fist of an adult; both were finely lobulated, resembling on section an ordinary gin-drinker's liver. The spleen was enlarged in both cases, that of the elder child very much so.

But little information could be obtained concerning the previous history of the younger child. Well in 1870, she suffered from cold and hunger during the German siege of Paris. The parents of the elder girl were temperate, and presented no evidence of syphilis; their child had measles at the age of three, and often complained of her stomach since. During the three years previous to her death she had frequent nose-bleed. When seven years old she had a mucous (typhoid?) fever; from this time her belly began to enlarge. She suffered from indigestion, diarrhœa, and occasional slight tenesmus. Her abdomen became larger during an attack of jaundice lasting two months. The girl had never had intermittent fever. She had lived most of her life in a damp basement.

1 Progrès Médical, March 20, 1875; from Medical Times and Gazette, May, 1875, page 472.

Dr. Cazalis considered that cold and damp might be deemed an important element in the development of cirrhosis in children.

The cases seem to show that this affection may occur in children, independently of heart-disease, syphilis, or the abuse of stimulants.

Exfoliation of the Mucous Membrane of the Bladder. — Mr. Bell[1] showed the specimen to the Medico-Chirurgical Society of Edinburgh. Three months previous the patient had been delivered of a still-born child ; about a month afterwards Mr. Bell was consulted concerning incontinence of urine. At the mouth of the urethra, which was largely dilated, there was detected what seemed to be a tumor. The fingers could be passed between the bladder and this in all directions. The mass was finally detached and withdrawn. It was found to be the whole mucous membrane of the bladder, coated with phosphates. The patient made a good recovery, though there is still a little incontinence of urine if she walks about much.

PAGET'S CLINICAL LECTURES AND ESSAYS.[2]

EVERYTHING which emanates from Sir James Paget's pen is sure to attract attention. The demands of an immense consulting and fashionable London practice having latterly diverted him from pathological pursuits, his occasional lectures nowadays deal chiefly with practical subjects. Sagacious clinical observation, rather than study and research in the laboratory and among books, characterizes this admirable volume, which reflects almost exclusively the mind of its author. Mature practitioners will perhaps appreciate the clear tone of its ring better than beginners, but both will derive an excellent lesson from the caution, bred of experience, which prominently reveals itself on almost every page, and especially will it prove instructive to those who are always eager to " do something," in or out of season.

Its list of contents is a striking one. The fifty pages on Strangulated Hernia are full of practical wisdom. The lecture on Sexual Hypochondriasis is a judicious discussion of this difficult question ; and the Notes for the Study of some Constitutional Diseases an excellent specimen of the author's contemplative writing. The Calamities of Surgery, Stammering with other Organs than those of Speech, Nervous Mimicry, Cases that Bone-Setters Cure, are other titles which indicate the originality of the varied subjects.

Mr. Howard Marsh, who, Sir James says in his preface, " has done what he could to amend the chief of his defects," in a brief appendix and scattered foot-notes adds a certain amount of references and cases in support of the author's views. Most of the lectures and essays are reprints; but the evidences of revision and addition are numerous, and nothing suggests the idea of an attempt at mere " book-making." It is a valuable contribution to permanent medical literature.

[1] Edinburgh Medical Journal, 1875, ccxxxviii. 935.
[2] *Clinical Lectures and Essays.* By SIR JAMES PAGET, Bart. Edited by HOWARD MARSH, F. R. C. S. New York : D. Appleton & Co. 1875.

HEATH'S MINOR SURGERY.[1]

THIS little book appeared originally in 1861, and was specially adapted by the author to the wants of the "dressers" and "house-surgeons" of the London hospitals. The work performed by these individuals is such as every medical student is desirous to learn and every young practitioner ought to be familiar with. In writing, therefore, with a well-defined object in view the author has succeeded in avoiding many imperfections which are common to books of this kind. The range of subjects is not too great, and each one is treated in a concise manner, but clearly and full enough to be of practical value. Descriptions of antiquated methods of treatment, apparatus, and bandaging have been carefully avoided, while the writer has shown his appreciation of what a student wants to know by introducing quite a variety of topics not strictly belonging to such a book, which may also be said to contain in addition to the usual instruction a great deal of excellent advice. There are a few subjects, indeed, which we hardly think necessary, such as the conduct of the house-surgeon or pupil in the operating theatre; there are, on the other hand, useful chapters on case-taking and on post-mortem examinations, by reading which students would certainly be benefited. The wood-cuts are fair and not too numerous, and although they are rather in accordance with the methods of English than of American surgeons, the changes that could be made are of no great importance. The fact that Mr. Heath's little book has reached a fifth edition, and that the last one has been carefully revised, is, we think, a sufficient guarantee of its value.

SMITHSONIAN REPORT, 1874.

THE Smithsonian Institution, as appears from its last report, is steadily pursuing its gigantic labors. Gigantic they may fairly be termed when we consider the wideness of their range and the efficiency with which they are executed. The museum at Washington has been enriched by many valuable additions during 1874. Among the more important contributions to the department of mammals we may mention the nylghau, the manatus, and the sun-bear presented by P. T. Barnum. A specimen of the sea-lion of Patagonia has been received from Dr. Burmeister, of Buenos Ayres. Henry W. Elliott has procured a series of skins and skeletons of the fur-seals. Doctor Gabb has furnished complete collections of nearly all the known mammals of Costa Rica, in great number. A series of the seals of Newfoundland was received from Rev. M. Harvey; and Captain Scammon has contributed additions to the series of cetaceans of the Pacific coast, especially that of California. The fish collection is a special feature of the institution. Every summer Professor Baird, with able assistants, devotes himself to perfecting the collection, and various agents are constantly on the lookout for rare and curious spec-

[1] *A Manual of Minor Surgery and Bandaging.* By CHRISTOPHER HEATH, F. R. C. S. Fifth Edition. Philadelphia: Lindsay and Blakiston. 1875.

imens. According to the report, by means of the various fresh fishes thus obtained, the series of casts of the food-fishes of the United States, commenced a few years ago, has been greatly extended during the past season; this now numbering over three hundred specimens, painted carefully from nature, and representing fishes and cetaceans, some of them of nearly a thousand pounds' weight. This collection of casts is said to be unique in this country, and to be only represented on a smaller scale by that of Mr. Frank Buckland, in London, aud that of the natural history museum of Trinity College, Dublin.

One of the greatest favors that the Smithsonian Institution confers on the community is the carrying on of the system of exchanges of publications between the leading societies of the Old World and those in this country. Expressage must be paid in this country to and from Washington as the case may be, but after that, owing to the liberality of the principal transportation companies, the packages are sent to and received from the limits of the civilized world free of expense, and pass through all custom-houses free of duties and unopened. We quote from the report to show the extent of this interchange.

NUMBER OF FOREIGN CORRESPONDING INSTITUTIONS.

Sweden	20	Belgium	110
Norway	24	France	274
Iceland	2	Italy	169
Denmark	27	Portugal	20
Russia	160	Spain	12
Holland	65	Great Britain and Ireland	357
Germany	622	South America	40
Greece	7	West Indies	7
Turkey	11	Mexico	10
Africa	23	Central America	1
Asia	42	British America	27
Australia	27	General	5
New Zealand	13		
Polynesia	2	Total	2146
Switzerland	69		

"During the past year 4326 packages, each containing several articles, have been received from abroad for distribution to institutions and individuals in this country.

"One hundred and forty-one boxes, averaging seven cubic feet each, with a total weight of 29,600 pounds, were sent abroad by the institution, during the year, namely, to Germany, 40; England, 30; Sweden, 5; Norway, 3; Denmark and Iceland, 4; France, 11; Russia, 7; Holland, 5; Belgium, 5; Australia, 11; Italy, 3; Cuba, 2; Brazil, 3; Liberia, 1; Egypt, 1; Canada, 10.

"The total number of separate parcels contained in these boxes was about 10,000."

The report contains the account of some explorations and surveys in the territory of the United States, and includes also a number of scientific papers. Among these are many translations of papers, eulogies especially, read at foreign societies, of which we own we cannot see the propriety of the reproduction. There are also a number of observations on American antiquities of various degrees of merit; many containing much that is interesting, but few much that is really new.

MORTALITY FROM PHTHISIS.

Dr. GLEITSMANN, of Baltimore, has prepared and published an elaborate essay concerning the statistics of mortality from pulmonary phthisis in the United States and in Europe.[1] His little book is rather dull reading for the average physician, for it embraces a series of tables which serve as a text for the author's comments ; compositions of this nature possess very little fascination to any except the plodding student of vital statistics. The discriminating reader, whether he be fascinated or repelled by the array of figures here presented, cannot but observe that the writer has used his data legitimately, to point to certain conclusions, and that he has not abused them to bolster any chimerical notions conceived beforehand.

The author has analyzed the mortality statistics of sixty-five American cities for the year 1873, and has compared them with the returns of the Registrar-General of England with reference to the deaths from consumption. He has also placed the records of twenty-five life insurance companies under contribution for facts relating to the mortality from phthisis. Oldendorff's tables have likewise been appealed to for the sake of a comparison between American and German statistics. Painstaking as all this labor has been, we cannot but regard its results as only measurably valuable, inasmuch as it embraces too short a period (a single year), and gives figures relating to population and mortality which are partial and approximative. To be really and permanently useful, such a work should embrace many years of time and great extent of territory. So far as it goes, however, Dr. Gleitsmann's book confirms the conclusions already reached by other laborers in the field of vital statistics, namely, that the deaths from consumption comprise about one eighth of the whole mortality ; that most of the deaths occur in the spring ; that the female decedents exceed the male ; and that the period of life between the ages of twenty and thirty years suffers most severely.

COCHITUATE WATER.

THE unpleasant odor and taste of the water supplied to the citizens of Boston have been the cause of numerous complaints, and naturally of much anxiety as to the sanitary effects likely to be produced by the impurities which give rise to these disagreeable features.

As to the source of these impurities there are several theories. The first and most probable is the decomposition of the vegetation upon a large extent of the bottom of Lake Cochituate. This vegetation has been allowed to spring up by the exposure to the air of two hundred acres or more in the southern division of the lake, which always takes place in very dry seasons.

[1] *Statistics of Mortality from Pulmonary Phthisis in the United States and in Europe.* By WILLIAM GLEITSMANN, M. D. Baltimore : Turnbull Brothers. 1875.

The vegetable growth, when covered with water of sufficient depth, dies, and in decaying imparts to the water a large quantity of organic matter which usually gives it a certain amount of color, odor, and taste, disagreeable but not necessarily noxious.

The same condition of the Boston water has been noticed after similar extended droughts, such as those of 1854 and 1872. In 1872 many referred the unpleasant taste to the connection made between Farm Pond and Lake Cochituate, and the consequent introduction of the Sudbury River water, but it is far more probable that it was caused by the previous exposure of about two hundred acres of the bottom of the lake, as at the present time.

Another explanation is that the water which has been lying at the bottom of the lake during the summer, and which is " said to be almost in a putrid state," has been raised on account of the cooling of the surface water, and is now being distributed. Granting this to be the fact (which, however, we by no means admit), the same condition of the water would be noticed every autumn, which is not the case.

Still another theory is that the Brookline reservoir is in a very filthy condition. Were this the cause of the difficulty, the disagreeable taste would be perceived only in those districts which are supplied with water from this reservoir. We learn, however, that the complaint is general and not limited to any particular portions of the city.

Too much care cannot be taken to insure a pure and abundant supply of drinking-water for cities, and we are pleased to be able to state that all possible means are being taken to secure this object. As soon as the report of the medical commission upon the sanitary qualities of various sources of water supply for Boston was made, measures were immediately taken to utilize the water of Sudbury River in accordance with the recommendation of that commission. As, unfortunately, the completion of the plans will require several years, the connection between Farm Pond and Lake Cochituate has in the mean time been reopened, to prevent a water famine. Probably, therefore, since the city has obtained complete control of the Sudbury River from the legislature, and has now decided permanently to use its water, there will never be a repetition of the present state of affairs, the falling of Lake Cochituate to such an extent as to expose a large area of the bottom to the action of the atmosphere being readily prevented by the temporary introduction of the Sudbury River water.

THE CORRECT TABLE OF EXERCISES AT THE HARVARD MEDICAL SCHOOL FOR THE FIRST TERM OF 1875–76.

OUR readers may remember that we criticised, a short time ago, a table that appeared in the New York *Medical Record*, purporting to give the order of exercises at some of the leading medical schools for the present year, inasmuch as the order at Harvard had not then been determined. The editor of the *Record* replied that the table had been received from the secretary, and implied that we could not show any errors in it.

The table of exercises at Harvard which the *Record* published was that of last year, and it was undoubtedly true that we could not then show how inaccurate it might be, as the following correct table has only just appeared.

FIRST YEAR — FIRST TERM.

	MONDAY.	TUESDAY.	WEDNESDAY.	THURSDAY.	FRIDAY.	SATURDAY.
9	Histology.	Laboratory.	Laboratory.	Histology.	Laboratory.	Laboratory.
10	Histology.	Laboratory.	Laboratory.	Histology.	Chemistry. R.	Physiology. R.
11	Physiology. L.	Physiology. L.	Chemistry. L.	Laboratory.	Physiology. L.	
12	Laboratory.	Laboratory.	Laboratory.	Laboratory.	Laboratory.	Museum.
1	Last 11 weeks, Anatomy. L.	Anatomy. L.	Anatomy. R. 1st 8 weeks Anat. L. last 11 weeks.	Anatomy. L.	Anatomy. R.	
5	Prac. Anatomy. After Jan. 1.	Prac. Anatomy. After Jan. 1.	Prac. Anatomy. After Jan. 1.	Prac. Anatomy. After Jan. 1.	Prac. Anatomy. After Jan. 1.	

SECOND YEAR — FIRST TERM.

	MONDAY.	TUESDAY.	WEDNESDAY.	THURSDAY.	FRIDAY.	SATURDAY
9	M. G. H. Med. Vis.	B. C. H. Med. Vis. Bost. Disp.	Clin. Medicine. L.	M. G. H. Med. Vis.	Bost. Disp.	Chemistry. R.
10	Aus. & Per.	Clin. Surg. L. After Dec. 1. Aus. & Per.	Aus. & Per.	Aus. &. Per.	B. C. H. Surg. Vis. Aus. & Per.	M. G. H. Surg. Vis. Aus. & Per.
11	Clin. Surgery. L.			Materia Medica.	B. C. H. Op.	M. G. H. Op.
12	Path. Anat. L.	Chemistry. L.		Materia Medica.		Museum.
3	Path. Microscopy.	Path. Anat. R.	Path. Anat. L.	Path. Microscopy.	Path. Anat. R.	
4			Surg. R.	Clinical Conf.		
5	Prac. Anatomy. Till Jan. 1.	Prac. Anatomy. Till Jan. 1.	Prac. Anatomy. Till Jan. 1.	Prac. Anatomy. Till Jan. 1.	Prac. Anatomy. Till Jan. 1.	

THIRD YEAR — FIRST TERM.

	MONDAY.	TUESDAY.	WEDNESDAY.	THURSDAY.	FRIDAY.	SATURDAY
9	M. G. H. Medical Visit Eye & Ear Inf.	B. C. H. Med. Vis. Bost. Disp.	Clin. Medicine. L.	M. G. H. Med. Vis. Eye & Ear. Inf.	B. C. H. Ophthal. & Otology. Bost. Disp.	Dis. of Nerv. Sys.
10	Theo. & Prac. L.	Clin. Surgery. L. After Dec. 1.	Dermatol. Clin.	Theo. & Pr. L.	B. C. H. Surg. Vis.	M.G. H. Surg.Vis.
11	Clin. Surg. L.		Surgery. L.	Surgery. L.	B. C. H. Op. Dis. of Children.	M. G. H. Op.
12	Obstetrics. L.	Till Dec. Surgery. L.	Obstetrics. L.	Obstetrics. R.	Venereal Dis.	Museum.
1		After Dec 1, Dis. of NerV. Sys.				
3		Theo. & Prac. R.			Theo. & Prac. R.	
4	Therapeutics. L.	Dermatology. L.		Clinical Conf.	Therapeutics. L.	
5	Otology.					

DR. JOHN HUGHES BENNETT.

THE profession of Great Britain has lost one of its most prominent members by the death of John Hughes Bennett, late professor of the institutes of medicine at Edinburgh. He died on September 25th, at the age of sixty-three, a few days after an operation for stone in the bladder. He was in all respects a remarkable man, a deep thinker and good practitioner, who united scientific and practical attributes to a degree rarely seen. He was an original investigator of great enthusiasm and keenness, who endeavored to draw practical deductions from facts or theories that to others were ends in themselves. His conclusions were, no doubt, not always sound, and he was by no means free from prejudice, but much of his work will live after him. He was an excellent teacher, endowed with the rare talent of making alike attractive and profitable to his class both his theories and his experience. Many may criticise much that is to be found in his Practice of Medicine, but no one can read it without being impressed with the vigor of the author. In microscopy he was an opponent of the cellular doctrine in its entirety, holding that granules were the really active element. In his Practice he says, "As to development, the molecular is the basis of all the tissues. The first step in the process of organic formation is the production of an organic fluid ; the second, the precipitation in it of organic molecules, from which, according to the molecular law of growth, all other textures are derived, either directly or indirectly."

In 1857 he was the leader of the reform party in the celebrated discussion on venesection, and contributed probably more than any other man to the decline of the practice. It is proper, however, to remember that he was the opponent only of its general and indiscriminate use, and had no desire to have it numbered among the lost arts. He did good service also by protesting against the excessive use of mercury. It is, we believe, acknowledged that he was the first to recognize the combination of symptoms known as leucocythæmia.

We give some account of the case of this distinguished man, interesting in itself, which we take mostly verbatim from Mr. Cadge's account in *The British Medical Journal.*

" By slow degrees his general health failed, he grew thinner, looked pale, and lost strength. A few years ago it was discovered that he had diabetes ; but this disappeared without any great rigor of treatment, and has not been thought or known to have recurred, except occasionally and very slightly. . . . Very recently, however (in August), sugar was again found ; and I have before me a paper containing observations on the urine made three times daily during the first half of September, 1875, from which it is shown that, while the specific gravity and the quantity of the urine were but little, if at all, above the natural standard, sugar appeared and disappeared in a quite irregular and intermitting way. . . .

" If," says Mr. Cadge, " in this long interval between the first and last clear recognition of diabetes, the urine was but seldom examined, and, when examined, chanced to be free from sugar, it seems probable that glycosuria, in one of its intermittent and milder forms, existed throughout, and was the true and chief cause of the emaciation and debility which, on any other hypothesis, it has been found so difficult to explain. . . .

" Be that as it may, his health continued to decline. The last three winters he passed in the south of France, with some benefit, possibly, to his bronchial and laryngeal affection, but apparently without any effect on his general state. For many years Dr. Bennett had suffered from occasional attacks of gout, and he was liable, too, to lithic acid deposit in his urine ; occasionally, for several years, he had experienced some slight impediment and irritation in making water, which he thought to be due either to slight stricture or to prostatic enlargement. From time to time a simple catheter was passed, but no stricture was discovered. Last winter, at Nice, he had rather more vesical irritation than usual. . . .

" In July he came to Norwich, looking more emaciated, pale, and ill than I had ever seen him. On carefully sounding, a stone was readily felt, apparently of some size; the bladder was capacious and healthy, and could retain nearly half a pint of urine ; the prostate was slightly enlarged ; the urethra very sensitive and irritable ; the urine was clear, acid, specific gravity 1020, and contained no albumen. He was much depressed by the knowledge that he had stone, but his innate force of character came to his aid; he looked the difficulty in the face, and was prepared at once to undergo treatment. . . . He returned to Norwich in September, and the question of operation, lithotomy or lithotrity, presented itself. Either must be attended with the greatest hazard in one so worn and unhealthy; but the thought of doing without operation was simply intolerable, and not to be considered. In favor of lithotrity were the fair quietude and healthy condition of the bladder and urine ; but there were serious drawbacks. Dr. Bennett was a man of high spirit and courage ; but his courage fitted him rather to encounter one great risk than to endure the wear and tear of repeated operations, frequent use of instruments, and the probability (made more probable by the presence of glycosuria) of troublesome cystitis. The size of the stone alone could decide the point; and, to ascertain this, Mr. Clover kindly came down and administered nitrous oxide, followed by ether; while, with the lithotrite, I found that the stone measured one and a half inches by one inch. Such a stone as this was fairly within the compass of lithotrity in an otherwise favorable patient; but, in this case, I had not a moment's doubt that lithotomy, if carefully and accurately done, notwithstanding its greater immediate risk, afforded the best chance of complete recovery. In this view the patient readily acquiesced, and on the following day, September 16th, I removed the stone by lateral lithotomy, assisted by Mr. Crosse, Dr. Beverley, and Mr. Hooker. The nitrous oxide and ether were again used by Mr. Clover, with admirable effect; there was never a movement of the patient, nor the least headache or sickness afterwards. The operation was easy and satisfactory. The transverse artery of the perinæum was large, and spurted freely; it was easily tied when the stone was removed; the blood was so thin, and so little disposed to coagulate, that every little vessel continued to ooze, and I deemed it best to plug the wound round a silver tube rather than allow any quantity of blood to be lost. The stone was composed of lithic acid; it measured one and a half inches by one inch, and weighed one hundred and ninety-three grains. No more blood was lost, and urine passed freely afterwards. He suffered considerable aching pain in the wound for some hours; but it was gradually checked by half a grain of morphia introduced into the rectum at the time of operation, and twenty drops of Battley by the mouth two hours after. At night he turned cautiously on one side, took twenty grains of chloral, and had some hours' sleep. Pulse 90. . . .

" I need not record minutely the daily progress of the case. Suffice it to say that for four or five days there was a good prospect of speedy recovery; he took food plentifully and was in good spirits, and everything went on well so far as concerned the pelvis and bladder; the urine was easily caught and was clear, but loaded with sugar, with a specific gravity of 1030 to 1035. By degrees, however, the cough and expectoration became more frequent; and this, with the frequent spasm and larger amount of urine secreted, distressed him and prevented sleep. Opiates by the mouth or bowel relieved for the time, but were apt to be followed by sickness; chloral did not act well, and signs of increasing debility showed themselves. The pulse continued from 90 to 96, but became weaker and weaker. Aphthous patches gathered on the tongue and throat, and made swallowing difficult, and thus the prostration went on, and death from sheer exhaustion took place on the 25th, the tenth day after the operation.

" Post-mortem examination, forty-eight hours after death. The body was emaciated; the surface pale and bloodless. The blood was thin, and transuded through the vessels and stained the tissues. Only one small clot in the right ventricle of the heart was met with. The bladder was perfectly healthy; its muscular walls were rather thin and dilated; its mucous membrane was pale and smooth. The prostate gland was enlarged to the size of a small apple; it projected somewhat like a cornice into the bladder, and on this projecting part there were traces of slight ecchymosis beneath the mucous membrane. The lithotomy wound was clean, and so slight that, looking from the bladder, none could be seen, and on closer scrutiny it was found that the knife had only divided the mucous membrane and had scarcely reached the left lobe ; this doubtless explains the power of the bladder to retain urine the moment after the tube was removed. . . . On raising the calvarium, a soft tumor was discovered situated on the right side of the head, about an inch above the ear, between the dura mater and the bone. It was about the size of a hen's egg, and projected toward the brain, so as to produce a deep pit or hollow, into which it fitted. The convolutions were flattened and pressed down, but not otherwise altered ; no softening; no congestion. The dura mater covering the tumor was somewhat thickened. The parietal bone was thickened and hypertrophied around the circumference of the tumor ; over it there was thinning by pressure and absorption, and at one point, about the size of a shilling, all trace of bone had disappeared, and it was replaced by fibrous membrane. The tumor had a cystoid character, with a distinct investing membrane, and its contents consisted of a blackish pulpy material resembling the interior of a recent aneurism, or more closely of a myeloid tumor. Under the microscope there were seen cells of various descriptions, plates of cholesterine, fatty granules, and altered bloodcorpuscles. The brain itself was anæmic, but not, on the whole, unhealthy ; it weighed forty-seven ounces. The optic thalami, corpora striata, pons Varolii. and medulla oblongata had a somewhat shrunken, atrophied appearance, and were perha, s harder and tougher than usual."

MEDICAL NOTES.

— The annual meeting of the American Public Health Association will begin at Baltimore on November 9th, and will continue four days. Judging from the programme we should think four weeks would be inadequate to the proper discussion of the many important questions that are to be brought up. It is in the nature of things that there should be much loose and unprofitable talk, but we see many names that assure us that the meeting will not be without results. The association has been very happy in its choice of officers, and, we believe, is in excellent condition.

— Dr. Robert T. Edes has been appointed professor of materia medica at the Harvard Medical School, and Dr. William L. Richardson instructor in clinical midwifery.

— The St. Louis *Clinical Record* contains a remarkable case of brain lesion. A man named Waters, living near Leavenworth, Kansas, died from morphia a short time ago, and as it was known that he had had a habit of running wires and even nails through his own skull during his former residence in the penitentiary, a careful autopsy was performed. Two openings were found in the skull, one, which the prisoner was known to have made with a brad-awl, near the inferior posterior angle of the right parietal, and another near the superior posterior angle of the same bone. A wire was found in the brain. It had been introduced through the upper opening, and just missing the superior longitudinal sinus had pierced to the base of the brain a little in front of the fissure of Sylvius. It is stated that the corpus striatum was not wounded. A nail, one and three fourths inches in length, was found lying beside the wire. Although wires had been removed during life from the lower aperture, no trace of their course was discovered. Though the patient had shown a suicidal tendency he did not appear insane, except for this habit, and could do his work with correctness and understanding.

— The English medical journals are full of the introductory lectures at the various medical schools of London, and we may expect shortly a number of the same at various schools in this country. We regret to find that the rowdyism which appears to be a part of the show continues unabated in several London hospitals. A scene that would disgrace any legislative body seems hardly an edifying one to be the first for the new students to take part in. These lectures are and must be twice-told tales to the members of the profession, and if they are merely subjects of mirth to the neophytes, whom they should impress, we think they might as well be abolished. Everything that was once new has been said till it is old, everything brilliant till it has become stale, and everything sound till it at least appears silly. Moreover, it were well that the student should learn at his first entrance into the profession that he has devoted himself to a calling of work rather than of words.

— Recovery from a compound comminuted fracture of the entire left side of the os frontis is reported by Dr. E. VonDonhoff to the *American Medical Weekly*. The patient, a boy, fell some fifty feet, from the top of a three-story wall. The left side of the frontal bone was crushed in, and the eye of the same side was held as in a vice between the supra and infra orbital ridges. The boy was comatose and bleeding from the nose, mouth, and injured orbit. A projecting fragment of bone, about the size of a silver quarter, was removed by the fingers; an elevator was then introduced and the remaining fragments pushed into position. The patient soon revived, and made an uninterrupted recovery. The treatment was the application locally of cold compresses, and internally the administration of bromide of potassium.

— A case of triplets complicated with double uterus is reported by A. G. Duncan, M. B., to the *British Medical Journal* of September 18, 1875. Dr. Duncan was called to see a patient in her fifth pregnancy on December 25, 1873. She was eight and a half months advanced, and was troubled because she was different in shape and size from what she had ever been in previous pregnancies. Examination showed the abdomen to be wide, large, and falling forward. There was a well-marked depression from above downwards, and a little to the left side. This depression was a distinct division between two tumors, the one on the left being the larger. Fœtal heart-sounds could be heard in both, and the diagnosis of a double impregnated uterus was made. December 27th, at seven P. M., the os was fully dilated and the head presenting in the first position. Soon after, a healthy female weighing six pounds, and a little later another female child of nearly the same size, presenting by the breech, were born. A double placenta came away. There was now the well-contracted womb in the lower part of the abdomen on the right side, but the left-hand tumor remained. In six hours another female child, weighing over seven pounds, appeared. After the separation of the placenta the tumors were of about equal size. After recovery of the patient an examination showed that the external os was single, the opening being much elongated from side to side, but on tilting it forward the divided septum was distinctly seen. A uterine sound could be introduced into each cavity, and the septum felt by the introduction of the finger.

— Another epidemic of typhoid fever, whose origin is attributed to the distribution of infected milk, has occurred at Jarrow, in England. According to the report of the Health Officer, Dr. Spear, as furnished to *The Sanitary Record* of September 18, 1875, the district had been tolerably free from the disease for some weeks, when suddenly on August 13th he found that it had invaded houses in all parts of the town. Between August 3d and 19th no less than thirty-four cases occurred in twenty different families. The houses were, with two exceptions, clean, and to nothing in them or their surroundings could this outbreak of fever be attributed. As house after house was visited it was found that the milk-supply was obtained almost invariably from the same source. On visiting the farm from which the milk came it was found that six of the farmer's family were sick with typhoid fever. The water used in the dairy was derived from a well situated about eighteen yards from a privy and cess-pit, the latter being simply a hole dug in the ground, and not in any way paved or otherwise protected. This had been in existence for years, and in it the discharges of the fever patients had lately been deposited. There could be no question that soakage had been going on into the well from the privy and cesspit. A quantity of the well-water that had been standing in the dairy for two days was quite putrid. It was quite unfit for domestic purposes, and contained, on analysis, free, saline and organic ammonia. Analysis of the milk showed it to be of poor quality, but not necessarily adulterated by the addition of water. One consumer complained that the taste of the milk was excessively disagreeable, and another that it soured very quickly. It is not, however, necessary to prove the fraudulent adulteration of the milk, for it has been shown in other cases that the washing of cans with polluted water is sufficient to contaminate it. All the arrangements of the farm were found to be of a disgusting kind. There was direct communication between the dairy and a room in which some of the fever patients were lying, and the dairy was used as a wash-house, where clothes of the sick had been washed. The fever had been in the family about a fortnight before the outbreak occurred in the district.

Dr. Spear thinks that if the facts are well considered no one will venture to say that the outbreak of disease fell so heavily on the farmer's customers by mere coincidence. At least eighteen other farmers and dealers send on an average an equal quantity of milk into the district, and yet their names were scarcely mentioned in the course of the inquiry. Of the twenty-seven families supplied from the farm in question, eleven suffered, and from the moment the supply was cut off from the town, and proper sanitary measures instituted, the spread of the disease was stayed.

THE OTHER SIDE.

MESSRS. EDITORS, — Your article the other day on the metric system suggests a few remarks, which I hope you will be kind enough to publish.

It is well known that this system, attractive as it is at first sight, has never been entirely popular even in the country of its birth, and that the old denominations of weights, measures, and currency are still in common use in France, especially among the masses and in the rural districts.

The reason is that the natural method of subdivision is not by decimating, but by halving and quartering. If you wish to divide a string, an apple, or a bar of soap, it is very easy to cut it into halves or quarters or eighths or sixteenths by the eye with a good degree of accuracy; to divide it into thirds, fifths, or tenths is extremely difficult, and requires nice measuring and weighing. Now tradesmen, grocers, apothecaries, and the like always divide first by the eye and then verify with the scales. Our present system, confused as it is, is in conformity with this natural method of subdivision, hence its popularity and convenience.

This defect of the decimal system has always been felt, even in arithmetical notation. Hence a duodecimal system of notation has often been advocated by mathematicians in place of the decimal one now in use. The number 12 has four factors, 2, 3, 4, and 6, while 10 has only two, 2 and 5. It is evident that calculation would be facilitated by such a notation.

Our present system of weights and measures is a duodecimal system based, as all the world knows, on the Roman *as* and its twelve *unciæ*. It is universally known both in Europe and in America. It has stood the test of two thousand years. It is an old friend. Let us spare it.

We know the national fondness for innovations; let us remember that there is another " great nation " which has a similar weakness, and that French experimentations are not always attended with the most imposing results.

We have no time to criticise the nomenclature of the new system or its utter inconsonance with natural and preëxisting standards.

Perhaps enough has been said to show that there are objections to it, not only practical but scientific and mathematical.

With great respect,   E. T. W.

WEEKLY BULLETIN OF PREVALENT DISEASES.

THE following is a bulletin of the diseases prevalent in Massachusetts during the week ending October 23, 1875, compiled under the authority of the State Board of Health from the returns of physicians representing all sections of the State: —

The summary for each section is as follows: —

Berkshire : Bronchitis, influenza.

Valley: Typhoid fever, influenza, bronchitis, rheumatism. Diphtheria has increased. Springfield reports typhoid fever very prevalent.

Midland : Typhoid fever, influenza, bronchitis, rheumatism. Diphtheria is increasing again, and scarlatina is more prevalent.

Northeastern : Influenza, typhoid fever, scarlatina.   Scarlatina is especially prevalent in the cities and towns in the eastern part of Essex County.   Gloucester reports diphtheria.

Metropolitan : Bronchitis, typhoid fever, influenza.   Diphtheria has subsided. Scarlatina has increased.

Southeastern : Typhoid fever, influenza, bronchitis.   Diphtheria continues along the South Shore, but it is declining.   Scarlatina is increasing.

In the State at large, influenza and bronchitis prevail extensively ; their coincidence with the epizoötic catarrh is noteworthy. ˙ Diphtheria and scarlatina have increased.   The diarrhœal affections have very nearly disappeared.   The prevailing type of disease is mild.

F. W. DRAPER, M. D., Rej ,ıi'rar.

COMPARATIVE MORTALITY-RATES FOR THE WEEK ENDING OCT. 16, 1875.

	Estimated Population.	Total Mortality for the Week.	Annual Death-Rate per 10(0 during Week.
New York	1,060,000	487	24
Philadelphia	800,000	326	21
Brooklyn	500,000	216	22
Chicago	400,000	139	18
Boston	342,000	162	25
Cincinnati	260,000	95	19
Providence	100,700	49	25
Worcester	50,000	14	15
Lowell	50,000	25	26
Cambridge	48,000	19	21
Fall River	45,000	15	17
Lawrence	35,000	14	21
Lynn	33,000	11	17
Springfield	31,000	13	22
Salem	26,000	11	22

Normal Death-Rate, 17 per 1000.

SUFFOLK DISTRICT MEDICAL SOCIETY.— Stated meeting, Saturday, October 30th.

Dr. A. Young : Oxygen as a Corrective in the Anæsthetic Use of Chloroform, and as an Antidote in Asphyxia.

Dr. B. Joy Jeffries : Report on Cases of Cataract Operations.

Dr. J. R. Chadwick : Extirpation of the Uterus by Abdominal Section.

Members of other State and District societies are cordially invited.

THE Boston Society for Medical Observation will meet Monday, November 1st. Dr. Swan will read a paper on a case of Painful Tumor near the Cæcum.   There will be a discussion on depositing the library with the Boston Medical Library Association.

BOOKS AND PAMPHLETS RECEIVED. — Therapeutics, Materia Medica, and Toxicology. By H. C. Wood, Jr., M. D.   Second Edition.   Revised and Enlarged.   Philadelphia : J. B. Lippincott & Co. 1876. (For sale by A. Williams & Co.)

Human Physiology for Students and Practitioners. By John C. Dalton, M. D.   Sixth Edition.   Revised and Enlarged.   Philadelphia : Henry C. Lea. 1875. (For sale by A. Williams & Co.)

Two Thousand Years After ; or a Talk in a Cemetery. By John Darby.   Philadelphia : Claxton, Remsen, and Haffelfinger. 1876. (For sale by Lockwood, Brooks, & Co.)

THE BOSTON
MEDICAL AND SURGICAL JOURNAL.

VOL. XCIII. — THURSDAY, NOVEMBER 4, 1875. — NO 19.

REPORTS OF SIXTEEN CASES OF CATARACT OPERATIONS.[1]

BY B. JOY JEFFRIES, M. D., OF BOSTON,

Ophthalmic Surgeon to the Massachusetts Eye and Ear Infirmary, the Carney Hospital, and the New England Hospital for Women and Children.

LAST season I published in the JOURNAL[2] the records of one hundred and five cases of cataract operations, in seventy-one of which I used Graefe's operation for other than congenital, soft, or traumatic cataracts. To these I have now to add the records of sixteen more cases, being those which I have done since last season. The resulting vision in all comes within the range of success, and they therefore bring up the percentage. The relations of the family physician, the ophthalmic operator, and the surroundings of the cataract patient, I discussed in my previous article, and will say nothing further here on these topics.

The success I have met with I must attribute to the employment of Graefe's method of operating, from which I have varied only as the individual case required. Whilst in some or many of these eighty-seven cases I could have used the old flap operation with equal success, on the other hand, Graefe's operation alone was in place in all. I have not yet seen reason to depart from it, as I believe it gives me the largest number of successful operations. I was taught the old flap operation in Europe. Graefe's method came into use after my return, and I adopted it as soon as I became convinced of its superiority from its adaptability to all cases of cataract extraction.

In looking over my cases I can realize how valuable this method is, for I recognize many in which I should hardly have dared attempt any other. I have not thought it good ophthalmic surgery to try to prove by practice or precept in what way *other* than Graefe's modified linear extraction a cataract could be removed, but rather by the steady use of it, as most in place in all cases, to give my patients the best chance so far as the operation was concerned. That cataracts can be removed, and successfully, by various cuts through the cornea, I know and admit,

---

[1] Read before the Suffolk District Medical Society.
[2] Boston Medical and Surgical Journal, October 1, 1874.

but to me Graefe's operation still seems the safest and, as time shows, the most useful.

My friend Mr. Carter, in his recent work, has expressed these relations so practically and clearly that I can best serve my own purpose by quoting them at some length here. After explaining how Graefe was led to his operation and discussing the subsequent introduction of various forms of spoons, he says, " From this time onwards the history of cataract extraction bears a great surgical analogy to the history of ovariotomy; for just as one by one the causes of death have been eliminated from the latter operation by careful study and successive setting aside of the conditions which tended to the production of a fatal result, so in like manner the causes of failure have been eliminated from the former. Von Graefe then strove to combine an incision so small that it should produce little risk of corneal sloughing with one so made and so situated that it should permit the exit of the lens without injurious pressure. The result was that method of ' modified linear-extraction ' which was the last of his great contributions to the art he loved so well. But in order that Graefe's incision should avoid the cornea, and should at the same time preserve the direction of a plane passing from the margin of the cornea through the centre of the eyeball, it became necessary that its extremities should lie very near to the ciliary region ; and hence arose the danger already mentioned of inflicting an injury liable to be followed by cyclitis and irido-choroiditis in the eye which was operated upon, and by sympathetic ophthalmia in its fellow. In order to avoid these risks, many operators prefer a somewhat more extended incision in an anterior plane, not, as in the old method, in a plane parallel to the iris, but in one which, although inclined with reference to the iris, would not pass through the centre of the globe. In this preference I myself concur, and perhaps the best rules for making such an incision are those which have been laid down by M. de Wecker. I do not think, however, that an experienced operator will allow himself to be very closely bound by any rules of procedure, but he will vary every operation a little, in accordance with the size and prominence of the eye, the position of the cornea, and the estimated size of the hard nucleus of the lens."

As to various innovations proposed by one or another, Mr. Carter is quite outspoken, and with what he says I must agree. " During the period," he remarks, " when real and important changes were being effected in the methods by which cataracts were removed, the surgeons engaged in the work had many followers who made changes which for the most part were only apparent. It is hardly possible for two pairs of human hands, especially if endowed with different degrees of skill, to execute all the steps of a complicated operation precisely in the same way ; and so it came about that each of several operators found it more convenient to himself, more suited to the requirements of his own eyes and fingers, to deviate in some minute point of detail from the practice of somebody else, of whom, nevertheless, he was in the main an imitator. Of such changes there were none really worthy of record, or which possessed more than a fleeting or personal interest. They mostly suggested themselves as natural correctives to some kind of manual incapacity, and will suggest themselves again, as it were instinctively, to those who share the defects of dexterity in which they had their origin."

As to the various transverse corneal incisions for cataract-extractions, I am agreeably surprised to find Mr. Carter so entirely agreeing with my own views and experiences. He says, " Transverse corneal incisions stand self-condemned on *a priori* grounds. They have the single recommendation that it is very easy to make them, and they might perhaps be attempted with advantage by a benevolent traveler who was sojourning among a savage tribe, or by an ophthalmic surgeon upon whom the infirmities of age were creeping, or by one who was prevented by the natural quality of ambi-sinistrousness from employing better methods with ordinary prospects of success. Even in such cases Lord Melbourne's pithy inquiry, ' Could n't you have let it alone ?' would be likely to suggest itself to reasonable men. As a matter of first principles, an incision through the front of the cornea must in a large proportion of cases be followed by adhesion of the iris to some part of the cicatrix ; and adhesion of the iris, even if vision is for a time restored, entails a perpetual liability to the occurrence of destructive morbid changes. Moreover, again in a large proportion of cases, such an incision must be followed by alteration of curvature during the healing process, that is to say, by such a distortion of the cornea as to interfere seriously with vision. We see this every now and then in clean corneal wounds made accidentally by broken glass or by some sharp instrument, and in which the lens has escaped injury. It was seen still more frequently a few years ago, when flap-extraction was commonly performed, in the cases in which that operation had been badly done. On all the above grounds I have abstained from seeking any personal experience of transverse corneal sections, feeling that they cannot be said to fall within the boundaries of legitimate surgical experiment."

REPORTS OF SIXTEEN CASES OF OPERATION FOR CATARACT.

No.	Age.	Sex.	General Health.	Quality and Duration of Cataract.	Functional Examination.	Method of Operating; Incidents; Anæsthesia, in all cases by Ether; Remarks; After-Treatment.	Duration of Treatment.	Resulting Vision and Date of Record.
1	83	M.	Good.	Hard, more than ripe. O. S.	All normal.	Graefe upwards. Very large lens. Patient had done so well with previous operation on the other eye that after the wound healed in 48 hours he took off the bandage and got up and went about, opening inner angle of wound in which tag of iris is. This has given no trouble one year later.	18 days.	1 year. V. = 15-100. Sn. 5½.
2	71	F.	Fair.	Senile. O. S.	Good.	Graefe up. Normal. Patient very restless, and bandages kept on with difficulty.	21 days.	1 year. V. = Sn 3½. V. = 20-70.
3	57	M.	Feeble.	Senile. O. S.	Normal.	Graefe up. Vitreous fluid, and flowed at completion of cut. Lens sank and removed with spoon. Did well till 9th day, when patient had an attack of neuralgia and conjunctivitis from being sent into a cold ward by mistake. The case, however, did well, and vision improving when discharged.	37 days.	37 days. V. = 20-50. Sn. 6½.
4	48	M.	Good.	Senile. O. S.	Good.	Graefe up. Quite normal, considering the posterior synechia.	16 days.	16 days. V. = 20-100. Sn. 1½.
5	58	F.	Feeble.	Senile. O. D.	Very convex cornea, and spots on it from ulceration.	Graefe up. Normal, except the thin and very prominent cornea fell in quite flaccid, which did not prevent healing normally.	21 days.	21 days. V. = 20-100. Sn. 3.
6	48	M.	Good.	Senile. O. D. of No. 4.	Good.	Graefe up. Normal, except much cortical left, as patient was irritable under ether.	17 days.	17 days. V. = 20-100. Sn. 2½.
7	42	F.	Good.	Traumatic. 6 months. O. S.	Good.	Graefe up. Normal.	11 days.	11 days. V. = 20-70. Sn 4½.
8	73	M.	Good.	Senile. Hard. Overripe. 10 years. O. S.	Good.	Graefe up. Normal, except considerable blood, and a large but flat lens emerged through a wound made large on purpose. Patient did very well till 12th day, when inflammation came on and some small pieces of cortical proliferated. Patient had senile delirium. Pulled off bandages constantly, and found on floor pulling off clothes. The mass in anterior chamber became absorbed under atropine, leeches, etc. In 4 months most of pupil cleared. The case did well beyond expectation.	25 days.	4 months. V. = 8-60. J. 12.

No.	Age	Sex		Diagnosis		Operation and Remarks		Result
9	70	M.	Good.	Senile. Hard. Overripe. O. S.	Good.	Graefe up. Large amount of cortical, showing lens was liquefying.	14 days.	14 days. V.=15-30.
10	66	M.	Good.	Senile. Hard. O. D.	Good.	Graefe up. Normal. Either minute tag of iris or pigment in inner angle of the wound.	14 days.	37 days. V.=20-50. Sn. 1½.
11	65	M.	Good.	Senile. O. S.	Good.	Graefe up. Normal. Considerable soft cortical. Patient constantly interfered with bandage.	21 days.	21 days. V.=20-70. Sn. 2.
12	64	F.	Fair.	Senile. Overripe. O. S.	Good.	Graefe up. Eye very deep set. A hard, smooth lens escaped, quite clear of cortical.	17 days.	25 days. V.=20-70. Sn. 3½.
13	45 to 60	F.	Fair.	From old irido-choroiditis.	Good.	Graefe up. Upon pressure a large, pretty firm mass escaped through the cut, with a cup shaped depression on its anterior surface. On pressure again another mass came, the size of a nucleus, but of no firmer consistency than the former. Resulting vision is no better on account of former choroiditis.	16 days.	30 days. V.=20-200.
14	65	F.	Good.	Senile. O. D.	Good.	Graefe up. Normal.	14 days.	14 days. V.=20-70. Sn. 1½.
15	66	F.	Fair.	4 years. From old choroidal trouble.	Good.	Graefe up. Against orders patient had eaten; he vomited during ether, requiring its suspension. Operation rendered difficult. Long-continued ciliary redness.	44 days.	46 days. V=8-40. Jäger, 8.
16	60	M.	Good.	Senile. 2¼ years.	Good.	Graefe up. Normal. Twice, without apparent cause, a little blood in anterior chamber.	21 days.	21 days. V.=20-80. J. 6.

EXTIRPATION OF THE UTERUS BY ABDOMINAL SECTION.[1]

BY JAMES R. CHADWICK, M. D.

ON May 28, 1875, I was called to Mrs. C., a patient of Dr. Kingsbury, of Holbrook, with a view to the removal of an abdominal tumor. She was fifty-four years of age, had had a child and a miscarriage in early life. She was in good health until a tumor appeared in the left side of the abdomen, and uterine hæmorrhage set in, about six years ago. The flow of blood persisted uninterruptedly for three years; during the last three years it recurred profusely at intervals. The growth of the tumor had been slow but continuous. Menstruation had ceased eighteen months before. The patient was fairly nourished, but was gradually losing flesh and strength. She had been confined to the house for nine months, owing to constant pain in the abdomen, apparently caused by the pressure of the tumor. Latterly she had been subject to frequent attacks of headache, vomiting, and convulsions, the latter apparently of hysterical nature.

Examination. The girth at the umbilicus was thirty-four inches; half-way between this point and the pubes it was thirty-seven inches. The lateral symmetry of the abdomen was perfect. A firm, perfectly round tumor was felt, rising two inches above the navel and resting upon the brim of the pelvis. Bimanually the mass was recognized as being unmistakably the body of the uterus, enlarged by a fibroid growth. Three inches obliquely above and to the left of the navel was a body as large as a small potato, projecting from the surface of the uterus. It was either an enlarged ovary or a second fibroid. The abdominal walls were very lax, and freely movable over the tumor. The cervix was immediately behind the pubes but could be readily displaced to the hollow of the sacrum by inserting the left hand above the fundus and tilting it forward. The uterine sound could not be introduced more than an inch. All other organs and functions of the body were normal; the heart's action, however, was quite irregular, intermitting every fifth beat ; the pulse was of fair strength.

In my opinion there was no possibility of removing the tumor per vaginam, owing to its size, and I was timid about undertaking the abdominal operation, with its great risk, on account of the weak action of the heart. I consequently declined interfering, in spite of earnest solicitations, until all other means for the relief of the patient's sufferings had been tried.

It is needless to specify the various remedies resorted to without avail during the summer ; let it suffice to say that at the end of three

---

[1] Read before the Suffolk District Medical Society, October 30, 1875.

months the condition was unchanged, except that under the administration of quinine the intermittence of the heart had become much less frequent. Actuated by the following considerations, I finally consented to operate, provided Dr. Knight failed to discover evidence of organic lesion of the heart: the woman's sufferings in one way or another had been so great during the past year that she had not been out of the house, had had no enjoyment of life, and had been of no service to her friends; there seemed to be no chance of relief by other measures; the patient and her friends fully realized the danger of the operation, and yet claimed it persistently. The prognosis I gave was that the chances of recovery or death were equal; this was a little more favorable than is shown by the sixty odd operations that have up to this time been placed on record, but many of these were done in very desperate cases, without suitable instruments, whereas the local condition in my patient was the very best that could be hoped for; she was, moreover, calm, hopeful, and came of good and healthy stock.

Dr. Knight reported as follows: " I found on examination occasional intermittence of the heart. It was difficult to determine its size on account of fat and the large size of the mammary gland. The sounds were of fair strength, the pulmonic second sound, however, being more distinct than the aortic. There was a systolic souffle heard over the ensiform cartilage, not propagated far away. There is no proof of serious organic disease."

I operated in Boston on Saturday, September 18, at ten A. M., with the assistance of Drs. Lyman, Ellis, Nichols, J. Homans, Sinclair, and Boardman. With the patient under the influence of ether, I made an incision eight inches long in the median line of the abdomen, lifted the enlarged uterus out of the abdominal cavity, and found entire freedom from adhesions as expected. I next affixed a Wells' clamp to the cervix and broad ligaments, but fearing that the latter might not be properly held by the clamp, I passed a double whip-cord through the cervix and tied it on either side so as to include the broad ligaments. The body of the uterus, containing the fibroid, was then cut away. In spite of my precautions the left broad ligament slipped from out both clamp and noose; the large vessels ramifying in it sank into the pelvis and bled considerably before they could all be secured. The woman's pulse at this time became imperceptible, but soon rallied under the influence of repeated subcutaneous injections of brandy. I sponged out the peritoneal cavity until it was entirely free from blood, brought the clamp into position without much tension upon the pedicle, closed the wound with silk sutures, applied the common support of cotton-wool secured by adhesive plaster, and put the woman to bed in a rather prostrate condition. The operation lasted a little over an hour.

The patient rallied from the state of depression in the course of two hours; she had some pain during the afternoon, requiring morphine; there was a little gentle vomiting. Pulse 125, temperature (vaginal) 100°. Beef-tea and brandy enemata were administered.

Sunday, September 19, A. M. Pulse 140, temperature 1005°.; slight vomiting arrested by ice-pill in a teaspoonful of brandy; quinine. Four P. M., pulse 165, temperature 101.2°. No pain; sweating, retching.

From this time the pulse gradually fell until it reached the normal on the fourth day; while it was elevated there was no intermittence, but as it sank, the old irregularity again manifested itself, and became so marked on the sixth day that I was repeatedly unable to count fifty beats in the minute. The temperature fluctuated between 101.6° and 102.2° until the sixth day, when it began to sink.

The clamp fell off on the sixth day, as did most of the sloughing end of the pedicle. The wound was cleansed and disinfected with salicylic acid most thoroughly every four hours. There was at no time any abdominal tenderness, distention, or even flatulence. The bowels responded to enemata on the fourth day. The urine was drawn with a catheter every one or two hours. All the abdominal sutures except the one next to the pedicle were removed on the seventh day.

On the seventh day the pulse was normal; the temperature had fallen to 101°; the tongue was clean; the appetite was good; the skin felt naturally; the slough had all come away from the pedicle, which was suppurating nicely, and drawing together; the bowels were acting freely; there was no peritonitis or flatulence. I felt that my patient had escaped all the natural dangers attendant upon the operation.

At eleven o'clock Mrs. C. had a slight chilly sensation running down her spine; the temperature and pulse, however, had not risen. In the afternoon she complained of sore throat, which grew worse toward night, but did not arouse my suspicions, as the pulse was only 80 and the temperature had actually fallen half a degree since morning. By midnight it became evident that tetanus had set in. The respiration became so difficult that, dreading lest the abdominal wound should be torn open by the straining, I supported the abdominal walls by fresh broad strips of adhesive plaster, but in spite of this precaution my fears were soon realized. After a severe paroxysm, I found a large mass of intestines protruding from the wound; it was with the greatest difficulty that I finally succeeded in replacing them within the abdominal cavity and sewing up the wound again.

Toward morning the breathing was so labored that at my request Dr. Lyman performed tracheotomy with much temporary relief. The patient lingered, with but slight benefit from enemata of chloral, and died near the end of the eighth day.

An *Autopsy*, made by Drs. Fitz and Cutler and myself, demonstrated that all the internal organs were perfectly healthy. There was no trace

of lymph in the peritoneal cavity except in the vicinity of that part of
the wound which had been forced open twenty-four hours before death.
There was not a drop of serum or a trace of blood or lymph in Dong-
lass's pouch. I have here the pedicle, made up, as you see, of the cervix
uteri and right broad ligament; the cut layers of the left ligament are
here plainly visible, bounding this long denuded surface of cellular tissue,
which was taken up from the floor of the pelvis. You will notice that
the peritoneum up to the very edges of this surface, as well as entirely
around the cut surface of the pedicle, is free from all signs of inflammation. The pedicle had evidently been firmly united in its whole circumference to the muscular layer of the abdominal walls.

Nothing could more fully corroborate the perfect success of the operation *per se*, as indicated by the clinical history, than the condition
found at the autopsy.

The specimen, removed at the operation, weighed about four pounds,
was oval in shape, measured twenty-two or twenty-three inches in its
greatest circumference, and had projecting from its surface two or three
potatoid tumors, one of which had been recognized during life ; they
were ordinary fibroids of dense structure. The left ovary was the seat
of a small fibroid. The uterine cavity passed up posteriorly to the principal mass for the distance of seven inches, as had been discovered at
one time in the course of the summer, when the os had been dilated
with sponge-tents and the sound passed up to the fundus. An incision
into the large tumor in the anterior wall of the uterus showed that it
was of a coarse trabeculated structure, with interstitial spaces lined with
a delicate membrane. The whole mass was inclosed within a capsule,
which was readily enucleable from the encompassing uterine walls.
Only a comparatively thin wall of uterine tissue interposed between
the tumor and the cavity of the uterus.

In conclusion, I feel justified in claiming that the result in this case,
although fatal, should not depreciate the operation in the eyes of the
profession, but should encourage them to adopt the opinion of Péan,
who, after operating in twenty cases with fifteen recoveries, asserts that
the danger is no greater than in ovariotomy. The cause of death here
was one that is common to all surgical operations, great or small, and
can in no way be regarded as a danger peculiar to the extirpation of the
uterus.

RECENT PROGRESS IN OPHTHALMOLOGY.

BY O. F. WADSWORTH, M. D.

Embolism of the Arteria Centralis Retinæ. — Although many cases
have been reported with this heading, the diagnosis has been till lately
only in a single case verified by autopsy. Recently several cases have
been published in which an anatomical examination was made.

I.[1] A man aged fifty-eight, while sitting quietly in his chair, suddenly and totally lost the sight of the right eye without pain, headache,
or giddiness. Seven days later the eye was externally normal ; the
media were clear ; the vision was wholly gone. The disk was much
obscured by a white halo. The retina was rather hazy throughout,
much more so at the disk than at the equator. The macula was marked
by a dark reddish dot, surrounded by a white hazy halo, shading off
gradually. The retinal arteries were reduced to very fine lines. The
retinal veins as they emerged from the disk were about half the normal
size and increased gradually up to the first bifurcation; each of the
branches arising here began as a very fine trunk and increased to the
next point of division, and this appearance was repeated everywhere.
On the halo around the macula, the minute venous branches were remarkably evident. There was a loud double aortic murmur. The
effusion in the retina was in eleven weeks absorbed, the disk had become
very white, the arteries were very fine, the veins rather larger than the
arteries, especially toward the equator. Four months after the loss of
sight the patient died. Very extensive disease of the aortic valves was
found. The right optic nerve was somewhat shrunken. The central
vein was patent but smaller than normal. The artery, as a tube, was
no longer in existence; its former position was clearly indicated, however, by a well-defined circular mass of concentrically arranged fibrous
tissue adjacent to the vein.

II.[2] A clerk, aged fifty-four, while standing at his desk lost the sight
of the left eye suddenly. " There was a kind of bright mist before it,"
but it was not quite blind. Four days later, Mr. Wordsworth saw
him and diagnosed " œdema of the left retina and embolism of the
arteria centralis retinæ." Very distinct mitral and aortic systolic bruits
were heard on auscultation. Three months later the patient had symptoms of acute glaucoma, and he described only " a diamond shape " of
light as remaining at the temporal side. Iridectomy was followed by
temporary relief of pain, enlargement of the visual field, and improvement of sight so that he could count fingers. Three or four weeks
later there came on great congestion of the eye, pain, and loss of sight.

---

[1] Priestley Smith. British Medical Journal, April 4, 1874.
[2] Nettleship. Ophthalmic Hospital Reports, viii. 1.

The globe was excised. All the chief retinal vessels, both arteries and veins, contained blood, and in both sets of vessels the column was frequently broken, leaving small empty spaces. This appearance, at least in the veins, was probably due to post-mortem coagulation and shrinking. The principal veins in the retina were somewhat engorged, but became suddenly diminished in size on the disk. The column of blood in the arteries was smaller than that in the veins, and their walls appeared whiter and thicker, a change due probably to simple contraction. On the disk the main upper and lower divisions of the artery were obscured by a white structure, but two moderate-sized branches dipped into the disk a little distance from its margin. There were a few small hæmorrhages and glistening white deposits in the retina. Sections through the nerve showed the main terminal branches of the central artery plugged by a fibrinous mass, somewhat organized. Behind this was a more recent deposit, made up of fibrine and white blood corpuscles, which had, as it formed, cut off the blood current from the remaining arterial branches. The appearance of the most posterior portion of the thrombus, as well as of that of the blood in the branch which was given off farthest back, made it probable that blood had flowed through this branch not many days before the eye was removed. Nothing was found to explain the glaucomatous symptoms.

III.[1] A man of fifty-eight, a patient in hospital on account of partial paralysis of the left extremities, which was supposed to be the result of embolus in the right hemisphere, suddenly became blind of the left eye one night as he sat on the chamber-pot. The eye, examined within twenty hours, was externally normal ; the media were clear. The disk was pretty well defined, and of the normal color. The arteries on the disk were empty, scarcely recognizable, but they could be followed some distance on the retina. The retinal veins resembled dark bluish-red, pretty thick lines, less winding than normal, and with occasional breaks in the blood column. The region of the macula and toward the disk presented a slight grayish opacity. The macula was not distinguishable. At a spot corresponding about to the lower edge of the macula, a thick, dark-red line, the length of half the diameter of the disk was seen. The following day an irido-choroiditis, with chemosis of the conjunctiva, œdema of the lids, and some exophthalmus, had commenced to develop. The retina was more opaque ; its vessels were much in the same condition. In the course of two weeks the inflammation had begun to subside, and slowly disappeared. Four months from the attack, the vitreous had become transparent. There was atrophy of the disk and retina, and large patches about the disk on which the choroid was atrophied. Three thin vessels ran on the retina from the disk. In the retina were a few small hæmorrhages. Toward the periphery of the

[1] Schmidt. Archiv für Ophthalmologie, xx. 2.

fundus the changes were less, and more vessels could be seen. The
patient died eleven months from the occurrence of blindness. There
was an old hæmorrhage in the right hemisphere. The heart was
much enlarged, the wall of the left ventricle thickened, the aortic
valves atheromatous. The left opticus was decidedly smaller than the
right. The arteria centralis retinæ in a large part of its course in the
nerve was filled with a hyaline mass, in one place at least showing
signs of organization. Very soon after the entrance of the artery into
the nerve it gave off a considerable branch which ran parallel with it
toward the globe. This branch also was from a point near its origin
filled with a mass similar to that in the main artery. Within the eye,
at the parts in which the inflammatory changes had been greatest, the
retina and choroid were so fused as to form but one thin membrane,
and here the specific elements of the retina had disappeared and it was
changed into fibrous connective tissue. In the more peripheral parts
the tissues were better preserved, and here, in correspondence with the
ophthalmoscopic appearance, the blood-vessels were more numerous
and larger. At the point where the arteria centralis was given off
from the ophthalmic artery, and in some of the fine arteries in the
neighborhood, there were signs of thrombi, and this would accord with
the supposition that the irido-choroiditis which developed was in consequence of embolic stoppage of ciliary arteries.

IV.[1] A woman aged fifty-four, after a fright, became suddenly blind
of the left eye. The following day a large fresh hæmorrhage at the
macula lutea of this eye, and many small hæmorrhages, some old, and
in both eyes, were seen. There was a large central scotoma in the
left field of vision. The retinal vessels and the disk appeared normal.
A murmur was heard with the systole of the heart at the apex. Vision
improved, and after three months the patient could read 17 Jaeger. A
month later vision again failed, and there was found atrophy of the
disk, with the arteries obliterated at the disk, but containing blood at
the periphery. The atrophy increased. Death occurred some fourteen
months after the loss of sight. There was insufficiency of the bicuspid
valve. The arteria centralis in the nerve was small, and filled with a
partly homogeneous, partly granular substance. The eye was not removed, however, till sixty hours after death, in the summer, and the
history and appearances would seem to point at least quite as strongly
to hæmorrhagic retinitis as to embolism. The diagnosis can be hardly
considered other than doubtful.

V.[2] A woman of sixty, while quietly sitting, suddenly became blind
of the left eye. Five years before, an apoplectic attack had been followed by permanent paralysis of the left side. When the blindness

---

[1] Sichel. Archives de Physiologie, iv.
[2] Popp. Inaugural-dissertation. Erlangen, 1875.

came on there was no pain nor other symptom. Ophthalmoscopic examination gave the "characteristic appearances of embolus of the central artery of the retina, as it has been described by v. Graefe and Liebreich." No more minute account of the symptoms is given. There was marked insufficiency of the mitral valve. Two years and a half later the patient died, and in the heart was found great dilatation of the left auricle and insufficiency of the mitral valve, while the arch of the aorta presented much atheromatous roughening. The arteries at the base of the brain were much sclerosed and dilated. The left optic nerve was thin and atrophied, but careful examination showed nowhere obliteration or narrowing of its vessels, nor was there anything to point to the possibility that the supposed embolus had again become pervious.

VI. Loring[1] gives five cases which had been regarded by himself and others as of embolism, but in which their further development led him to doubt the correctness of the diagnosis. In the first case there was an anatomical examination.

A woman aged sixty-two, while standing still, experienced a sudden loss of sight of the right eye, without other sensation than that of commencing faintness. During the three weeks which elapsed before she presented herself, vision in this eye was limited to distinguishing between light and darkness, though with slight and transient occasional improvement. The disk appeared rather injected than pale, the arteries were not much diminished in size, the veins were greatly distended. There were three comparatively recent hæmorrhages in the retina. No pulsation of arteries or veins could be produced by pressure. About the macula there was a milky opacity of the retina, and a bright cherry spot at its centre. A month later the arteries appeared about the same, the veins were less distended, and narrowed toward the nerve; the opacity about the retina had disappeared, and the hæmorrhages had been absorbed. Soon after there was a glaucomatous attack, with hæmorrhage. Two months after the first attack there was another attack of glaucoma, and the eye was excised. No embolus was found, but there were thrombi in some of the vessels of the choroid; some signs of proliferation in the lamina cribrosa. The patient died a year and a half later. She had enjoyed good health till three or four months before her death, when symptoms of phlebitis began in the left leg and gradually increased, and at this time signs of heart-disease were found. No heart trouble could be made out at the time the eye was affected.

It has been often asserted that the diagnosis of embolism cannot be correct unless there is very decided diminution of the retinal vessels, and that therefore many of the cases reported as embolism must be rejected. In support of the opposite view, it has been urged that a more or less ample collateral circulation might soon be established through

[1] American Journal of the Medical Sciences, 1874, page 313.

the vessels which enter the papillà and disk from the anastomosing ring of ciliary arteries in the sclera around the nerve, and from the choroid. The anatomical investigations of Leber do not support this idea, however ; he reiterates in his more recent publication on the subject that such communication is a very contracted one. It is by no means certain that in any case collateral circulation of any amount is established, but Schmidt, in relation to this point, calls attention to the recent investigations of Schwalbe.[1] Schwalbe states that from the central artery, soon after it enters the nerve, a branch of considerable size is given off, which, gradually diminishing, runs forward parallel with the arteria centralis as far as the sclera, giving off branches to supply the nerve-bundles in its course. In Schmidt's case this branch was present, but plugged. He suggests that in case of sudden stoppage of the flow of blood through the central artery, the pressure in this side branch would be naturally much increased, and it would therefore be in a more favorable condition to afford a collateral supply of blood to the retina than the ciliary arteries, in which stopping of the arteria centralis would have but little influence on the pressure.

In the case reported by Nettleship no details of the ophthalmoscopic appearances are given, so that it is impossible to say what the condition of the vessels, as to size, etc., was soon after the attack. It is probable, however, from the state of things found in the eye after removal, that they contained, some of them at least, a considerable amount of blood. Loring's case seems to furnish negative evidence against the existence of embolism without contraction of the vessels. The case reported by Sichel is too doubtful to be taken as evidence.

The opacity about the macula, with red patch at the fovea, described as a characteristic sign of embolus, is observed also in other affections. Magnus[2] states that with embolus this opacity only appears late, and if it is present in the first few days it is evidence of hæmorrhage into the optic nerve. Schmidt's case disproves this, as the opacity was found twenty hours after the loss of sight. Here the red spot at the fovea was wanting; perhaps the disturbance which showed itself as an irido-choroiditis within the next twenty-four hours was already sufficient to cause opacity also of the thinner portion of the retina at this spot, or of the choroid behind it.

(*To be concluded.*)

[1] Handbuch der Augenheilkunde, i. 346.
[2] Die Sehnerven blutungen, page 50.

PROCEEDINGS OF THE SUFFOLK DISTRICT MEDICAL
SOCIETY.

R. H. FITZ, M. D., SECRETARY PRO TEMPORE.

SEPTEMBER 25, 1875. The vice-president, Dr. C. D. HOMANS, in the chair.
Limited Responsibility. — DR. T. W. FISHER read the following paper : —
" This term is applied by alienists and medical jurists to those forms of
mental unsoundness which do not wholly destroy the patient's legal responsibility. The law as well as public opinion has not been in favor of nice distinctions in this matter, and the legal tendency is towards entire responsibility
when a person is not decidedly and manifestly insane. The stubbornness of
facts has, however, gradually forced the admission of the above term into general use. The case of Arthur O'Connor, who two or three years ago was arrested for an attempt to shoot the Queen of England, is a good illustration of
the way in which this legal prejudice usurps the place of justice. In spite of
Dr. Tuke's evidence that this boy was insane, court and jury made indecent
haste to show their loyalty by a conviction for murder. Recently pardoned
by the clemency of the Queen, the boy has given unmistakable evidence of
continued homicidal tendencies and of undoubted insanity, and has been sent
to an asylum.
" The criminal laws are based on the moral responsibility of the criminal,
though in a very rude way, since the degrees of moral accountability are many
and obscure. The idea that the insane are sometimes morally responsible
seems to be new to the public, judging from newspaper discussions in cases in
which insanity has been alleged as an excuse for crime. Of course the insane
are often responsible for their acts, and know it, and are thereby subject to
moral and disciplinary treatment in hospitals. If it were not so, no appeal
could be made to their sense of propriety, or feeling for right and wrong, or
desire for improvement in conduct. This responsibility, however, is largely
limited in most cases by disease, placing the patient somewhat in the attitude
of a child towards those in authority, and the physician *in loco parentis.*
" All the insane except the utterly demented, or acutely maniacal or delirious.
know that they are considered to a certain degree unaccountable for their acts.
The knowledge is very seldom taken advantage of as an excuse for violence
or crime, though it is not an uncommon line of argument for a reasoning lunatic to adopt. The insane act usually either upon impulse or from delusion,
and in neither case does the question of their irresponsibility often occur to
them. If acting from impulse they do not stop to reason ; or if they act from
delusion, they believe themselves to be both in the right and fully responsible
for their acts, whatever others may think of them.
" The case of George Blampied, of England, recently quoted,[1] is no exception to the above rule. It is dangerous to infer perfect self-control because
the patient shows it in reference to certain of his acts. Blampied could be bought
off by tobacco from committing minor acts of violence, not resulting directly perhaps from morbid impulse, but was helpless to resist under other circumstances.

[1] Boston Medical and Surgical Journal, August 26, 1875.

Last week I was called to testify in a case of homicidal impulse where the evidence was no stronger than in the case of Blampied. The district attorney and the judge admitted the existence of insanity, and the jury acquitted the prisoner in their seats.

"The law practically does recognize many degrees of responsibility for the same crime, as in the case of minors. First offenses incur light punishments, and principals are more severely dealt with than dupes and accessories. There is a certain degree of leniency exercised towards offenders who give evidence of extreme ignorance or a low grade of intellect. In prisons there is always a milder discipline for the large class of epileptics and weak-minded prisoners, upon whom punishment has no reformatory effect.

"These distinctions are easy to make when feelings of prejudice and resentment towards the criminal have not been excited. If, however, an atrocious murder has been committed, especially if a number of unpunished murders has previously excited public indignation, we often feel an instinctive desire for the immediate extermination of its author. The criminal is held to be as bad as his crime. Instead of putting ourselves in his place, we put him in our own place, and attribute to him the same degree of guilt we should expect to feel at having deliberately committed the same crime.

"The above feelings have evidently possessed the public mind to a large degree in the case of Jesse Pomeroy, now under sentence for murder. This boy, by his own confession, is guilty of a series of shocking crimes at which nature revolts. At the age of twelve years he was sent to the State Reform School for the torture of young children in a manner showing utter insensibility to their sufferings, and in some cases evident satisfaction. He was pardoned by the culpable leniency of the trustees, and soon after, at the age of fourteen years, committed two murders upon children, the details of which are well known.

"The first thing that strikes an alienist in reading the evidence in the above case is the apparently motiveless character of the acts, and the fact that they belong, by family resemblance, to that class of acts often committed by boys, and sometimes by girls, who are either morally deficient or morally insane. These acts are most frequent about the age of puberty, and depend in some cases on a state of cerebral erethism induced by masturbation. They comprise every variety of vicious and outrageous conduct, such as theft, running away from home, intoxication, self-abuse, cruelty to animals, obstruction of railroad trains, setting of fires, torture of children, and sometimes homicide or suicide. Every physician knows some such case, and is satisfied of the partial absence, at least, of moral accountability, in spite of the apparent intellectual soundness.

"I will take as illustrations three instances of boy torture, selected from the daily papers within a few weeks.

"The first is that of Harry Rogers, of San Francisco. When eight years old he was fond of flaying and cutting puppies and chickens, carefully avoiding any vital part. At the age of eleven or twelve he shockingly mutilated a child three years old by cutting it with a sharp bone, making no less than nineteen wounds, and nearly cutting off its right ear. He generally confesses his misdeeds, and says he cannot help them. He is equal in education to other boys of his age, and has no marked peculiarities of appearance.

" The second case recently occurred in Newton. A boy eighteen years old took a younger boy into the fields, and compelled or induced one of his comrades to go also. The younger boy was stripped, tied hand and foot, and then cut in various places in a deliberate manner. A young girl accidentally passing was forced to come and look at the naked and mutilated boy. When he was released and allowed to dress, he made a rush at his tormentor with his pocket-knife, but was knocked down with an axe-helve.

" The third case recently occurred in a small village near Florence, in Italy. Four children had mysteriously disappeared, when Carlo Grandi, a carpenter's apprentice, twenty-three years of age, was discovered in the act of killing a fifth victim. He had dug a grave in the yard of his shop, and had attempted to bury alive a little boy about ten years old. He decoyed him into the hole, covered his head with an apron, heaped a basketful of gravel on him, and stifled his outcries by gagging him with the handle of a chisel. On searching the yard the graves of three other children were found. No motive could be assigned for these acts.

" Cases of moral imbecility or insanity in minors, from their evident need of moral treatment and discipline, have usually been sent to reformatory institutions when coming within the operation of the law. This has been the course taken even when homicide has been committed. A boy named Shehan, aged fourteen years, was sent to the Westboro' Reform School from Franklin, Mass., a few years ago, for stoning and drowning a young companion, simply, as he said, that he might ' see the little devil kick in the water.' The same boy put stones on the railroad track. Every hospital for the insane has a few specimens of this kind. I recently certified in the case of a young girl who had set three fires in her mother's house before being suspected as the incendiary.

" The Pomeroy case has excited so much feeling that it is almost impossible to judge it fairly. The public pressure for his execution is strong in some quarters, and the medical profession is not free from the infection. But if the morbid element is seen and admitted in other cases of this class, why deny its existence in this one simply on account of the number and atrocity of the acts committed ? These acts are a most important part of the evidence for or against insanity, and the more unnatural and motiveless they appear, the stronger the evidence of some morbid impulse to account for them. What could have been the motives, for instance, which incited Pomeroy to force one of his victims to repeat after him the Lord's Prayer, closing it with a vulgar word ? Or in another case to kindly draw the subject of his tortures home through the streets of South Boston on a hand-sled ?

" I have seen Pomeroy but once, and that was since his sentence. He recounted his horrible deeds without reluctance and with perfect *sang-froid*. In some of the details his memory seemed at fault, though he admitted the probability of all the evidence against him. He was unable to give any reason for his conduct except the usual one that he felt that he must do as he did. He confirmed the testimony of his school-mates that he was subject to sudden and violent headaches, but did not claim to have had one at the time of his acts. He did not claim to have been insane, and yet did not see how he could have done as he did in his right mind.

" The evidence of self-abuse was plainly written on his countenance, as well as in his hands, which he kept concealed at first. On seeing that I observed them he asked what was the matter with them. They were purple, cold, and clammy to a degree seldom seen except in old cases of dementia with masturbation. He at first denied but afterwards admitted the correctness of my inference. He also admitted that he had practiced the habit for years, and particularly at the periods when his crimes were committed. At the Reform School he read some medical book on the subject, which checked the practice for a time. He has recently written to some friend, as the sheriff informs me, warning him against the habit.

" Mania from masturbation is a well-characterized form of insanity, being set down as a distinct variety in Dr. Skae's classification. It affects all three departments of the mind. The attention and memory are weakened and the judgment impaired. There is a state of vanity, conceit, and love of notoriety, change, and adventure in direct contrast to the dullness, passivity, and love of solitude noticed before the mind is actively affected. Sometimes great restlessness is observed, with a tendency to go from place to place without motive, to run away from home on some wild, impracticable errand, in hopes of making a fortune or becoming famous, with inability or indisposition for continuous employment of any kind. The moral sense is blunted, and vicious courses new to the individual are entered upon. The will is weakened not only in reference to the habit in question, but as shown in fickleness of purpose, and in sudden yielding to impulses of an erratic or dangerous character. Under the cerebral conditions induced by this habit there is a tendency to mental spasmodic action, as well as to epileptic vertigo and convulsions.[1]

" All the experts without exception who examined Pomeroy before his trial considered him weak-minded ; all but one were sure he was insane and at least but partially responsible at the time of the homicides ; two of them suspected the presence of epilepsy in an obscure form. The diagnosis of masked epilepsy is often difficult. The patient can give no clear account of his condition at the time of attack, and when epileptic vertigo is so often ignored by ordinary observers, it is not strange that the signs of this mental epilepsy, as it might be called, are generally misunderstood. In these cases a brief attack of mania, or of semi-consciousness, in which the patient wanders long distances and does strange things, takes the place of vertigo or convulsions in persons disposed to epilepsy. If the test of complete forgetfulness of what has occurred be applied in the case of Pomeroy, he was not epileptic. This is still a mooted point, and I believe the want of memory is sometimes but partial.

" The case shows many of the characteristics of mania from masturbation. Conceit and love of notoriety are especially prominent in his recent foolish and inconsistent retraction of his numerous confessions, in which he argues in a confused way the impossibility of his having committed any of the crimes with which he is charged ; alleges that he confessed to keep his mother out of jail, and that he imposed on the doctors who examined him with false state-

---

[1] Since writing the above, I have learned that young Walworth, the New York parricide, has been examined by a commission of experts, who have decided that he was a victim of this form of insanity, and he has been removed from prison to an asylum. T. W. F.

ments about his head symptoms. This piece of special pleading is compounded of lies, quibbles, and slang jokes put together in a sort of mock legal manner. He is evidently tickled at his own ingenuity. The press have made much of this retraction, but the waste basket of any insane hospital would furnish similar copy in abundance. The only point worth noticing is that while denying the commission of the crimes which he had freely confessed over and over again, for months, and to many different persons both before and after conviction, he argues with apparent sincerity that if he did commit them he must have been insane. He is evidently willing to take what advantage may accrue from this plea, as it is natural that he should, whatever his real belief may be.

" Whether he is at present insane is a distinct question from his probable condition at the ages of twelve and fourteen, the time at which the acts were committed. This is a point which continually escapes the attention of the press when discussing the case. The mental status of a boy undergoing imprisonment, trial, and conviction for murder must in ordinary cases be profoundly influenced by those circumstances, and it is one of the significant facts in this case that Pomeroy is not more affected. He does not have that realizing sense of the situation which might be expected. Puberty has also changed his physique as well as his mental condition since his arrest.

" His attempted escape has been thought to indicate the skill of a hardened and experienced criminal. It does not, however, show much judgment, as its success was an impossibility. It was a feeble imitation of such examples as abound in the cheap literature of the day. In hospitals for the insane such attempts are expected as a matter of course in the case of many boys and young men, not too maniacal or demented to control their actions. Incited by the restlessness of immaturity, and sometimes by a morbid love for such notoriety as even failure would afford, they make repeated and often ingenious efforts to escape. Repeated failure, and the certainty of capture and return, does not deter them. A little common sense would have convinced Pomeroy, not only of the impracticable nature of his plans, but of the inevitable prejudice such an attempt, in addition to his false retraction, would create in the mind of the public.

" Upon all the evidence obtainable, I am satisfied of Pomeroy's present mental unsoundness, as well as of his partial if not complete irresponsibility at the time of the commission of the crimes with which he is charged. This evidence is meagre, depending as to the acts on his own imperfect recollections and unreliable statements and on those of little boys half-dead with fright at the time. There is no doubt of the existence of head-symptoms of some kind. He was known at an early age to be guilty of cruelty to animals. He twice ran away from home before the age of twelve, bought fire-arms, and took cars for the West to fight the Indians. He was fond of reading stories of savage warfare. It is not improbable that impressions made in this way in his youth, under the stimulus of puberty and the excitement of constant self-abuse, with its accompanying impairment of will-power, developed into morbid, fixed ideas, and these ideas passed uncontrolled into the horrible acts of torture and murder which have startled the community.

" This development of a fixed idea from some vivid impression in early life is well shown in a case quoted from Marc, by Bucknill and Tuke.[1] A lady when young had been present at an execution, and conceived a desire to be placed in a similar position. Her religious scruples restrained her for a long time, but on witnessing another execution her morbid fancy was so stimulated as to overcome all self-control, and she murdered a person against whom she had no dislike, for the sake of being hanged in public.

"The authorities which I have consulted — about a dozen in all — agree that these motiveless crimes of young people are due to mental disease of some form, either congenital moral imbecility, moral insanity, masked epilepsy, or uncontrollable impulse, from disorder of the brain connected with puberty, menstruation, or self-abuse ; and I believe the case of Pomeroy, if all the facts were known, would prove no exception. It may be said that it is impossible to estimate the amount of self-control existing in any given case ; but in hundreds of cases of mental disease with impulsive acts of violence, where there is no motive for prevarication, the patient's assertion that he ' could not help it,' expresses probably the exact truth. Such acts are done without appreciable motive and against the patient's best interests. The physician is often appealed to by persons so afflicted, to put them under restraint and save them from the consequences of their impulsive acts. A recent patient of mine, a boy with a record indicating moral insanity, said to his mother one day, ' Have n't I behaved well to-day?' and without further conversation threw a heavy stone at her. He was immediately alarmed at her narrow escape, and cried out ' Why did n't you dodge it? Why, I might have killed you!'

"It may be claimed that though but partially responsible, the public safety requires the execution of Pomeroy, both for the extermination of a dangerous moral monster and for the sake of deterring others from similar acts. Imprisonment will sufficiently protect the public, and it is not likely his execution would have any deterrent effect whatever. If it would, his hanging might be desirable if not warranted. The effect would be more likely to resemble that of smothering an hydrophobiac. The dread of that process, in addition to a natural horror of the disease, has no doubt induced many cases of imaginary hydrophobia. In the same manner the publication of the details of murder, rape, executions, insane homicides and suicides, and tales of assassination and crime, in the newspapers, spreads an infection which, taking root in the congenial soil of a disordered and enfeebled brain, brings forth a ghastly harvest. The contagiousness of hysteria and suicidal impulse is well known to the profession, and this contagion of homicide is of similar character. It seems to me, on the whole of greater importance to society that the causes which conduce to the growth of such moral monstrosities should be understood, than that a few specimens should be hung, as the French say, ' pour encourager les autres.' "

Dr. D. F. Lincoln asked the reader's opinion as to the probable effect of the hanging of Pomeroy upon other children of a similar stamp.

Dr. Fisher thought it would have no effect whatever.

Dr. S. G. Webber had been interested in the case of Pomeroy with reference to the assumption, by others than the reader, of an epileptic condition.

[1] On Insanity, page 199.

The previous history of the boy showed an obscure attack of sickness in 1871, with subsequent occasional headaches, and the torturing of children from time to time. He thought it important that all these conditions ceased during the boy's stay at the Reform School. If the condition were allied to epilepsy, such an interruption would have been very unlikely. Further, there seemed to be too much contrivance in his plans for them to have been of an epileptiform character. Dr. Webber thought the main point to be whether Pomeroy's motives were similar to those actuating sane boys, or the reverse. The former seemed to him to be the case. The reasoning power was apparently retained, there was no evidence of his being prompted by delusions, and the various acts seemed to lack all the elements existing in the various kinds of insane conduct.

As to his moral nature, it is well known that in individuals there is every degree even to almost complete absence of moral feeling, and yet the person may be considered as perfectly sane. Even if we admit that Pomeroy may have possessed a low degree of moral feeling, his education, his surroundings, his ideas derived from trashy stories (he himself stated that reading Indian stories led him to torture boys in imitation of the Indians), all this, with a disposition to cruelty which gained strength the more it was indulged, would seem to have been sufficient motive for his acts.

The circumstances attending the acts cannot be regarded as a proof of sanity, although the acts may be sane. His attempt at breaking jail might be regarded rather as an attempt at notoriety than as an evidence of insanity. Though Dr. Webber had not seen the boy, and had had but little experience in insanity, yet he had carefully read the testimony, and judging from this alone, Pomeroy did not seem to him to be insane, nor did his acts appear motiveless, as has been argued by the counsel for the defense.

DR. FISHER stated that the suddenness of the impulse could not be considered of special value in forming an opinion, as it is a characteristic of the insane to delay as well as to act quickly. This is evident in the cunning hown by insane suicides, who will often conceal their delusions, even appear to be recovering ; thus endeavoring to disarm suspicion, they will suddenly seize upon an opportunity when it arrives. The murder of the girl in Pomeroy's case was certainly a sudden, impulsive act.

DR. WEBBER thought the only evidence of his insanity was derived from the acts. These furnish evidence so far as they go, but there should be other evidence which should rather be strengthened by the acts. Possibly Pomeroy's future may give additional light, and the view of his insanity be thus corroborated.

DR. J. J. PUTNAM thought that the discussion as to the sanity or insanity of Pomeroy, regarded from the scientific point of view, was to a certain extent an aimless one, because no exact scientific definition of insanity could be given. Every man is in some degree insane and irresponsible, inasmuch as he occasionally commits acts as it were involuntarily, which he wonders at. and for the committing of which he blames himself. The law, on the contrary, is obliged to give a more or less absolute though arbitrary definition of insanity, and Dr. Putnam agreed with Dr. Fisher in thinking that the mental characteristics of Pomeroy and the history of his acts fairly placed him in the class of those whom the law agrees to call insane. At the same time he thought it could not be said that the execution of Pomeroy would do more harm than good, in consequence of its helping to inflame the morbid tendencies in the class of persons of a similar disposition to his own. Although this would no doubt occur to some extent, it seemed to Dr. Putnam to be more than counterbalanced by the fact that the execution would have a salutary influence upon the larger class of ordinary malefactors, who needed to be shown that on the whole punishment was the regular consequence of misdemeanor, and therefore, so long as the jury and a majority of the community had pronounced him guilty and liable, he favored the carrying out of the sentence.

Dr. Fisher did not regard the case as epileptiform. The feeling of relief after the act was no evidence of such a condition, since after the accomplishment of an act, the insane patient frequently manifested such a feeling

Dr. Webber stated that it had occurred to him that Pomeroy's desire seemed to have been to torture, and that the murders were accidental.

Multiple Cystoid Myxoma of the Chorion. — Dr. Haskins showed the specimen, which had been removed from a case seen by him in consultation. The patient had been well till some five weeks ago, her catamenia having been regular. Since then there had been occasional slight flowing, irregular appetite, vomiting at times, and progressive emaciation. She was unmarried, and denied the possibility of conception. When he saw the patient she had been flowing profusely, was very pale and feeble ; her pulse was 150. The uterus was enlarged to about the size at the fifth month of pregnancy. The os was found to be dilated slightly. The finger was introduced into the uterus, its contents were detached and came immediately away, following an expulsive pain. The uterus then contracted.

Poisoning from Snake Bite. — Dr. A. B. Hall reported two cases, those of a woman and her husband, who were in the habit of handling snakes at a public exhibition recently given in this city. The woman was seen twenty minutes after having been bitten by a viper, the skin in the vicinity of the wound then being of a greenish hue. He made an incision, cauterized the wound thoroughly with lunar caustic, and ordered whisky to be given freely. On the following day he was informed that his prescription had been fully carried out. The lymphatics of the arm were then swollen. After a week complete recovery had taken place.

The husband was soon after bitten by a rattlesnake ; he adopted the whisky treatment and recovered after the lapse of a week.

MEDICAL NOTES.

— Dr. Tissier reports, in *L'Union Médicale*, the case of a girl now seven years old who was born with two teeth. She has always been healthy, both during the time of her nursing and after weaning. She had all the front teeth when six months old, and her first set of teeth still remains entire.

Usually, the reporter remarks, the precocious eruption of teeth is due to some pathological condition of the gums, causing ulceration of the dental follicles and the eruption of the teeth ; but in this case the child has always been well, and has kept her teeth without accident. Moreover, the teeth with which she was born were the two upper middle incisors, whereas, usually, the eruption of the middle lower incisors precedes that of the upper.

— We are in receipt of the new circular of the Medical School of Maine announcing the beginning of the next term on February 17, 1876. The following changes have occurred since the last course. Dr. Burt G. Wilder has become professor of physiology, Dr. Jenks, of Detroit, has resigned the chair of diseases of women, and Professor Mitchell has been appointed lecturer on that branch in addition to his own professorship. Dr. Gerrish will give, during the coming term, a short additional course of lectures on public health.

— The cold-water bed as a new method of reducing temperature is recommended by H. D. Felton, M. D., in the *Medical Record* of October 3, 1875. In the case of a patient in the fourth week of typhoid fever, whose temperature was 103.5°–104°, Dr. Felton made use of a water-bed, constructed from a rubber air-mattress, with inlet and outlet at opposite ends, to which he coupled a rubber hose, one pipe being attached to the aqueduct faucet and the outlet conveying the water from the house. His patient lay upon the bed eighteen days, the water being renewed every five hours. It was found that at the time when the temperature of the atmosphere was 62°, and that of the hydrant water 68°, the water in the bed, after remaining unchanged seven hours, was 79°, an increase of seventeen degrees over that of the atmosphere, and of eleven degrees above that of the aqueduct water; therefore the patient imparted eleven degrees of heat to a barrel of water in seven hours, and still his temperature remained at $102\frac{3}{4}°$.

LETTER FROM PHILADELPHIA.

MESSRS. EDITORS, — After a summer of almost unprecedented good health, and a consequent small death-rate, Philadelphia has begun preparations for a new winter. The daily journals have made you familiar with the immense fruit crop with which southern cities have been blessed since June. The unusual abundance of peaches in particular has enabled even the poor to enjoy this delicious, healthful fruit without stint. To its effects I believe we chiefly owe the low death-rate and the comparative freedom from the ordinary summer complaints.

The two regular medical schools opened last week with large classes. Thus far the Jefferson class numbers four hundred and thirteen students, the University class about three hundred. How long this disproportion will last is uncertain. The University, with its hospital and laboratories, presents large and tempting inducements ; but, as I have before remarked, students prefer to live in the main town, and West Philadelphia is a long walk from the boarding-houses. This trivial circumstance seems to carry weight. Professor Gross delivered the inaugural at the opening of the Jefferson school. His subject was the Medical Literature of America. In a future letter I mean to give you some interesting extracts from this valuable address.

At Wills's Eye Hospital last week two new pavilion wards were dedicated by appropriate services. Addresses were made by the chairman of the hospital committee (General Collis), and by Mr. William Welsh, president of the board of city trusts, who described the construction, heating, and ventilating of the new buildings; finally, Dr. A. D. Hale, chief of the surgical staff, gave an interesting surgical history of the hospital, and of the remarkable improvements in the art and science of ophthalmology which have been made during the existence of the institution. By the erection of the new wards the number of beds for resident patients has been doubled. The cost of these structures has been taken from the principal of the hospital funds, with the belief that the citizens of Philadelphia, who exhibit the most untiring generosity toward charities of this nature, will make good the deficit. A portion has already been donated. The new wards have been erected on ground which belongs to the hospital, and they stand about twenty-five feet from the main building. Each ward is ninety feet long by twenty-two wide, and has a ceiling fifteen feet high. Like all pavilion-wards they have but one story. The north end of each is divided into a vestibule and three rooms. The nurse will occupy one room; the other two will be devoted to bathing, washing, and other conveniences. They are thoroughly ventilated, and have the latest improvements in sewerage. The floors of these rooms are covered with Pelletier cement; the windows here, as throughout the building, are double glazed, and those in the end rooms have solid inside shutters to retain the heat during the winter months. Externally, Venetian blinds serve a contrary purpose in summer. The wash-room has streams of water instead of wash-basins. Each patient is here provided with a hook for his towel, and another for his clothing, which will thus be kept out of the sleeping apartment. In each of the large wards there are twenty beds, with an air-space of twelve hundred cubic feet for each patient. Seventeen windows on the sides and ends of each building will afford ample summer ventilation. Those on the sides are not opposite each other, as is customary, but alternate. This arrangement, it is thought, will prevent stagnant air-spaces in the wards. The outside Venetian blinds will exclude heat and glare, and permit ventilation during the nights of warm weather; they will also prevent injury by rain when the windows are open. The inner surface of these blinds is covered with wire gauze, which will protect patients from currents of cold air by diffusing the latter, and will also exclude troublesome insects. The plaster on the walls and ceilings is of hard sand finish; the sills are of slate, and in the wards there are no inside shutters or curtains to absorb unhealthful exhalations. In winter tepid fresh air will be introduced through convenient heaters, which are placed at each end of the wards. By the same means the patients will be supplied with radiant heat. The gaseous products of combustion are conducted by iron pipes from each heater into the centre of the two large ventilating chimneys which refresh each ward. Rarefied air in these ventilating shafts will induce a rapid current from the wards, the impure air escaping by openings in the cold external walls near the floor, and thence through ducts under the floor and into the warm shafts. Large flues also lead into these shafts near the ceiling of the wards. They are intended for summer use, when the temperature of the wards is too high and external air cannot be safely introduced. The ward floors are composed of single layers of yellow pine boards. This simplicity, it is hoped, will prevent absorption of poisonous effluvia and collections of vermin. The only objection to single floors is their chilliness. This objection has been removed in this case by an arrangement which will keep the air-space between the floor and the brick pavement beneath at an uniform temperature. The stone foundations and basement walls are capped by a horizontal layer of North River flagging, which will check the upward movement of moisture which rises from the ground through ordinary stone foundations and into brick walls by capillary attraction. The floor-joists rest upon this flag-stone coping, and do not enter the brick walls, as is usual. By this means they are ventilated, and kept free of dampness and liability to decay. External grated openings will, in summer, ventilate the space beneath the floors. These openings will be closed in winter, but it is thought, since the sun will shine upon the opposite side of the buildings during the day, that sufficient change of air in the sub-space will be caused by currents induced throughout the hollow space between the walls of the building. This space opens into the roof-ventilator. The outer walls are of hard brick, the inner of soft. The hard outer brick will resist the weather, the inner will prevent condensation of moisture. The air-space between the walls ventilates the roof and cellar, and will act as a non-conductor to external heat in summer, to internal warmth in winter. Cedar shingles cover the roofs; they are the most expensive covering, but are a better non-conductor than either slate or metal.

The loft is plastered under the rafters; the ceiling on its upper as well as its lower surface. The wards are thus interiorly protected in this portion by a triple non-conductor. The building materials are of the best stock. Including plumbing and heaters, the cost of the two wards will be $5500, to which may be added $2000 for furnishing, paving, and fencing the ground plot. The surgeons of the hospital now control four sections, of twenty beds each. The hospital has heretofore been overcrowded, and the new wards were much needed. The last three yearly reports of the institution show a steadily increasing demand upon its acommodations. In 1872 there were treated 2876 out and in patients; in 1873, 3504; in 1874, 3809. Wills's Hospital was founded in 1823 by means of the legacy of James Wills, a Quaker grocer, who, with the exception of a few small legacies, gave his entire fortune to this object, stipulating only that the hospital should adopt his name.

In many particulars the new wards resemble the pavilion-wards of the Presbyterian Hospital, which I described in detail fifteen months ago. Yet in many other respects they differ from the latter, and since this style of ward is creating an increasing interest among hospital committees, I have ventured to give you this somewhat lengthy description.

A few evenings ago the Pennsylvania Association of Dental Surgeons held its annual meeting. This association was organized in December, 1845, and has ever since been in active operation, holding monthly meetings for the consideration of all matters relating to dentistry and collateral subjects. Standing committees investigate questions of interest to dentists, and from time to time make reports. At the meetings of the association essays are read, special cases in practice are considered, each subject is discussed, and ideas are compared; mutual instruction and the elevation of the art of dentistry being the aim and end of the association.

At the meeting of the Pathological Society this week, one of the members presented for inspection a human foot, upon the outer surface of which, directly after its forcible removal from the leg by a railway crush, he had rubbed one drachm of dry salicylic acid. He then exposed the foot to the sun and weather for eighteen days. At the end of this time he cut into the member, found it perfectly sweet, the skin soft and pliable, the muscles unchanged both in color and in consistence, and hence he recommended the acid as an economical preservative. Since salicylic acid is soluble in not less than three hundred parts of water, the rationale of this conservative effect was asked for. The experimenter could not give it, but considered the healthy condition of the foot an obvious argument in favor of the process, whatever that might be. Dr. Tyson thought the action of the acid might be explained by the abundant presence in the blood and serous fluids of phosphate of soda, which substance renders salicylic acid very soluble. Dr. H. Allen then suggested that since the new theory of decomposition claims that it is caused by bacteria, the acid might have preserved the foot simply by protecting it from these animalculæ. The subject of the possible value of this acid as a preservative agent was then referred to a committee for investigation.

A promising young scoundrel of gentlemanly appearance, perhaps a student, one day last week supplied the morning papers of Philadelphia with false information of the death of Professor Charles A. Stillé, Provost of the University of Pennsylvania. Obituary notices of a highly complimentary character were published by the morning press, but before evening the information proved to be a hoax. The societies of the university are making earnest search for the miserable youth who forged the report. Professor Stillé has reason to be gratified by the warm and friendly words of the press in connection with himself, but the public are highly indignant over this outrage.

As a coincidence, I may mention that a Philadelphia physician, in July last, at the request of the editor of the *Philadelphia Medical Times*, wrote for that journal an obituary notice of Professor Traube, of Berlin, news of whose death was primarily derived from the *Allegemeine Zeitung*, of Vienna. Having been well acquainted with Professor Traube and his family, he also wrote a letter of sympathy to the surviving members. He has just received a verbal message from them to the effect that they had received his letter, and that he would appreciate their silence when informed that Professor Traube *is not dead.* Medical and secular papers in Germany and elsewhere published biographical and very friendly notices of the professor. But this is the *second* time that he has met with this painful experience. It is not then surprising that he feels annoyed and depressed by it. Professor Traube, however, knows nothing of the embarrassment of those who have written the obituary notices. The Philadelphia physician just mentioned finds only a slight compensation for his somewhat awkward dilemma in the appreciative and affectionate character of the obituary which he so unsuspectingly wrote. X.

PHILADELPHIA, *October* 16, 1875.

THE METRIC SYSTEM.

MESSRS. EDITORS, — Your correspondent E. T. W., in the JOURNAL of October 28th, calls our present system of weights and measures *duodecimal.* We fail to see in what respect it is so. He speaks of our tables and of the duodecimal system of notation in such a way as to lead us to infer that the principle is the same in both. This is calculated to convey an entirely wrong impression. The system of notation he refers to is that in which the figure 1 (or the first figure used in numeration, whatever sign may be chosen therefor) followed by 0 has the value of twelve units, and not of ten as in the decimal system. In this sense the duodecimal system does not exist at all ; much less could it exist in our tables, and yet any one unacquainted with the meaning of the term would suppose from the wording of his article that it did exist in the latter.

Let us now see if our tables are duodecimal in any sense. In the only other sense of the word, a duodecimal is a number belonging to a series all of which are multiples of 12, or the scale of which is 12. A table of weights and measures is in this sense duodecimal when the units therein progress by 12's. We will examine our tables (we can do it with the aid of an arithmetic) and see if they progress by 12's.

I find the first table usually given in our school-books to be that of Federal currency. Here we have four 10's ; there are no duodecimals, but decimals in *every* sense of the word ; decimals, to which your correspondent so warmly objects.

The next table is that of liquid measure. In this we find two 4's, three 2's, one 63, and one 31½. Here again there are no 12's, but instead a 63 and a 31½, neither of which can be halved or quartered, a process for which your correspondent finds our tables so admirably adapted.

Next comes the table of avoirdupois weight. This contains two 16's, one 28, one 4, and one 20. Still no 12's, but instead one multiple of 10.

In this way, if we go through all the tables, we shall find every variety of number, with a good share of fractions thrown in for ornament. But how many 12's are there ? We will count them.

I have before me fifteen different arithmetics taken at random from a much larger collection.

In no two of these are the tables exactly alike in form and number. I find them most complete in Walkingame's arithmetic, an old work. Not including the four 10's in the table of money, nor the numbers in that of English money, these tables contain one hundred and fourteen numbers. Among these appear nine 3's, four 5's, two 7's, five 8's, one 10, three 20's, six 30's, three 40's, one 50, three 60's, two 100's, one 640, one 1120, six 31's, one 1728, one 1½, one 5½, one 7½, one 13½, one 31¼, one 272¼, nine 2's, and eleven 4's. And how many 12's? Only four ! And two of these used for the same thing, namely, to express the relation between the ounce and the pound in two different tables.

Only four 12's with one hundred and fourteen numbers which are not 12's. Adding to the numbers given in these tables those in other arithmetics, but not included in this, we have one hundred and twenty-eight, of which, by the way, six are 10's, and twenty-six are integral multiples of 10.

Such are the tables which your correspondent sees fit to call duodecimal.

But he may object that these four 12's are oftener used than many of the other numbers. One, for instance, in the table of long measure, where it expresses the relation between feet and inches. True; it occupies here a very important place. *Consequently* our engineers have long since given it up; given up the only 12 in this table, and divided the foot no longer into 12 parts, as before, but into 10. This, too, they have done knowing that they thereby subjected themselves to the inconvenience of being at variance with their neighbors. Such is the importance which practical men have given to the decimal.

E. T. W. implies that there is one other defect in the metric system. While the decimal ratio is infinitely more favorable to calculation than any other in use, for the daily purposes of life he prefers the binary subdivision He would halve and quarter things. So would we. There is no need on this account to reject the decimal. We may employ both, and we do employ both. Does your correspondent remember ever having seen a half or a quarter of a dollar? Has he ever seen half a dime, or a five-cent piece? He may cut his soap as well as his dollars into halves and quarters, and call the pieces a half or a quarter metre long. History will show him, if he will only take the trouble to consult it, that the metric system has received by law in France, and in Germany in the act of January 26, 1870, its regular binary subdivisions. There are by this law in use $\frac{1}{2}$, $\frac{1}{4}$, $\frac{1}{8}$, $\frac{1}{16}$, $\frac{1}{32}$, $\frac{1}{40}$, and $\frac{1}{80}$ litre pieces, and so with the gram and metre.

In our own tables, however, there are, according to Walkingame, thirty-two numbers which cannot be divided by 2, an inconvenience which never occurs in the metric system.

" In small dealings, the convenience of buyers and sellers is best consulted when the multiples and sub-multiples of quantities correspond with the multiples and sub-multiples of coins. If a pound of any commodity costs twenty-five cents, it would better suit all parties who use the Federal currency if we could divide the pound evenly into five parts than it does now to divide it into four. Nothing is more certain than that quantities bought and sold, and the instrument of purchase and sale, should be subject to the same law.[1]

As to whether or not the duodecimal (or duodenary) or the octonary system of notation will ever supplant the decimal is a matter of speculation into which it is unnecessary to enter here. In the published proceedings of the American Pharmaceutical Association for 1859 is an exhaustive and very interesting report on the subject, of about forty pages, to which we would refer your correspondent E. T. W. In the mean time, since the world actually uses the decimal system of notation, and *we* use the decimal system in our table of money, let us adopt it also in our other tables.

As for our having received our tables from the Roman *as*, this one statement, made with pride by your correspondent, certainly *sounds* correct. But if hitherto it has been our disgrace and our misfortune to endure for two thousand years a ridiculous jumble of weights and measures, which can point to nothing better than an *as* for its origin, it is high time, now that wiser nations have set us the example, to adopt this decimal system, model of beauty and simplicity, born of science, and proud to count as its originators the most famous savants of the world. J. P. P.

BOSTON, *October* 30, 1875.

[1] See pamphlet on The International or Metric System, published by Hurd and Houghton.

MESSRS. EDITORS, — Your correspondent E. T. W., in arguing in favor of what he is pleased to call "our present system" of weights and measures, really suggests the strongest reason for abandoning it. This is to be found in the importance of establishing conformity between our method of numerical notation and our system of weights and measures.

It may be perfectly true that "the natural method of subdivision is not by decimating, but by halving and quartering," but inasmuch as the arithmetic of all civilized nations is established on a decimal basis, the practical question for us to consider is whether we shall change our arithmetic to suit our weights and measures or change our weights and measures to suit our arithmetic. Of the two courses there can be no doubt that the latter offers the less violence to the mental processes of the civilized world.   H. P. B.

BOSTON, *October* 29, 1875.

MESSRS. EDITORS, — So far as our own profession is concerned, the only practical difficulty about the metric system consists in accustoming ourselves to writing prescriptions decimally. An occasional half-hour, however, in practice will soon convince any one that the change is easy. Much may be done by your own excellent journal by giving us, especially in the department of Recent Progress in the Treatment of Disease, an occasional prescription written with the old and new systems side by side for comparison. For example, on page 157, volume xcii., —

		Approximately.	
℞ Potassæ chloratis	. . . .	8	℈ ij.
Aquæ destillatæ	. . . .	225	℥ vij.
Syrupi rubi idæi	. . . .	25	℥ vj.

This is indeed an *innovation:* so also were vaccination, ether, steam-engines, obstetric forceps, and telegraphs, but none the less useful as *innovations*.

A decimal system has its chief advantage in its simplicity, for its operations are conducted by the simple shifting of a point to right or left, as in Federal money.

Another advantage is in the disuse of the old signs ℈ and ℥, which were so likely to be confounded when carelessly or hastily written. It is a fact that the similarity of these signs has resulted in the loss of human life.

The allusion of E. T. W. to the use of the old system in the "rural districts" of France reminds us that in the "rural districts" of New England potatoes are still sold at *four and sixpence* a bushel, cloth at *two and threepence* a yard, and laborers are paid at *nine shillings* per day, instead of 75 cents, 37½ cents, and $1.50. It is needless to state that this argument is almost *too rural*.

The old Fahrenheit thermometer, with its unmeaning standards of 32° and 212°, ought also to be numbered with the things of the past, and give place to the Centigrade or decimal thermometer, based upon a standard of common sense.   SAMUEL W. ABBOTT.

WAKEFIELD, *November* 1, 1875.

Another correspondent suggests that the new system could best be made familiar to the profession by a new edition of the Dispensatory, with the weights given according to the metric system with their equivalents in the present system in brackets. We fear that such a publication can hardly be expected before July 4th.   EDS.

WEEKLY BULLETIN OF PREVALENT DISEASES.

THE following is a bulletin of the diseases prevalent in Massachusetts during the week ending October 30, 1875, compiled under the authority of the State Board of Health from the returns of physicians representing all sections of the State: —

The summary for each section is as follows: —

Berkshire: Bronchitis, influenza, typhoid fever.

Valley: Typhoid fever, influenza, rheumatism, bronchitis. ·South Hadley reports measles and diphtheria.

Midland: Typhoid fever, influenza, bronchitis.

Northeastern Typhoid fever, influenza, bronchitis. Lynn reports diphtheria and German measles; Lexington reports measles "mild and abundant;" Gloucester returns diphtheria " on the increase and severe."

Metropolitan: Typhoid fever, bronchitis, diphtheria (mild), scarlatina (mild). The two latter have increased considerably.

Southeastern: Influenza, typhoid fever. Very little sickness. A few towns report diphtheria.

In the State at large there was a subsidence of all diseases except diphtheria. The order of relative prevalence is as follows: typhoid fever, influenza, bronchitis, rheumatism, diphtheria, scarlatina, pneumonia, diarrhœa, measles, croup, dysentery, whooping-cough ; the last seven are low in the scale.

F. W. DRAPER, M. D., Registrar.

COMPARATIVE MORTALITY-RATES FOR THE WEEK ENDING OCT. 23, 1875.

	Estimated Population.	Total Mortality for the Week.	Annual Death-Rate per 1000 during Week.
New York	1,060,000	457	21.5
Philadelphia	800,000	315	20.5
Brooklyn	500,000	205	21.3
Chicago	400,000		
Boston	342,000	154	23.4
Cincinnati	260,000		
Providence	100,700	35	18.1
Worcester	50,000	15	15.6
Lowell	50,000	16	16.6
Cambridge	48,000	16	17.3
Fall River	45,000	12	13.9
Lawrence	35,000	11	16.3
Lynn	33,000	14	22.1
Springfield	31,000	4	6.7
Salem	26,000	8	16.0

Normal Death-Rate, 17 per 1000.

THE BOSTON
MEDICAL AND SURGICAL JOURNAL.

VOL. XCIII. — THURSDAY, NOVEMBER 11, 1875. — NO. 20.

CASES OF DIPHTHERIA.[1]

BY E. N. WHITTIER, M. D. (HARV.)

B COURT projects in a southerly direction, on the line of twenty feet above mean low tide, from C Street into the rear of estates and tenement houses on D Place and E Street. The house in which the outbreak which forms the subject of this paper took place is the last in the court, and is an old-fashioned, poorly ventilated, two story wooden structure, having in its rear two vaults belonging to estates on E Street. Within a few feet of and below the level of the sitting-room window is the open ventilator of a large privy, very offensive at times. Across the end of the house a narrow passage-way separates it from the rear of tenement-house yards, cess-pools, and vaults on D Place. In the court and immediately in front of the house in question the sewage from the large block of houses in the court, and from those on the southerly side of C Street unites, and flows into an old-fashioned plank drain, which, undermined by rats and rotten from age, passes almost directly under the corner of the house in its course to the main drain on E Street. A few days before the first case of diphtheria in this series was brought to my notice this drain had been opened because of an obstruction in it, and remained imperfectly closed for four or five days, immediately under the windows. The children played in and about the place, attracted by the workmen and by the novelty of the proceedings.

The family sitting-room seemed to have been an after-thought on the part of some owner of the property; it had no cellar under it, and the kitchen sink-spout discharged part of its contents into the earth under the floor; the remaining portion of the sink-washings flowed across the cellar bottom towards the sewer.

A hollow plug, partly destroyed by rats, permitted the free ingress of sewage, and several times earlier in the season the tide had backed the contents of the sewer up into the cellar, once to a depth of nearly eighteen inches, and had left the cellar bottom saturated; the leaking sink-drain had maintained the point of saturation thus obtained.

In the cellar was a layer of rotten plank covered by new plank; the

---

[1] Read before the Boston Society for Medical Observation, October 4, 1875.

cellar bottom in part was little better than dock mud. In one corner of this cellar was the family water-closet, not particularly offensive, but still an important factor in the result we have to consider. In the autumn of 1874, at the time when the infant (Case IV.) was born, there were six cases of scarlet fever at the same time in this house, with two deaths. I understood the cause of death to be scarlatinal diphtherite.

CASE I. A boy, five years and six months old, in the afternoon of July 24th was seized with vomiting, and complained of feeling cold ; during the evening he grew feverish ; he vomited several times before morning; he complained of headache and pain in the back. During the 25th he was very listless, slept a great deal, ate but little, and towards evening was more feverish, complaining of pain as before ; he became very restless and somewhat delirious during the night, and in the forenoon of the 26th, the mother, thinking his neck was swollen, sent for me. I saw him early in the afternoon.

He was very pale ; pulse 126, feeble ; respiration 24 ; temperature in the mouth 102.4°. The glands of the neck on either side were enlarged and tender ; the breath was extremely offensive. The tongue had a thick yellowish coat. A grayish-white exudation was seen involving the tonsils on either side, covering the right side of the uvula, extending up in an arch on the hard palate from the left tonsil, and in patches scattered over the posterior wall of the pharynx. But little of the surface in view was unaffected. The tonsils were not very much enlarged. The boy complained but little of pain. Deglutition was not much impaired ; occasionally some drink was thrown out of the nostrils. Up to this moment so slight had been the throat symptoms that the parents, intelligent people, had thought the swollen glands alone were at fault. The nostrils, reddened about their margins, were the seat of a thin muco-purulent discharge.

The whole affected surface was attacked with nitrate of silver, the tonsils, particularly the right one, breaking down in every direction, a gangrenous mass. As much of the exudation as could be removed showed the apparent enlargement of the tonsils to be in great part due to successive diphtheritic layers superimposed and mixed with pus and blood. Fomentations were applied. Two grains of quinine were given every two hours; brandy, beef-tea, broken ice, and iced coffee were also administered. The patient was put to bed and strict seclusion enjoined. The throat was washed out every two hours with a mixture of potassium chlorate and honey.

During the night and the following day the patient was less troublesome ; he took large quantities of nourishment. At night the pulse was 116. The tongue was more coated, the whole aspect less favorable. Examination showed new points of exudation, the pharynx being nearly covered. Another application of nitrate of silver was made ; otherwise no change was made in the treatment.

In the morning of the third day (28th), while his throat was being swabbed, the patient vomited shreds of membrane which left the surface of the tonsils nearly clean ; the probang removed nearly all the exudation from the soft palate, the palatine arches, and a large portion from the walls of the pharynx. The previous night had been most distressing; delirium was present, and there were one or two involuntary discharges. Pulse at midnight 140. The extremities were cold and damp. At the time of the evening visit the lad was much improved, but the mother told me that the next younger child, a girl of four, had been vomiting and seemed very weak ; that she had eaten nothing, and was in bed nearly all the afternoon.

Extreme pallor was most marked in the appearance of this second case. The pulse was 112. The patient complained of pain in her head and ears, and in back of her neck. There was no difficulty in swallowing. The voice was a little husky. The surface of the tonsils, the arches of the palate, and the uvula and greater part of the wall of the pharynx were deeply injected. The surfaces of the tonsils particularly were studded with minute, semi-opaque points, separate and in groups, pellicular in appearance. The child was at once set to eating broken ice ; stimulants were ordered, with quinine, and occasional strong coffee iced. The morning of the 29th showed a firm white exudation over the right tonsil, with detached points of exudation on the pharyngeal surface and on the right side of the uvula. Before night similar appearances had developed upon the left tonsil. The same course of local treatment was pursued here as in the first case.

Evening visit on the 29th brought to my care Case III., that of a feeble child of little more than two years. There was occasional vomiting from the earlier part of the day, with loss of appetite and slight fever. No particular glandular enlargement was observed, but there was a distinct deposit on the right tonsil, and scattered opaque points on the palate and pharynx. The same course of treatment was adopted, save the ice ; that the child would not touch. This night was a very trying one : No. 2 was in a most pitiable stupor ; No. 1 was raving and tossing, and towards morning vomiting occasionally ; No. 3 resented all attempts to afford relief.

The morning of the 30th dawned yet more darkly. Case IV., that of an anæmic, teething baby, nine months old, developed; this child had been vomiting and very fretful during the latter part of the night, and the right tonsil was the seat of an exudation crowning its projecting summit; the remaining portion of the palatine surface was deeply injected and studded with opaque points. The same course as with the other children was adopted. This morning Nos. 1 and 2, so far as local evidences of diphtheria were concerned, were much improved; there were only minute points of new deposit. Their throats were easily kept clean by means of a sponge and mixture of potassium chlorate and honey; No. 3 was unchanged; No. 4 received an application of nitrate of silver.

In the morning of the 31st, it was reported that No. 1 had been vomiting during the night; there had been frequent epistaxis, and loose, very dark discharges. General œdema was present. There was some cough. A few purpuric spots were seen on the body. By evening, blood changed by the fluids of the stomach made up the greater part of the matters vomited. With but little variation other than their increase these symptoms continued until the 3d of August, when the child died, without affording any indications of local extension of the disease, but rather of systemic infection. No autopsy was obtained.

The remaining children made good recovery, all the indications of the primary diphtheritic lesion disappeared, convalescence was well established, and out-door exercise was permitted; but on August 13th, ten days after the death of No. 1, No. 4 was seized with capillary bronchitis. On the 14th cough became more tracheal and intense; symptoms of laryngeal obstruction grew rapidly more marked. Emetics, steam, hot applications, afforded no relief, and at noon of the 15th, the child's respiration being 50, the pulse 146, the extremities cold, and the lividity extreme, tracheotomy was done by Dr. Porter because of the impending suffocation. The parents of this child were not offered much hope of a favorable result from tracheotomy, but they were told that at least there should be substituted for a painful, a painless death.

Great difficulty was met with in the introduction of the tube; at last only the inside canula of the smallest tube could be inserted, the trachea was so narrowed by inflammatory products. Looking upwards into the larynx one could see the free ends of a densely formed membrane, cone-like, " which," says Bretonneau, " attached by its base and having its tracheal points free, becomes a valve the horrible mechanism of which is perfectly completed. At the period of inspiration the valve elongates and extends itself, unfolding and allowing the air to pass when deeply and strongly inspired; while at the moment of expiration, the free extremity of the valve, being pushed back, opposes an insurmountàble obstacle to the passage of air outwards; thus retained, the air is imprisoned without giving place to fresh air, and hence sudden asphyxia is caused." With this child the tube anticipated this result; the pulse improved, lividity gave place to color, and respiration returned to nearly the normal rate. The patient partook freely of nourishment and stimuli with iron, and by night was sitting up in her crib; she passed the next day and succeeding night with the utmost comfort, annoyed only by cough, which had begun to increase in frequency and force ; at last she refused nourishment, sank rapidly, and died without a struggle near the close of the second day after the operation, yielding to the broncho-pneumonia which some of the earlier observers (Guersant, Daviot, and Trousseau) strongly insist is the most frequent and dangerons complication of convalescence, sometimes developing tracheal diphthérite as secondary to the catarrhal process affecting the air-passages.

The disturbance is as yet too recent to enable me to say that these children have escaped the sequelæ of the various forms of paralysis. No. 2 had limited paralysis of the muscles of one side of the neck, No. 3 of the palatal muscles, and now is under treatment for convergent strabismus.

Etiology. This has been one of the most obscure parts of the study of diphtheria. Broadly stated the disease is governed by the same law that rules the zymotics. Though not highly contagious, " and in the scale of infectiousness far below scarlet fever, it is still communicable from the sick to the healthy, and it appears highly probable that it may be originated *de novo* by filthy emanations from sewage and cess-pools." The literature of the subject, particularly that in the English language, is teeming with reports of cases in which those combinations of conditions which are called local and atmospheric, and which are required to develop the disease, are assigned the greatest prominence. It is classed by highest authority among the filth-diseases. Sanderson [1] says, " It is not possible to avoid the conclusion that it is due to local causes, and would have been prevented in particular instances if the nuisances had been abated." At the last meeting of the British Medical Association, Dr. Ross said that not density, but dirt, had to be guarded against, and defects of construction, particularly the defects arising from bad foundations. Dr. Johnson [2] says, "Diphtheria in all its forms and varieties is as certainly as typhoid a disease of filth origin." I think, therefore, that we may accept as demonstrated that in very large numbers of cases the relation between diphtheria and unsanitary conditions obtains as much force as that between typhoid and its similar unsanitary conditions.

Contagion. König says that diphtheria almost always spreads by contagion, and he cites a case of the disease arising from use of a knife which had been employed, I think, for tracheotomy. Bahrdt records that diphtheria of a wound of the hand gave rise to tracheal diphtheria on the second day. It is very easy to find abundance of proof of its contagious nature in cases where all other appreciable causes or means of transmitting the disease are absent. Trousseau's auto-inoculation, and its negative results, upon which so much stress has been

[1] British Medical Journal, 1873.
[2] British Medical Journal, September 18, 1875.

placed by non-contagionists, have but little weight to counterbalance the multitude of fatal cases similar to those of Valleix, colleague of Trousseau, of Adams in 1864, and more lately those of Lady Amberly and her child, which last year were the subject of so much excitement in England, and called forth this statement from one of the best English authorities : [1] " This is the point. Diphtheria is a communicable disease, like scarlatina. Its spread may be at times wholly accounted for by its infectious or contagious properties, but in any case the proclivity to the disease may be enormously increased by defective drainage or other sources of air-contamination." Oertel defines it as a miasmatic, contagious disease.

The same writer, supported by a multitude of observers, boldly declares that without spheroida bacteria there can be no diphtheria, demonstrates their presence in the most superficial patches, and follows them into the canaliculi of bone denuded by the diptheritic process, detects them in immense masses as emboli and the cause of metastatic abscesses, and asserts that the intensity of toxic influences increases with the number of these organisms. One of the last meetings of the Pathological Society of London was wholly taken up with the consideration of the germ theory of disease. Dr. Bastian's address was a most candid review at great length of the present state of knowledge on this point. The discussion which followed, participated in by most prominent men, is compared by the English journals to the fruitless theoretical discussions of the French Academy, and the verdict rendered, more familiar to English than to American ears, concerning this whole subject is, " not proven."

When Home, in 1765, seized upon the Scotch word croup, which had been used to designate a group of diseases attended with noisy breathing, and engrafted it upon the medical literature of his day, he could have had no conception of the hot contest which at the present day is waged to establish both the identity and the dissimilarity of croup and diphtheria. This war of words has been by no means barren of results ; since the contributions to the literature of diphtheria have been so complete that as an outgrowth we have the question, not what is diphtheria, but what is croup? Competent observers declare that a careful analysis of Home's cases of croup is conclusive that he had under observation laryngeal or tracheal diphtherite. Johnson says that we must discard the word croup, or, as a compromise, I suppose because it cannot be safely let loose alone, it must be associated with a distinct prefix : spasmodic croup, the neurosis ; inflammatory croup, catarrhal laryngitis, rarely fatal, excited by exposure to cold, non-contagious, never associated with the formation of a coherent false membrane ; diphtheritic croup, laryngeal diphtheria, membranous croup, a specific

[1] Lancet, July, 1874.

contagious disease often occurring as a complication of measles or scarlet fever.

Treatment. I cannot venture to vex your patience with even the briefest allusion .to many of the various forms of treatment now in vogue. Of course, the division is made into local and general. Local measures range from nothing, or next to nothing, to extirpation of affected tonsils. The oldest advocates of the active use of nitrate of silver (lapis infernalis) are still to be found among its firmest friends ; but or late there have been great accessions to the ranks of believers in the virtues of the stronger astringents, and I find the testimony almost universal that the pernitrate, persulphate, and perchloride of iron are of the greatest value as local applications. Cleanliness, by means of washes, gargles, and disinfectants, is of next importance. Rest in bed, careful attention to ventilation, and, as early as can be, removal from the vicinity of the origin or cause of the disease, are very necessary measures.

General treatment embraces all the measures known to aid the patient to withstand the encroachment of the disease and to sustain the vital powers. Quinine and iron in doses strangely large are given, apparently absorbed, and with most satisfactory and beneficial results. Alcoholic stimulants should be resorted to with great boldness.

All therapeutic measures should have reference equally to the time being and to the probable course of the disease and the strength of the patient, and these measures must be persistently prolonged, for the period of convalescence ordinarily assigned has not yet been found free from the dangers of relapse ; not even when once the surfaces in easy view have been cleared of the deposit, can we with great confidence assert that this or that near day, when reached, will place the patient out of danger, since too often when the progress of the disease has been most encouraging, death may suddenly threaten from impeded access of air. Progressive recession of the thoracic walls may show that the cause of the obstruction to the entrance of air is increasing, and should admonish the physician that the moment of greatest promise for the successful performance of tracheotomy, this most important resource, will soon pass by. " I do not stand alone," says Trousseau, " in preaching that there is an imperative duty imposed on the practitioner of performing tracheotomy, a duty as obligatory as tying the carotid when that vessel has been wounded, and though death quite as often as recovery follows the operation." Mr. Spence, in his recent address on surgery before the British Medical Association, says repeated failures to save life by this operation must not discourage the practitioner ; perseverance is certain of success ; the operation should be resorted to early, before the strength of the patient shall' have been undermined in the fruitless struggle for air. Mr. Buchanan, of Glasgow, in his address on tracheotomy in croup and diphtheria, is more conservative in his views, and says, "When medical treatment is proving of no avail, and death from suffocation, not from exhaustion, is imminent, it is the duty of the practitioner to perform tracheotomy." I choose rather the position taken by Millard, that the indication for tracheotomy is the predominance of the symptoms of asphyxia over all the patient's other symptoms; "I would follow the indication which is most urgent, and would make the dying child breathe, thus acting notwithstanding the apparent hopelessness of the case, because there is no absolute certainty of its hopeless nature." Barclay [1] says that it does not materially increase the risk of fatal issue.

Had Bretonneau, dismayed by his disappointments in 1818 and 1820, refused to make the third attempt in 1825, the first well-authenticated successful case would have been much longer postponed, Trousseau could hardly have followed the example of his master, and the force of his first series of two hundred cases, in assuring the success of this operation, would have been lost. The gain in the percentages of success during these fifty years has been such as most effectually to silence opposition. Trousseau in his first series attained twenty-five per cent; in 1854, a little more than seventy-seven per cent. Without very great exertion, I have succeeded in finding the records of sixteen hundred and thirty-six cases, with an average of success of thirty-three and one eighth per cent.

NOTE. Since the above paper was presented, diphtheria has again broken out in the same court. Case V., that of a lad eleven years of age, made a good recovery after nine days' illness. Case VI., that of a gentleman forty-one years of age, died after an illness of four days.

A CASE OF MENIÈRE'S DISEASE.

BY JAMES J. PUTNAM, M. D.

WELL-MARKED cases of auditory vertigo, of the severer, typical forms, not being very common, I have thought it worth while to report the following, although it cannot be said to throw any new light upon the pathology of the disease. The case was observed recently in the out-patient department of the Massachusetts General Hospital.

The patient is a day-laborer, of Irish descent, about twenty-five years old, and, in all respects except that now in question, apparently in perfect health. For the past twelve years he has been subject to a feeling of dizziness, of varying intensity, accompanied with noises in the left ear,

[1] Holmes's System of Surgery, iv. 513.

sometimes also in the right, which he likens to the sound of a storm, with wind and rain. The patient thinks that he can mark the very day and moment when these symptoms first attracted his attention, since he remembers that he was leaning over his kitchen fire at the time, and that the skin of the face itched severely, inducing him to rub it, an incident to which he seems inclined to impute a causal connection with his trouble. From that date the sense of giddiness has been almost constantly present, though it is only recently that it has actually incapacitated him for work. It is increased by stooping forward, and he then also complains, at times, of a feeling of pain in the right side of the forehead. Besides this moderate, persistent giddiness, which of itself frequently causes him to walk with an uncertain gait, he has had, from time to time, special exacerbations of the same sensation, of two or three minutes' duration (according to his own account), attacking him without warning, sometimes while he was at his work, sometimes even while he was sitting in a chair or lying in bed. At such times he loses his balance, staggers, if standing, and, if he cannot find means of supporting himself, falls to the ground, as he has actually done some nine or ten times in all. It is impossible to learn with accuracy, as the patient is uneducated and stupid, whether or not the severer attacks of vertigo are attended with loss of consciousness, but so far as he knows he has never been convulsed at such times, and with the lighter attacks loss of consciousness does not seem to have occurred. He reports that when the vertigo is severe, outside objects seem to whirl around ; but in describing the direction and character of their apparent motion with his hand he made it revolve at one time from left to right, at another from right to left. The direction in which he falls also appears to be variable ; once it happened in such a manner that his nose struck directly upon the ground, and once he fell backwards from a chair on which he was sitting astride.

When I have seen the patient sitting at rest in a chair, his head has generally been turned somewhat to the right and downward, and has frequently been seen to oscillate with a fine motion, a fact to which he himself called my attention, though not until I had already noticed it. From time to time the head, or the whole body, gives a sudden jerk, as if the patient had been startled, a symptom which Charcot also has observed. His face wears an expression of distress, and he occasionally draws a long, sighing inspiration.

Besides the more or less constant vertigo, he suffers frequently, especially in the morning, from nausea, from which he sometimes seeks relief by inducing vomiting ; and in connection with the severer attacks there is often spontaneous vomiting of a greenish or yellowish fluid.

Some time after the original onset of his trouble, the patient noticed that the left ear had become somewhat deaf ; at the present time he can hear the ticking of a watch with that ear at a distance of one half an inch only, while with the other it is heard at two feet. He thinks, nevertheless, that the hearing has been better lately than it was some time ago, which is interesting in connection with the statement of Charcot that the vertigo sometimes diminishes as the hearing becomes more impaired. The reverse of both conditions apparently obtains here.

Dr. H. L. Shaw, who kindly examined the patient for me at the Massachusetts Eye and Ear Infirmary, reported signs of chronic catarrhal inflammation of the middle ear, with calcareous deposits on the membrana tympani, and other old changes in the neighborhood.

It is well known that a variety of lesions of the auditory apparatus, whether produced experimentally or due to disease, may give rise to vertigo, often of definite and peculiar types,[1] and that clinically this occurs in connection with affections of the middle ear as well as with those of the labyrinth; though in the former case probably through a secondary affection of the labyrinthine organs. The results of the gross lesions produced by disease are, however, as a rule too complicated to throw much light upon the nice physiological problems involved in the matter. Investigations as to the relative ease with which vertigo and the tendency to incline the head to one side could be excited by the application of galvanism respectively to the left and to the right mastoid process gave only negative results, partly on account of the inability of the patient to observe his symptoms with accuracy.

RECENT PROGRESS IN OPHTHALMOLOGY.[2]

BY O. F. WADSWORTH, M. D.

Conium in Disease of the Eye. — Curtis [3] has published a very interesting paper on the action of conium and especially its influence in blepharospasm. Its notorious character for irregularity of action is to be referred to want of care or skill in gathering the plant, or to faulty methods of preparation. Like many other drugs which cause paralysis, conium has a predilection for certain nerves, and the nerves earliest and most affected by it are those which supply the muscular apparatus of the eye. The symptoms of progressive muscular paralysis which it produces begin in the ocular muscles. One great point in its favor is that it produces no disagreeable after-effects.

Not the least interesting, if not the most instructive, part of the paper

------

[1] For an excellent description of Menière's disease, with references to the literature of the subject, see the London Medical Record for April 22 and 29, 1874, and May, 1875.

[2] Concluded from page 530.

[3] New York Medical Record, 1875, pages 353 and 369.

is the ingenious comparison drawn between the giddiness and nausea produced by conium and that of seasickness. On shipboard the spot toward which the eye or foot is directed changes its position while the movement of eye or foot is being made, and when the movement is completed the desired goal has not been reached. When one is under the influence of conium, surrounding objects are indeed stationary, but the muscular innervation judged necessary to make a' given movement proves insufficient to accomplish it on account of the partially paralyzed condition of the muscles, and the effect upon the sensorium is the same as if the object toward which the movement was made had changed its place. In either case there is giddiness and consequent nausea.

The blepharospasm which accompanies many affections of the conjunctiva and cornea, and sometimes of the iris, aggravates the original trouble and is often exceedingly obstinate. That not simply the orbicularis, but also the third nerve, is implicated is shown by the contracted condition of the pupil, its resistance to the action of atropine, and the rolling up of the eye when the lid is forcibly raised. Probably, Curtis thinks, all the ocular muscles may be involved. In such an affection, conium, having a special influence on the muscles of the eye, is particularly indicated.

An account of the case of a man of twenty-three years, with iritis, diffuse inflammation of the central part of the cornea, and great blepharospasm, is given in detail. For five days, treatment with atropine, warm applications, and rest in a dark room was of no avail. Then forty minims of Squibb's fluid extract of conium brought relief in half an hour ; and for the first time in twelve days the patient could open his eyes. This effect lasted four hours. The next day thirty minims gave relief for two hours, and a second dose of thirty minims was even more successful. Three hours after the last dose, and after all general symptoms due to the drug had passed off, the man walked boldly with open eyes to the full light of a window. Now first did the iris begin to dilate. Three days longer he did well with one dose daily ; then the drug was omitted and pain and spasm recurred, but yielded again as soon as hemlock was readministered. A month later an operation to break a posterior synechia brought back the former symptoms. Again atropine, etc., failed to relieve, but conium was as promptly efficacious as before. In another case, Curtis found that conium did not produce the desired result. Two cases are referred to, however, treated by others at his suggestion, in which the drug acted promptly.

Disinfecting Treatment of Corneal Ulcers. — The affection known as hypopion-keratitis, ulcus corneæ serpens, etc., is now very generally considered as an infected traumatic keratitis.

Dilute chlorine water and solutions of quinine or of carbolic acid have been employed as disinfectants, dropped into the conjunctival sack, but without pronounced effect. Horner [1] has instituted a more energetic treatment with, as it appears to him, very encouraging results. He applied diluted chlorine water with a camel's-hair pencil directly to the ulcer. Though this treatment was employed in only a limited number of cases (fifteen), yet, having had a large experience with other methods, the author was surprised at the rapidity with which the progression of infiltration ceased, and the hypopion was absorbed, as well as at the favorable condition of the eventual cicatrix. In cases where the ulcer is already very extensive, however, this means is insufficient, and Saemisch's slitting through the whole ulcerated portion is necessary.

Choroiditis and its Influence on Vision. — Bergmeister [2] made use of the extensive material in Arlt's clinic to obtain some definite ideas as to the relation between the different ophthalmoscopic appearances seen in choroiditis and the amount and character of the disturbance of vision. He reviews the various anatomico-pathological changes which have been described in choroiditis, and is obliged to admit that different as these changes may be, the variations in the ophthalmoscopic picture depend far less on the diversity of the anatomical processes than on the resulting condition of the pigment of the epithelial layer and of the choroidal stroma. It even appears to him doubtful if an exudation in the stroma of the choroid can ever be diagnosed as such by the ophthalmoscope.

He divides the pathological changes into two classes, those which may run their course, at least to a certain degree, without implication of the retinal elements, and such as, starting in the choroid, directly endanger the integrity of the retina. To the latter class, so far as the objective appearances are concerned, must be added certain affections which are confined to the retina and epithelial layer.

Clinically he makes four divisions. The first comprises the ordinary atrophic forms characterized by changes in the amount of pigment, without visible exudation. These may be unattended with disturbance of vision so long as the visible changes are confined to a zone situated between the equator and the posterior pole of the eye. The prognosis depends mainly on the tendency of the disease to advance in one or another direction. If the progression be to the neighborhood of the papilla, vision will be affected either by interference with the circulation in the nerve, which may lead to atrophic degeneration, or by the formation of opacities in the posterior part of the vitreous. If the disease extend forward beyond the equator, then loss of vision will accompany opacity of the anterior portions of the vitreous.

A second division consists of the cases in which defined circumscribed

---

[1] Monatsblätter für Augenheilkunde, xii. 432.

[2] Archiv für Ophthalmologie, xx. 2.

exudations on the surface of the choroid may be seen with the ophthalmoscope. These cause local interferences with vision which manifest themselves as scotomata and are accompanied by photopsia, chromopsia, and metamorphopsia. The amount of visual impairment here depends chiefly on the situation of the exudations, and is most marked when they appear in the region of the macula lutea.

A more rare but very grave form of choroiditis is characterized by the formation of extensive white exudation at the posterior pole of the eye, about the disk, and especially at the macula. This is attended by diffuse infiltration of the outer layers of the retina and more or less implication of the whole uveal tract. Often it is due to syphilitic taint. It may follow long-existing, disseminated choroiditis, or may occur as an acute inflammation. With it, vision is most severely affected ; the optic nerve may undergo atrophic degeneration ; the exudation is with difficulty absorbed, if at all, and a central scotoma may persist.

Finally there is pigmentation of the retina in connection with progressive choroidal atrophy, which, advancing from the equatorial zone toward the posterior pole, causes narrowing of the field of vision and, generally, hemeralopia ; while, even when the opticus early assumes the appearance of atrophy, central vision may long remain intact.

New Method of Operating for Cataract. — While the introduction of Graefe's operation has caused much greater security as to immediate bad result than the flap method, there has been at the same time a little loss in the excellence of the optical result, owing to the necessity of removing a portion of the iris. On the other hand, the attempt to make a linear section in the cornea diminishes the chance of rapid healing, and leads in many cases to prolapse of the iris or anterior synechiæ. Led by these considerations, De Wecker[1] has devised an operation which he thinks fulfills the following desiderata : (1.) The section should be placed in the best conditions for coaptation and cicatrization ; it should be at the junction of the cornea and sclera. (2.) The wound should allow easy and complete exit of the lens, without the need of enlarging the pupil. (3.) Attachment and prolapse of the iris should be avoided as much as possible. (4.) The price of a considerable number of failures, as in the flap operation, should not be paid for the sake of securing certain advantages.

The section, made by a knife half the width of the old cataract knife, divides the upper third of the cornea at its junction with the sclera, without forming a conjunctival flap. After allowing the lids to close, and covering them with a cold sponge for a moment, the capsule is divided in the usual manner. The lens is forced out by gentle pressure from below through the lower lid, while at the same time the upper periphery of the iris is pushed backward by a thin hard-rubber spatula, in such a

[1] Annales d'Oculistique, lxxiii. 264

way as to free it from the lens. Fragments of cortical which may be left are removed by gentle rubbing from below upward through the lower lid. During this manœuvre no heed need be taken of prolapse of the iris, but when the pupil is clear the iris is pushed back into place by the rubber spatula. Then two or three drops of a one-half per cent. solution of neutral sulphate of eserine are instilled, and after waiting five minutes till the myotic has acted and there is no tendency to prolapse of the iris, the compressive bandage is applied. It is well to look at the eye one or two hours after the operation, and re-instill the eserine if myosis is not marked. The myosis thus produced endures some twenty-four hours, long enough for the wound to close, and afterward recourse may be had to atropine, if necessary, without fear of prolapse.

Wecker does not state how often he has done this operation. If its results are better than those he has given for 1873 and 1874 by a method a little modified from Graefe's (429 cases of simple senile cataract: 1.7 per cent., total loss; 13 per cent., $V = \frac{20}{20}$; 28.5 per cent. more, $V = \frac{2}{3}$), it must be very nearly perfect.

Congenital Fistula of the Lachrymal Duct. — Steinheim[1] observed this unique anomaly in a girl fourteen years of age. On the outer third of the right upper lid, four or five lines from the edge, a little funnel-shaped opening, lined with hairs resembling the eyelashes, ran upward under the skin. From this opening tears continually trickled, and fell in large drops over the cheek. The inner opening was so hidden under the skin that even after removal of the hairs it could not be seen, but a fine sound could be passed in two or three lines. Compression of the opening by forceps, one arm of which was passed under the lid, showed that the duct ran upward and outward. This condition had, according to the father, existed from birth. No other abnormity of the lid or of the lachrymal gland could be discovered. The fluid was clear, without mucus, and had a salty taste. Unfortunately, a portion which was collected for chemical analysis was lost, and the girl was not again seen.

PROCEEDINGS OF THE OBSTETRICAL SOCIETY OF BOSTON.

JUNE 12, 1875. The president, DR. HODGDON, in the chair.

Hypospadias. — DR. HOSMER reported the case. In the last week in May he was called to a primipara. The child was born with the cord tight about its neck. The genitals appeared to be those of a female with the external labia a good deal swollen. The next day after the child's birth, Dr. Hosmer found it to be a case of hypospadias. The penis was very short, and almost en-

[1] Monatsblatter für Augenheilkunde, xiii. 303.

tirely concealed between the large folds of the scrotum. Where the skin of the abdomen turned upon the penis there was a fold like the edge of a prepuce. The common integument continued almost to the apex of the glans. At the end of the penis there was a slight depression but no channel. Raising the penis there was seen a funnel-shaped cavity bounded by the penis and sides of the scrotum; this became narrower and narrower and was lost in the urethra. The superior wall of the urethra did not run out upon the penis.

Dr. CHADWICK referred to the case of a patient seventeen or eighteen years of age whom he had seen in hospital. In this case the urethra ran out upon the penis and acted as a frænum, causing especial pain during erection, the penis remaining much curved.

Dr. INGALLS, speaking of the treatment, mentioned a case reported in a medical journal in which the surgeon took the stylet from an elastic catheter and forced it into the tract of the urethra, where there was a semblance of a canal.

Dr. HOMANS said the trouble is that the portion abnormally open cannot be closed, and therein lies the chief objection to operative interference, an objection rarely overcome. In one case, that of a child three years old, there was an opening at the bottom of the glans. The child had phymosis, an operation to relieve which disclosed the other defect. No attempt was made to remedy this, but there was no trouble from it. The testicles and scrotum were normal. In answer to a question Dr. Homans said he thought hypospadias was very rare.

Dr. SINCLAIR said he had seen four or five cases, in most of which the opening was at the base of the glans, the most common site. The majority of these patients were subjects of gonorrhœa.

Dr. HOSMER mentioned a case which he saw a few years ago, of a healthy male child in which the orifice of the urethra was just in the line of the corona at the base of the glans.

Dr. HOMANS said he had recently seen a child weighing eleven pounds at birth, the brother of a child with hypospadias. Two or three days after the child's birth, he found at the lower extremity of the sacral region, just between the folds of the nates at the upper part, an opening which was discharging pus, and a little above it a red spot. With probe and knife a seton was introduced. There was no bunch of hair or other peculiar contents; it was merely an abscess which in the course of a month healed up. The labor was easy and natural.

Pulmonic Syringe. — Dr. CHADWICK stated that he was called, the night previous, to a woman with hæmorrhage from carcinoma uteri. He prepared an injection of solution of perchloride of iron and water in equal parts, but as the syringe did not work he unscrewed the top, extracted the piston, applied his mouth to the barrel, and blew with success. The syringe was a Vienna one, of rubber, light, with small nozzle capable of fitting into a catheter.

Acute Albuminuria of Pregnancy. — Dr. RICHARDSON reported the case of a primipara twenty-four years old, who had entered the Boston Lying-in Hospital three weeks previously, and two weeks before her confinement. At the time of her entrance the urine was found free from albumen, and otherwise perfectly normal. The labor began in the evening. At this time the patient passed her water, which was found to contain a slight amount of albumen. At four A. M. next day she could not micturate, and four or five ounces of urine were drawn by the catheter and found to contain a large amount of albumen, together with epithelial casts. At 7.30 the urine was very scanty, only about an ounce and a half. It was loaded with albumen and contained very numerous casts. The patient, who had previously shown a good disposition, now became ugly and cross. She was drowsy and restless, and complained of terrible headache. The catheter drew less than half an ounce of urine. At eleven A. M. the forceps were applied. At four P. M. six or seven ounces of urine were passed. This contained a large amount of albumen, but the casts were much diminished. The next morning, twenty-four hours after delivery, ten ounces of urine were obtained, which showed simply a trace of albumen. That afternoon the urine was wholly free from both albumen and casts. The patient had not had a bad symptom since, and was now making a good recovery. The specific gravity of the urine varied from 1018 to 1024. There was very slight œdema of the feet. When the forceps were applied the head had passed the superior strait and had entered the pelvis. The os was two thirds dilated, and was very soft and dilatable. The labor had been going on very gradually and slowly till about seven or eight A. M., and from that time the pains seemed to die away. The patient was etherized for the operation. The placenta was adherent at one spot over a surface as large as a silver half-dollar, and all around the site of adhesion were thin plates of calcareous degeneration.

Arm Presentation. — DR. TUCK reported the case of a German girl, nineteen years old, primipara, who entered the lying-in hospital two months since. Her report on entrance was that on a Friday night labor pains began, on Saturday night the waters escaped. The pains continuing, she went out on the following Monday morning to consult a physician, who sent her to the hospital. She went down in the horse-car, standing ; she was unable to sit down. On examination a whole arm was found external to the vulva. She was delivered by version, without ether, of a dead child. She was discharged well at the end of ten days.

Artificial Dilatation of the Cervix in the Obstinate Vomiting of Pregnancy. — DR. SINCLAIR referred to cases recently reported by Dr. Copeman. Dr. Copeman was called to a patient six months advanced in pregnancy. In endeavoring to break the membranes he failed after two or three efforts. He retired for an hour to consult, and in the mean time the vomiting had ceased. The patient did well without furthur interference. In another case, a pregnancy of two months, abortion was proposed, and the cervix was dilated with the same result. In another patient, eight months along, a like effect resulted from the same treatment. Graily Hewitt, in commenting upon the above cases, says that vomiting due to version or flexion of the uterus is removed by dilatation. He says he has accomplished the same thing by elevating the womb. Dr. Sinclair had had a case in Charlestown, of a woman who had been vomiting from the sixth week to the fourth month. She was put in the knee and elbow position with good effect.

DR. MINOT reported a case in which a sponge tent stopped the symptoms completely, much to the indignation of the woman, who had hoped to abort. In another case, seen with Dr. Clarke, Dr. Minot had applied tincture of iodine. Dr. Putnam, in consultation with Dr. Clarke, proposed removing the contents of the uterus, and a sponge tent was inserted for the purpose. The vomiting stopped. In a case seen with Dr. Buckingham, the dilatation had no effect whatever in stopping the vomiting, and the patient died.

DR. SINCLAIR said he imagined there was no great danger of producing abortion by the process of dilatation spoken of. In the cases reported there is no mention of subsequent examination to see whether the os closed again.

Difficult Labor. — DR. WELLINGTON reported the case. The day before the meeting, he had seen, in consultation with Dr. Norris, a woman aged thirty, in her fourth labor. The three previous labors had been protracted. The first was natural, but lasted three or four days. The second and third were terminated by instruments after two or three days' duration. On the present occasion the pains had been present from Wednesday morning till Friday night, when Dr. Wellington arrived. The waters had come away at about noon. The anterior part of the head rested on the pubes, the posterior fontanel was directly backwards. The pains were hard, pressing down a little the front of head and the posterior part. The patient seemed to be in fair condition. Dr. Wellington suggested giving the head a quarter turn. This was attempted but without success. The forceps were next got on, with difficulty, but with no effect. Turning was next proposed. The pelvis was small, and the sacral prominence considerable. Turning was performed without much difficulty. The body was small, but the head proved an obstacle. The face was in the hollow of the sacrum. The child was dead. Each attendant pulled till he was tired. Finally a towel was twisted about the neck and both operators pulled, the finger being retained in the child's mouth, and the head came. The difficulty of this case was the concurrence of the long diameter of the head with the short diameter of the pelvis. Dr. Wellington had had but one case before like this. He could not rotate the head to get it right in either case, and in both the head was above the brim of the pelvis.

DR. SINCLAIR reported a case of difficult labor which he had recently seen. Labor had continued twelve hours. The waters had come away. The forceps failed. The prominence of the sacrum was very marked indeed. The head had not entered the strait. By pushing up one part and pulling down another, Dr. Sinclair got hold of an extremity, but the head stuck. Firmer pressure over the pubes, however, aided in forcing the head through. The child was born apparently still, but breathed after half an hour.

DR. WELLINGTON said he was recently called to a woman, three months in the family way, who was flooding. The vagina was full of clots. The uterus was enlarged. The patient was faithfully plugged. The next morning, on removing the plug the os was found pretty well dilated, the ovum not extruded, and the patient was again plugged. The next morning the ovum was gone, and nothing was ever seen of it. The hæmorrhage ceased and the patient did well.

Rupture of Vagina. — DR. FRANCIS said he was called to see an Irish

40

woman who had been in labor two or three days under the care of a homœopath. An examination showed a transverse rent of the vagina, through which the child had passed wholly into the abdominal cavity. The hand in the uterus detected no rupture there, and found the afterbirth in its normal site. The child was extracted without the least difficulty, and a loop of intestine, apparently colon, followed. The woman had been in violent pain all night and all the next day until four P. M., when the pain suddenly ceased, about two hours before Dr. Francis saw her. The report was that she died two or three hours after delivery.

Hæmoptysis with Polypus Uteri. — DR. HODGDON gave the case of a stout lady, fifty years old, who had not menstruated for fourteen or fifteen months, and who was attacked with hæmoptysis. There were no physical signs of disease in the chest. Vaginal hæmorrhage occurred shortly afterwards, and a polypus half as large as the thumb was found projecting somewhat from the os uteri. The patient was plugged. After two or three days Dr. Hodgdon twisted off the polypus and the hæmorrhage ceased. There was no cough and no recurrence of hæmoptysis.

DR. SINCLAIR remarked that a considerable artery is sometimes found near the base of a small polypus, and instanced the case of a patient in whom the loss of blood was unusually large after the operation for removal.

Supernumerary Nipples. — DR. RICHARDSON described the case of a colored woman, forty years old, the mother of eleven children, a recent patient at the lying-in hospital. Her breasts were enormously large, and on the left were two distinct nipples, the lower nearer the median line than the upper, and separated by a strongly marked transverse furrow. When the breast was full, nursing from one nipple drained only a portion of the breast, and then the other nipple could be nursed. There was, as far as could be made out (the woman was very black), but one areola to the two nipples. The right breast was perfectly normal.

The Decomposition of Coagula. — DR. SINCLAIR asked how long clotted blood might remain in a cavity without undergoing decomposition. He said he had known such a condition to exist five weeks.

DR. MINOT mentioned a case in which the blood had remained essentially unchanged four or five weeks.

Mammary Abscess. — DR. TUCK inquired if acute disease were liable to occasion abscess of the breast in a nursing woman, and alluded to a recent case of severe pneumonia during which the milk, which had previously been abundant, disappeared without trouble.

DR. MINOT said he had a patient who omitted nursing three weeks after labor, in consequence of typhoid fever, and who was able to resume after the fever had disappeared.

Extensive Injury without Miscarriage. — DR. HOMANS reported the case of a pregnant woman a considerable portion of whose abdominal surface was scalded with boiling water. She was carried to the hospital and it was thought she would die. But she recovered and did not miscarry. Patients who are burned to the extent of a third or more of the abdominal surface generally die, whether pregnant or not. The present is an exceptional case.

Hæmatocele. — Dr. WELLINGTON gave a case of hæmatocele which occurred two years ago. There was a sudden discharge through the rectum of dark coagulated blood, with recovery.

Dr. MINOT said that the authorities, as for example Thomas and Barnes, are decidedly averse to puncturing.

Dr. WELLINGTON referred to a case in which he was consulted by Dr. Marcy, of Cambridge. The advice was 'to let it alone. The tumor disappeared by absorption in six months.

Dr. MINOT mentioned a case of Dr. Merrill's, in which a large opening was made. The cavity was syringed out with a solution of carbolic acid in water, thus avoiding the difficulty which would result from opening the cavity and admitting air upon a putrescible mass without the process of cleansing. In a large number of cases, Dr. Minot remarked, the tumor seems to be outside the peritoneum.

Hysterotomy for Fibroid Tumor. — Dr. CHADWICK said he wished to consult the society as to the propriety of performing hysterotomy in the case of a large fibroid tumor of the uterus, and gave the particulars of the case and statistics of the operation. Dr. Chadwick also reported two cases of uterine fibroid, complicated with pregnancy.

Dr. ABBOT gave the case of a woman aged thirty-five, who has had a very large tumor of the kind for ten or twelve years past, who used to flow tremendously at first, at times menstruating regularly, and who is very much better than she was ten years ago. Dr. Abbot mentioned also the case of a woman who had had a fibroid tumor of the size of an orange, attached to the base of the uterus, and who with this complication had had two or three labors.

Dr. WELLINGTON reported the case of a woman who ten years ago had a large fibroid tumor which filled up the abdomen considerably. Recently the tumor was found to have considerably diminished. The patient had not passed the climacteric period.

TRANSACTIONS OF THE PHILADELPHIA COLLEGE OF PHYSICIANS.[1]

THIS volume presents unusual attractions in the very full and interesting report on the autopsy of the bodies of the Siamese twins. The account of the examination is given by Harrison Allen, M. D., professor of comparative anatomy and zoölogy in the University of Pennsylvania. It is remarkably full and complete in consideration of the fact that the autopsy was not begun until two weeks after the death of the subjects, and that but limited incisions into the abdominal cavities and connecting band were permitted. The illustrations aré numerous and clear, and give a very satisfactory idea of the anatomical relations, the important features of which are already familiar to the readers of the JOURNAL. In regard to the cause of death of Chang, as the

[1] *Transactions of the College of Physicians of Philadelphia.* Third Series. Volume the First. 1875.

head could not be examined it remained uncertain whether there existed a cerebral clot. Eng died, it is supposed, in a state of syncope induced by fright, " a view which the over-distended bladder and the retraction of the right testicle would appear to corroborate." Dr. William H. Pancoast gives some remarks on the surgical considerations in regard to the propriety of an operation for the separation of the twins. Two colored plates accompany this paper, showing diagrammatic views of the uniting band. Other similar cases are referred to ; in only one, however, was an operation for severing the band successfully performed : this was done by Dr. Fatio in 1689.

A case of adenoid (Hodgkin's) disease is reported by Dr. Hutchinson, and is accompanied by a copious bibliography, although we suspect that the latter includes examples of more than one form of disease. The case is a valuable contribution, however, to a subject about which there still exists much confusion in the minds of many scientific men.

Dr. J. Ashhurst, Jr., contributes the first of a series of articles on the conservative surgery of the larger joints, on excision of the elbow-joint. We are somewhat surprised at the high rate of mortality, four out of the eight cases reported having died. In three out of the four in which recovery took place the normal motions of the part were restored.

Dr. Keen's experiments on the laryngeal nerves and muscles of respiration in the body of the criminal Heidenblut are given here, and also a report on the use of nitrite of amyl in various forms of spasm, and on its value as an aid to diagnosis, by S. Weir Mitchell, M. D. This drug was used successfully by Dr. W. S. Forbes in a case of acute tetanus, the account of which is given here.

Dr. J. Ewing Mears reports a case of encysted dropsy of the peritoneum in which suppuration had occurred and abdominal section was performed, with recovery. There are a number of other carefully prepared and valuable papers.

The Transactions are published in a style much superior to that customary in this country. The volume is an elegant one in its appearance, and its contents are certainly highly creditable to the college.

THE METRIC SYSTEM.

WE are much gratified by the attention that our statement of the claims of the metric system has attracted, and we hope that all our readers will give the subject serious thought, so that when the time comes to throw their influence one way or the other they may have decided opinions. If there is anything of importance to be said for or against it, that has not appeared in the JOURNAL, we beg that it be brought to our notice, as we think that a full discussion is very desirable, and while we believe that it will make more plain the merits of the system, we wish its disadvantages also to be fully exposed. After much reflection we believe that the only serious objection is the difficulty of familiarizing ourselves with the new system, and we admit that we do not know how great that may be. We are not sanguine enough to suppose that the passage of a law would cause the old system to be thrown aside like a suit of old clothes on the night of July 3d, and put a new one at our bedsides for the next morning; the change must of necessity be gradual, but a great deal may be done by the profession to hasten it. The rapidity with which the "new chemistry" is superseding the "old" illustrates how effective a lever is education. The "old" has been quietly discarded in the colleges, and the present students know nothing of it. So it is, though to a less extent, with the metric system; the preparatory and professional schools, by sending out young men thoroughly trained in it, can force us to adopt it in self-defense, and there form in time will spread through all classes. We are nothing less than revolutionary in our ideas, and we are quite free to admit a reluctance to throw away tools which, bad as they may be, have served us as they served our predecessors. We should be sorry to see our old friend, the mile, deposed from the place it holds in daily life in favor of the kilometre, though in legal and geographical documents it may be necessary. We have a lingering regard even for the ounce, though as we write we do not know precisely which one we mean, and this is surely a commentary on the clumsiness of our present systems, and is convincing evidence that we would not discard them from any caprice, but because they have been tried and found wanting.

MEDICAL NOTES.

— Dr. Robert Somerville, in an article in the *Edinburgh Medical Journal* of August, 1875, on the hydrostatics of the catheter, calls attention to the fact that in cases of retention of urine, particularly those in which the bladder is paralyzed, and the patient lies upon his back, the outer end of the instrument is at a higher level than that of the base of the bladder, and therefore this organ cannot without assistance, as by external pressure, expel all its contents. The hydrostatic pressure of the column of urine in the catheter is considerable, and to overcome this resistance by external pressure through the abdominal walls, and to keep the end of the catheter depressed, may require a force which cannot be used without injury to the bladder. He therefore recommends that the catheter should be converted into a siphon, either by making the outer extremity end in a curve, and attaching to it a flexible tube, so that the cathether shall form the short arm and the tube the long arm of the siphon, or by having a curved metal tube, to which the flexible tube is attached, slipped on to the end of an ordinary catheter. The advantages of this arrangement are (1) it is clean and convenient; (2) it completely empties the bladder; (3) it reduces the irritation of the mucous membrane of the bladder by the catheter to the minimum; (4) it avoids the temptation, when the urine has ceased to flow, to raise the patient into an erect or semi-erect position — a proceeding never devoid of danger with a metallic catheter in the bladder.

— We learn from the *Berliner klinische Wochenschrift* of October 4, 1875, that Professor Traube will soon return to Berlin and resume his various duties. It is suggested that the false reports concerning his condition which have appeared from time to time in political journals may have been inserted intentionally.

— At a recent session of the French Association for the Advancement of Science, M. Léon Tripier read a paper on the pathogeny of knock-knee, which is published in *La France Médicale* of September 29, 1875. It has been usual to consider this affection as having an habitual connection with rachitis, but M. Tripier has observed that very young patients affected with knock-knees do not show old or recent traces of rickets, and that both limbs are not always affected. In eight or nine tenths of the cases observed by him no traces of rickets were present, and more than half had only one knee affected. Moreover, where a double deformity was present there was always a difference in the amount of the deformity of the two limbs, a point which the writer considers of great importance.

The author's researches have shown that knock-knee appears particularly at the periods which correspond with those when the normal increase of the skeleton is most rapid. It is a law complementary to those laid down by M. Broca relating to the appearance and development of rachitic lesions, and by M. Ollier regarding the unequal development of the extremities of the long bones. From sections of the bones of a great number of subjects of different ages, and from measurements of the intermediate cartilage, that is, that between the shaft and the ends (increase of height), and of the diaphysis at the middle and the two extremities of the bones (increase in breadth), M. Tripier has found that knock-knee appears especially between three and five years of age, — sometimes a little earlier, — but most often between fourteen and seventeen, or at the time of the solidification of the skeleton, from twenty to twenty-five years for males and a little earlier for females. His researches having shown him that at these periods the increase of the intermediate cartilage at the inferior extremity of the femur is especially augmented, have led the author to ask whether this fact does not afford sufficient explanation of the appearance of so great a number of knock-knees unaccompanied by any old or recent symptoms of rickets. This being admitted, it remains to consider why, when both knees are affected, one is less so than the other.

The disease appears most frequently in bakers, cooks, locksmiths, and carpenters; in a word, in those whose work compels constant standing. In the erect posture we do not naturally incline equally on both feet; we bear our weight more upon one limb than upon the other. Thus the centre of gravity of the side which bears the weight passing with regard to the femoral line more to the outside than to the inside, and this pressure coming on one side at the time when the growth is taking place most rapidly, accounts for the inequality in the development of the lesion.

Experiments made upon young rabbits and kittens, bent pins being used to hold their bones in unnatural positions, confirmed the author in the views he had entertained regarding the disease in question. He attempted to make observations upon those employed in various factories where both sexes are compelled to work standing, but insuperable difficulties prevented any satisfactory investigations.

In conclusion, the author recommends for the malady a tonic treatment, and various mechanical contrivances for the correction of the deformity. He does not favor the disjunction of the epiphysis, a plan proposed and carried out by M. Delore. If he had a very rebellious case, he would prefer to make very fine subcutaneous punctures into the intermediate cartilage on its inner side, and then put the limb into an immovable apparatus. Thus he would hope to arrest the increase of the side where it was most marked, and to reëstablish the equilibrium; nevertheless the danger is great where the joint has to be penetrated.

LETTER FROM NEW YORK.

MESSRS. EDITORS, — With the beginning of October, the profession here may be said to really commence their winter's work; the medical schools open, the many societies begin their meetings, and every one is expected to be " at home," ready for such services as he may be called upon to perform. If you turn to the hospitals you find the wards and operating theatres again crowded with students at the visiting-hours, and clinical instruction going on as smoothly as though there had been no intermission. In connection with the matter of schools, a letter from New York that failed to notice the new building erected during the past summer by the trustees and faculty of the University Medical College would be doing a great injustice to that prosperous institution. Last spring the trustees purchased a lot of sixty feet by one hundred feet, opposite the entrance to Bellevue Hospital, on which they have erected a handsome building devoted to the purpose of medical education. They have endeavored to make it as complete and perfect as possible, having placed in it every conceivable improvement, due attention being paid to the comfort of both teachers and students.

The structure is four stories high, and is built of Philadelphia brick with Belleville stone trimmings. After passing through a handsome corridor, flanked on either side by polished marble columns, you enter a hall sixteen feet by one hundred, covered with white marble tiling, and running the whole length of the building, broken only at its farther end by a wide staircase leading to the lecture-room on the second floor. On either side of this hall, and opening into it, are, first, on your right as you enter, the dean's room (which strikes one as being too handsomely furnished for the purpose); opposite, is a large reception-room for students, so that they can have no excuse for lounging about the hall; there are a room for the clerk and a room containing the museum of Professor Darling, and several smaller ones for various purposes. The second floor is devoted mainly to a large lecture-room, fifty by sixty feet, capable of accommodating five hundred students; it is furnished with upholstered chairs with iron frames, similar to those used in concert-halls, and so arranged that the students are not raised as much above the lecturer as is sometimes the case. Behind the lecturer, and communicating with the amphitheatre by folding doors, is another room containing electric, physiological, and chemical apparatus, where the professors can arrange for their lectures, and thus save much time. The rest of the story is divided into private rooms for the professors. The third floor is devoted to the private laboratories, ophthalmoscopic and laryngoscopic rooms, etc. On the fourth floor is a well-lighted and well-ventilated dissecting-room, containing about forty tables; opening from this are some private rooms devoted to the same purpose. The rest of the story is given to Dr. Arnold, professor of physiology, and consists of five rooms communicating with each other and containing all the requisites of a well-equipped physiological laboratory, not omitting a room for dogs, cats, and the like. There is also a photographic room in the building, under the supervision of Dr. Piffard. As an improvement upon the old way of summoning students by ringing a bell or sounding a gong, the whole building is furnished with a system of electric bells, connecting the janitor's office with every other room; by this means, each professor is notified a short time before his hour for lecturing arrives. The whole building is heated by steam, and thoroughly ventilated and lighted. The cost of the lot and building is not far from one hundred thousand dollars, and it certainly reflects great credit on the trustees and faculty. Another lecture-room would have added much to the convenience of the building. The interior is finished in black walnut and oak.

Dr. Alfred C. Post has resigned the professorship of surgery and has been made emeritus; Dr. John T. Darby has been appointed in his place. The number of students attending lectures this year is not as large as it was last year, although the university has a larger class.

The profession has met with a great loss in the death of Dr. Krackowizer, which occurred on the 23d of September at his summer residence at Sing Sing; his disease was peritonitis following typhoid fever; he was fifty-five years old. He came to this country in 1850, settled in New York seven years later, and soon established for himself a reputation as a surgeon not only among his own countrymen but among American practitioners. In 1867 he was appointed one of the surgeons to the New York Hospital.

In 1874, when the Bellevue Hospital staff was reorganized, he was appointed on the original board, but resigned the present year, because he thought that the commissioners had broken faith with the profession. His death causes a vacancy in the attending staff of the New York Hospital, and as the new building will probably be ready for the reception of patients next year, there is considerable competition for the place. Heretofore, those who have held one or more hospital positions have always stood the best chances to get others, the principle seeming to be that the more a man has the more he should get; consequently these positions are filled by comparatively a few men. It is not an uncommon thing to find a physician or surgeon attached to two or even three hospitals.

The Presbyterian Hospital started with the rule that they would not give an appointment to any one holding an active position in another institution; but one of their recent appointments was in violation of this rule. It has been intimated that the same plan would be hereafter adopted in appointments to the New York Hospital, and it now remains to be seen whether school influence is strong enough to prevent it. The *Medical Record* has had some editorials on the injustice of a comparatively few men monopolizing all the best positions in the hospitals, and draws attention to the fact that one hundred college men hold three hundred and six hospital appointments, of which one hundred and sixty are active and one hundred and forty-six consulting.

The Commissioners of Charity and Correction have at last yielded to the pressure and have placed a hospital under the control of the homœopaths, and they are as pleased as a child is with a new toy. The hospital is situated on Ward's Island, opposite Ninety-Eighth Street, in the East River, and has accommodations for about four hundred patients. They are to receive one third of the cases coming under the care of the commission, Bellevue and Charity hospitals receiving the rest. Whether there are many purely homœopathic practitioners in the city is doubtful; a gentleman at the head of the Homœopathic Medical School here is reported to have said in reply to the remark made by one of the commissioners that he supposed that the requisition for quinine would be small, " By no means. You will find our requisition as large as that of any of your other institutions."

We do not seem to get rid of diphtheria here; the lowest mortality for any week during the past summer was thirty-five, and it has been as high as sixty. Within the past few days I have heard of several cases. It now looks as though we were going to have another epidemic of it during the coming winter. No cause has been assigned for its prevalence unless it is bad trapping and sewerage.

The trouble at the Presbyterian Hospital is still unsettled. The board does not seem to have any definite policy, and there is evidently a want of harmony of action among its members. They are certainly not improving the condition of affairs by procrastination.

New York, *October* 24, 1875.

STRAW IN THE STOMACH.

Messrs. Editors, — In the case reported before the Boston Society for Medical Improvement, and published in the Journal of October 14th, it should have been stated that the masses in the stomach were each four and one half inches long and two and one half inches in diameter. The one in the duodenum was four and one half inches long and one inch and a half in diameter; how it could have passed the pylorus it is difficult to conceive. The masses were said to consist of "straw, twigs, twine, tea-leaves, etc., resembling the hair-balls that are sometimes found in the stomachs of cattle." A few small twigs were seen, but the masses consisted mainly of straw; the one nearest to the cardia being cemented by a dark, dirty-looking substance, but from this last the two others were comparatively free. The structure was therefore loose, and very different from the hair-balls, which are generally very compact.   ****

Boston, *November* 3, 1875.

DUODECIMAL ARITHMETIC.

MESSRS. EDITORS, — The note on the metric system over my initials seems to have produced a strange excitement. I have but a word to add on the facility with which a duodecimal numeration in arithmetic might be introduced.

It is as easy to count by dozens as by tens. It is as easy to say " one gross " as " a hundred and forty-four ; " it is as easy to say " eight dozen and four" as " one hundred." We might call the great gross a *primo*, its square a *secundo*, its cube a *tertio*, and so on.

Then as to notation. We should require two new characters for ten and eleven, as x (ten), ℥ (eleven) ; twelve would be written *10*, twenty-four *20*, thirty-six *30*, etc., and read one dozen, two dozen, three dozen, and so on. The intermediate numbers would be read thus : twenty, *one dozen and eight ;* thirty, *two dozen and six*; forty-seven, *three dozen and eleven*, and so on.

To avoid confusion the new numerals, when used, could be written in italics, or dotted over the top like the i and j.

Such a numeration would greatly facilitate calculation. The science of arithmetic would be revolutionized. Take the multiplication table. The twos, threes, fours, sixes, and twelves would become perfectly regularized, as much so as the twos, fives, and tens now are. The eights would come round regularly with every second dozen, the nines with every third dozen. This leaves only the three prime numbers, five, seven, and eleven (ten being the multiple of five), for the irregular ones.

The reduction of decimal numbers into duodecimals would be effected by dividing by twelve and its powers. Thus one hundred divided by twelve gives *eight* and *four* over, written 84, and read *eight dozen and four.* Two hundred divided by one hundred and forty-four (one gross) gives *one* and fifty-six over ; this remainder divided by twelve gives *four* and *eight* over ; combining we have 148, *one gross, four dozen, and eight.*

The converse would be effected by simply adding together the given number of grosses, dozens, and units.

It is evident that this species of arithmetic might be introduced without any great " violence to the mental processes of the civilized world." (H. P. B.) We do not think the change necessary, but if we must have a change, let us make the true and radical one ; let us first reform our arithmetic, then we can construct a system of weights and measures on a *really* scientific basis.

One correspondent (J. P. P.) says the metrical or decimal system is " born of science." I should say of sciolism. It is a relic of the savage custom of counting by the fingers, and its substitution for the present (confessedly imperfect) duodecimal system is simply a reversion to barbarism.

And such I believe will be the ultimate, though perhaps remote, verdict of mankind.   Truly yours,   EDWARD T. WILLIAMS, M. D.

4 CENTRE PLACE, ROXBURY, *November* 5, 1875.

A NEW NIPPLE SHIELD.

MESSRS. EDITORS, — The importance of protecting the nipples from injury and friction during normal lactation, and especially if there is the least tendency to soreness, is well recognized.

The shield made by Codman and Shurtleff, and shown in the accompanying cuts, half size, presents no novelty, but is found, after experiment, to be of the right shape, size for the average, and material. It is made of box-wood, very light, destitute of odor, and easily cleansed; the largest diameter is two inches; five eighths of an inch is the inside diameter, and it is three fourths of an inch high.

The shield should be worn at all times, except while the infant is nursing, so as to entirely prevent the chafing and pressure of the clothing.

NORTON FOLSOM, M. D.

BOSTON, *November* 1, 1875.

WEEKLY BULLETIN OF PREVALENT DISEASES.

THE following is a bulletin of the diseases prevalent in Massachusetts during the week ending November 6, 1875, compiled under the authority of the State Board of Health from the returns of physicians representing all sections of the State : —

The summary for each section is as follows : —

Berkshire : Influenza, bronchitis.   Very little sickness reported.

Valley : Typhoid (and remittent) fever, influenza, bronchitis.   All diseases except typhoid fever have diminished.

Midland : Influenza, bronchitis, typhoid fever, rheumatism, diphtheria.

Northeastern : Typhoid fever, influenza, bronchitis, rheumatism.   A Lynn observer reports "twelve cases of typhoid fever from two bad wells, and as many from a bad drain."

Metropolitan : Bronchitis, diphtheria, typhoid fever, influenza, scarlatina, pneumonia.   The noteworthy feature is the decided increase in the prevalence of diphtheria; four fifths of the physicians report its prevalence.

Southeastern : Influenza, bronchitis, rheumatism.

In the State at large the prevalent diseases stand related as follows : influenza, bronchitis, typhoid fever, diphtheria, rheumatism, scarlatina, pneumonia, croup, whooping-cough, diarrhœa, measles, dysentery, cholera infantum, cholera morbus.   The last seven are very low in the scale.

F. W. DRAPER, M. D., Registrar.

COMPARATIVE MORTALITY-RATES FOR THE WEEK ENDING OCT. 30, 1875.

	Estimated Population.	Total Mortality for the Week.	Annual Death-Rate per 1000 during Week.
New York	1,060,000	482	23.6
Philadelphia	800,000	275	17.9
Brooklyn	500,000	201	20.9
Chicago	400,000	113	14.7
Boston	342,000	161	24.5
Cincinnati	260,000	108	21.6
Providence	100,700	35	18.1
Worcester	50,000	12	12.5
Lowell	50,000	20	20.8
Cambridge	48,000	26	28.2
Fall River	45,000	18	20.8
Lawrence	35,000	10	14.8
Lynn	33,000	15	23.6
Springfield	31,000	11	18.4
Salem	26,000	7	14.0

Normal Death-Rate, 17 per 1000.

BOOKS AND PAMPHLETS RECEIVED. — A Practical Treatise on Fractures and Disloca-tions. By F. H. Hamilton, M. D. Fifth Edition. Revised and Improved. Philadelphia: Henry C. Lea. 1875. (For sale by James Campbell & Co., Boston.)

Catalogue of Dartmouth College, 1875-76.

Transactions of the Minnesota State Medical Society, 1875.

Printing for the Blind. Report of a Committee of the American Social Science Associa-tion, at Detroit, May, 1875. Boston. 1875.

, Transactions of the New Hampshire Medical Society, at Concord, June, 1875.

The Relations of the Urine to Diseases of the Skin. By L. Duncan Bulkley, M. D. (Reprinted from the Archives of Dermatology.) New York: G. P. Putnam's Sons. 1875.

Two Cases of Exophthalmic Goitre associated with Chronic Urticaria. By L. Duncan Bulkley, M. D. (Reprinted from the Chicago Journal of Nervous and Mental Diseases.) New York: G. P. Putnam's Sons. 1875.

Lectures on Syphilis and some Forms of Local Disease affecting principally the Organs of Generation. By Henry Lee, Professor of Surgery at the Royal College of Surgeons of England. Philadelphia: Henry C. Lea. 1875. (For sale by A. Williams & Co.)

Peritonitis. By Professor Alfred Loomis. A Series of American Clinical Lectures. Vol. I. No. IX. New York: G. P. Putnam's Sons. 1875.

Fever and Ague. By Dr. John H. Weir. (Read before the Madison County Medical Society.) Edwardsville, Ill. 1875.

THE BOSTON SOCIETY FOR MEDICAL OBSERVATION will meet Monday, November 15th, at eight o'clock. Dr. Beach will report a series of surgical cases.

RESIGNED AND DISCHARGED. — B. Joy Jeffries, Surgeon First Corps of Cadets, M. V. M., October 16, 1875.

THE BOSTON
MEDICAL AND SURGICAL JOURNAL.

VOL. XCIII. — THURSDAY, NOVEMBER 18, 1875. — NO. 21.

—————

A NEW INSTRUMENT FOR THE READY AND EFFECTIVE USE OF THE DOUBLE CURRENT IN THE TREATMENT OF SUPPURATING CAVITIES AND IN PELVIC DRAINAGE.

BY GEORGE H. BIXBY, M. D., OF BOSTON,

Surgeon to St. Elizabeth's Hospital for Women.

IN the course of a somewhat extended experience in the treatment of the surgical diseases of women, an unusually large number of cases of pelvic abscesses, retro-uterine hæmatocele, and intra-uterine tumors have come under my observation. In a review of the clinical history of the two first-mentioned affections and of the means employed in their treatment, I find that while in a few instances a single evacuation by aspiration or otherwise was sufficient to obliterate the suppurating cavity, the majority of cases required the use of stimulating and disinfectant injections. The employment of the different forms of double catheters and drainage tubes hitherto in use was most unsatisfactory, in my hands at least, the treatment being in some cases unsuccessful and in others unnecessarily prolonged. Among the difficulties encountered I will mention, first, the liability to displacement, and, owing to the lax condition and the change in the relations of the tissues, the extreme difficulty attending reposition, attempts to restore the instrument not unfrequently proving unsuccessful, even after prolonged and tedious manipulations, thus necessitating the establishment of a new opening; second, the tax upon the strength of the patient and the demand upon the time and patience of the surgeon. I recall the histories of several cases in which, from a tardy recognition of the disease, surgical interference was delayed, and the poisonous effects of the discharge were so marked that the interruption of the treatment, even for a few hours, was followed by grave symptoms of septic poisoning; and notwithstanding the imperfect appliances at my disposal, upon vigorous resumption of the treatment an amelioration of the symptoms took place immediately. It is evident from these facts that the displacement of any appliance for maintaining a patent aperture, the subsequent closure of the aperture, and the interruption of the treatment, even for a short time, become under all circumstances serious affairs. In view of these difficulties, and encouraged by the recent discussions and by the acceptance on the part of the profession of the theory that blood-poisoning is the most frequent cause of death after abdominal and pelvic operations, as well as a possible cause of the so-called puerperal fever, I have been led to the suggestion of a new instrument for the application of an old but most useful surgical principle in the treatment of such affections. The instrument, which I shall denominate the *double trocar*, consists of a canula ten inches long and one fourth of an inch or less in diameter, straight or curved according to its particular use. A horizontal septum divides its cavity into two equal chambers, the inferior extremity of each being, fenestrated to the extent of an inch. Superiorly each chamber is connected by a branch, the afferent and the efferent, with rings and guard for retention. Into this double canula there fits a flexible double trocar attached to a common handle, and answering for both the curved and the straight canula. When the trocar is inserted and forced home, the two extremities come together in sufficiently close apposition to form a single point. A piece of rubber tubing two or three inches in length attached to the afferent branch forms a convenient coupling for the nozzle of the syringe, and the efferent is lengthened to the desired extent by the same means. The copious and uninterrupted current and the

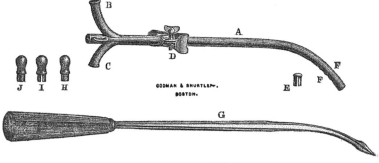

A. Canula.
B. Efferent branch.
C. Afferent branch.
D. Guard.
E. Probe point.

F F. Fenestræ.
G. Double trocar.
H J. Efferent and afferent stoppers.
I. Central stopper.

absolute immunity from the admission of air, obtained by the use of the fountain syringe, render that instrument, or an apparatus constructed upon the same principle, absolutely indispensable to the use of the double canula.

It is claimed for the double trocar that, while it has all the advantages of the single instrument, it possesses the additional advantage of establishing at the same time a complete appliance for the double current. It is claimed also, that from the copiousness of the current obtained by means of this instrument it has all the advantages of a large opening, without the dangers of hæmorrhage, and with less risk of self-inoculation.

This instrument is recommended in the following conditions : —

With straight trocar and canula :

I. Pelvic abscess.

II. Retro-uterine hæmatocele.

With straight canula alone and blunt point :

III. Pelvic abscess and hæmatocele, when a free opening is preferred and when there is a multiple sac.

With the curved instrument :

IV. Pelvic drainage after ovariotomy and abdominal operations.

With straight canula alone :

V. The uterine cavity after the removal of intra-uterine and interstitial uterine fibroids.

VI. The uterine cavity in acute puerperal endometritis, offensive post-partum vaginal discharges, for the application of cold and of astringents in post-partum hæmorrhage, and for the treatment of the female bladder.

I. *Pelvic Abscess.* — At the opening of this paper I stated that with rare exceptions a single evacuation, by whatever means, was not sufficient to destroy the pyogenic membrane of a pelvic abscess ; therefore the existence of pus in the pelvic cavity was an indication for the immediate commencement of the protracted treatment.

Pelvic abscesses are most often unilocular ; cases with multiple sacs, however, do occur. In case of doubt as to whether we have to do with a unilocular or a multiple abscess, by evacuating completely with the aspirator the subsequent presence or absence of fluctuation is easily determined by a careful examination.

The method of operating now considered, being a substitute for the free opening, does not differ materially from that laid down in the text-books ; but at the risk of being prolix I shall describe it in detail, with some modifications. The patient, etherized and with a bandage passed around the waist, is placed upon the left side across a bed or upon a table ; the limbs are sharply flexed, or, if preferred, in the lithotomy position. The uterus, if not anteverted, which is more often the case, should be so placed, if it be possible ; if necessary it should be held in that position with a sound.[1] The diagnosis is then confirmed with an aspirator, the depth required to reach the fluid being carefully noted.

Since a complete or even a partial evacuation in a unilocular cyst would cause it to become flaccid, and would render further operative interference exceedingly difficult if not dangerous, the least possible amount of fluid drawn the better. The most prominent part of the tumor hav-

---

[1] During the past year I saw a case of pelvic abscess in which the uterus was retroverted and bound down by adhesions. I have no doubt that the inflammation and subsequent suppuration were due to efforts employed to separate them.

ing been ascertained, and the seat of the pulsation of large vessels avoided, the trocar, with concealed point and armed with the guard and with both rubber tubes in place (the afferent closed with a stopper, the efferent tied in a single knot), is introduced into the vagina upon the finger of the left hand and placed firmly against the tumor. With the left hand in the vagina, controlling the extremity of the trocar, the puncture is made in downward direction with a firm but steady force. The peculiar impression imparted as the instrument passes into the cavity is quite unmistakable. The previous arrangement of the tubes prevents a sudden escape of the fluid. The trocar is now withdrawn sufficiently to conceal its point, the guard secured against the vulva, and the tapes for retention applied. The last step is best effected by passing them through the staple, around the limb, under the bandage around the waist, and finally tying or, what is better, buckling the extremities together in front. The patient being on the left side, the right tape of course is first applied, and will serve to retain the instrument until she is turned upon the back, when the other is adjusted. If the operation is performed with the patient on her back, of course both tapes are put in position at once. The patient is now placed upon the back, near the edge of the bed, and the left tape adjusted. We may evacuate the abscess at once, but the better plan is to attach to the afferent branch the tube of a fountain syringe charged with a disinfecting solution, and suspended or held six feet above the bed, at the same time untying the knot in the efferent branch and placing its extremity in a vessel on the floor beside the bed. The trocar is now withdrawn without fear of displacement, the central opening of the canula is closed with a stopper, the stop of the syringe is opened, and the contents of the abscess are forced out by the strong current.

We have now in position a convenient and ever ready appliance for the use of the double current, with little risk of displacement, of easy application by the most inexperienced attendant, and with slight annoyance to the patient. The frequency of the application should depend upon the nature of the discharge and its effect upon the system. I have usually commenced the treatment with three daily applications and one at midnight. Under all circumstances the application should be copious. The efferent current should be frequently interrupted, the cavity thus filled, and contact with every part of it secured. After a fair trial of the usual disinfectants I have returned to the use of a five per cent. solution of carbolic acid (two drachms to sixteen ounces of glycerine, soap, and water) as by far the most efficacious.

II. *Retro-Uterine Hæmatocele.* — Since the investigations of M. Nélaton the surgical treatment of this affection has been confined to those urgent cases in which the life of the patient was imperiled from a distention that threatened rupture into the peritoneal cavity. The cases under my observation were of this character. In all, the treatment was by a primary free opening, followed by disinfecting injections. The discharge, at first sero-sanguinolent, became putrid, demanding protracted and unremitting attention. Owing to the great tendency to close in spite of repeated dilatations, the method of treatment was reduced virtually to an opening of the size made by a large trocar. The patients recovered, but not until many weeks had elapsed, the most alarming symptoms of blood-poisoning frequently occurring. Notwithstanding the recommendation by most authorities of a free opening in the treatment of this affection, I am disposed to attach much importance to the method above suggested in connection with the treatment of pelvic abscess, for the reason that, as the aspirator indicated in all my cases, the contents of the cyst are composed, even in the late stages, not only of coagula but of a large amount of sero-sanguinolent fluid. After what seemed to be a complete evacuation after the free opening, the cavity continued to secre·e for weeks a purulent, offensive discharge, as if from a pyogenic membrane. I am convinced that the entrance of air through such an opening was sufficient to break down and liquefy the coagula. That this process was materially expedited by the copious double current there can be no doubt.

III. *In Pelvic Abscess and Hæmatocele,* after free opening, the use of the straight canula with probe-point in connection with the fountain syringe, in the manner to be described when the treatment of the uterine cavity is discussed, will be found to render invaluable service.

IV. *Pelvic Drainage after Ovariotomy.* — When the operation has reached the stage prior to that of the closure of the wound, after applying a bandage around the body, the surgeon passes the left hand into the pelvis along the pedicle until it reaches a point in the reflexion of the peritoneum opposite Douglas's fossa, and with the right hand introduces the trocar into the vagina, armed with its guard, its afferent and efferent tubes adjusted, and its point concealed. With bimanual manipulation the extremity of the instrument is placed against Douglas's cul-de-sac, as low as possible below the uterine connection, without impinging upon the rectum, and held firmly in position. An assistant pushes the trocar through the vaginal septum, its passage being guarded and controlled by the operator's left hand, still in the pelvis. This done, the point of the trocar is concealed by a slight withdrawal, the instrument tilted upward and forward, and the extremity of the canula protected by a probe-point.[1] The guard and tapes are adjusted as in pelvic abscess, and the trocar is entirely removed.[2] Of the use of the double current in pelvic drainage, special mention will be made later.

---

[1] After introduction, Dr. Kimball reverses the curved canula.

[2] The straight canula with probe point introduced through the wound into the pelvis at the time of the operation, and reposed in the angle of the wound, would, it seems to me, admirably carry out Professor Peaslee's method of drainage, having also the additional advantage of the double current.

For the conception of the idea of drainage in the after-treatment of ovariotomy, and its first application, the profession is indebted to the genius of Prof. E. R. Peaslee of New York, who first employed it through Douglas's fossa. For the further development and perfection of this method, the credit belongs to Dr. Gilman Kimball of Lowell. This, I think, is fully substantiated by the following brief history. In 1846, Dr. Handyside, of Edinburgh, after tying the pedicle, passed the ligatures through Douglas's fossa into the vagina. In 1849, Dr. March, of Albany, *suggested* the idea. Professor Peaslee, not aware of this, did the same in 1854. The object of this procedure, as in the above cases, was simply to dispose of the ligatures. *In 1855, in a case of ascites complicated with an ovarian cyst, Professor Peaslee passed an elastic catheter from the vagina up into Douglas's cul-de-sac, expressly for purpose of drainage.* The method of passing the ligatures through the cul-de-sac of Douglas, as inaugurated by Dr. Handyside, was employed again in 1866 by Dr. J. F. Miner, of Buffalo, by Dr. Gilman Kimball in 1867, and still later (I believe in 1871) by Dr. William Warren Greene, of Portland. The object of the operation in the three last cases was *to establish drainage.* In 1868, Dr. Kimball modified the operation by lodging the ligatures in a canula introduced *per vaginam* into Douglas's cul-de-sac. More recently he again modified it, bringing the ligature outside of the wound (except when the clamp was used) passing the canula into Douglas's fossa and allowing it to remain as long as it served to conduct off any matter that had accumulated in the pelvic cavity. Pelvic drainage has been frequently employed since, and the subject has been discussed by able authorities at home and abroad.[1] A complete history of this important subject would far exceed the scope of this paper. I cannot, however, resist the opportunity to vary somewhat its descriptive character, by submitting without comment the condensed histories of a few cases from the literature of the subject (confining myself to three authorities), as illustrative of the primary and secondary indications and applications, and of the results of pelvic drainage after ovariotomy.

The following is the *first case on record of primary drainage* through Douglas's cul-de-sac, by Prof. E. R. Peaslee, of New York.[1] " This was a case of ovarian tumor complicated with ascites, one hundred and six pounds of fluid withdrawn by a previous tapping. In anticipation of con-

---

[1] Prof. E. R. Peaslee: Diseases of the Ovaries, pages 437, 438; American Journal of Obstetrics, August, 1870, pages 509, 510; American Journal of the Medical Sciences, January, 1856. Dr. Gilman Kimball: Boston Medical and Surgical Journal, May 28, June 11, August 6, 13, September 17, 1874. Mr. Spencer Wells: Diseases of the Ovaries, 1865, page 393, 1873. Dr. Skene, Brooklyn: New York Medical Record, October , 1873. Dr. J Marion Sims: New York Medical Journal, December, 1872, April, 1873. Dr. W. W Greene, Boston Medical and Surgical Journal, lxxxiv. 137. Mr. Thomas Keith: Transactions of the London Obstetrical Society, v. 62; also his cases Nos. 36, 39, 59, 81, 101 and 103. Dr. J. F. Miner: Buffalo Medical and Surgical Journal, June, 1866, September 1866.

[2] Ovarian Tumors, pages 510–518. American Journal of Obstetrics, August, 1870.

tinned secretion from the distended peritoneum, after operation a gum-elastic catheter was passed by the vagina through Douglas's cul-de-sac into the peritoneal cavity, and tightly corked. Patient did well until fifth day, when symptoms of septicæmia appeared, and on removing the cork a small amount of fœtid fluid escaped.   Injected a quart of luke-warm water through the tube into peritoneal cavity, and allowed as much to flow back. On repeating this, the patient remarked, ' I feel as refreshed as if I had taken a bath,' and became bright and natural. Septicæmic symptoms would, however, return in eight or twelve hours.   Injections of artificial serum composed of one or two drachms of common salt to the pint of pure water ; later, solution of the liquor sodæ chlorinatæ, from one to two drachms to the pint of water, alternately with the salt and water, was employed two or three times daily for seven days, when, there being no longer any odor of decomposition in the fluid obtained through the tube, the latter was removed." Result, recovery.[1]

The following are abstracts of Dr. Kimball's cases from 1867 to 1875, giving the indications for application and results of primary drainage ; these include the first cases in which the ligature was lodged in a canula and also the first cases in which the canula was used alone.

CASE I. Single ovary. Complications : chronic adhesions, anteriorly, parietal, omental, and colon ; laceration of peritoneum ; escape of contents into peritoneal cavity.   Pedicle : short and thick ; tied in two parts ; cut close ; dropped into pelvis.   Method of drainage : ligatures passed through posterior uterine cul-de-sac and out by the vagina. Symptoms : excessive vomiting, relieved upon escape of putrid discharge from vagina ; no further interruption to convalescence.   Result, recovery.

CASE II.   Single ovary.   Complications : ascitic fluid, chronic adhesions, parietal and omental.   Pedicle : slender, ligated.   Drainage : ligature passed through Douglas's fossa.   Symptoms : third day, pain in abdomen ; vomiting ; quickened pulse ; prostration.   The same day free offensive discharge per vaginam.   Result, recovery.

CASE III.   Single ovary. · Complications : ascitic fluid ; adhesions anteriorly, parietal and omental.   Separation followed by free hæmorrhage, ligature required ; several shreds of peritoneum and omentum ligated and removed.   Pedicle : short, slender, ligated.   Drainage : ligatures passed out through vaginal cul-de-sac.   Symptoms : favorable till eleventh day, when signs of tetanus appeared ; abundant flow of bloody serum immediately after operation, and continued to a greater or less extent throughout ; was offensive and fœtid on the second day.   The fact that there were no signs of septicæmia proved the value and success of the drainage, and without the accidental com-

---

[1] Professor Peaslee has used drainage in every case of ovariotomy since 1855, in which there was anything to drain from the peritoneal cavity after that operation ; but he has always, since then, preferred to drain through the abdominal wound, and not by the cul-de-sac.

plication, recovery would have very likely resulted. Result, death from tetanus, twentieth day.

CASE IV. Single ovary. No pedicle; tumor attached and identified with entire broad ligament, and portion of the fundus uteri; breadth of mass, six inches; division into six parts, each embraced in a separate ligature, uterus cut through, its centre having been transfixed by strong ligatures and tied separately. Drainage: passage of the latter ligatures through canula in vaginal cul-de-sac. Symptoms: indications of peritonitis after twenty-four hours, namely, vomiting, tympany, continuing three days, when a free flow of bloody serum began from the canula. Immediate cessation of above symptoms. Later, discharge offensive, nature improved by the use of disinfecting injections through the canula. Canula removed after eight days; discharge continued, but gradually diminished and ceased at the end of ten days. Result, recovery.

CASE V. Single ovary. Complications: tapping previous to operation; ascitic fluid; rupture of the cyst; prolonged operation; adhesions parietal and omental, portions of omentum removed. Pedicle: tied in two parts, dropped back. Drainage: ligatures passed through Douglas's fossa through a canula. Symptoms: first day, pulse 130–140, abdomen somewhat distended, slight pain. Third day, pulse 130, no pain, no tympany; P. M., pulse 140, dark discharge from vagina, the first since operation. Fourth day, morning, pulse 132, no vaginal discharge; six A. M., vaginal discharge returned; twelve M., discharge continued; two P. M., tired and nervous, slight discharge from the vagina, bowels distended, clammy sweat, cold feet. Fifth day, A. M., discharge from wound slight, distention continued, return of heat to extremities; P. M., two ounces of foetid discharge from vagina. Eighth day, discharge more abundant, pulse 130. Tenth day, ten ounces sero-purulent, dark-colored, offensive fluid from peritoneal cavity, symptoms more alarming. Twelfth day, pulse 110, offensive discharge continued from abdomen and vagina, incision not inclined to heal soundly. Fifteenth day, pulse 100, discharge from abdomen diminished and less offensive, vaginal discharge continued. Result, recovery, after protracted convalescence.

CASE VI. Single ovary. Complications: tapping previous to operation; adhesions parietal and omental; profuse hæmorrhage from the same; portions of omentum cut away and stump reposed in incision; escape of fluid into cavity. Pedicle: tied in two parts; dropped. Drainage: ligature passed by a canula through Douglas's fossa. Symptoms: two days after operation, discharge of bloody serum; ceased on the third and did not return; symptoms favorable up to fourth day; then became alarming, such as pain, distention, nausea, vomiting, and quickened pulse. In absence of surgeon, nurse passed a female catheter into left iliac fossa and removed ten ounces of fœtid fluid; immediate relief. Result, rapid disappearance of threatening symptoms, speedy recovery.

CASE VII. Both ovaries. Complications: burst cyst; escape of contents into peritoneal cavity; adhesions general and to viscera. Pedicles: both slender, short; cut close to tumor; dropped back. Drainage: ligatures twisted together, passed through Douglas's fossa, through a canula. Symptoms: first day, A. M., slight pain in abdomen; vomiting occasionally as before operation. Second day, nausea; pulse 110; no discharge through canula. Third day, slight discharge. Sixth day, pulse 112; vomiting continues; slight distention; discharge from vagina abundant and offensive. Later, escape of discharge through incision, that from vagina in no way diminished; antiseptic injections through canula and into abdominal cavity produced no favorable effect upon the quantity or quality of the discharge; continues unabated. Result, death from septicæmia, twelfth day.

CASE VIII. Single ovary. Complications: ascitic fluid; none escaped into cavity. Pedicle: broad, thick; clamp. Drainage: angle of wound, and ligature passed through vaginal cul-de-sac through canula. Symptoms: first day after operation, bloody serum passing freely from canula. Fourth day, pain in the bladder; discharge from canula ceased. Sixth day, free discharge of offensive matter forced through the incision; injection through angle of the wound every few hours. Symptoms favorable. Convalescence interrupted by an attack of diarrhœa, lasting four days. Result, recovery.

The following are notes of other cases of Dr. Kimball, that came more or less under my observation: —

CASE I. Large cyst. One ovary. Complications: adhesions, parietal, omental; profuse hæmorrhage; walls everted. Pedicle: ligated, drawn up and reposed in the angle of the wound. Drainage: single curved trocar; cul-de-sac. Symptoms: escape of bloody serum twelve hours after operation. Third day, passage of rectal injection through canula, and later, fæcal matter. Canula removed. Pain, distention, restlessness, evidence of impaction of fæces, relieved by oil and afterward copious soap and water enema. Result, subsequently rapid recovery.

CASE II. Both ovaries, in a patient aged seventy. Complications: enormous distention; fifty inches; extensive adhesions to parietes, omentum, intestines, pelvis. Operation protracted; large portions of peritoneum and omentum ligated and removed; escape of fluid into cavity; tumor and contents weighed one hundred and fifty pounds. Pedicle: clamp and ligature; the last reposed in angle of wound. Drainage: canula through Douglas's fossa. Symptoms: bloody serum first two days; displacement of canula fourth day. No further discharge, no untoward symptoms. Result, slow but complete recovery.

CASE III. One ovary. Complications: œdema of extremities; great distention intensified by respiration; infiltration of walls of abdomen; burst cyst. After closure of the wound ascitic fluid welled up through angle of wound. Drainage: canula, cul-de-sac. Symptoms: abundant flow of serum for several days. No serious symptoms. Result, recovery rather slow but complete.

Mr. Spencer Wells's cases, showing secondary indication for drainage, are as follows : —

CASE I. Single ovary. Complications: tumor in connection; extensive adhesions to omentum and bladder. Pedicle: ligated and returned. Symptoms: third day, sharp pain, relieved after uterine discharge, resembling menstruation; continued well until ninth day. Later, sleepless night from pain and flatulence; typhus symptoms; dry tongue, dilated pupils, flushed face, drowsiness. An accumulation of fluid detected in pelvis per vaginam. Puncture with trocar, five ounces dark, bloody serum, ammoniacal odor, removed. Tenth day, pulse 112, 95, 92. Typhus condition aggravated, as discharge from vagina had ceased; examination revealed fluid still present in vaginal space. Puncture again resulted in removal of ten ounces of fluid; more putrid than that of the day before, and containing pus. Chassaignac's drainage tube passed through the two punctures forming a loop. Free discharge through tube for several days; rapid improvement. Tube removed twenty-eighth day; thirty-fourth day sat up; forty-second day left for home; one month later was in perfect health.

CASE II. Single ovary; no adhesions. Pedicle: clamped. Symptoms: second day, flatulent distention of abdomen; removal of clamp necessary; pulse 130. Fifth day, free discharge of dark, bloody serum from wound. Sixth day, discharge free, pulse 116. On ninth day, also on tenth and eleventh, discharge still fœtid, but more purulent. Twelfth day, patient very low; a soft swelling found behind the uterus. This was punctured through the cul-de-sac, giving escape to a pint of serum with blood and some pus. Thirteenth day, free suppuration from wound; P. M., a free discharge of fœtid pus by the vagina. She gradually sank, and died on the twenty-sixth day.

Post-Mortem. No signs of general peritonitis; bottom of Douglas's fossa and cavity holding three or four ounces of pus. The opening through Douglas's fossa made with trocar was quite closed. *It is to be regretted that a freer opening was not made and left open.*

CASE III. One ovary. Complications: adhesions, parietal, pelvic. Pedicle: ligated. Symptoms: forty-seven hours after operation stitches removed, wound seemed firmly united; nine P. M., attack of vomiting, escape of reddish serum from angle of wound. Fifth day, pulse 140, abdomen tympanitic, evidently containing fluid. Evidence of fluid high up behind the uterus. Vomiting with prostration continued, and on sixth day pulse 160 ; a half-ounce of reddish grumous fluid from open angle of the wound. At midnight wound commenced discharging, and then the symptoms became more favorable. Seventh day, evidence of fœcal impaction ; relieved ; pulse fell at once from 160 to 130 ; discharge of curdy fluid. Eighth day, free discharge from the wound. Evidence of fluid behind the uterus still existing ; a trocar passed into Douglas's fossa gave vent to three and a half pints of black, fœtid, tarry fluid. Sixteenth day, trocar again introduced, and one pint of fluid discharged. Seventeenth day, canula replaced and more fluid escaped and continued to do so all night. On twenty-first day, discharge free, fœtid, yellow, and purulent; pulse 140. Twenty-fifth day, discharge continues ; canula withdrawn ; the flow ceased the next day. By probing the cavity one ounce of fluid removed. Result, death on twenty-ninth day.

Post-Mortem. Recto-vaginal pouch empty ; utero-vesical pouch filled with creamy pus ; pus found incarcerated between the coils of intestines, forming a large number of abscesses.

We come now to the consideration of the use of the double current in connection with drainage. As we have seen, the cessation of the discharge, which was invariably followed by alarming symptoms, was due to the obstruction of the canula. This was constantly proved, from the fact of its return after free injection. Upon examination of the canulæ that had been obstructed shortly after the operation, I found the closure to be due to hardened coagula, that required considerable force to detach. When the obstruction took place some days later, it was evidently caused by an accumulation of thick, tenacious, sero-purulent or ichorous matter, exceedingly difficult to dissolve and wash away with a single current.

From a careful study of the foregoing cases, we venture to offer the following suggestions. The canula in position as above described, as in pelvic abscess, the hose is attached to the afferent branch and the efferent tube is placed in a vessel beside the bed. The first few hours a sero-sanguinolent discharge usually flows of its own accord, but this being the usual stage for the formation of coagula, at least as soon as six hours after the operation a current of tepid water, slightly carbolized, should be allowed to make the circuit of the instrument, merely for the sake of insuring patency. If at the end of four or five days the fluid escapes in the same condition as when it entered, and there are no untoward symptoms present, in all probability the necessity for drainage has ceased, and the canula may be removed with impunity. Leaving the instrument in position a longer or shorter period, even after this stage its presence being, in my opinion, indifferent, must depend upon the

judgment of the surgeon. If, on the other hand, early after the operation, or even a few days later, we discover local or general signs of putrid accumulation, the injection should be copious, frequent, and highly
disinfectant, and the case treated precisely as one of abscess in any
other part. I see no reason why, by cutting off the efferent current
the entire abdominal cavity may not be thoroughly washed out.

V. *Treatment of the Uterine Cavity after the Removal of Intra-
Uterine and Interstitial Fibroids.* — If there be great danger from
blood-poisoning, when the exciting cause is situated in the cellular
tissue, how much greater must be the tendency when the nidus of infection is located in the cavity of an organ so rich in vessels and nerves
as the uterus. The uterus in patients enfeebled by years of constant
metrorrhagia tolerates most astonishingly the violent and protracted
manipulation often necessary in the enucleation of intra-mural fibroids,
but death results in a comparatively short time from the confinement
within its walls or cavity of the smallest quantity of putrid matter.
The cases are by no means rare in which death has taken place from
septicæmia, incident to a degenerating fibroid, and for want of a perfect
drainage for the removal of purulent and putrid matter, following the
removal of such growth by operation.

For the prevention of such unfortunate occurrences, from personal
experience the use of this instrument is most earnestly recommended.
The method of its application is as follows : The patient being on the
edge of the left side of the bed, the surgeon seats himself a little below
the pelvis. A No. 4 fountain syringe, previously charged with a disinfecting fluid, is suspended or held six feet above the bed. The hose
is coupled with the afferent branch of the canula. The canula is now
introduced into the patulous os, and held in position with the left hand ;
this done, the nurse arranges the bed-pan and places the afferent tube
(four inches long) of the canula in it. The suction extremity of a
Davidson's syringe is placed in the bed-pan, the other in a vessel at the
surgeon's feet. Everything being in readiness, the stop of the hose is
opened. As the fluid begins to enter the pan, having made the circuit of the canula and the uterine cavity, the surgeon simultaneously
commences with the Davidson's syringe to pump the fluid into the
vessel at his feet. In this manner any amount of the fluid can be employed without once overflowing the pan and wetting the patient, an
accident most annoying, not to say dangerous, since it necessitates an
immediate change of clothing. As in pelvic abscess, during the passage
of the fluid the current should be frequently interrupted, in order to
secure its contact with every part of the suppurating surface. In a
large and patulous uterus no danger need for a moment be feared. In
my cases this procedure occasioned a sense of fullness, but not the
slightest pain or discomfort. This treatment was employed in one of

my cases (twice daily by myself, and at midnight an injection through the drainage tube by the nurse) for eighteen days, the occurrence of menstruation being no contraindication. The quantity used was always profuse, not less than two and three quarts. Again I have to say that I relied mainly upon the employment of a solution of carbolic acid, two drachms to sixteen ounces of glycerine, soap, and water. Though the tumor enucleated was six inches in diameter, its removal leaving an enormous suppurating surface, from one end of the treatment to the other there was not the slightest evidence of septic poisoning, and the patient made a rapid recovery.

VI. *The Treatment of the Uterine Cavity in Acute Puerperal Endometritis and in Offensive Post-Partum Vaginal Discharges.* — For a clear and comprehensive view of the relations of puerperal fever to the infective diseases and pyæmia, I would in this connection call attention to the recent exhaustive discussions upon the subject at the instance of Mr. T. Spencer Wells, by the Obstetrical Society of London.[1] The editor of the *Obstetrical Journal of Great Britain* thus closes a short review of this memorable scientific contest:[2] "Now the profession may know what are the latest and most mature thoughts of the best obstetrical authorities in England,[3] upon a disease in which few indeed are not gravely interested. Every particle of evidence relating to it has been resifted and retested. The very term *puerperal fever* has had a struggle for its existence, and although the time does not seem to have arrived for its abolition, its right to exist is strongly denied by several. On many points there still remains much obscurity and difference of opinion. On others, again, there is a happy unanimity. All agree that the puerperal condition of a woman is one which renders her liable to be affected by influences which at another time might produce no serious mischief. A large majority of the Fellows believe that puerperal fever is caused by septicæmia, autogenetic or communicated. The very soul and strength of the discussion rests in this thought. Here is the idea which cannot be too vividly impressed upon the minds of all obstetricians and midwives. Upon its entire acceptance and proper apprehension depends the safety of the mother. An offensive post-partum vaginal discharge must not be permitted. It must be prevented by skillful management of the third stage of labor, by insuring efficient lochial drainage, and, if necessary, *by washing out the utero-vaginal canal with antiseptic fluid.* No one now doubts the communicability of the poison which exists in putrid lochia, or that the most minute quantity of it conveyed to a healthy puerperal woman

---

[1] Obstetrical Journal of Great Britain, May, June, July, August, 1875.

[2] Idem, September, 1874, pages 392, 393.

[3] The editor should have said also "America," since Prof. Fordyce Barker, of New York, took an active part in the discussion.

may produce in her a fatal complaint. A responsibility of a most serious nature attaches itself to all those who have in any capacity to deal with lying-in cases. A mystery hangs over the nature of this pyogenic fluid, but the laws which relate to its origin and propagation are sufficiently well known *to enable us to do much toward checking its generation and preventing the extension of its malignant action when begotten.*"

Notwithstanding their able opponents, so far as my experience goes I am disposed to place myself with the majority of the Fellows in regarding septicæmia, autogenetic or communicated, as the cause of so-called puerperal fever ; hence it has been my habit for years to employ disinfecting vaginal injections after every case of labor.

Again, as a further evidence of a growing interest in the subject, Dr. Grünewald, of St. Petersburg, details the measures which were adopted at the lying-in asylum in that city to prevent infection.[1] " Acting on the theory that some wound or laceration of the parts concerned in labor presented a nidus for the reception of the disease, attention has been directed toward these points, and the result has been happy. The most common starting-point was held to be the vagina or the os uteri. At these points the poison was absorbed, and the disease traveled onward along the planes of connective tissue. The rule observed was to examine every woman by the aid of a speculum immediately after labor. Every laceration or abrasion was then carefully attended to, and as soon as a morbid appearance, such as diphtheritic deposit or the like was noticed, a solution of carbolic acid and water (one part to twelve) was applied, or the sesquichloride of iron in a similar proportion. If the disease advanced and there were signs of endometritis, injections *were practiced by means of a double catheter.* The indications for intra-uterine injections were (1) retention of membranes, (2) retention and decomposition of coagulated blood, (3) lochiometra, (4) in any form of endometritis, and (5) in secondary hæmorrhage. In fact, it was customary to use a weak solution of carbolic acid (one part to four hundred) as an intra-uterine injection, in all cases, immediately after labor, by way of prophylaxis.

The necessity for the most thorough application of disinfecting measures at the slightest evidence of an offensive post-partum vaginal discharge being placed beyond question, the double canula and fountain syringe will be found an invaluable means for the accomplishment of this end. The method of application is the same as that employed in treatment of the uterine cavity after removal of fibroids.

VII. The method of application in the use of cold and astringents in *post-partum hæmorrhage,* being the same, does not require a separate mention.

VIII. In the treatment of *chronic cystitis in the female,* the canula

[1] American Practitioner, October, 1875, page 337.

is employed, with long efferent tube, as in pelvic abscess after simple puncture.[1]

Originality is here claimed for the double trocar only ; for the double canula is mainly an improvement upon those hitherto in use. The compactness of the instruments, available for so many different and important ends, renders it useful as well to the general as to the special practitioner. The double trocar is manufactured by Messrs. Codman and Shurtleff, of Boston, for whose patience and painstaking I desire to express my sincere obligations.

---------◆---------

RECENT PROGRESS IN OTOLOGY.

BY J. ORNE GREEN, M. D.

The Application of the Tympanic Catheter. — The tympanic catheter, first introduced by Weber-Liel in 1869 as a more direct means of making applications to the tympanic cavity, consists of a fine flexible tube with an opening either on its end or on one side close to the end, through which either air or fluid can be injected. This is inserted through an ordinary Eustachian catheter along the whole length of the Eustachian tube into the tympanum, and the application of either air or fluids made through it directly into the cavity. Politzer[2] gives the results of his extended experience in the use of the instrument, after several years' trial, as follows: for simple inflation of the tympanum with air he considers that the tympanic catheter is not as useful as the other methods of inflation, because from the minute calibre of its tube the stream of air loses much of its force from the friction in passing through and force enough cannot be exerted on the membrana tympani to overcome and relieve the abnorma ltension of the drum-membrane and ossicula. In cases of sclerosis of the tympanic mucous membrane and rigidity of the articulations of the ossicula, the injections of medicaments through the tympanic catheter offer no better results than those made through the ordinary Eustachian catheter. In cases, however, in which the tympanum becomes filled with inspissated pus or caseous matter, as in old otorrhœas with or without caries of the bone, but with perforation of the membrana tympani, which offer such a resistance that injections of water through the common Eustachian catheter cannot enter the cavity, Politzer has found the tympanic catheter an invaluable means of evacuation ; in such cases the tympanic catheter is inserted fully into the tympanum, and then a stream of warm water or an alka-

---

[1] The curved canula with probe point admirably answers the purpose of a double male catheter.

[2] Wiener medicinische Wochenschrift, Nos. 15 and 16, 1875.

line solution is injected against the mass till it softens and runs out through the meatus. The instrument is especially valuable in these cases when, as is not unfrequently the case, the meatus is so narrowed by chronic periostitis that all applications from the outside are impossible.

Again, in exacerbations of inflammation coming on in the course of a chronic otorrhœa with very severe pain, the tympanic catheter offers a means of douching the cavity with warm water, one of the most efficient agents for the relief of the pain and for subduing the inflammation ; when, in these cases, the Eustachian tube is much contracted, the tympanic catheter offers the only means of douching the cavity, but if the Eustachian tube remains fairly free the same douching can be accomplished through the ordinary Eustachian catheter. Another class of cases in which Politzer has found the tympanic catheter useful is that in which the membrana tympani has become attached to the inner wall of the tympanum in such a way as to divide the cavity into two distinct parts, so that inflation through the Eustachian tube can affect only the anterior half of the cavity ; in several cases in which a previous inflammation had produced such adhesions, a fresh inflammation filled the posterior cavity with fluid which could not be removed by paracentesis, because air could not be driven in behind the secretion owing to the adhesions; in these cases Politzer first performed paracentesis, and then inserted the end of the tympanic catheter through the meatus into the cavity, and by suction succeeded in removing the whole of the secretion.

Not only in tympanic affections has Politzer found this instrument useful, but also in diseases of the external meatus and the mastoid cells. When the external meatus has been very much narrowed by exostoses, it is often extremely difficult to remove masses of cerumen and of epithelium which form behind the contraction, because the stream from a syringe is unable to penetrate deep enough to float out the mass ; but by passing the tympanic catheter some distance into the mass an alkaline solution can be driven in so as to render it fluid, and then by syringing with warm water the whole of it can be removed. The same mode of procedure is useful for softening and removing collections of pus behind a narrow stricture of the meatus. In inflammation of the mastoid the delicacy and flexibility of the tympanic catheter especially adapt it for the removal of inspissated pus and caseous matter from the irregular cavities of the cells by very much the same process as that used for the meatus ; and the value of any instrument which will accomplish such removal can be appreciated when it is remembered that these masses not only interfere with the closing of the abscess cavity, but also directly cause, by their presence, ulceration and even purulent infection.

The application of the tympanic catheter in cases of serous and mucous effusion in the tympanum is spoken of in the next section of this report.

Movable Exudations in the Tympanum. — The term movable exudation
is used to indicate the more or less fluid serous or mucous secretions which
are found in the tympanic cavity as the result of an inflammation of its
mucous lining membrane, in contradistinction to the solid masses, such as
dried mucus, inspissated pus, or epithelial collections, sometimes found in
the cavity. These movable exudations are the product of an inflammation of the tympanic mucous membrane, usually too slight to have gone
on to the purulent stage, but their presence in the tympanum leads to
serious functional disturbance, and if allowed to remain for any length
of time may produce permanent changes which are incurable. They
may and usually do interfere with the conducting apparatus of the ear
by drawing the membrana tympani inwards, and, as Politzer has shown,
so increasing its tension that it cannot conduct the sound-waves properly; they also increase the hyperæmia of the original inflammation,
and cause fresh exudation. As the result of this we may have growths
of connective tissue in the tympanum binding down the ossicula, and
thus preventing their free vibration.

These exudations are sometimes absorbed spontaneously, but not infrequently remain for weeks and months unless removed by artificial
means. The certain diagnosis of many of them, which is one of the
triumphs of modern otology and dates only from about the year 1868,
has been quite thoroughly described by Schwartze, Politzer, and others,
and has been from time to time mentioned in these Reports, as new points
in diagnosis and treatment have appeared. The chief indication for
treatment is to get rid of the secretion as soon as possible, and thus relieve the constant hyperæmia which it keeps up. When the secretion is
thin and limpid this can generally be accomplished in some of the ways
which have been mentioned in previous Reports, by means of the air-
douche in some of its forms or by paracentesis of the drum-membrane ;
but when the secretion is thick and viscid its removal is always difficult
and often impossible by any of these methods.

In the last Report[1] a method of Gruber's was described, by which he
sucked out the exudation from the tympanum by means of a syringe,
the point of which was inserted into the cavity through a perforation of
the drum-membrane. The same method of evacuation had been previously used by Weber-Liel, without, however, any injury of the drum-
membrane, by inserting through the ordinary Eustachian catheter a
small elastic catheter which could be passed fully into the tympanic cavity,
and through which he claimed that the exudation could be withdrawn by
suction. Politzer[2] now gives his experience of the use of this flexible
tympanic catheter in movable exudations, and concludes that, in cases
in which the secretion is thin and limpid, the evacuation of the tym-

---

[1] JOURNAL, xcii. 590, May 20, 1875.

[2] Wiener medicinische Wochenschrift, No. 15, 1875.

42

panum is accomplished more thoroughly by paracentesis of the drum-membrane than by suction through the tympanic catheter, as the entrance of the Eustachian tube is at the upper portion of the tympanum, while the fluid lies in the lower portion of the cavity, and consequently the tympanic catheter can at the best reach and withdraw only the upper portion of the fluid. He says, however, that by inclining the patient's head in such a position that the Eustachian tube is perpendicular, that is, bending the head forward and toward the opposite side, the fluid flows toward the tympanic orifice of the Eustachian tube, and can be withdrawn much more completely ; in this position of the head he has, in some cases, been able to get a thorough evacuation of the cavity by means of the tympanic catheter. When the exudation is very viscid he has found the tympanic catheter of great service in evacuating the tympanum after paracentesis of the drum-membrane had been performed. In some cases, he says, the secretion was so viscid that not only did no evacuation follow paracentesis, but the air-douche by means of the common catheter was insufficient to force out any of the secretion ; by inserting the tympanic catheter fully into the tympanum, however, and then injecting the air, he was able, by means of the gradual increasing air-pressure, to effect a thorough evacution.

(*To be concluded.*)

———◆———

PROCEEDINGS OF THE BOSTON SOCIETY FOR MEDICAL OBSERVATION.

EDWARD WIGGLESWORTH, JR., M. D., SECRETARY.

JUNE 21, 1875.   *Treatment of Diarrhœa in Young Children.* — DR. J. P. OLIVER read the regular paper of the evening, his subject being the treatment of diarrhœa in young children. The paper has been published in full in the JOURNAL of July 8, 1875.

DR. ELLIS referred to the difference in coagulability between the casein of the milk of the cow and that of woman. When pure casein of each sort is treated by artificial digesting fluids, that from woman's milk dissolves readily, or with a little acetic acid; that from the cow's slowly. Goat's milk also coagulates too firmly. The best milks are the rarest, such as mare's milk. Dr. Ellis approved of gelatine with milk under certain circumstances, and also of Liebig's food, provided it is very accurately prepared.

DR. PORTER highly approved of Robinson's prepared barley for small children. This should be boiled twenty-five minutes before the milk is added.

DR. VOGEL stated that gelatine, with or without milk, was much used in Germany, especially in dysentery, and that the action of coagulating fluids was the same upon boiled and unboiled milk.

DR. C. P. PUTNAM said he considered the flour or meal of pease as quite nutritive. The coagulum of cream formed soon after milking is soft; that formed later is harder and less digestible. Bismuth with chloral hydrate every two hours often improves the condition of the bowels, but may interfere with the appetite. Dr. Putnam approved of Liebig's food. Six ounces of boiled pap is changed by half an ounce of digestive fluid into a liquid nearly as thin as vinegar, showing that much starch must have been converted into dextrine. In constipation, Liebig's food at night will often procure a natural discharge in the morning, and the amount need never be increased. When the mother's milk is scanty, Liebig's food is especially valuable as an adjuvant. As to the fact that Dr. Oliver had seen children gain when fed upon cream and barley, whereas they had not gained while using Liebig's food, it is true that children while gaining strength and health do not accumulate necessarily much fat, and in such cases a little oil or cream may be added ; or, when the digestion has become normal, other food may be substituted. Condensed milk answers in some cases, but often contains too much sugar.

Conservative Surgery. — DR. WARREN exhibited the cast of a foot upon which he had recently operated. By the falling of a weight the first, second, and third metatarsal bones had been destroyed, the distal ends of the tarsal bones injured, the joint opened, and the skin removed from the tarsus behind the metatarsal bone of the great toe. In opposition to Chopart and Lisfranc, Bryant says, " Save all you can ; " and in accordance with this advice the three metatarsal bones alone had been removed, leaving the two outer toes. The result had been very good.

Ovariotomy. — DR. CHADWICK then read a paper upon ovariotomy.[1]

Simulation of Bronchial Respiration. — DR. ELLIS referred to a statement made by him some months before in regard to the simulation of bronchial respiration. He spoke of the well-recognized fact that bronchial respiration may be transmitted from the throat, but it was also thought to originate in the bronchi. He was convinced, however, that the passage of air through the healthy bronchi never gave rise to such a sound. If care were taken during a full and rapid inspiration to avoid the production of any sound in the nares, pharynx, or larynx, no sound would be heard over the trachea or larger bronchi, where the so-called tracheal or bronchial respiration was very distinct when produced in the parts above.

It is so difficult to breathe without causing the vibration of the parts mentioned, that great care must be taken. Ordinary hospital patients with low intelligence seem to be incapable of doing it, and this difficulty is increased by those forms of thoracic disease which give us an opportunity to test the accuracy of the statement. Moreover, a third person is necessary to listen carefully at the mouth of the one who is breathing to be sure that no sound is produced there. To prevent such sound the walls of the external air-passages must be perfectly immovable.

A patient with chronic catarrhal pneumonia of the right apex, in whom there was the so-called bronchial respiration, was requested to inflate the chest and then remain perfectly immovable. At the moment when the chest was at rest, air was forced through a glass tube against the soft palate, producing a

[1] Vide JOURNAL of July 22, 1875.

blowing sound, which was heard as bronchial respiration by a person whose ear was applied to the chest.

If further experiments verify the views advanced, it will be shown that bronchial respiration is a sound conducted from the parts above the trachea in the same way as the voice, modified or intensified by the media through which it may pass.

DR. LANGMAID alluded to the fact that the bones of the head vibrate greatly, and advantage is taken of this to get harmonic notes in which the trachea, etc., take no part.

Ice-Bags in Croup and Diphtheria. — DR. C. P. PUTNAM spoke of the value of bags of ice applied to the neck in croup and diphtheria. These should be made of thin India-rubber by means of a cement of the same, and provided with stop-cocks to let off the air coming from the interstices of the ice. They should be narrow across the neck in front, and possess ears for the attachment of tapes. Such bags, of various shapes, may be employed also for many other purposes, and may be constructed upon the spot, if necessary. Dr. Putnam had noticed no depressing effects from their use, and for superficial inflammations preferred them to the jacket poultice. In the sore throat of scarlet fever he had found them to cause great relief as to symptoms, though he would not assert any change in the morbid processes from their use.

OCTOBER 4, 1875. *Diphtheria.* — DR. WHITTIER read a paper upon diphtheria.[1]

DR. KNIGHT mentioned some cases under the charge of Dr. Bowen, of Philadelphia, which recovered after the inhalation of sulphurous acid, while other cases in the same family, not so treated, died.

DR. MINOT said he thought that the topical use of nitrate of silver was at present condemned by many physicians of high standing. For himself, he believed in local applications, but preferred the salts of iron to those of silver. He had seen benefit from a dilute solution of muriatic acid applied by means of a swab. Permanganate of potassium also gives little discomfort, relieves fetor, and apparently promotes convalescence. The use of ice-bags is approved of by every one.

DR. INCHES said that the records of the temperature should always be carefully kept. He considered them of much value, they often even assisting in the diagnosis. Wet packs he held were of great benefit in the treatment. His favorite topical application was oxalic acid, eight grains to the ounce. He believed tracheotomy at times contra-indicated, and he had seen cases in which the cut surface became an ulcer.

DR. WHITTIER repeated that in his opinion tracheotomy was called for whenever asphyxia set in. Life might be saved, and it was our duty to try all measures for that end.

DR. WEBBER remarked that the mere relief to the patient, and perhaps even more to the friends around, was sufficient warrant for the operation.

DR. CHADWICK recalled twenty-three cases of tracheotomy performed for croup at the Massachusetts General Hospital. The average age of the cases which recovered was five years; of the cases in which the operation failed, two

[1] Vide JOURNAL of November 11, 1875.

and a half years. He thought that the operation was rarely, if ever, successful with children of two years of age or less.

Dr. Webber alluded to the question of drainage and sewerage as bearing upon diphtheria.

Dr. Stedman had never known tracheotomy to succeed upon a child less than three years of age. He had known of an epidemic of diphtheria in Dorchester in which drainage certainly could have played no part.

Dr. Jeffries spoke of two cases, interesting as bearing upon the question of contagion. At a home for children, a child convalescent from measles showed signs of diphtheria. No other sick child caught it, but one of the strongest and healthiest took it and died in about fifty hours. The other cases of measles were not affected by the diphtheria, but ran a normal course.

Dr. Minot related the case of a physician who threw off some eight inches of membrane like the finger of a glove. Some time subsequently he died suddenly, without warning. There was no opportunity for tracheotomy. Membrane was found below the glottis, and his death was attributed to strangulation, the piece dropping back after death.

Dr. Fitz referred to cases of embolus, paralysis of the heart, etc., which might cause death suddenly. He was inclined to doubt the propriety of attributing the death to suffocation from the presence of membrane in cases where none was found in the larynx. In cases of suffocation from pieces of meat partially swallowed and catching in the larynx, lividity remained after death.

Dr. Norton Folsom stated that he had seen cases of suicide by hanging in which either lividity or pallor was present.

Dr. Bolles remarked that where pallor was present the neck was found unbroken.

Diaphragmatic Hernia in a Child. — Dr. C. P. Putnam showed a specimen of diaphragmatic hernia in a child. The case will be published.

Cancer of the Rectum and of the Liver. — Dr. Bolles exhibited a cancer of the rectum, causing stricture and accompanied by cancer of the liver. Two years ago the only symptom had been persistent diarrhœa, which had since continued, the discharges recently numbering from six to twenty daily. Hæmorrhoids also existed. Before death there had been great pain in the right side and a pleuritic rub (to and fro sound) at the lower border of the lung on the right side, together with rapid, hitching respiration and high pulse. The rubbing of the liver against the wall of the upper part of the abdomen resembled closely the rubbing of a lung.

Urinary Calculus. — Dr. Porter showed a urinary calculus. P. P., aged three and a half years, was scalded two years since by the upsetting of a tea-kettle over his thighs and genitals. Since recovery he had been greatly troubled by dribbling of urine, and at times by stoppage of the stream. The symptoms have been more troublesome during the last three months. A metallic sound showed to the finger and to the ear a calculus in the bladder.

August 1st. The calculus was removed, under ether, by lateral lithotomy. A chemise catheter was passed through the wound into the bladder for the passage of urine, and hæmorrhage was checked chiefly by means of sponges packed about the canula. Few ligatures were applied.

August 13th. Twelfth day after the operation, the patient passed about half an ounce of urine through the urethra.

August 16th. Urine passed wholly by the urethra, the wound not being moistened.

The thirty-fourth day after the operation the patient was discharged, well. The calculus weighed twenty-four grains. It was oval in shape, and measured five eighths by one half by five sixteenths of an inch.

Colloid Cancer of all the Abdominal Organs. — DR. PORTER showed also a colloid cancer of all the organs in the abdomen. It originated from the ovaries, and the whole peritoneum was covered by small colloid cysts.

DR. FITZ spoke of this as a rare form. It was an alveolar cancer, composed of a fibrous stroma full of sage granules.

Salivary Calculus. — DR. PORTER then exhibited a salivary calculus. For two years a woman forty-two years old had noticed a tumor of her neck occupying the submaxillary triangle, and about the size of a horse-chestnut. It could be felt also in the mouth, and had been accompanied by pain for about three weeks. The tumor, on section, proved to be a hypertrophy of the submaxillary gland, and in its centre there was a small salivary calculus in a cavity containing pus.

Plans for Hospitals. — DR. NORTON FOLSOM showed plans for the new Johns Hopkins Hospital in Baltimore, and took occasion to speak of the evils in the construction of various existing hospitals: in regard to absence of ventilation and light, for instance, also with reference to the existence of "shoots" for dirty clothes. He referred to the necessity that the medical profession should look after matters which hospital boards are apt to neglect. He then read Mr. Hopkins's letters, which he regarded as models. The plans will be published in full in New York by the trustees of the Johns Hopkins Hospital, of Baltimore.

MEDICAL NOTES.

— At a recent meeting of the Clinical Society of London, Mr. Callender reported his experience in the use of salicylic acid as a dressing for wounds. He concludes that it is of value because it is odorless, and because wounds heal under its influence usually without local pain. Above a strength of two per cent. of the acid a solution acts as a local irritant and causes constitutional disturbance. It gives rise to more discharge than carbolic acid does, and its influence on a recent wound is not so efficacious against the occurrence of decomposition as is that of carbolic acid, chloride of zinc, or boracic acid. The repair of the wound is less active and the granulations are more flabby than when other simple or antiseptic dressings are employed. Mr. Callender therefore regards it as inferior to other antiseptic agents now employed.

— Gelseminum sempervirens as a remedy for cough is advocated by Dr. J. R. Thompson in the *British Medical Journal* of October 16, 1875. He has administered it recently to a large number of patients suffering from pulmonary disease (as, for example, chronic phthisis) as a cough sedative. The tincture is given in five-minim doses. When much bronchial irritation existed he has combined it with bromide of ammonium, tincture of squills, and syrup of codeia. He claims that his results show that gelseminum has a marked power in subduing cough, that it acts probably as a nervous sedative, that it is useful when other sedatives have failed, that it seldom produces any unpleasant general effect, and that the kinds of cough in which it may be administered with advantage are very varied.

— The use of nitrite of amyl in nervous headache is recommended by R. A. Douglas-Lithgow, in the *Lancet* of October 16, 1875. The writer's method is to place two drops on the palm of the patient's hand, and quickly diffusing them with the finger over the palmar surface, the patient immediately covers the mouth and nose with the hand, and inspires deeply and quietly. The patient should be seated while inhaling, as the peculiar effects of the remedy are produced almost instantaneously, and may occasionally alarm a nervous and hysterical female. These symptoms last but a short time, and with their cessation the pain almost invariably ceases. Two drops of the remedy may be given as a draught in water instead of by inhalation, but the results of the latter method are far more satisfactory.

Some of the symptoms which may occur during the inhalation of the amyl are, in addition to the invariable flushing of the face, great throbbing in the temples, "fluttering of the heart," and a feeling of breathlessness, as if one was "dying away." Some describe a sensation of "tingling from head to foot," and others have experienced pains in the limbs analogous to cramp, while in other cases objects seem to acquire a bright yellow hue, such as sometimes results from the use of santonine. The severer symptoms are, however, by no means common. The writer has never seen any serious results from the administration of the remedy which he recommends, but he thinks that, owing to the temporary palpitation of the heart produced in most patients, care should be taken in administering it in cases of organic cardiac disease.

— In a lecture on deodorizers and disinfectants, delivered by Dr. John Day to the members of the School of Science at Geelong, and reported in the *Medical Times and Gazette*, the lecturer stated that the great value of peroxide of hydrogen as a deodorizer was only just beginning to be understood. Dr. Day has discovered the presence of the agent, spontaneously generated, in a vast number of substances in daily use, such as all fats and fatty or expressed oils; nearly all perfumes; most, if not all, essential oils; kerosene, gasoline, and benzine, and deal and pine woods. In many respects gasoline is the best disinfectant with which he is acquainted. In addition to being highly volatile, it possesses the property either of generating peroxide of hydrogen, or of originally forming it and storing it up until brought into contact with any of those oxidizable substances for which it has an affinity. One of these two actions, he could not say which, takes place long after all the gasoline has passed away. When unglazed paper, or any porous substance, is brushed over with gasoline, it will at once give the reaction of peroxide of hydrogen, and continue to do so for a year or more. It is thus persistent in its action, which gives it an immense value over other disinfectants. He recommends that books, newspapers, and the like, which have been used by fever patients or kept in their apartments, be disinfected by brushing them over with gasoline. The most delicate wall-paper may be brushed over with it without injury, as may also articles of wearing apparel. The hands may be disinfected by brushing them over with the same agent and allowing them to dry in the air. The only drawback to its use is its inflammability.

— The following method of making and using pancreatic enemata is given by Dr. R. Fiechtner, of Basel. For an adult from two hundred to four hundred grammes should be used for an injection ; two thirds of this should consist of beef and one third of pancreas. The beef and pancreas must be quite fresh, free from fat and skin, and intimately mixed together ; a little warm water, under 39° C. (102.2° F.), is added. The enema should be administered by means of a strong syringe. If a common clyster syringe is used, a long elastic tube, or better still a stomach-pump tube, should be attached. By means of this the injection can be propelled far up without the risk of injuring the gut. In the author's cases the tube is always introduced to the extent of eighteen inches. The further the enema reaches the greater will be the extent of the absorbing surface, and the greater the rapidity of its absorption. Before resorting to the operation the bowel should be well cleaned out by an ordinary injection of water.

— The case of sudden death following thoracentesis reported by Dr. Legroux, and referred to on page 286 of the JOURNAL of September 2, 1875, has been the subject of an extended report of a committee to which it was referred by the Société Médicale des Hôpitaux. The paper may be found in full in *L' Union Médicale* of October 14 and 16, 1875. M. Legroux attributed the death of his patient to syncope resulting from cerebral anæmia, but the committee think that we are to attribute the fatal result to congestion of the lung, which, though not very intense, was sufficient to cause death. Undoubtedly the congestion existed prior to the operation, and this procedure is to be wholly exonerated from the catastrophe. The thoracentesis did not hasten the death of the patient ; it was powerless to prevent it.

— A fatal case of hydrophobia treated by jaborandi is reported in *Le Progrès Médical* of September 11, 1875. The case is chiefly of interest because of the cerebral lesions which were found at the autopsy. The cerebral meninges were healthy in appearance. The brain itself to the naked eye showed nothing abnormal except rather numerous puncta vasculosa. The other parts of the encephalon, namely, the medulla oblongata, the pons Varolii, and the cerebellum, were carefully examined after several days' maceration in Müller's fluid, and reported upon by M. Gombault. A marked alteration was found in the blood-vessels, which consisted in a considerable accumulation of leucocytes in the lymphatic sheath of the vessels. At some points these leucocytes were sufficiently numerous to completely conceal the vessel, and in some places to distend its sheath ; in others, on the contrary, the white globules, less numerous, were disposed in two parallel rows on each side of the blood-vessel. Here and there, at the bifurcation of the vessels, they formed round or fusiform masses. The accumulation of leucocytes in the perivascular sheaths was far from uniform in the different parts of the organs examined. The vessels of the cerebellum, of its pia mater and nervous substance, appeared absolutely healthy, and in the anterior part of the medulla and pons they were found in only a portion of the preparations. They were most numerous at the level of the floor of the fourth ventricle, especially at its inferior part and at the barbs of the calamus scriptorius.

M. Jeffroy remarked that the cauterization to which the patient had been subjected immediately after she was bitten by the dog could not have been very energetic, since it did not prevent the supervention of hydrophobia. He further said that he had at one time opportunity to examine the nervous centres of two individuals who died from this disease, and they presented lesions quite similar to those of the case just reported, although they were not so localized. The pia mater was much congested, especially on the convexity of the cerebrum ; all the capillaries were congested, a great number of red and white corpuscles were extravasated into the perivascular sheaths and into the meshes of the pia mater, without there having been a veritable hæmorrhage. The pons and medulla in their entire thickness and in the gray substance of the convolutions were likewise much congested.

M. Charcot said that as M. Gombault had only the pons and the medulla at his disposal to examine, and as the meninges were not sent to him, we ought not perhaps to attach too much importance to the localization of the lesions in the case under discussion.

— Dr. P. Aubert advocates, in the *Lyon Médicale* of October 17, 1875, the employment of nitrate of silver followed by metallic zinc as a means of cauterization. The method of application is to touch the surface to be cauterized first with the nitrate of silver, either in the form of a crayon or of a concentrated solution of the salt, and then directly afterwards to rub over the same surface a crayon of well scraped metallic zinc. Immediately the part touched becomes of a beautiful black color. It is claimed for this procedure that as a method of cauterization it is more efficacious than when the nitrate of silver is employed alone, owing to the action of the nitrate of zinc which is formed ; and that it is well worth our endeavor to try to substitute directly the nitrate of zinc, pure or mitigated, for the nitrate of silver, this last salt being expensive and soiling the articles with which it comes in contact.

— M. Laroyenne, of Lyons, calls attention to the employment of the actual cautery in tissues that have been rendered bloodless by Esmarch's method. The effects of the cautery are much more marked than when the circulation of the tissues is normal, and it is very easy in their anæmic state to destroy fungosities and to affect the tissues deeply. It is only when the rubber band is removed that the results of the cautery can be properly estimated.

"MYSTERIOUS (?) DISEASE."

Messrs. Editors, — I have recently investigated a case of "mysterious disease," and the inquiry has brought out so many facts illustrative of the dangers to which many of us who live in Boston are exposed, that I send them to you in brief.

Mr. —— lives on the slope of a hill about twenty feet higher than the level of its base, in the farther half of a double house. The neighborhood is a favorable one to health, and the occupants of the houses·are intelligent and of the upper class. Mr. —— himself has read much of the so-called sanitary literature of the day, and is a gentleman of wide general information.

There have been three cases of severe illness in his house ; one (fatal) of diphtheria, one of scarlet fever, and one of typhoid fever, all occurring at nearly the same time. In the last case, the patient had slept in the adjoining half of the house on account of the diphtheria in his own half, and was taken ill immediately upon his return home.[1] There was also one case of typhoid fever in the house directly opposite.

These cases all occurred before the recent impurities in the Cochituate water had been observed, and the three houses referred to are the only ones connected with the sewer running down the street on which they are situated.

External to them, there is some low land upon which one case of typhoid fever occurred; but I think that the influences which might produce disease there were too remote to affect the houses which we are now considering.

Mr. ——'s house is well-built and there are many arrangements for ventilation, etc., which show that the owner has thought of and tried to provide everything that is necessary to promote the health of the inmates. The faults of construction are many. Upon careful examination of the furnace, it was found that the heated air supplied to the dining-room during the day (from which it was shut off to warm the entry on the second floor at night) really came from the cellar and not from the external atmosphere. The air of the cellar, too, was liable to two sources of contamination beside the ordinary ones : first, the house-drain passed directly under its floor, and secondly, the floor of the vegetable-cellar, although well cemented, was four feet lower than the level of the water in a catch-basin for the surface-drainage in the yard, at a distance of only ten feet from the wall. (This catch-basin has since then been made as impervious as cement will make it.) The house-drain is very liable to be obstructed by grease, the sink having the ordinary bell-trap, with a " goose neck " in the leaden pipe in the cellar. The drain was of glazed earthenware. The water-closet in the cellar was entirely unventilated except by a small window, which is closed during the winter months. The water-closet in the second story was in the centre of the house and entirely unconnected with the external air except by a square wooden "ventilating shaft" running from the ceiling out through the roof. The soil-pipe had not been continued to the roof, and there was no ventilation in the proper sense of the word. In the back entry, there was a window in the roof, which served for ventilation in fair weather. The stairway leading up to the third story formed a direct channel of communication from the furnace-register, from the water-closet, and from a wash-basin, also in the entry, to the chamber where the most severe illness occurred, while a more indirect line existed from the water-closet in the basement up the back stairs, the heated and lighter gases following a natural law to reach the highest point accessible. The chamber in which the less severe cases occurred were subject to the same influences, but

---

[1] The ordinary period of incubation of typhoid fever is from five to eight days when the specific poison is conveyed through the lungs, and somewhat longer (probably from eight to twenty days) if introduced into the stomach.

to a less degree, as they were on the second story and therefore not so high. The water from the roof was discharged into the sewer by trapped pipes. A sewer about six hundred feet long and at a steep grade had been built in 1869 from the main sewer on —— Street and ending opposite Mr. ——'s house *without a manhole or any means for inspecting or flushing,* not even the water from the streets serving the latter purpose. The main sewer on —— Street, too, joined another from —— Street, which latter conveyed a large amount of sewage of an especially putrescible character from a large establishment near by. Added to this, the two manholes at the two points of junction referred to had large catch-basins underneath them and in the bottom of the sewer, which were always necessarily full of the worst kind of sewage; and, as if that were not sufficient, the sewers at this (the lowest) point, in case even of such a moderate rain as we had a few weeks ago, were entirely inadequate to carry off what was put into them, and sewage was actually forced into the adjoining houses through the water-closets (*not* those in the cellars.) At this low junction is the bulb of the retort where the gases are manufactured, free to pass up its neck into the three houses, that in which the most illness occurred being at the very top.

It is easy to see that an elevation of two degrees of temperature within the sewers, or a heavy rainfall, will cause a pressure which no traps or series of traps can resist. Had it not been that one, the lowest, of the houses had connected its rainwater spouts with the sewer without traps (an arrangement which is often not without serious objections, but in this case one of the best things that could have been done, as it served to protect in a measure three houses) the results would probably have been even much worse than they were.

I was asked what should be done. There certainly was a complication of evils. No matter how carefully these gentlemen used their wealth and intelligence to perfect the sanitary arrangements of their own houses, there was a condition of things external to them and which they were utterly powerless to remedy, which, to say the least, it was not pleasant to look in the face.

C. F. F.

BOSTON, *October* 30, 1875.

WEEKLY BULLETIN OF PREVALENT DISEASES.

THE following is a bulletin of the diseases prevalent in Massachusetts during the week ending November 13, 1875, compiled under the authority of the State Board of Health from the returns of physicians representing all sections of the State: —

The summary for each section is as follows: —

Berkshire: Influenza, typhoid fever, bronchitis.

Valley: Influenza, typhoid fever, rheumatism, bronchitis.   Springfield and Greenfield report diphtheria.

Midland: Bronchitis, influenza, typhoid fever.   Athol reports a case of meningitis.

Northeastern: Typhoid fever, influenza. Less sickness. Diphtheria has increased somewhat.

Metropolitan: Bronchitis, diphtheria, pneumonia, scarlatina, rheumatism. Diphtheria continues to prevail, but it has not increased since last week, if we may judge by the mortality and by the number of physicians reporting its prevalence.

Southeastern: Typhoid fever, bronchitis, scarlatina, and pneumonia more prevalent. Very little sickness.

In the State at large the prevailing diseases are bronchitis, typhoid fever, rheumatism, influenza, diphtheria, pneumonia, and scarlatina. Typhoid fever is most prevalent in the western sections ; diphtheria and scarlatina in Boston and its suburbs. F. W. DRAPER, M. D., Registrar.

COMPARATIVE MORTALITY-RATES FOR THE WEEK ENDING NOV. 6, 1875.

	Estimated Population.	Total Mortality for the Week.	Annual Death-Rate per 1000 during Week.
New York	1,060,000	455	22
Philadelphia	800,000	271	17
Brooklyn	500,000	245	25
Chicago	400,000	110	15
Boston	342.000	148	22
Cincinnati	260,000	106	21
Providence	100,700	38	19
Worcester	50,000	16	17
Lowell	50,000	19	20
Cambridge . . .	48,000	18	19
Fall River	45,000	13	15
Lawrence	35,000	12	18
Lynn	33,000	13	20
Springfield	31,000	10	17
Salem	26,000	7	14

Normal Death-Rate, 17 per 1000.

APPOINTMENTS. — By General Order No. 15, Series of 1875, A. G. O., Assistant Surgeon Robert Amory, First Battalion Light Artillery, M. V. M., is appointed a member of the Board of Medical Officers, organized by General Order No. 23, A. G. O., Series of 1874, to fill the vacancy caused by the resignation and honorable discharge of B. Joy Jeffries, Surgeon First Corps Cadets. As junior member of the board, he will act as recorder.

Dr. William L. Richardson, appointed Surgeon First Corps Cadets, *vice* Jeffries, resigned and discharged, passed a successful examination before the Board of Medical Officers, M. V. M., November 11, 1875. ROBERT AMORY,

Assistant Surgeon First Battalion Light Artillery M. V. M., Recorder of Board.

THE BOSTON
MEDICAL AND SURGICAL JOURNAL.

VOL. XCIII. — THURSDAY, NOVEMBER 25, 1875. — NO. 22.

SHALL WE REVACCINATE? [1]

BY FRANCIS F. BROWN, M. D., OF READING.

IN the JOURNAL for January 14, 1875, are statements by the honored president of the Massachusetts Medical Society in regard to revaccination, which, while not absolutely condemning the practice, are decidedly unfavorable to it. Dr. Cotting would " prefer the risk of variola to the chances of the dangerous inflammations and septic affections frequently developed by revaccination.' The *exceptional possibility of really taking vaccine disease a second time* (as any other disease is sometimes so taken) is the only justifiable reason for revaccinating any one. This liability is less than is generally admitted. In the thousands of revaccinations witnessed in others' practice and his own, he had never seen in such revaccinations more than half a dozen vesicles, if as many, which, the history untold, would be mistaken for vesicles of first vaccination." [2]

If I understand rightly, then, Dr. Cotting has seen no more than half a dozen cases of revaccination in his life-time which conferred any protection. From this it appears that, in Dr. Cotting's opinion, in those only who have had the vaccine disease the second time, as shown by the second vaccination running through the regular stages of the first, that is to say, in perhaps one case in a thousand, is the operation of any benefit whatever, while in the other nine hundred and ninety-nine it is worse than useless. " The injury," he says, " thus incurred by revaccination is beyond computation; it frequently impairs health for years or a life-time." Dr. Cotting, however, does not absolutely refuse to revaccinate, but he does not advise it, with this exception: after all the stages of a primary operation are passed, within say six months, he proposes it as a test of the first. If the probabilities of benefit are so slight as he states, and the dangers so great, we may properly inquire whether this test, even, is justifiable. Is a revaccination at the end of six months attended with any less danger than it is twenty years afterwards ?

[1] Read before the East Middlesex District Medical Society.
[2] This accords with my own observation.

The charges here made against this practice are two, namely, —

(1.) That it is dangerous.

(2.) That it is with rare exceptions useless.

I. That dangers do occasionally attend this operation is well known. Dr. Cotting writes that " the ' accidental revaccination ' was a serious matter to me. My arm has not yet recovered from the effects of it. A moderate varioloid would have been less damaging." Experience shows that " severe constitutional symptoms are out of all proportion more frequent in revaccination than in primary vaccination." Erysipelas sometimes follows; rarely, pyæmia and death. A fatal case was reported in the JOURNAL of May 29, 1873. The virus was from the patient's own child, a healthy one, but the patient's wife thought that the crust, which was used, was a secondary one, the original having been rubbed off. Whether this vaccination was performed by a physician is not stated. Dr. Ayer[1] had had a similar case, recovering after four weeks. But primary vaccination is not always free from similar unfortunate results. In the same connection Dr. Fifield reported a case of a child who died in two weeks from the effects of a primary vaccination. In the JOURNAL of January 23, 1873, are reported two fatal cases of vaccination; but whether primary or secondary is not stated.[2]

That revaccination frequently impairs health for years or a life-time is a rather startling assertion. It is a matter of regret that so sweeping a charge as this, as well as others in this report, is not sustained by some proof. Inquiry among the members of this society fails to discover anything to substantiate it. A not very extended examination of the literature of the subject leads me to the conclusion that the experience of the profession generally is like our own. If this is a delusion of ours it ought to be dispelled. We want the facts.

Making due allowance for all the possible dangers of the practice, I think it can be shown that they are not a hundredth part as great as those arising from its neglect. I doubt whether a thorough search can find a dozen fatalities due to revaccination during the last twenty years. On the other hand, the deaths from small-pox of those who trusted to a single vaccination amounted in Boston alone, during the epidemic of 1872–73, to several hundred. Moreover, the facts go to show that most of these deaths would have been prevented by timely revaccination.

II. Is revaccination, with infrequent exceptions, useless; that is, does it confer additional protection only on something like one in a thousand? If that is the case, statistics ought to show that the frequency and fatality of varioloid is nearly as great among the revaccinated as

[1] Loc. cit.

[2] I have lately learned that they were *revaccinations*.

among those vaccinated only once. The only figures that I have seen that at all seem to support this view are those in the report of Dr. Webb on the late epidemic of small-pox in Boston, which give the percentage of deaths in the hospitals of the vaccinated once as 19.55 and of the revaccinated as 17.85. There were six hundred and ninety cases of the former, however, and of the latter eighty-four, less than one eighth as many. This would at first sight seem to show that the mortality was nearly equal in the two cases *among those attacked*, but that the revaccinated had much less *liability* to the disease. But inferences from these figures are worthless, for two reasons : (1) We do not know the numbers in the two classes exposed to the contagion ; (2) the figures themselves are unreliable. Dr. Webb tells me that the only information as to the revaccinations of these patients was derived from the statements of the patients themselves ; so that what sort of a revaccination these eighty-four got, how many of the operations were successful, how many were performed after exposure to contagion of small-pox, and so on, we know nothing about ; we know only that these patients were said to be revaccinated. Moreover, I am informed by Dr. Webb that among persons known to be successfully revaccinated small-pox was extremely rare.

All other facts and statistics which I have seen support the view in which nearly all the highest authorities are agreed, namely, " that the liability to a subsequent attack of small-pox is almost incalculably diminished by revaccination." [1] Dr. Marson,[2] of London, who has had during the last thirty years fifteen thousand cases under his personal care, a majority of which, by the way, were post-vaccinial, states that " but very few patients have been admitted with small-pox into the small-pox hospital who stated that they had been revaccinated with effect ; and that those few have had small-pox in a very mild form." . . . " For just upon thirty years we have revaccinated all the nurses and servants, who had not had small-pox, on their coming to live at the small-pox hospital, and not one of them has contracted small-pox during his stay there." . . . " At a time when a large number of work people were employed for several months about the hospital, most of whom consented to be revaccinated, two only were attacked by small-pox, and these two were amongst the few who were not revaccinated."

In Würtemberg, in five years, there occurred among fourteen thousand three hundred and eighty-four revaccinated soldiers only one instance of varioloid, and only one among thirty thousand revaccinated civilians ; while in the same country, during the same years, there were sixteen hundred and seventy-four cases of modified and unmodified small-pox ; so that the escape of these forty-five thousand from contagion was not from want of exposure.

[1] Dr. West.
[2] Reynolds, System of Medicine, i. 209.   .

In the Prussian army, since the introduction of systematic revaccination, the annual deaths from small-pox, which at one time were one hundred and four, have not averaged more than two; and on analysis of the forty fatal cases that occurred in twenty years it appeared that only four were in persons who were said to have been successfully revaccinated.[1]

Since 1843 [2] " revaccination has been compulsory in the Bavarian army; since that date absolutely no cases of variola have occurred; while of cases of varioloid which from time to time appear, though in small numbers, there has not within this period occurred a single death."

" For twenty-one years [3] revaccination has been general in the Danish army, and for thirteen years in the Danish navy, and these two populations have almost entirely escaped contagion during several epidemics of small-pox. The practice of Sweden has been similar, and its results satisfactory."

In the report of the Board of Health of Philadelphia for 1872,[4] Dr. William H. Welsh, physician in charge of the Municipal Hospital, says, " Among twenty-three hundred and seventy-seven cases of small-pox admitted during the epidemic ' (sixteen hundred and twenty-nine of which were post-vaccinial), " only thirty-six are said to have been revaccinated, and of these four died. But by subjecting these cases to a careful analysis, we find as follows : seventeen were revaccinated at a distant period, some as far back as thirty-one years; five had not been revaccinated until after exposure; seven were said to have been successfully revaccinated but were unable to exhibit any cicatrices as the result; sixteen bore upon their arms very poor and uncharacteristic scars, some of which were scarcely visible; five presented fair cicatrices, and only three were able to show good cicatrices. Of the four cases which died, two occurred among those without cicatrices, one among those revaccinated after exposure, and one among those showing poor and uncharacteristic scars." All the cases which bore on their arms unmistakable evidence of successful revaccination suffered from the mildest possible form of the disease. Indeed, in three of the thirty-six it was doubtful whether the eruption was that of varioloid at all. (Notice that after taking out those revaccinated at a remote period and those revaccinated after exposure, we have left only fourteen cases after revaccination against sixteen hundred and twenty-nine cases after a single vaccination.) " Not a single person connected with the hospital who had been revaccinated contracted the disease; while on the other hand some three or four of the nurses who had

---

[1] Simon. Papers on Vaccination, pages 35 and 36.
[2] Ditto (published in 1857), page 170.
[3] Ditto, page 36.
[4] Page 80.

been affected by small-pox previously took the disease the second time."

Dr. Edward H. Janes[1] is authority for the following statements: " We shall find nothing more fallacious than the attempt to establish an invariable rule that vaccination will protect the system from variolous poison during a certain number of years." From March 20, 1871, to March 20, 1872, there were in New York city three hundred and thirty-seven cases of varioloid in children under five years of age, one hundred and thirteen of whom showed marks of vaccination. "Since this practice (revaccination) was adopted no case of small-pox has occurred among those who were revaccinated immediately after exposure to the contagion." And positive protection, he says, was afforded to all by the operation.

The following statements are from Dr. E. C. Seaton's last annual report to the local government board : [2] " The observations which were made during the recent epidemic afforded remarkable evidence of the value of revaccination, not merely in controlling the mortality from small-pox, but usually in preventing altogether the occurrence of the disease." " In every hospital report which has reached me, it is specially stated that not a single one of those officials (attendants in the hospitals in the Metropolitan Asylum district, amounting at one time to more than three hundred) who had been revaccinated before coming to take duty at the hospital contracted small-pox." On the other hand, a few cases of the disease occurred in nurses or servants who were not revaccinated ; one case was that of a nurse who had had small-pox previously, and one very modified case occurred in a nurse whose revaccination was not performed till after exposure to the infection. " The cases of small-pox which were admitted for treatment in the several hospitals in persons who had been successfully revaccinated were very few and very slight. In the hospitals of the Metropolitan Asylum Board, in which upwards of fourteen thousand eight hundred cases of small-pox were treated, there were but four cases in which there was good evidence of revaccination having been performed with effect, and those were all light cases. In Liverpool, says Dr. Trench, revaccination was found a constant and perfect protection against the small-pox. In the Newcastle-on-Tyne small-pox hospital, in which seven hundred and seventy-eight cases were treated, there were two in which revaccination was alleged to have been successfully performed (but without mention whether there were marks of such revaccination or not), one of them ten years and the other four years before the attack of small-pox ; both recovered. Into the same hospital eight patients were admitted who stated that they had had small-pox before ; five of

---

[1] Public Health Reports, 1873, i., pages 176, 177, and 178.
[2] Public Health : a Journal of Sanitary Science and Progress. London, October 2, 1875.

these were distinctly marked by it ; one of the three not marked died, the remaining seven recovered.

" In the Leeds Hospital there were four cases in which previous revaccination was alleged ; but in none of them was the evidence of revaccination conclusive. One of them, in which the revaccination was said to have been done at seven years of age, was fatal ; the other three cases were mild. There were three (fatal) cases of small-pox in persons believed to have had small-pox previously, but the evidence of the former small-pox is not stated. Similar infrequency and mildness of small-pox after revaccination was noted in the hospitals abroad. In the municipal small-pox hospital at Berlin, in which fifteen hundred and twenty-nine cases were treated in persons who had been vaccinated, only nineteen of these were in persons (all above thirty years old) who had been successfully revaccinated ; they were all of them cases of varioloid or of variolous fever without eruption, and none of them died. In the same hospital there were seven cases (three of them fatal) in persons who had previously had small pox. In the Baracken Lazareth, used also as small-pox hospitals, in the same city, in which eighteen hundred and five cases were treated in persons who had been vaccinated, seven only were in persons who had been successfully revaccinated ; of these, six had a mild attack, and one (a woman between sixty and seventy years old) had the hæmorrhagic form and died. In the hospital at Leipsic, out of fifteen hundred and four vaccinated patients, there were thirteen who had been successfully revaccinated in early life, all of whom recovered ; in the same hospital there were twenty-two cases in persons who had had small-pox, and of these, six died. In the hospital at Hamburg the cases in persons who had been revaccinated were more numerous, amounting to fifty-nine out of a total of twenty-two hundred and sixty-seven vaccinated patients ; and there were three deaths."

These facts and figures all tell the same story, and I know of none telling a different one. In view of them, what possible escape can there be from the conclusion that revaccination does, with rare exceptions, shield from small-pox the large numbers of those to whom a single (and perhaps a remote) vaccination is not a sufficient protection. Take a thousand adults vaccinated in infancy only ; what is their condition on exposure to this disease ? An unknown number of them, estimated by different writers at from one tenth to one half, would take the infection, some in a mild, others in a severe form ; and from five to twenty per cent. of those attacked would die. Revaccinate that thousand, how many would die from the effects of the operation ? Is it likely that one would ? How many would be sick enough to be confined to bed ? How many would have their health impaired for years or a life-time ? I appeal to the experience of the profession on this point. It is our duty to know the worst of any of our procedures, however justifiable. Many would have sore arms, no doubt, but they would not jeopardize their neighbors, at any rate. On the other hand, is it likely that even two out of that revaccinated thousand if exposed would take varioloid?

It is not contended that this practice will protect all; neither will variola. Thirty-eight cases of recurrent small-pox were witnessed by Dr. Webb in Boston during the late epidemic. Three had the disease twice within six months. One, a child of four, vaccinated in infancy, had the disease in March, recovered, only to die of it in October. Such cases show that there are persons so susceptible to the poison of variola that no number of vaccinations or previous attacks will protect them, especially during a violent epidemic.

Neither does a successful revaccination, "a good arm," *prove* that the person was susceptible to the contagion of variola. "The utility and necessity of revaccination stand not upon any speculative reasoning from the local effects it produces, but upon the broad grounds of observation and experience." [1]

Should we revaccinate often? For one I doubt the necessity of repeating the process every seven or any other fixed number of years. Whether vaccination in infancy, repeated at short intervals till no local effect is produced, gives any more permanent protection than a single vaccination, I do not know; does any one? Whether the effect of non-humanized kine virus is more lasting than that of the long humanized will require years of systematic observation to prove. At present I think two points are established: (1) a recently vaccinated or revaccinated person has an extremely small liability to small-pox; (2) vaccination performed in infancy diminishes in protective power as a person advances in life, and especially after the age of puberty.

In Philadelphia, during the late epidemic, one hundred and eleven post-vaccinial cases were admitted to the small-pox hospital under fourteen years of age, and their mortality was 11.71 per cent.; fifteen hundred and eighteen post-vaccinial cases were admitted over fourteen years of age, and their mortality was 17.32 per cent. This renewed susceptibility to small-pox increases up to an undetermined period, perhaps to about middle life.[2]

If I were to lay down rules, I should say, —

(1.) Vaccinate in infancy.

(2.) Revaccinate at least once in after-life, and if but once, preferably not far from the age of puberty.

(3.) Revaccinate always on exposure to small-pox, unless it has been done recently with success; also, when danger of exposure is great, as when the disease is in the same tenement.

---

[1] Seaton.

[2] Eighteen is, according to Mr. Marson, the age at which post-vaccinial small-pox begins to be chiefly noticeable.

(4.) In case of persons who mingle much with all sorts and conditions of men, if a successful trial has not been made within eight or ten years, I should be in favor of revaccination, and when an epidemic of small-pox prevails should certainly advise it.

RECENT PROGERSS IN OTOLOGY.[1]

BY J. ORNE GREEN, M. D.

The Examination of the Ear by Polarized Light.— The examination of the eye by means of polarized light was introduced by Coccius years ago, but was given up as it was found that the tissues of the eye were so transparent as to render any such aid to their examination unnecessary. The tissues of the ear, however, have not such perfect transparency, and Hagen and Stimmel[2] by a slight modification of Coccius's apparatus have been investigating the appearances of the ear under polarized light, and claim that by this means they have a valuable aid to the diagnosis of certain anatomical changes in the middle ear and membrana tympani. They say that under polarized light the delicate glistening usually seen over the whole membrana tympani entirely disappears; the light-reflex on the lower anterior segment is changed so as to appear of a bluish-white color, and any other reflexes, either on the drum-membrane or from fluid in the meatus, are absorbed. Certain parts of the drum-membrane are found also to disappear entirely, while other parts are rendered much more transparent; the posterior upper segment, especially, disappears under polarized light, so that the long process of the incus, parts of the stapes, and the outline of the promontory are distinctly seen. This disappearance of parts of the drum-membrane was found also to occur, even if the membrane was considerably thickened, and Hagen claims in this way to have been able to see abnormal adhesive bands and pseudo-ligaments within the tympanic cavity.

Marked thickening of the drum-membrane and calcareous deposits do not disappear, but come out more prominently under polarized light; the same is true of ecchymoses in the membrane, but their exact position, whether on the surface or within the tissue, can be easily determined. These are the chief results of these investigations, and of course a long series of investigations is necessary to determine the appearances of all parts of the ear, both in health and in disease, under polarized light. The authors express the hope that the power which polarized light possesses of rendering certain tissues transparent will be found useful

---

[1] Concluded from page 592.
[2] Berliner klinische Wochenschrift, No. 48, 1874.

not only in the study of the physiology of the ear, especially of the movements of the separate ossicles, but also in the treatment of diseases of the middle ear. The apparatus as now constructed, however, has not the free movements of all its parts and the ease of manipulation which are desirable in an instrument intended for daily use.

The Action of Quinine upon the Ear. — The direct effect of quinine upon the ear is so well known that it seems wonderful that we have no more accurate knowledge of how this effect is produced. It has been claimed in Germany that the effect of quinine was to cause contraction of the blood-vessels and consequently anæmia ; this view was denied, however, by Von Graefe, as contrary to his clinical experience ; and it has been rejected by many others also, especially by those who have seen much of aural disease, as wholly inadequate to explain the phenomena which they observe in practice. That quinine can directly aggravate an existing inflammation of the tympanum has been shown by Roosa [1] and others, and that this effect could be produced by anæmia is wholly inconsistent with our knowledge of the process of inflammation ; that quinine can also produce deafness from its specific action upon the ear, whatever that may be, is also now quite generally acknowledged. Roosa in a paper on the diseases of the internal ear [2] asserts that the effects of quinine upon the ear were due to congestion ; and Hammond [3] takes the same view and publishes the result of an experiment on himself. These experiments are continued further by Roosa, [4] and although they are but few in number they confirm so thoroughly the theory of congestion and not that of anæmia as the effect of quinine on the ear that they are given in full. The subjects of the experiments were medical men in good health, the observer was Dr. Roosa.

Dr. H., vision normal, $\frac{20}{30}$; refraction emmetropic ; pulse 90 ; ocular conjunctivæ white, decidedly free from hyperæmia ; palpebræ congested at outer and inner canthus. No tinnitus aurium ; membranæ tympanorum entirely free from evidence of blood-vessels. At 8.30 p. m. Dr. H. took ten grains of sulphate of quinine ; at 9 p. m. the ocular conjunctivæ were congested at the outer and inner canthus, and the palpebral conjunctivæ were markedly congested over the whole surface ; there was no change in appearance of the drum-heads.

At 10 p. m. the head feels full ; left ear rings ; auricles burn ; face is decidedly flushed ; auricles are red, especially the lobe of the right, where there is a localized congestion so marked as to resemble an ecchymosis. There is now a vessel seen along each malleus. The optic

---

[1] Diseases of the Ear.
[2] Transactions of the American Otological Society, 1875.
[3] The Psychological and Medico-Legal Journal, October, 1874.
[4] American Journal of the Medical Sciences, October, 1874.

papillæ are pinkish from apparent enlargement of the lateral vessels. At 10.30 P: M. the right drum-head is very much injected along the handle of the malleus and its upper margin ; the left one is less red, but still shows vascular injection. Both papillæ are pink, the left more so than the right ; face flushed, eyes suffused, ocular conjunctivæ decidedly congested, slight headache, tinnitus in both ears. At 11 P. M. the redness of the auricles is diminishing, especially the circumscribed spot on the lobe of the left one ; the face is still flushed ; tinnitus continues ; no headache ; some exhilaration ; drum-heads still injected along the malleus. Vision normal.

Dr. E., aged twenty-four ; hearing distance normal, $\frac{40}{40}$, on each side ; refraction emmetropic. No tinnitus aurium ; the drum-heads are free from vessels and normal in appearance ; optic papillæ normal. At 11.05 A. M. Dr. E. takes ten grains of sulphate of quinine ; at 11.35 there is a very fine vessel along the right malleus ; no change in the left. At 12.30 there is some redness at the periphery of the left drum-head, but the vessel on the right has disappeared. At 1 P. M. the redness has disappeared on both sides. No change is observed in the optic papillæ, and there is no tinnitus and no sense of exhilaration.

Dr. C., aged twenty-five ; refraction myopic $\frac{1}{12}$; $V = \frac{20}{20}$; drum-heads absolutely free from congestion ; no vessel on or along the malleus ; optic papillæ both flushed. At 10.16 A. M. takes fifteen grains of sulphate of quinine. At 11 A. M. a vessel is seen along the malleus of the right membrana tympani, but the membrane itself presents no change ; there is slight vertigo. At 11.30 A. M. there is a sense of heat and tingling over the whole surface of the body, and a sense of fullness in the ears and head. The hands are tremulous, and the subject gives general evidence of nervous excitement. The handles of both mallei are injected ; there are sounds of a high note in the ears, and the ears feel warm. At 12.30 P. M. the injection of the mallei is disappearing, as are the vertigo and tremor.

From these experiments it will be seen that the administration of quinine was followed in each case by a decided congestion of the blood-vessels of the malleus within an hour ; in two of the cases there was very marked tinnitus aurium accompanying this congestion, while in the other case, that in which the congestion was the least, there was no tinnitus. The blood-vessels which were found congested in these cases are known to be intimately connected with the vascular system of the middle ear, and the vessels of the middle ear are in direct connection with the circulation of the labyrinth, so that a congestion of any one of these systems is sure to be communicated to the other systems ; and inasmuch as the amount of tinnitus is proportionate to the degree of congestion observed in the malleus, the conclusion seems reasonable that the specific effect of quinine upon the ear is the result of congestion and not of anæmia.

In practice the result of these experiments is of great importance in showing the risk, appreciated for a long time by a few but not generally known or recognized, of giving quinine either as a tonic or for any other purpose during an inflammation of any part of the ear.

Iodoform in Chronic Suppuration of the Middle Ear. — Dr. Rankin [1] reports good results from the insufflation of iodoform in powder in some cases of chronic suppurative inflammation of the middle ear which had obstinately resisted other methods of treatment ; and Dr. Mathewson [2] reports that very satisfactory results have been obtained by this remedy by himself in these cases. The ear should be first thoroughly cleansed and dried, and then the iodoform be applied in powder to the inflamed mucous membrane every day or every other day.

Inflammation of the Mastoid Cells without Affection of the Tympanum. — An inflammation of the mastoid cells, not secondary to an inflammation of the tympanum, is of such rare occurrence that the possibility of such a thing has been denied by some authors and the rarity of its occurrence acknowledged by all. Such a case is described by Dr. Pierce [3] in a man aged twenty-two, who after suffering for two months with colds in the head and slight pains in both ears was attacked with severe pain in the right mastoid and down the neck. The mastoid became red, swollen, and œdematous, but examination showed the membrana tympani, although somewhat thickened, entirely free from any congestion. An incision of the mastoid tissues and poulticing gradually relieved the existing inflammation there, but at no time were there any symptoms or appearances of inflammation in the tympanum proper.

Subcutaneous Injection of Strychnia for Nervous Deafness. — Stimulated by the good results claimed by Professor Nagel, of Tübingen, as the result of subcutaneous injections of strychnine in amaurosis and amblyopia, Hagen [4] has tried the same treatment in case of nervous deafness. After the treatment of a considerable number of such cases, he claims to have obtained good results from the injection over the mastoid process of a one per cent. solution of nitrate of strychnia ; the injections were given twice a week. The minutiæ of the cases are not given, but are promised later ; he merely states that the good results obtained were undeniable.

[1] New York Medical Journal, May, 1875.
[2] Transactions of the American Otological Society, 1875.
[3] The Lancet, January 2, 1875.
[4] Centralblatt für die medicinischen Wissenschaften, No. 36, 1875.

HAYDEN ON DISEASES OF THE HEART.[1]

THIS treatise is an exhaustive compilation of theories and facts which have been propounded or established in relation to the heart, especially since the time of Laennec, supplemented throughout with observations and opinions of the author, modestly expressed. It shows very extensive reading and familiarity with English and French medical literature. The book is too large, and it would have been well shortened by condensing the experiments and opinions of others, and by leaving out the details (except tables and summaries) of the author's own cases, which occupy two or three hundred pages.

One hundred and fifty-five pages are devoted to the anatomy and physiology of the heart, and to the phenomena of the heart's action in relation to its modification by disease. Then follow about one hundred and fifty pages on the physical signs of disease of the heart. Dr. Hayden holds that the primary and essential though remote cause of cardiac murmurs is friction of the blood-current against the walls or passages where the murmurs arise, and does not believe that valvular murmurs can arise from modified tension-property of the valves, irrespective of afflux or reflux blood-currents, as has been thought by Da Costa, Oppolzer, Bamberger, and others.

Dr. Hayden classifies murmurs as presystolic, systolic, post-systolic, pre-diastolic, diastolic, and post-diastolic. He dwells upon the usually presystolic time of the murmur of mitral obstruction, and gives credit to Dr. Austin Flint, after M. Fauvel, for correctly appreciating this.

On the subject of apex diastolic murmur, the author leaves his experience rather doubtful. On page 191 he says, " A veritable apex diastolic murmur is undoubtedly 'rare,' as Hope describes it. I have met with only two examples of such murmur, and Dr. Stokes informs me he has met with another." In a note at the foot of page 206 he says, " I have not met with an example of diastolic apex murmur in the strict sense, but Dr. Stokes has mentioned to me a case," etc. On page 693 is reported a case which bears among other headings this one : " diastolic murmur and quasi presystolic murmur at the apex." In this case there was also a loud double bellows murmur at the base. " Both murmurs (aortic) were transmitted some distance towards the apex, but were nearly lost at the seat of the apex beat ; " at the apex " the first sound was prolonged and associated with a murmur of quasi presystolic rhythm. In this situation, likewise, a loud bellows murmur took the place of the second sound, and was distinctly audible at the left axilla." It was found, on autopsy, that " the mitral orifice was somewhat less than the ordinary size, admitting only the tips of two fingers. The mitral valves were competent, and in all respects normal save that at the attached margin and on the auricular aspect there was a circlet of warty vegetations of about the size of a duck-shot ; they were soft, partially transparent, and smooth on the surface. The aortic valves were slightly thickened and shriveled at the free edge ; they admitted of axial reflux." Dr. Hayden felt sure that there were two diastolic murmurs, and not one transmitted, on account of there be-

---

[1] *The Diseases of the Heart and of the Aorta.* By THOMAS HAYDEN. In Two Parts. Philadelphia: Lindsay and Blakiston. 1875.

ing two points of maximum intensity of diastolic murmur, that is, one at the base and another at the apex. In commenting on this case he says, "It is, indeed, the only genuine example of the kind which has come under my notice ; " but, still further on, after mentioning the absence of a second sound at the apex in the case, and hence the difficulty of exactly fixing the time, he says, " According to the view now stated, the murmur was in reality not diastolic but post-diastolic in rhythm, having been misinterpreted owing to the absence of the ordinary chronometric standard, namely, a second sound."

Of post-systolic murmur the author has noted five examples. In three of these the murmur was confined to the area of the apex, and in two of this number was non-organic in cause, traceable in one to excessive tobacco smoking, and in the other, a female, to nervousness, and associated with nervous palpitation. In the third case in this category there was organic disease of the mitral valve. In one case only was the post-systolic murmur basic and due to trivial alteration of the aortic valve (shown post mortem).

Dr. Hayden has met with only one example of prediastolic murmur; it occurred at the base, and disease of the aortic valves was found post mortem.

Of post-diastolic murmur the author has observed eleven examples; four were located at the apex, and seven at the base. In only two was there an autopsy; in both of these the murmur was basic, and organic disease of the aortic valves was found.

Of tricuspid constriction three cases are given. There were two centres of pre-systolic murmur (mitral constriction being also present) ; in two of these cases post-mortem examination showed the constriction.

Most auscultators will be surprised, we think, to read that Dr. Hayden " has not met with a single example of diastolic aortic murmur which was audible even faintly in the carotid or subclavian arteries." [1] However, the reader will find further on that the author has met with at least one instance of it, for in the record of case No. 25 [2] he says, " Of these the diastolic murmur was relatively louder ; it was transmitted through the ascending aorta, but with diminished intensity, and (for a diastolic murmur a very unusual circumstance) likewise into the great arteries of the neck."

In discussing hypertrophy the author does not seem to present quite clearly and strongly enough the fact of hypertrophy of the right ventricle in case of mitral lesions. And in discussing the accentuation of the pulmonic second sound in connection with mitral lesions [3] he says, " I am safe in asserting that not one half of the cases of indubitable disease of the mitral valve which have come under my notice have presented " it ; but in another place [4] it is stated that " the two former [presystolic and systolic murmurs] are usually, but by no means invariably, associated with accentuated second sound in the pulmonary artery."

Cheyne-Stokes respiration existed in twenty-nine out of sixty-four cases of fatty degeneration of the heart, but Dr. Hayden regards the fatty degeneration as only accessory in the production of this symptom, the essential condition being, in his opinion, dilatation and loss of elasticity in the aorta, " with which,

[1] Page 237.   [2] Page 539.
[3] Page 136.   [4] Page 232.

however, fatty change of the heart is almost invariably associated." In another case he says, "Judging from my personal experience, such as it has been,
I feel bound to regard it [Cheyne-Stokes respiration] as pathognomonic of
the conditions of the aorta just mentioned."

We think Dr. Gee will be rather surprised to find the opinion (from which
Dr. Hayden dissents) that in case of serous effusion in pericarditis the liquid
accumulation takes place in the first instance at the base of the heart, and
around the roots of the great vessels, attributed to him alone, inasmuch as he
(Dr. Gee) shares his faith with Skoda, Oppolzer, Bamberger, Niemeyer, and
others.

Dr. Hayden has been unable to use the binaural stethoscope "on account of
the difficulty of keeping it steadily fixed in the ears, and the rustling noise
which it consequently produced, together with the irritation to the ears thence
arising." We wish that he might try one of American manufacture.

On the whole the book strikes us favorably, but it may be much improved
by condensation in another edition. Some inconsistencies of statement, like
those indicated above, may be due to the length of time over which the preparation of the volume extended (nine years). The paper and type are excellent.

----◆----

RUTHERFORD ON PRACTICAL HISTOLOGY.[1]

This unpretending little book by the new professor of the institutes of
medicine at Edinburgh will be a great acquisition to students of histology.
It is a clear and concise guide, telling the beginners what to look at, where to
get it, how to prepare it, and how to study it. In examining a microscopic
object the student is told to note the shape, size, border, upper and under surface, color, transparency, contents, and the effect of reagents. He is also urged
to draw what he sees. We are glad to read a work on this subject in which
we are spared a tedious description of various microscopes and two or three
chapters on optics. Dr. Rutherford's ideal instrument is simplicity itself, and
the few instructions he gives for its use comprise all that is essential. We are
glad to see that in England the school of microscopists who are searching for
facts is taking the place of those who work merely for demonstration. As a
crowning merit the world "diatome" is not to be found in the book.

In some minor points we must be permitted to differ from the author. We
think that he attaches too much importance to the camera lucida, as the skillful
draughtsman can make a good drawing and the poor one can express an idea
very well, especially if he practices, without it. We are surprised to find
Valentine's double-bladed knife recommended, as we thought that its useless-
ness was generally acknowledged. Dr. Rutherford writes enthusiastically of
the advantages of his freezing microtome, which certainly would appear to be
very valuable. The list of objects to be studied is long and very judiciously
chosen, with the exception perhaps of the retina and internal ear, which we

1 *Outlines of Practical Histology.* By William Rutherford, M. D., F. R. S. Philadelphia : Lindsay and Blakiston. 1875.

think the student will find difficult. A defect in this part of the work is that the author often quite arbitrarily designates the animal from which a tissue is to be taken; thus for the study of a transverse section of a nerve he recommends the sciatic nerve of a cat, and so may put to inconvenience the student who does not yet know that many other animals would do as well. Among the methods of preparation is one for skin, by Dr. William Stirling, which we believe is quite new : [1] "Mix 1 c. c. pure hydrochloric acid with 500 c. c. water at 38°C. (100° F.), and add 1 gramme pepsine. After keeping the mixture at 38° C. for three hours, shake it thoroughly. Stretch a piece of skin of man or dog, as fresh as possible, over the mouth of a dialyzing jar, and tie it firmly round the jar to keep it stretched. Digest the skin in the above fluid at 38°C. for a period varying from two to eight hours, according to the size and age of the skin. Young skin digests more quickly than that which is old. It is advantageous to use only about 100 c. c. of the digestive fluid at one time, and to change the fluid every second hour if the piece of skin be large, in order to remove the peptones, and thereby facilitate the digestive process. After partial digestion place the skin in water for twenty-four hours. In this it becomes swollen and transparent. It can then be hardened in the ordinary fluids and stained with logwood or carmine. By the above process the white fibrous tissue wells up and becomes extremely transparent, thus permitting of a clear view of the other tissues." Many other methods little known to others than experts are clearly given. Even the experienced histologist may derive some valuable hints from this book as to the method of conducting a course, but to the student, for whom it is written, it will be of the greatest service.   T. D., JR.

TWO THOUSAND YEARS AFTER.[2]

A NEW literary and philosophic *tour de force* by this graceful writer is pretty sure to command attention. The object of the essay is to show the fallacy of materialists in holding "that man has no different part or state assigned him than belongs to matter and force at large." The argument is carried on in a conversation between Socrates and some of his disciples, two thousand years after their demise. It is a reproduction of the old Greek style of instruction, which, it appears, consists on the part of the philosopher in leading the doubting pupil on by a series of difficult questions to a point where the weakness of his position is evident. Cebes, who serves as a lay figure, receives terrible punishment, but comes up smiling till he gets his final quietus. Though this style is not to our mind the most attractive, it is made interesting by the skill with which it is handled.

[1] Page 38.

[2] *Two Thousand Years after; or, Thoughts in a Grave-Yard.* By JOHN DARBY, author of *Thinkers and Thinking*, etc. Philadelphia: Claxton, Remsen, and Haffelfinger. 1876.

LECTURES ON DISEASES OF THE NERVOUS SYSTEM.[1]

So much valuable work has been done within the past few years towards clearing up the pathology of the nervous system, that each new writer has an advantage over his immediate predecessors in being able to bring up new evidence on one side or the other of the important discussions of the day. Realizing this fact we took up the book now before us with a feeling of pleasure, thinking that we should find in it, we will not say reports of original scientific investigations, but a careful and analytic statement of the latest results obtained by others. We must, however, confess to a feeling of disappointment as we lay it down.[2] It is a volume of lectures which were no doubt interesting and valuable to the students who heard them, but which as a contribution to the literature of the subject of which they treat have no *raison d'être.* The laborious scientific investigations through which alone our knowledge of the pathology of the nervous system can make real advance are but meagrely quoted, and instead of them we find a collection of statements, mainly clinical, often interesting, but too often inaccurate, insufficient, and dogmatic. We do not complain that the lectures when delivered to medical students did not contain detailed accounts of microscopic and physiological observations, but that in these days, when exact science is beginning to assert itself in medicine, and when our shelves are covered with books that we have not time to read, it should have been thought worth while to publish another fat volume of elementary lectures.

The author himself says of the book in his preface that he "cannot claim for it originality either as to its facts or as to its theories," and as it certainly does not contain anything like a complete survey of the scientific field, and as it is not a concise handbook, it is plain that it adds to the world's solution of science in literature a disproportionately large amount of menstruum.

In support of the charge that the book contains many inexact and insufficient statements, we will mention a few of them. At page 257 the author explains the fact that the extensor muscles of the fore-arm are preëminently affected in lead-poisoning, by assuming that on account of their (supposed) relatively greater functional activity in the case of painters, they would receive a more abundant blood-supply than the rest of the muscles of the arm, and therefore a larger share of the poison. No proof is given that either of these statements is correct ; nor does that explanation cover the cases of lead-poisoning in persons not painters. Neither is it mentioned that Hitzig, in 1868, showed some reasons for thinking that this disproportionate affection of the extensors is due to *insufficiency* of the venous circulation in those muscles, or that Bärwinkel maintained that it is due to insufficiency of the arterial circulation, or that others have brought forward strong evidence against both theories.

---

[1] *Lectures on Diseases of the Nervous System.* By JEROME BAUDUY, M. D., Professor of Psychological Medicine and Diseases of the Nervous System in the Missouri Medical College. Reported by V. BIART, M. D., revised and edited by the author. Philadelphia : J. B. Lippincott & Co. 1876.

[2] It is significant that among the twenty writers to whom the author expresses his grateful acknowledgment as having quoted freely from their works, the only German mentioned is Niemeyer.

In speaking of progressive muscular atrophy he says, " In France, atrophy of the anterior gray cornua of the spinal cord is considered the common and constant anatomical characteristic; an hypothesis which I need hardly say is more than doubtful." We do not ourselves affirm that this hypothesis is absolutely proved, but it is just now certainly a favorite theory with a large proportion of neuro-pathologists the world over.

In the chapter on the diagnosis of cerebral tumors, not a word is said of the frequency with which optic neuritis accompanies them.

If the book could have been cut down to include a few only of its present chapters, especially those on cerebral meningitis, it would have been much more useful and interesting than it is as it stands.

PROCEEDINGS OF THE MIDDLESEX SOUTH DISTRICT MEDICAL SOCIETY.

C. E. VAUGHAN, M. D., SECRETARY.

THE semi-annual meeting was held at North Cambridge, October 13, 1875, DR. G. J. TOWNSEND presiding.

Exophthalmic Goitre. — DR. WALCOTT read notes of a case of Basedow's disease, or exophthalmic cachexia, seen four years since. The patient was a girl of thirteen, and tall for the age. She was nervous and restless, dreaming at night. The skin was sensitive. Pulse 100 to 110. The pupils were dilated and brilliant, the sight unaffected. The thyroid body was enlarged, and considerable pulsation was observed in carotids and jugulars. The precordial dullness was increased.

During the next year the catamenia appeared. The symptoms became more pronounced. The patient was more nervous and impatient, and unable to study. She had taken iodine by the advice of another physician in the interval. On the whole, she was not much worse. The tumor was slightly larger, but the respiration continued unaffected. The patient is now in a Southern city, and growing worse. Iron has been of some benefit.

This disease was first described by Basedow, and subsequently by Graves and Trousseau. The most marked symptoms are prominence of the eyes and enlargement of the thyroid body. Arterial palpitation is generally noticed early. There is a cardiac souffle, prolonged into the great vessels. Precordial dullness may or may not be increased. The sight is not often affected. In the course of the disease we find progressive anæmia, anasarca, general cachexia, and death. The heart is generally enlarged. Increased vascularity of the choroid is found. The disease occurs most frequently in males from twenty to twenty-five years of age.

DR. MARCY mentioned the case of a book-keeper, aged twenty-four. He first noticed cardiac irregularity four years ago, and was seen by Dr. Marcy one year ago. Then the first cardiac sound was prolonged, the eyes were prominent, and the right lobe of the thyroid body was the most enlarged, show-

44

ing marked pulsation. Pulse 100, rising under excitement. The treatment consisted of quinine and digitalis, with rest. The patient is now well enough to attend to business.

DR. HILDRETH saw a case several years ago in which no benefit was derived from iodide of potassium and cod-liver oil.

DR. SULLIVAN had seen a case of recovery under iron and arsenic.

DR. WILLIS had a case in which the respiration was spasmodically affected, about every fourth inspiration being accompanied by a kind of shriek.

Cystitis in a Nursing Woman. — DR. SULLIVAN reported a case of easy labor with good recovery, followed six weeks later by dysuria and strangury, succeeded by a flow of pus from the bladder. The patient was treated for seven months by tonics and injections without benefit. Weaning was followed by relief, and the subsequent resumption of nursing by a return of the trouble. Another similar case recovered upon the removal of the child from the breast.

Arrested Development. — A case of this condition in a child was reported by DR. TOWNSEND. Two or three fingers of each hand were undeveloped, each terminating in a small tumor like a huckleberry. The right foot was well formed excepting the toes. The left leg was normal until, near the malleoli, it appeared as if a catgut had been twisted about the bone. The foot was a shapeless mass, with rudiments of toes, and was removed. The inner malleolus was wanting, but the fibula was so prolonged that it was thought advisable to remove the end by bone forceps.

DR. DRIVER stated that he had delivered a woman of an anencephalous foetus, the head as usual not dilating the os readily. The child lived some days.

DR. G. C. PIERCE, of Ashland, said that he had recently had a similar case. The deficient bone was supplied by copper-colored skin. The edges of the bones caused the mother much pain.

DR. HODGDON remarked that he had always found a large amount of liquor amnii in such cases, and that the labor was not difficult after the rupture of the membranes.

DR. L. R. MORSE some years ago had four such cases in four months. In all there was a large amount of liquor amnii. The labor was quick in three.

Mastitis in a New-Born Infant. — DR. McDONNELL reported a case of inflamed breasts in an infant two days after birth. Next day there was an oozing of serum from the breasts, followed by a bloody discharge from the vagina.

DR. TOWNSEND said he had seen hæmorrhage from the bowels and the vagina in a cyanotic infant, which, however, did well.

DR. HOLMES had seen two similar cases.

"DEATH FROM ETHER."

WE abridge the following statement from the *New York Herald* of November 22d. A man, fifty-four years of age, went to the homœopathic college in New York, on Saturday the 20th inst. " He was complaining of pain in the left upper jaw extending to the head, with great nervous prostration. There were four openings in the jaw, all discharging fœtid pus. On introducing a probe, caries of the upper jaw was found, and the patient was advised to have the bone removed." " IIe was placed under the influence of ether and *laid on the table*" (the italics are ours). " A physician was constantly feeling the patient's pulse while the ether was being given." An "incision was made into the upper jaw, and four teeth extracted." The operator was " about to extend the incision when he noticed the face of the patient become blue. Artificial respiration and the galvanic battery were applied, but they were unavailing ; he was dead."

The reputation of ether, in doses even of a pound or two, has been hitherto pretty good. It has been tried on patients with hearts variously fatty. It will be difficult to persuade us that two and one fourth ounces of this hitherto beneficent agent has proved so suddenly fatal, without any previous gradual diminution of the pulse. It should be conclusively shown that the patient died of nothing else. *This patient, so far as we can judge, died of asphyxia from blood in the trachea.* In the first place, after he was etherized, he was laid on his back. An " incision " was made in the jaw, and time enough elapsed to extract four teeth. Dead bone always makes the soft parts vascular. There was ample time for blood to fill the trachea. Until it is shown that there was no blood in the fauces and trachea this must stand as the cause of death. The autopsy is silent on this point. The suddenness and the lividity both belong to asphyxia and neither to etherization. In the Massachusetts General Hospital, operations on the mouth are usually done in the erect posture, with special attention to keeping the fauces clear of blood.

MEDICAL NOTES.

— A very remarkable case of ossification of muscles was lately presented before the New York Pathological Society by Dr. E. P. Gibney. The patient, still alive, was a girl of ten years, who some months ago suffered from diphtheria. The symptoms of ossification had been present for seven or eight months. The latissimus dorsi, scaleni, and erectes spinæ muscles were those affected, but the disease was, as is usual in these rare cases, progressive. The most remarkable case of this kind occurred in Dublin. The skeleton, now in the museum, shows a distorted and bony representation of many of the chief muscles of the body. The erectores spinæ, pectorals, gluteals, and latissimi dorsi were among the most affected.

— We are happy to announce that a new charity, the Hospital for Women, has been opened and is already in successful operation. In some respects it is similar to the New York State Woman's Hospital, and is designed only for the treatment of those diseases peculiar to women. The hospital is situated at 16 East Springfield Street, has accommodations for twenty beds, and was opened for the reception of patients on the second day of November. Eight beds are now occupied. The institution is supported by churches and by individual charity, governed by a board of trustees and the medical staff. Its objects are to give relief to some of the many poor women who crowd our dispensaries and public charities, and who require operative treatment which cannot be given them at those places; many will be benefited also who have not proper hygienic surroundings or who could not have the necessary nursing or care at their own homes. It is hoped, moreover, that this institution may be a field for the more careful clinical study of these cases. The hospital is to be considered fortunate in obtaining the services of the Episcopal Sisterhood of St. Margaret, whose noble work has been so well known in connection with the Children's Hospital.

The following is its list of officers : —

Board of Trustees: Benjamin E. Bates, President; Joseph W. Woods, Secretary; Edwin H. Sampson, Treasurer; Edwin F. Waters, Rev. E. E. Hale, Rev. Dr. Vinton, Rev. Phillips Brooks, Rev. Treadwell Waldon, Rev. Dr. A. R. Baker. Medical Staff: W. H. Baker, M. D., Visiting Surgeon. Consulting Board: D. H. Storer, M. D., W. W. Morland, M. D., A. D. Sinclair, M. D., J. P. Reynolds, M. D. And by Correspondence: J. Marion Sims, M. D., E. R. Peaslee, M. D., T. Addis Emmett, M. D., T. Gaillard Thomas, M. D.

Applications for admission to the hospital may be made to Dr. Baker at his office, 6 Beacon Street, every day, or at the hospital, Thursdays, at three P. M.

— We understand that renewed efforts will be made at the coming session of Congress to obtain the passage of the bill increasing the rank of surgeons in the army. The matter is sufficiently familiar to the profession to need no comment, for we all know how great is the merit of the medical corps of the army, how severe yet excellent their work, and how small the reward ; but it is greatly to be desired that these facts should be made so evident that Con‧ gress cannot overlook the justice of the claim.

— An attempt to explain the emaciation of consumption is made by Edward Williams, M. D., in a paper published in the *Medical Press and Circular* of October 27, 1875. It has been noticed that when in phthisis the apex of the right lung is alone affected, loss of flesh is not observable. When emaciation occurs it appears to be due to the deficient supply of chyle to the venous system. When the left lung becomes the first affected, emaciation more speedily shows itself in consequence of the thoracic duct opening into the left subclavian vein and becoming more immediately subject to the mechanical pressure of the disorganized lung. The impeded passage of the blood through the right side of the heart causes engorgement of the descending jugulars and left subclavian vein, and the engorged veins, pressing on the outlet of the thoracic duct, also prevent the flow of chyle into the venous system. Hence the inference that the emaciation occurs in consequence of a sufficient supply of chyle not being able to find its way into the venous system on account of the mechanical obstruction referred to above.

— According to Dr. Knapp, says the *Medical Press and Circular*, the arsenic-eaters of Upper and Middle Styria have discovered that arsenical food has much to justify it, and that taken in reasonable quantities its poisonous effects are very slow. They say that it prevents illness, furthers their wish to look rosy and healthy, is a remedy against difficulty of breathing, and assists the digestion of indigestible food. A poacher told Dr. Knapp that he acquired courage by the habit. The appearance of the arsenic-eaters is healthy and robust; and the author thinks only robust persons can become accustomed to the practice. Some of them attain a great age. The dose is at first very small, and is gradually increased, the largest quantity eaten in his presence being fourteen grams (three and a half drachms). The intervals at which the arsenic is taken vary — every fortnight, every week, twice or three times a week. Arsenic was formerly, and perhaps is now, taken in this country to improve the complexion; and in some skin diseases it is prescribed in large doses and for long periods of time. On the other hand, we hear of persons being poisonously affected by infinitesimal doses, as in arsenic-poisoning from wall-papers. The difference is doubtless due to the different way in which the drug reaches the system. In poisoning from wall-papers it is taken directly into the blood from the lungs, and poisons passing into the blood by subcutaneous injection or by inhalation have a much more powerful effect than when absorbed through the digestive tract.

— *The Medical Times and Gazette* reports the treatment at Guy's Hospital of several cases of diseased joints by sulphuric acid. Three patients were thus treated, all of whom were suffering from advanced pulpy degeneration of the synovial membrane of a joint; and in one case a condyle of the femur was also necrosed. Four joints in the three patients were operated upon; in one the ankle-joint, in one the knee, and in one the knee and wrist-joints were the seat of disease. The mode of operating was simply to make one or more incisions into the joint, let out any flaky or puriform fluid which might be present, and then stuff strips of lint, soaked in one part of the sulphuric acid of the shops with two of water, into it. The parts were then covered with carded oakum and a bandage, and the limb was fixed on a splint. No great amount of pain, it is said, can be produced by the operation, for one of the patients seemed quite comfortable and without any sign of suffering when seen about half an hour after recovering consciousness from chloroform.

— A case in which injection of strychnine into the bladder for paralysis of that organ was attended with success is reported by W. E. Tarbell, M. D., of Kinkiang, China, in the *Medical Record* of November 13, 1875. The patient, after a difficult labor, was unable to pass her water, and for twenty days subsequent to delivery the catheter had to be employed twice a day. Strychnia and other remedies were administered by the mouth during this period, but failed to restore power to the bladder; at length Dr. Tarbell made a solution of strychnia of one grain in two ounces of water (six centigrams in six deciliters), of which he injected into the bladder one drachm (three and six tenths cu. centim.) in half an ounce (fifteen cu. centim.) of tepid water, three times a day. After the third injection a copious voluntary flow of urine came on, and the patient was no longer troubled with retention.

— The treatment of patent urachus is discussed in a paper by J. J. Charles, M. D., which is published in the *British Medical Journal* of October 16, 1875. The urachus extends from the apex of the bladder to the umbilicus. It retains the tubular character of the allantois up to about the thirtieth week of fœtal life, and its cavity is in great part obliterated a short period before birth, though to a variable extent. From this fact it is easy to understand, more especially in cases where the obliteration at birth is less complete than usual, that any obstacle to the flow of urine from the bladder may give rise to undue distention of that viscus, to the dilatation of the slender cavity in the urachus, and to the discharge of urine from the umbilicus. The most rational mode of treatment in such cases is to remove any obstruction that may exist to the flow of urine by the ordinary passage. In the cases of patent urachus on record the treatment has been directed solely to the contraction and closure of the aperture at the umbilicus by the actual cautery or by plastic operation ; but such attempts have proved abortive. To Professor Redfern is to be ascribed the credit of recommending circumcision.

In a case reported by Dr. Charles of a boy about a year old, the umbilical cord fell off at the usual time, but urine was discharged ever afterward at the umbilicus. The urine was passed with difficulty by the urethra. No tumor was visible at the umbilicus, the prepuce was long, contracted, and adherent to the glans. Tincture of perchloride of iron had been applied to the umbilical aperture to produce contraction, but without avail. Dr. Charles then operated for the phymosis by slitting up the prepuce. After that very little urine came from the umbilicus, and when the patient was last seen there was scarcely any appearance of ulcer or opening of any kind.

— A case of deposition of the ova of a fly in the nasal fossæ is reported in the *Philadelphia Medical Times* of October 30, 1875, by Assistant Surgeon W. F. Buchanan, U. S. A. He was called to a woman aged eighty, who was experiencing terrible suffering. Her son stated that two nights previously a fly had got into her nose while she was sleeping, and that she now had worms in her nose. The constitutional disturbance was great, but no worms could be seen. Two days later there was great pain in the head, face, frontal and maxillary sinuses. The patient was delirious, her face was swollen, her eyes were closed by tumefaction, and there was a slight purulent discharge. Several maggots had appeared at the anterior nares, and one or two had been removed. Two days later the woman's general condition was much the same ; meanwhile maggots had continued to be discharged, and an opening had been caused by them through the soft palate and on the bridge of the nose. The orifices were injected with a solution of carbolic acid. In a day or two the patient began to improve, and then to rapidly recover. A portion of the anterior part of the soft palate of the size of a silver quarter of a dollar sloughed out, but afterwards presented a healthy appearance, and seemed to be closing. There were in all about three hundred and twenty-five large maggots discharged.

— Recently at a meeting of the Medico-Chirurgical Society, as reported in the *Edinburgh Medical Journal* for September, 1875, Dr. G. W. Balfour gave an account of three patients who had been much benefited by the use of large quantities of raw onions, which had acted as a diuretic. The first case was that of a woman who had suffered from large white kidney and constriction of the mitral valve. Her abdomen and legs had been tapped several times, but after using the remedy given above she had been free from dropsy for two years, although still suffering from albuminuria. Of the other two, one suffered from cardiac disease, cirrhotic liver, and ascites ; the other had ascites depending on tumor of the liver. In both these cases the remedy had been given with good results. Both had been previously tapped, and purgatives and diuretics alike failed to give relief. Finding that the fluid was steadily reaccumulating, the patient had recourse to onions. Under their use the amount of urine passed rose in a few days from ten ounces (three liters) to a hundred ounces (thirty-three liters).

SURGICAL OPERATIONS IN THE MAINE GENERAL HOSPITAL.

[REPORTED BY E. E. HOLT, M. D.]

Hæmorrhoids. — J. E. K., aged sixty-eight, a railroad employé, was admitted August 28, 1875, with the ordinary history of piles; he had a pendulous mass, of the size of a man's fist, around the margin of the anus, which had begun to degenerate. He was unable to pass his urine, which was smoky and was made turbid by heat and nitric acid. Dr. Gerrish thought that there was more albumen present than could be accounted for in the blood, which probably came from the kidneys, bladder, and urethra; he also found pus and epithelium, the latter being renal. It was decided that operative measures would best relieve the hæmorrhoids and the irritation along the urinary organs.

September 1st. The bowels having been moved freely and the patient put under ether, Dr. Weeks dilated the sphincters and ligated the piles.

September 8th. The tied masses sloughed off. The urine was clearer. The bowels, which had been kept constipated by opium, were freely moved by warm-water injections and castor-oil.

September 25th. A dejection was accompanied by severe hæmorrhage, which was checked only by repeated enemata of dilute solution of sub-sulphate of iron. The fæcal discharges were now involuntary, and excessive purging occurred occasionally. The patient was able to pass a little urine twice, which is now free from blood and albumen. He took opium, nux vomica, quinine, and tincture of iron three times daily.

October 2d. The patient has gradually obtained perfect control of the bowels, and passes his urine freely. Discharged, well.

Cheiloplasty. — W. S. B., aged forty, was admitted August 23, 1875, with cancer of the lower lip, the disease having commenced six years ago. He has had it burnt out several times by "cancer doctors," so that now the four incisors are in view, and what is left of the lip is thickened and indurated. His father and two uncles were treated for cancers about the face.

August 27th. Sulphate of quinine (one grain) with tincture of the chloride of iron (fifteen drops) has been given three times daily and the bowels have been freely moved. The patient was etherized and Dr. Weeks, assisted by Professor Greene, who suggested this mode of operation, made an incision from each corner of the mouth down the whole length of the chin, including every part of the cancer and indurated tissue in a V-shaped space. This was removed and two horizontal incisions were made through the entire thickness of the cheek, outward from either corner of the mouth, for an inch. The flaps thus formed were dissected up from the jaw as far as the angle, so that they could easily be brought together in the median line ; they were held in position by silver and silk sutures. The mucous membrane and skin of the lip thus apposed were stitched together by fine silk sutures. Two triangular pieces, the bases of which corresponded with the horizontal incisions made from the corners of the mouth, were removed from the cheeks above ; the edges were brought together and held by silver and silk sutures, and the whole was dressed in dry cotton.

September 2d. No pain. The patient is very comfortable, and has taken beef-tea, milk, and egg-nog, readily, through a tube. The wound healed entirely by the first intention. The first suture was removed on the third day and all the rest before the fifth day.

September 14th. On the 3d, a severe erysipelatous inflammation began in the left cheek and thence spread upwards over the face and head, accompanied by high fever. This attack was subdued by appropriate treatment, principally by large and repeated doses of tincture of the chloride of iron, and the patient was discharged with a lip so perfect that at a short distance it appeared entirely natural.

It is believed that this mode of operation, originally proposed by Professor Greene in this class of cases, is far superior to any other, as there are no surfaces to heal by granulation, mucous membrane is supplied in its normal place, there is no tension of the parts, and the patient soon regains movement of the lip, with very little deformity.

Perineorraphy. — Mrs. J. H. A., aged fifty, was admitted September 20th, with complete rupture of the perinæum; she had only slight control of the bowels, and was subject to profuse metrorrhagia, in which the tampon had to be used to save her life. Her disability was caused by a prolonged labor thirteen years ago, in which instruments were used. She has had two children since that time, with precipitated labors.

September 21st. The bowels having been thoroughly moved by castor-oil, and ether having been administered, Dr. Weeks proceeded first to restore the sphincter muscle, by denuding the edges and bringing them together by silver sutures according to Sims's method, so thoroughly demonstrated and illustrated with practical results by Dr. Emmett. The second part of the operation consisted in vivifying the two lateral surfaces of the ruptured perinæum, and bringing them together by silver and silk sutures. The urine was drawn, the wound dressed with dry cotton, and the patient put to bed, morphia being administered hypodermically to quiet and relieve pain. The diet consisted of milk, beef-tea, and toast.

October 6th. Union of the wound by first intention was obtained ; there was no suppuration except along the line of the sutures, the first of which was removed on the fourth day and all the rest before the sixth day after the operation. The bowels were kept constipated by opium till the fifteenth day, when they were freely moved by warm-water injections and castor-oil. The patient had perfect control of the sphincter muscles.

October 16th. Discharged, entirely well.

THE AMERICAN PUBLIC HEALTH ASSOCIATION.

[FROM OUR SPECIAL CORRESPONDENT.]

MESSRS. EDITORS, — The American Public Health Association is a sober, painstaking body of disinterested sanitarians, who for four days sit patiently listening, through the long hours of daylight and evening, to learned — often dry — discourses, and waste no time on late suppers, as so many of our medical associations do. It is difficult to divest one's self of the idea that this is really a medical convention, so prominent are the doctors in every department of it. It is therefore a matter of some disappointment to find them meeting together without eating together, after the approved fashion of the American Medical Association; but it may be that in this respect they wish to inculcate a new code of dietetic precepts, even if they suffer martyrdom in the act. What other profession or occupation than our own would calmly sit down to discuss plans for diminishing their pecuniary receipts, a result which the prevention of sickness by improved sanitary measures must assuredly accomplish sooner or later? Imagine a body of unselfish legal practitioners assembled to devise methods for elevating the moral tone of the community, so that legal advice would be no longer necessary! Solidity is a prominent characteristic of this association, but a solidity that must in time make a permanent impression for good. It has hardly a humorous phase in any form ; the gentlest murmur of a smile was once or twice almost audible after some quaint expression in a paper devoted to some profound question of sanitary science, and the only laugh that agitated the auditors was elicited after the presentation of the paper by Mr. Jackson S. Schultz, of New York, on the utilization of animal and vegetable refuse. This gentleman spoke of the great expense incurred by New York city for a useless system of conveyance of its garbage and other refuse to the sea, hundreds of tons of valuable food for swine being weekly towed out to the ocean and cast overboard. It was proposed by the writer that an island in Long Island Sound should be chosen as the place of deposit of this valuable mass of refuse matter from all the hotels and dwelling-houses of New York, and that as many hogs should be placed there as were necessary to devour it. Fat dead animals (one hundred horses die weekly in New York) should also be converted into nutritious food for the hogs. Dr. Hunt, of New Jersey, said he had no doubt that hogs would eat city garbage and dead horses, but who would eat the hogs? It was like drinking the milk of swill-fed cows. Mr. Schultz said that if the doctor was eating pork at all, he was now eating that sort ; to which the latter replied that he would go then to Gehenna, turn Jew, and eat no hog at all. Who knows whether in good time the Sound lines to Boston may not hold out as an inducement for the patronage of wavering tourists the fact that they will pass *en route* (root?) this fragrant isle of the sea, at a time, perhaps, when in nautical phraseology a sow-west wind may be wafted from it?

A notable fact at this meeting was the absence of members of the boards of health of some of the larger cities. The worthy secretary of the association fitly represents the health interests of New York, even if he should be their solitary champion on such an occasion. But what were Philadelphia and Washington doing, while these measures for sanitary improvement were being discussed at Baltimore? The health officer of the first-named city, who is chairman of an active political organization, could have scarcely recovered from the excessive labor of folding election tickets during the previous week, and the board of health was too much agitated on the subject of keeping its proceedings from the public eye, — a conclusion finally resolved upon by this model sanitary board, — to take part in matters of such vital moment as those in which the sanitarians of the whole country were participating in a sister city. Besides, did not this body last year scrupulously abstain from any part in the cordial welcome which all other lovers of human progress extended, in spirit if not in person, to the association at its meeting in Philadelphia? Of the Washington board, we noticed Dr. Bliss, of cundurango memory, present at the first day's session, we believe, unofficially. Ought not these boards to be foremost in every such sanitary movement, or at least modestly to seek admission for their representative men into the ranks of an association all of whose objects are in the highest degree worthy of their study and attention? It was expected that Philadelphia would be chosen for the next place of meeting, the date of which should be fixed at some time, say September, during the holding of the centennial exposition ; but Boston was selected, and the second week of November as the date.

There was general unanimity in the proceedings, with little or no clashing ; but then, there was so little discussion indulged in that clashing was almost an impossibility, except in the written expression of views. Most of the speakers advocated proper systems of drainage and sewerage as great desiderata, but one gentleman argued against deep-soil drainage, inasmuch as it had been in some instances the exciting cause of epidemics, by bringing to the surface poisons contained in the soil. He doubtless believed with the Scripture, that "trouble springeth out of the ground," a quotation which lost its freshness after being indulged in by two or three of the writers on sewerage. The rules of the association should at all meetings be strictly enforced, and no paper should be allowed to occupy the attention of this body for more than thirty minutes, or preferably twenty. Some of the papers presented were not strictly of a class to be read at a meeting of a sanitary association ; such should hereafter be carefully sifted from the rest by a process of exclusion practiced before the time of meeting. Nothing of merely local interest should be allowed a place on the programme, unless its applications admitted of indefinite extension.

Of the good results accomplished by this association, much must be of a silent and for a while unseen nature, penetrating into the plans of the architect, the builder, and the administrators of the interests of cities. General Vielé was right in saying that there is not one man in ten thousand who can tell whether or not the soil-pipe of his residence has a trap connecting it with the street sewer, and that there is not one instance in a thousand where such a trap is in existence, and that no trap or other contrivance has yet been invented to prevent the gases of an unventilated sewer from penetrating into the house's along its route. Can such facts as these be published so universally without awakening a lively sense of responsibility somew1ere? Can the authorities lend a deaf ear to all the questions of faulty hygiene which are associated with school life and the training of children? Will not some practical improvement result from the agitation of theories — even if they be only theories — of ventilation? Many of the questions discussed were entirely out of the usual range of medical practice and reflection. It is with the view of hereafter exciting an interesting discussion on such extra-professional topics that there should be urged upon this association the propriety of seizing upon every available opportunity to add civil engineers and men of good, sound, practical business ideas to their list of membership. Their absence may have been the cause of the silence that almost invariably reigned after the reading of a paper, for the medical men were afraid to handle topics that were somewhat beyond their powers of treatment, though not by any means beyond their comprehension. It has not been my object to refer to the individual merits of the papers presented, which have been so lavishly spread before the public, but rather to point out some of the methods in which the interests of the association can be enhanced, and its practical usefulness extended. Its future must be prosperous and its kindly influences wide-spreading, for it is concerned in the perpetuation of nature's first law, self-preservation.

BALTIMORE, *November* 13, 1875.

WEEKLY BULLETIN OF PREVALENT DISEASES.

THE following is a bulletin of the diseases prevalent in Massachusetts during the week ending November 20, 1875, compiled under the authority of the State Board of Health from the returns of physicians representing all sections of the State: —

The summary for each section is as follows: —

Berkshire: Bronchitis, influenza, pneumonia, rheumatism.

Valley: Bronchitis, influenza, typhoid fever, pneumonia. South Hadley Falls reports a "severe epidemic of measles."

Midland: Influenza, bronchitis, rheumatism, typhoid fever. Spencer reports " scarlatina unusually malignant."

Northeastern: Bronchitis, scarlatina, typhoid fever. Diphtheria has increased. Lexington reports an " epidemic of measles."

Metropolitan: Bronchitis, pneumonia, diphtheria, scarlatina, rheumatism. Less diphtheria reported.

Southeastern: Typhoid fever, bronchitis, influenza. Not much sickness reported.

In the State at large, bronchitis, influenza, typhoid fever, rheumatism, pneumonia, diphtheria, and scarlatina comprise the prevailing diseases. Bronchitis and influenza are everywhere present; diphtheria and scarlatina are most prevalent in and around Boston; typhoid fever is reported mainly by the western sections.　　　F. W. DRAPER, M. D., Registrar.

COMPARATIVE MORTALITY-RATES FOR THE WEEK ENDING NOV. 13, 1875.

	Estimated Population.	Total Mortality for the Week.	Annual Death-Rate per 1000 during Week.
New York	1,060,000	486	24
Philadelphia	800,000	286	19
Brooklyn	500,000		
Chicago	400,000	128	17
Boston	342,000	169	26
Cincinnati	260,000		
Providence	100,700	52	26
Worcester	50,000	19	20
Lowell	50,000	16	17
Cambridge . . .	48,000	18	19
Fall River	45,000	22	25
Lawrence	35,000	9	13
Lynn	33,000	14	22
Springfield	31,000	10	17
Salem	26,000	16	32

Normal Death-Rate, 17 per 1000.

BOOKS AND PAMPHLETS RECEIVED. — Transactions of the Medical Society of the State of Pennsylvania, 1875.

Medico-Chirurgical Transactions. Published by the Royal Medical and Chirurgical Society of London. Vol. LVIII. 1875. (In exchange.)

On the Treatment of Venereal Disease by Salicylic Acid. By George Halsted Boyland, M. D. (Extracted from the American Journal of the Medical Sciences.)

Outlines of Practical Histology. By William Rutherford, M. D., F. R. S. E. London : T. and A. Churchill ; Philadelphia : Lindsay and Blakiston. 1875. Pages 72. (For sale by James Campbell).

Addison's Disease. The Croonian Lectures for 1875. By Edward Headlam Greenough, M. D., F. R. S. Philadelphia : Lindsay and Blakiston. 1875. Pages 212. (For sale by James Campbell.)

Review of Professor Palmer's Statement respecting Homœopathy in the University. (Reprinted from the Detroit Review of Medicine, October, 1875.)

Homœopathy in Michigan University. (Reprinted from the same journal of September.)

Report of the Board of Health of the City and Port of Philadelphia to the Mayor for the year 1874. Philadelphia. 1875.

Are Carbolic Acid Disinfections useful in Yellow Fever ? By Dr. Y. R. LeMonnier. From the New Orleans Medical and Surgical Journal, November, 1875.

Opium Eating. An Autobiographical Sketch. By an Habituate. Philadelphia : Claxton, Remsen, and Haffelfinger. 1876.

The Student's Guide to Human Osteology. By W. W. Wagstaffe, F. R. C. S., Assistant Surgeon to and Lecturer on Anatomy at St. Thomas's Hospital. Philadelphia : Lindsay and Blakiston. 1875. (For sale by A. Williams & Co.)

Phthisis. A Series of Clinical Lectures. By Austin Flint, M. D. Philadelphia : Henry C. Lea. 1875. (For sale by A. Williams & Co.)

SUFFOLK DISTRICT MEDICAL SOCIETY. — The regular meeting will be held on Saturday next, at 7.30 P. M. Papers will be read as follows : —

Dr. E. Cutter, Nascent Chloride of Ammonium in Bronchitis.

Dr. F. I. Knight, Systolic Murmurs at the Apex of the Heart.

Dr. E. Chenery, Experience in the Treatment of One Hundred and Fifty Cases of Diphtheria.

Dr. E. Cutter will exhibit a battery for electrolysis.

ı THE BOSTON
MEDICAL AND SURGICAL JOURNAL.
VOL. XCIII. — THURSDAY, DECEMBER 2, 1875. — NO. 23.

A CASE OF LESION OF THE MEDIAN NERVE WITH REFERENCE TO THE DISTRIBUTION OF THAT NERVE.[1]

BY S. G. WEBBER, M. D., OF BOSTON.

THE distribution of the nerves of the ıand to the fingers has recently attracted considerable attention. One of the best descriptions of the final distribution of the cutaneous brancıes of the median, ulnar, and radial nerves has been given by L. Gustave Richelot.[2] He removed the skin and subcutaneous tissues from the ıand, and tıen followed the nerves by dissection from witıin outwards. He also reports cases of injuries wıicı confirm the results obtained by his dissections.

In the *Archiv für Psychiatrie und Nervenkrankheiten*[3] is an article by M. Bernıardt on the same subject and giving essentially the same results as tıose above alluded to. In a case reported by ıim in wıicı the median nerve was injured, he found tıat on the back of the ıand the wıole of the last two pıalanges of the index and the median finger were affected, and also the radial side of the same pıalanges of the ring finger. In this latter respect tıere is a difference between his case and tıat of my patient.

Henle[4] describes the distribution of the finger-nerves. He states tıat on the palmar aspect the ulnar nerve supplies the tıree medial finger sides, the median nerve the seven lateral. On the dorsal aspect the ulnar supplies one ıalf, the five medial sides; the otıer ıalf, the five lateral sides, is supplied by the radial nerve. It is in the tıumb alone tıat the dorsal nerves are distributed under the nail; in the otıer fingers tıey end at the middle pıalanx, and the distal pıalanx is supplied by brancıes from the palmar nerves. As to the most sensitive portion of the fingers, tıat ıaving the most abundant nerve-supply, the distal pıalanx, the dorsal surface of the tıree medial finger sides is supplied

[1] Read before the Boston Society of Medical Sciences.
[2] Archives de Physiologie, normale et pathologique, No. 2, 1875, page 177. This paper has been referred to in the Report on Anatomy; see the JOURNAL, page 281, September, 1875.
[3] Vol. v., No. 2, page 555.
[4] Handbuch der systematischen Anatomie des Menschen, iii. 499.

by the ulnar, the five next by the median, the two radial, or thumb, by the radial nerve.

The drawings on page 504 of Henle represent the median as distributed to the dorsum of only the last phalanx of the index and middle fingers and the radial side of the ring finger.

Létiévant has, however, made the most exhaustive study of this subject.[1] He describes the limits of the patch of anæsthesia produced by division of each of the three nerves, and considers the causes which operate to render the borders of the patches more sensitive than the centres. He also studies the motor lesions depending upon such divisions. In regard to the region of the hand over which the sensibility is altered after division of the median, he shows that the limits may vary; sometimes the radial side of the median finger and sometimes the radial side of the ring finger being the extreme limit of the change on the palmar side; on the dorsal aspect sometimes the last phalanx of the thumb is affected. The varying statements made by different authorities are easily explained by variations in the subjects examined.

The following case, which was seen at the room for nervous diseases of the Boston Dispensary, illustrates well the distribution of the median nerve.

James S——, shoemaker, on Saturday had a hard day's work stitching boots. When he awoke on Sunday he found that he had lost the power of moving his right hand, and there was pain in the palm of the hand and in the fingers. The previous night he had slept heavily; he could not tell in what position the hand was when he awoke. On Monday morning he came to the dispensary. The pain was described as of a tingling, pricking nature, such as is felt when the ulnar nerve is hit at the elbow. The parts affected were the radial side of the palm of the hand, the palmar aspect of the thumb, and of the index and median fingers, and the radial side of the ring finger; on the back of the hand, the dorsum of the last two phalanges of the index and median fingers. The same pricking sensation was felt in a line up the centre of the palmar side of the fore-arm as far as the elbow, and ending just by the side of the tendon of the biceps.

As to motor disturbance there was much trembling of the hand, the cause of which, whether merely mental agitation or nervous lesion, was not clearly evident. The motions of the hand in flexion, extension, and rotation were slowly performed, but were still possible. Whether there had been decided improvement in this respect since the occurrence of the lesion was not learned.

Létiévant's explanation of the preservation of motion after injury to the median nerve is interesting. He says, " This paralysis with atrophy does not, however, abolish certain motions which belong properly to the affected muscles. Thus, the pronators are paralyzed, and yet pronation

---

[1] Traité des Sections nerveuses. 1873.

is possible. The wrist is flexed, although the palmaris longus and brevis are paralyzed and atrophied. All the fingers can be flexed in all their phalanges, and yet the flexor sublimis and proprius, and half of the flexor profundus, have lost their power of contracting."

This is Létiévant's explanation of these motions. Pronation is performed by the muscles which rotate the shoulder inwards, and by some of the flexors of the fore-arm on the arm, and the weight of the hand assists. Flexion of the wrist is performed by the flexor carpi ulnaris. Flexion of the first phalanges is accomplished by the interossei ; of the last two phalanges of the little and the ring finger by the half of the flexor profundus innervated by the ulnar nerve ; of the median by the tendinous expansion which the muscular fibres of the ring finger send to it, and by which the flexion of these two fingers is associated. The extensors of the metacarpus produce the flexion of the last two phalanges of the index finger and the last phalanx of the thumb, by drawing on the tendons of the paralyzed flexors.

In the case above described the lesion was not so serious as to have necessarily abolished all action of the muscles supplied by the median, though their action must have been at best very weak.

The muscles were faradized, and the motions of the hand immediately became freer ; especially was improvement noticed in the middle and index fingers, but it was most marked in the middle.

The etiology of the lesion is somewhat uncertain. It is possible that during the night the head pressed upon the nerve at the bend of the elbow ; yet it is doubtful whether this could be sufficient to give rise to the symptoms, as the nerve is so situated that it is protected from pressure by an object of the shape and size of the head. There was no history of a blow or other pressure upon the course of the nerve. The hard work sewing boots on Saturday would call into use the pronators and flexors. It may be that this overwork of the muscles supplied by the median caused irritation and exhaustion of that nerve. Or it may be that the prolonged use of the pronator radii teres caused an irritation of the nerve at the point where it passes between the two portions of that muscle at the elbow ; this would perhaps be the most reasonable explanation, in view of the fact that the pain followed accurately the course of the median nerve to the elbow and there stopped.

A CASE OF INTUSSUSCEPTION: RECOVERY.

BY B. F. SEABURY, M. D., OF ORLEANS, MASS.

SEPTEMBER 21, 1875, D. S., aged forty-nine years, generally very healthy, was suddenly attacked, at one o'clock A. M., with severe pain in the left iliac region, extending down the thigh ; retraction of left testicle and retching, without vomiting, accompanied the seizure. The pain was deep-seated, and increased on firm pressure; there was but slight tenderness or fullness of the part, but the pain was persistent and almost intolerable. The symptoms indicated, as I supposed, the presence of a calculus or of some other hard substance in the left ureter; I prescribed opiates in full doses, local hot-baths, etc., till relief should be obtained, and a full dose of castor-oil to be taken next day. I suggested careful inspection of the urine through the next two or three days.

September 22d. The patient was somewhat relieved, but still suffered considerable pain and discomfort in the left side; a slight tumefaction was detected. No effect followed the cathartic; I prescribed a much larger dose, to be followed by injections of soap and water in full amount, and repeatedly, if necessary.

September 25th. No operation from bowels. The patient suffered little pain, but had slight nausea and occasional vomiting. There was no increase of the tenderness or fullness over the seat of the disease. The pulse was a little accelerated and the tongue slightly coated. From the first there was very little thirst or febrile action. Tenesmus occurred whenever injections were administered. Nothing had been detected in the urine, which was of the usual quantity and appearance. Suspecting the nature of the case, cathartics were now discontinued; the warm bath (for half an hour) and persistent use of injections of soap and water, in as large quantity as could be forced into the bowels, were directed.

October 9th. The condition of the patient continued much the same up to this date. Not a particle of fæcal matter, nor anything indicating a natural passage through the intestines, had been detected. The use of the warm bath twice daily, the injections of warm water in as large quantity as the patient could bear, and of castor-oil with a tablespoonful of oil of turpentine, mixed with a pint of warm water, the inflation of the bowels, the application of tincture of iodine over the seat of pain, liquid diet only and in small quantity (even from the first), all these measures were diligently persisted in, but to no purpose.

On the 5th of October something was discharged which the nurse described as a skinny substance, mixed with quite a large clot of blood and about three inches long; unfortunately it was thrown away, but in answer to my questions the nurse said it looked very like a piece of intestine. This discharge was attended with an unusual amount of pain and tenesmus.

In the evening of October 9th, eighteen days from the time of the attack, I was summoned because the patient had had a dejection of a very unusual kind; on careful examination I found a portion of intestine, evidently a part of the ileum, in a partially decayed condition, and measuring, as I and others judged, not less than fourteen inches in lengti. Tiis disciarge was unaccompanied by any fæcal matter; tiere was no blood, and no larger quantity of mucus tian usual, but the stool was attended witi a greater amount of tenesmus tian common. The patient immediately expressed iimself greatly relieved of the feeling of weigit in the bowels, as of " someting tiat ougit to come away."

From tiis time tiere was no return of tiat peculiar feeling, and very little pain or tenesmus; small portions of fæces began to appear, but in form " very like siavings or ribbon, appearing as if the mass had been forced tirougi a very small place," as the nurse described it. The fæces retained tiis form, in some degree, nearly two weeks; but at tiis date (November 6) ticy are nearly normal. The bowels iave become regular, the dejections are not painful, and do not require muci effort. The general iealti of the patient has rapidly improved, his appetite and digestion are very good, and at tiis time, forty-six days from the time of attack, he considers iimself quite well.

A CASE OF PROLONGED GESTATION.

BY FRANK WELLS, M. D.,

Professor of Obstetrics and Diseases of Women and Children in Cleveland Medical College.

MRS. M., a lady of great intelligence, had sexual intercourse witi her iusband on August 27, 1874, two days after the completion of her montily period. On the following day her iusband was called away by business, wiici detained iim from iome until the existence of pregnancy had declared itself to his wife by the cessation of the catamenia. She quickened in the early part of January, 1875, and naturally expected to be confined about the 3d of June, for wiici period she engaged her nurse. Labor did not come on, iowever, until June 26th, nor was it completed until the following day, exactly tiree iundred and four days from the date of sexual congress.

The birti, wiici was a tedious one, necessitating the application of the forceps, was ciiefly ciaracterized by the almost entire absence of liquor amnii, only sufficient being disciarged to make upon the sieet a stain of the size of a silver dollar. The ciild, wiici weigied eigit and one ialf pounds, looked as tiougi it had been in a measure macerated in the amniotic fluid, its skin being loose and wrinkled, and the epidermis peeling off in strips. At tiis date (November, 1875), the ciild (a boy) is iealtiy and vigorous, and weigis eigiteen and one ialf pounds.

The case is remarkable, not only for the long continuance of the gestation, but also for the undoubted evidences of the absorption of some, at least, of the liquor amnii tirougi the cutaneous surface of the fœtus. Tiat tiis must iave been the case is indicated by the fact that as late as the eighth month the child was quite freely movable in the uterine cavity, which shows that at this time there must have been some fluid in which it could float ; and still further by the absence, during gestation, of all painful motions of the child, which would undoubtedly have been felt, had the solid contents of the womb come in direct apposition to the uterine walls, without the medium of a protecting fluid.

RECENT PROGRESS IN DERMATOLOGY.

BY JAMES C. WHITE, M. D.

The Relation of the Urine to Diseases of the Skin. — Dr. L. D. Bulkley,[1] of New York, in a paper upon this subject read before the New York Academy of Medicine, gives his conclusions drawn from the examination of the urine in a large number of cases (five hundred and twenty-three) of skin disease, including eczema, acne, psoriasis, urticaria, ichthyosis, and purpura. In eczema he divides the changes in the urine into two classes : those indicating acid dyspepsia with varying specific gravity, or with persistent abnormal acidity and high specific gravity ; and those in which the urine is not only acid but deposits uric acid or urates. In acne the urine was usually acid, its average specific gravity $1023\frac{1}{4}$, and its changes those of dyspepsia, including urates, uric acid, and an increase of phosphates. From these observations he regards the urine as a most important element in the study of dermatology, giving not only indications of great therapeutical value, but also conclusive evidence of the falsity of the doctrine that diseases of the skin are generally of a local origin. He goes so far, even, as to state that not in one of the cases of skin disease examined was the urine found normal.

There can be no question as to the intimacy of the physiological relations between the kidneys and the skin in health, or of infrequent changes in the tissues of the latter when its circulation is surcharged with products which the kidneys have failed to eliminate, or of common disturbances in both in certain constitutional affections. That the skin may exceptionally be examined as a means of diagnosis in renal disease or in certain changes in the urine is a fair conclusion from these facts, but they do not warrant the conclusion that diseases of the skin are capable of producing such disturbances of the excretion of the kidneys as to be recognized by analysis, or that they are but the expression of certain central or constitutional disorders, simultaneously exhibited by tissue changes in the integument and chemical modifications of the urine. The relations of the urine to diseases of the skin must be most carefully studied and all possible chances of error excluded, before any

[1] The Medical Record, May 1, 1875.

conclusions can be drawn from them affecting the question of the relations of the skin disease to the general economy.   Dr. Bulkley's observations do not seem to have been conducted in this manner, if his
paper is fairly represented in the report of the proceedings of the society.   He analyzes the urine of five hundred patients with skin diseases
and discovers certain changes in it.   These changes are certainly of
a trivial character in the main, and such as occur in the most various
and unimportant conditions of the economy.   They can in no way,
we believe, be regarded as characteristic of the cutaneous affections
in which they are recorded by him as occurring.   Take his analyses in acne, for instance : observations were made in fifteen cases ; in
these the urine was found acid, the specific gravity $1023\frac{1}{4}$ on the average, and " the urinary changes more commonly those of dyspepsia,
including urates, uric acid, etc., and the presence of an abnormal
amount of phosphates."   Are not these results the same as would be
gained from the analysis of the urine in a large porportion of cases
taken as they occur in any hospital ward, among which there was not
a disease of the skin ; or such as would be obtained by no means infrequently in the examination of the urine from the same number of apparently healthy people ?   My own experience in the study of the
urine in health and disease tells me that they are, and that I can see
in them nothing characteristic of the cutaneous diseases in which they
may have been found, or indicative of any " systemic disturbance "
which can be considered as intimately connected with them.   Dr.
Bulkley does not state, moreover, whether in these fifteen cases of
acne dyspepsia did not co-exist as the possible cause of the changes in
the urine ; digestive derangements, according to his views, being closely
connected with the etiology of this and other cutaneous affections.

That disturbances in the functions, and pathological changes in the
tissues, of the skin may be associated with or even caused directly by
disorders of the inner economy cannot *à priori* be denied ; but we must
not apply to the solution of this question methods of observation or
reasoning which would not be allowable in investigating the natural
history of the diseases of other parts of the human frame.   The skin is
a very complex structure, and has the same right to be independently
diseased as any other organ or tissues of the body.   That it is more or
less intimately connected with other systems of the economy there can
be no more doubt than that the same blood flows through them and it
in common ; but that its diseases are in any way necessarily more intimately dependent upon this or that mysterious systemic disturbance,
or still more shadowy changes in the blood, or causes of a " constitutional " origin, than those of other organs, — the lungs, liver, or kidneys,
for instance, — there are no substantial grounds for believing; except such
as are the result of rigorous observation alone.   In no branch of pa-

thology has there been such unwarranted substitution of prejudice and empty theorizing for such investigation as in dermatology. Independent and simple observation has been made almost an impossibility in some nations and schools, owing to the atmosphere or haze of imaginary diatheses which has surrounded it. It is well, then, to call to our aid in its study the exact science of chemistry, if its teachings are not misinterpreted; but we fear that little will be learned, through its application to the urine, of the causes or therapeutics of skin diseases.

Since the above was written, Dr. Bulkley's paper has appeared in full in the October number of his *Archives of Dermatology.* It is a long one, and contains, apparently, mention of everything hitherto written upon the subject, in addition to his own investigations and conclusions, which are fairly enough stated in the report of the society. It fails, however, to show that the urinary changes in question are the result of the cutaneous changes they accompany. The paper brings together much interesting material, and illustrates the writer's indefatigable industry.

Molluscum Contagiosum. — Dr. Cäser Boeck, of Christiania, communicates [1] the results of his investigation of the anatomy of this very peculiar affection. Ordinarily regarded as a disease of the sebaceous glands, it is known that Virchow considered its starting-point to be the hair follicle, while Retzius maintained that the epidermis is the seat of the disease. Peculiar bodies have long been recognized as a constant and characteristic microscopic feature of the growth, which are supposed to be the contagious element of the affection, and which have been regarded in their histological relations most variously by different observers. If some of the matter from the gland-like structure of the growth be squeezed out through the opening in its centre, these bodies will be found in great abundance, more or less round or oval in shape, sharply defined, transparent, and of a fatty lustre. Boeck concludes, as the result of his study of them, that they are not foreign bodies, not the products of an endogenous process, but only cells of the rete which have undergone a peculiar metamorphosis of protoplasm, the nature of which he does not comprehend. That they must be the bearers of contagion seems to be accepted in want of any other plausible theory to explain the facts of transference of the affection from child to nurse, from one to several playmates, from the genitals of one sex to those of the other in connection, and by direct experiment. The cells, if they be the guilty bodies, must have the power of multiplying themselves by subdivision upon another host, or of inducing by contact healthy cells to take on the same pathological process. It is Boeck's opinion, too, that molluscum is not an affection of the sebaceous glands, but of the rete mucosum.

[1] Vierteljahresschrift für Dermatologie und Syphilis, 11 Jahrg., erstes Heft.

The Inoculation of Varicella. — Professor Steiner[1] reports his experience in ten cases in which he has practiced inoculation of the clear watery fluid taken from freshly developed varicella vesicles. Eight of the ten succeeded, that is, they were followed by the development of varicella, and never of variola. Of these, five had been vaccinated, and three not. In all, the duration of what he calls the stage of inoculation lasted eight days. Four times the eruption appeared without any prodromata. The highest temperature, as a rule, coincided with the eruption; the defervescence was rapid and complete. The course observed after the inoculation was ordinarily the following: on the third day nothing was to be seen at the point of insertion; on the fourth a gradually increasing febrile movement began, with distinct evening exacerbations and morning remissions. There was decided reddening of the mucous membrane of the mouth and throat before the appearance of the eruption. This followed on the eighth day, and the disease ran its ordinary course.

Etiology of Infantile Eczema.[2] — Dr. R. W. Taylor, of New York city, discusses in this paper, which has also been published in a separate form, the question of the relations of eczema to the general economy. He first considers the effect which certain "diatheses," the rheumatic and scrofulous, may have in predisposing to its development in the infant. The manifestations of the former are so tardy in their evolution that, as he believes, it cannot affect the skin in infancy; while with regard to the latter no more intimate connection can be shown than in the greater tendency to inflammation it impresses upon the integument in common with all the tissues of the body. In cases of this origin the disease is extensively distributed, deeply seated, of purulent form, obstinate, and more than usually disposed to relapse. With regard to the question of transmissibility from parents to offspring of a tendency to eczema, he is of the opinion that this can be accepted without believing in such theories as the handing-down of blood-conditions or diatheses, certain parts of the organism being perpetuated in an abnormal state, as shown in inherited xeroderma, for example. Local debility, therefore, and not hereditary morbid dyscrasia, is to be regarded as the explanation of this class of cases, an inherited tendency to local disease awaiting any sufficient exciting cause for its manifestation.

Another question considered by Dr. Taylor is the relation between the disease and other cutaneous affections in children. Eczema, as a sequela of vaccination, of the exanthemata, etc., or in a relapsing form, he would explain on the theory that inflammatory processes of the skin, whether simple or specific, induce a tendency to a similar process

---

[1] The Medical Record, October 23, 1875, from Rundschau, August, 1875.

[2] American Practitioner, June, 1875.

in the future by ingrafting a peculiar morbid condition upon the cells, blood-vessels, and nerves of the part; that eczema, likewise, more especially of severe form, " localized to one spot, ingrafts a tissue tendency therein to a subsequent similar attack ; and also that this affection of one part of the tegumentary membrane predisposes to a greater or less degree the whole to the same morbid process, which is manifested either by its direct extension from the original focus or by its beginning spontaneously at some point more or less remote from its origin." Even with this tendency, he is of the opinion that in rare instances only does the affection arise spontaneously, and that in the vast majority of cases in infants it starts from local sources of irritation.

Anal Eczema. — Vérité, in *La France Médicale,*[1] gives an excellent account of this most common and troublesome affection: Vesicles are rarely observed on account of their early absorption, he thinks, and the moisture of the parts he attributes to glandular secretion, not to eczematous discharge. His description of the intensity of the accompanying pruritus and the consequent changes is very characteristic: patients press aside the nates to get at the mucous surface, and not only rub and scratch it, but introduce two or three fingers into the rectum for several minutes, thus producing a titillation which is followed by a slight serous discharge, succeeded by relief and sleep. This habit, difficult of renunciation, is dangerous in proportion as it is accompanied by pollution. The consequent changes are analogous to those which are characteristic of passive pederasty ; an infundibulum is formed, fissures and crests ensue, and the semi-spherical concave is transformed into a plane which extends from one ischiatic projection to another. Thickening of the tissues and excessive pigmentation are often observed. Alkalies internally and the application of ferric sulphate are advised.

The Management of Eczema.[2] — Dr. L. Duncan Bulkley republishes in pamphlet form under this title an essay read before the American Medical Association in 1874. For presenting it in this more accessible form to the profession he could have offered no better motive than the following : " If he shall have assisted any in their attempts at mastering this protean malady, and shall have aided in removing its treatment from the rut of Fowler's solution and zinc ointment, . . . the writer will be amply repaid for his labor." He begins with a brief account of the pathological anatomy of eczema, and defines it to be a catarrhal dermatitis in its early stages, but would apparently restrict the definition to cases arising from unknown causes, as he states that the eruptions which are produced by most external agents, rhus, arnica, soaps, etc., are not eczema, although dermatitis. That these agents, and others, are capable of giving rise to graver forms of inflammation than the

1 Chicago Medical Journal and Examiner, September, 1875.
2 The Management of Eczema. New York : G. P. Putnam's Sons. 1875.

usual tissue changes of this disease, there can be no doubt, but that they often do so is beyond our observation. The appearances produced by the rhus poison, for instance, in surface manifestations, subjective symptoms, and course, are in a great majority of cases wholly those of acute eczema, and, although generally stamped with certain characteristic though trivial peculiarities, present ordinarily no greater deviations from the average type than occur in a series of idiopathic cases. Their cause is often overlooked for this reason, and cases not unfrequently present themselves where even the most experienced observers are unable to determine whether the eczema be of this extraneous origin or not. Farther on the author admits the influence of local agents in the production of the disease, for he refers to the eczema caused by pediculi, the itch insect, heat, water, sugar, lime, and other chemical agents. He is strongly inclined, however, to adopt the diatetic view of causation, inasmuch as these eczemas of local origin are inclined to run an acute course without subsequent chronic infiltration of the skin, proving, as he thinks, a failure to find the system in a condition to sustain the cutaneous manifestations, when their direct cause is removed. This condition he regards as some unknown blood change, deranged cell action, congenital defect, perverted innervation, or the like, with special emphasis on the first named, as further manifested in the paper on the urinary changes in this affection, above noticed. What are these sets of words but confessions that the causes of idiopathic eczema are almost wholly unknown, not yet within the range of demonstrative reasoning, in which respect it is like most diseases of the skin, like most diseases in general?

·With regard to the management of eczema Dr. Bulkley's views are largely influenced by these theories concerning its etiology. Starting with the assumed doctrine that the fact of local disease necessarily proves constitutional disease, he considers that it is absolutely necessary to employ internal treatment addressed to the system at large, and that the effects of external remedies are but local and in a great measure temporary. The medicines which he finds to be requisite are treated of under these heads : cathartics, diuretics, alkalies, tonics, and sedatives. The first he uses sparingly at the beginning, but cautions against their abuse. Diuretics, he thinks, are " positively demanded in a goodly proportion of cases," because the cutaneous capillaries are irritated by the circulation of effete products through them. Under this head he includes alkalies as of the utmost importance, as he considers eczema to be largely the result of over-acidity, as shown by the acidity of the urine and by the presence of acid dyspepsia, the " almost universal vomiting of infants with eczema " (?) being, he thinks, an effort of nature to get rid of the acid. Under tonics he gives the first place to cod-liver oil, its effect in the proper cases being " magical." Of arsenic he says that he rarely gives it, although it may assist at times and give permanency to the cure. Among sedatives he strongly recommends chloral for the relief of nocturnal itching, and includes with them tar and carbolic acid given internally.

But Dr. Bulkley does not neglect local treatment, although he makes it subordinate. He gives the most particular directions as to the different classes of remedies to be used in the acute and the chronic stages of the disease. They are, however, mostly those of the German school, modified, as he thinks to be necessary, for the more delicate American skins, and therefore need no special comments here. In his Analysis of One Thousand Cases of Skin Disease [1] occurring in dispensary practice, he calls attention to the satisfactory results he has more lately obtained by the use of tannin ointment (one drachm to the ounce), and subnitrate of bismuth (half a drachm to the ounce) in ointment. Domestic soft soap he also advises in place of sapo viridis. Its unequal strength, however, makes its action very uncertain.

That there are often faults of the general economy or disorders of special organs and functions in patients with eczema, no one would deny, or the importance of removing them so far as possible by proper means. That they are generally or necessarily present, as shown by legitimate evidence, or that, when present, they can be demonstrated in most cases to be the cause of the disease, are questions upon which very different opinions from those of Dr. Bulkley are held by the best of observers, the correctness of which, we think, may be most clearly shown by the practical test of applying their principles to practice. That our author treats eczema most successfully by his skilled use of local remedies and universal internal medication, we doubt not; so do others who believe and practice differently.

Étude sur la Dermatite exfoliatrice généralisée.[2] — This article is founded upon the observation of three recent cases in St. Louis Hospital which, the writer thinks, find no place in the lists of ordinary affections of the skin. According to his conclusions, epidermal exfoliation shows itself as an important element in many cutaneous affections, but it is rare, except in scarlet fever, to see it develop simultaneously over the whole surface of the body and in the form of large scales. The universal distribution of the exfoliation, together with the enormous size of the scales, is sufficient to characterize the disease as a special affection under the name of dermatite exfoliatrice, and to distinguish it readily from such squamous affections as psoriasis and pityriasis. Several cases described by Wilson, the cases called herpétide exfoliatrice by Bazin, and others described under the title pemphigus foliaceus, pityriasis rubra, etc., seem to him to deserve the same name. He recognizes two varieties

---

[1] American Practitioner, May, 1875.
[2] Émile Percheron. Paris. 1875.

of the disease. The first is characterized by a very abundant and persistent exfoliation with a rapid renewal of the epidermis, and embraces several varieties, according as the cutaneous affection is accompanied, or not, by grave general symptoms, and according as it is developed primarily and persists as such throughout the whole course of the eruption, or in the course of some other affection of which it is in some way a modification. In the second the exfoliation is of less importance, and perhaps should be regarded as the last stage of an erythematous affection. In order to give an idea of its rapid course and mild character, it might be called dermatite exfoliatrice pseudo-exanthématique. He thinks that it would be premature, with the few facts in our possession, to pronounce upon the nature of the affection, but that it is not always the same.

(To be concluded.)

HAMILTON ON FRACTURES AND DISLOCATIONS.[1]

THE excellent and comprehensive treatise of Dr. Hamilton is too well known to require extended comment. In examining it we are impressed with a criticism which applies to most last editions of medical works. A good deal is added and little taken away. It is often said of a long sermon that it would be improved by boiling down, but this process occupies time, which we can hardly expect from a large practitioner with extended occupations. The evil resulting from a want of this kind of revision is very obvious. Each edition becomes more and more a collection of desultory facts at each issue less digested. In the present work examine, for example, the chapter on treatment of the fractures of the thigh. It contains, as we infer, everything that has been said or done by every practitioner, at least in the United States, for the last forty or fifty years, with wood-cuts of the apparatus employed by them. As a store-house of history it has its value; but to a student or practitioner who desires to know what is the best treatment for a fractured thigh its value is less apparent. Every surgical practitioner has a hobby by means of which he produces results as good as those of any other practitioner or as are known to science. This means that certain principles are common to all methods and certain features essential to all apparatus. We desire to see these common and essential elements of treatment and apparatus emphasized and made so accessible that the practitioner who runs may also read. In a word, the criticism we have to make upon this excellent work of Dr. Hamilton is that it lacks that perspective which brings important facts into the foreground. It is a Chinese picture of surgical practice, in which every object obtrudes its claims with equal force upon the observer. Such a work leaves for the reader that business of selection and appreciation which legitimately belongs to the writer.

One more example will suffice. In this community it is believed that the

[1] *A Practical Treatise on Fractures and Dislocations.* By FRANK HASTINGS HAMILTON, A. M., M. D., LL. D. Fifth Edition. Philadelphia: Henry C. Lea. 1875.

impacted fracture of the neck of the thigh-bone is, to say the least, one of the most common of those occurring in adults about the hip.[1] It is a source of constant error in diagnosis, and sometimes of litigation. It is liable to be overlooked as a sprain, or to remain in doubt while the patient is lame ; and yet its signs are so far pathognomonic that it is hardly too much to say that this most common fracture need never occasion doubt. We look in vain in Dr. Hamilton's book for any such identification as this of the impacted fracture of the neck of the thigh-bone. In reading his chapters no one would suspect its frequency, its importance, or the certainty with which it can be diagnosticated.

We observe a few omissions. In so exhaustive a work we should expect some notice of the V or W fractures of the tibia, so often accompanied by serious injury to the ankle-joint, described so minutely in past years by several French authors as well as in the pages of the JOURNAL.[2] Nor do we see any account of Suersen's apparatus for fractured jaw, which has been employed with satisfactory results by surgeons in this city. But where there is so much that is good we may well refrain from criticism. We commend the work to our readers as the best treatise extant in connection with this subject, and we trust that its distinguished author may find time in future editions to increase its value by condensing its details.

DALTON'S PHYSIOLOGY.[3]

THE statement of the author in the preface to this edition that " the additions and alterations in the text . . . have resulted . . . in an increase of fully fifty per cent. in the matter of the work," gives a very inadequate idea of the labor involved in the preparation of the volume. The character of the book has been radically changed, large portions of it having been entirely rewritten. The new matter has been added with great judgment and discrimination, and the student now finds in this work clear and concise statements of the present condition of our knowledge in nearly all the principal departments of physiology. The most important additions are in those chapters which relate to the nervous system, and particularly to the nerve-centres. A very good general account is here given of Hitzig's observations on the localization of motor centres in the cortex cerebri and of the confirmation of his results by a committee of which the author was a member. As chapters in which the improvement over former editions is most marked may be mentioned those on respiration and on animal heat. In the latter chapter the recent observations of Senator on heat-production are appropriately recorded. The portion of the work devoted to the physiology of reproduction has been enriched by a full and well-illustrated account of the formation of the blastodermic layers,

----

[1] Bigelow on the Hip. 1869.

[2] Nouveau Dictionnaire de Médecine et de Chirurgie, xix. 526. Richard, page 67. Folin and Nélaton. R. M. Hodges, M. D., Boston Medical and Surgical Journal, new series, vi. 102.

[3] *A Treatise on Human Physiology.* By JOHN C. DALTON, M. D. Sixth Edition. Philadelphia : Henry C. Lea. 1875.

as well as by some additional information on the subject of infusorial animalcules and their relation to the question of spontaneous generation.

In comparing this edition with that preceding it, one is struck by the entire omission of the chapter on the spleen ; nor is this omission made good by any reference to that organ in other portions of the work. It is true that we are lamentably deficient in positive knowledge of this viscus, but this hardly seems a sufficient reason for ignoring the subject altogether. The physiology of the vaso-motor nerves is also rather too hastily disposed of. This subject has of late years been investigated so extensively, and with such good results, that it seems to deserve rather more notice than can be bestowed in the three pages which the author devotes to it.

In spite of these defects it may be safely said that the work will take very high rank as a text-book of physiology. In fact, it would be difficult to point out any book in the English language so well adapted to meet the wants of medical students.   H. P. B.

WOOD'S THERAPEUTICS.[1]

THE first edition of this work was so recently reviewed in the JOURNAL that an extensive notice would now be superfluous. We are pleased to find that many of the errors in the first edition are corrected in the second edition ; and also that Dr. Wood has taken great pains to carefully revise those of his conclusions which are not supported by more recent contributions to the literature of therapeutics. In view of its clinical importance we would call the attention of our readers to what the author says of the antipyretic action of quinia :[2] "The drift of our present clinical evidence seems to indicate that quinia exerts in febrile disease a decided antipyretic action, which is especially manifested during those stages of disease in which the natural tendency is towards a lowering of temperature. . . . As an antipyretic the drug should be used whenever there is serious elevation of temperature, except it be in cases of simple inflammation of the brain or its membranes." This conclusion is somewhat different from that expressed in the first edition. .

Among the additions to the list of drugs caffein, the alkaloid of coffee, may be noted ; and very properly, it would seem, Dr. Wood has included under this head also a description of thein, the alkaloid of tea. The medical world is probably not yet willing to allow that either caffein or thein will produce the same effects as the hot infusion of coffee or tea, and perhaps if Dr. Wood had confined his description to the hot infusions of tea, and other vegetable "food substitutes," he would have been induced to place these substances under the head of stimulants rather than antispasmodics. However, the description of the therapeutical effects and uses of caffein are in accord with the light of modern investigations. We may notice the following words, which will hardly tend to add confidence with regard to the use of this remedial agent: "To predict in any case what its influence will be, in the present state of our clinical knowledge, is impossible."

[1] *Therapeutics, Materia Medica, and Toxicology.* By H. C. WOOD, M. D., Professor of Botany, etc., in the University of Pennsylvania. Revised Edition. Philadelphia : J. B. Lippincott & Co. 1876.
[2] Page 71.

It may also be noticed that in this second edition of his work Dr. Wood has rearranged his classification. He has included in Part I. what in his former edition was placed under the head of Part II. In order, however, to make his classification more systematic, he divides the materia medica into —

" 1. Those substances which act on the solids and fluids of the body.

" 2. Substances which act externally to the body."

He includes in Part II. " remedies which are not drugs." These latter he describes under the head of forces, in which he includes caloric, cold, and electricity.

Dr. Wood has evidently exercised a good deal of discretion and bestowed much labor in revising the first edition, and nowhere else can we find such an accumulation of original work of investigators in the field of physiological research as in this book.

We can hardly forbear to remark that a careful perusal would seem to show that physiological investigation has certainly achieved more exact progress than clinical experience. It is rather a cause for regret that we have not more careful observers of the results of clinical experience with drugs, so that the same tests might be applied at the bedside as are now done in the physiological laboratory. We might then feel assured that the practical utility of drugs in disease had attained a rapid progress. As it is now, the medical student commences his combat against disease with rather a confused idea of the value of medicines. Indeed, he can better describe the pathology than the medicinal treatment of disease.

————◆————

PROCEEDINGS OF THE BOSTON SOCIETY FOR MEDICAL IMPROVEMENT.

F. B. GREENOUGH, M. D., SECRETARY.

AUGUST 23, 1875. *Diphtheria.* — DR. C. P. PUTNAM spoke of seven cases of diphtheria which had been under his care, in a tenement house in the rear of Cambridge Street. Of these, four were fatal. In three there was an eruption resembling that of scarlatina, but differing from it in not making its appearance in patches, as is usual in scarlatina at the outset; it consisted of small dots and it spread downward over the body like that of the eruption of scarlatina. Three of the children, who had had scarlatina last winter, did not have this eruption. One of the cases, a girl six years old, had when first seen little white spots on the tonsils, and next day diphtheritic patches; on the second day the eruption appeared, and lasted four days. The deposit on the tonsils increased somewhat, and there was some redness of the fauces. At this time some enlargement of the cervical glands was noticed on the side of the neck. The patient was doing well otherwise, apparently, and on the tenth day she was sitting up, dressed and sewing. On the eleventh day, during the morning she seemed rather heavy, but made no special complaint. Her appetite was poor and her feet were somewhat œdematous. In the afternoon she became restless, moving from one seat to another. A little before five P. M., she exclaimed that she wanted to see the doctor. At this time no dyspnœa or change of color was noticed, but the patient seemed more restless. Suddenly she called out, "For God's sake, bring the doctor," and died. During the time that the eruption was present the urine was examined once, and found to be slightly albuminous. Dr. Putnam supposed that death was due to d ph-theria and not to scarlatina, and thought that the case was interesting, from the fact of sudden death's taking place without any dyspnœa. No record of the temperature was taken in this case, but in that of a younger child (three years old) in the same family, who also had the eruption, and who also died suddenly, it had been 102.5° at the onset. In this case the eruption preceded the diph-theritic throat. Dr. Putnam asked if other gentlemen had seen cases of diph-theria where the death was sudden without any dyspnœa.

DR. ABBOT said that he thought such cases were not so very rare. He mentioned one, in which a gentleman who was thought to be convalescent was up and about the house. He lay down on a sofa and died without any pre-monitory symptoms. A child six years old, in the same house, with a diphthe-ritic deposit in the throat, died suddenly while sitting up and dressed.

DR. JACKSON expressed a doubt whether the eruption in these cases was really that of scarlatina.

DR. FITZ said that Dr. Robinson, of New York, had attempted to prove that sudden death in diphtheria was due to the formation of a clot in the heart, but that he was not supported by his autopsies in this theory.

DR. PORTER spoke of the case of a young lady supposed to be convalescent from diphtheria, who died instantaneously while going up-stairs on her return from a drive. He had performed tracheotomy twice in cases of diphtheria. In one the mucous membrane of the trachea was so inflamed and œdematous that only the inner tube of the smallest tracheotomy-tube could be introduced. In both cases the patients died, although the dyspnœa was relieved. In an-swer to a question whether the operation was ever successful he said that cases of recovery after tracheotomy were reported. We know, moreover, that chil-dren have recovered without the operation, and it is reasonable to suppose that at least as many would get well after it.

DR. PUTNAM asked, with reference to Dr. Jackson's remark concerning the nature of the eruption, if any member had seen the so called eruption of diph-theria, a uniform blush preceding the deposit. In this case, the eruption re-sembled that of scarlatina, although there were no patches, and it spread over the body as that of scarlatina does. The papillæ of the tongue were enlarged, but the tonsils were not to any great extent. The locality in which these seven cases occurred was a crowded tenement house, the cellar of which was damp and musty, and was used to store fruit which was used in a bakery on the premises. The water-closets seemed to be in good order. The most "asthenic" cases occurred on the ground floor, and these, when moved to up-per rooms, improved.

Dr. Putnam showed several specimens of diphtheritic membrane in various solutions.

There were two specimens of the natural membrane unaltered; one of some of the membrane in lime-water, which was partially decomposed, the fluid looking opalescent; one in strong lactic acid, which was nearly dissolved, the fluid being perfectly clear; and lastly, one in an aqueous solution of sali-cylic acid, which seemed to have, as it were, tanned the specimen.

Syphilitic Placenta. — Dr. Fitz reported the case and showed the placenta, which came from a patient of Dr. Foster. The fœtus was a macerated one of about five months. The mother had had frequent abortions, but no syphilitic symptoms in the intervals; it was probable that the husband had been infected.

The changes in the placenta consisted of a thickening and opacity of its uterine surface, which presented yellowish patches alternating with others of a grayish-white color. Beneath these were nodular masses, corresponding in color and of a relatively homogeneous appearance; the yellow nodules were more dense than the gray ones. The membranes were also thickened, opaque in spots, and of a yellowish color. The changes in the placenta were due to a thickening and increased formation of the placental villi, with cell formations in them, and an eventual fatty degeneration.

Fränkel, who specially described these changes in the placenta as resulting from syphilis, considered them as indicating that the ovum had been directly infected by the father, when there was no evidence of disease on the part of the mother. That these changes in the placenta are due to syphilis is confirmed by the condition of the bones of the fœtus, which present the changes described by Wegner. The fact of there being no sharp dividing line between the bone and cartilage is of great value as a diagnostic sign.

Dr. Jackson asked if these changes had been noticed in other placentæ.

Dr. Fitz said that somewhat similar appearances resulting from hæmorrhage, fatty degeneration, fibrous thickenings, etc., had been found in placentæ, but that it was only recently that the connection between this special form of change and syphilis had been appreciated.

Dr. Ellis said that he had often in the past seen such placentæ, but that he had not been aware of their significance.

Dr. Jackson asked if it were a well-established fact that syphilis was a cause of repeated abortions.

Dr. Fitz thought that it was.

Dr. Williams said that it was certainly very common, where a child was seen with hereditary syphilis, to hear a history of repeated previous abortions on the part of the mother.

Dr. Greenough said that of the great number of married women who came under his care at the Boston Dispensary, and who were suffering from syphilis, a very large majority gave a history of repeated uncompleted pregnancies.

October 11. *Foreign Body in the Eye.* — Dr. Williams reported the case. The patient, a boy, was first seen in August, 1874, with a history of a piece of a percussion cap having been blown into the eye in June. Examination showed a scar of the cornea, and a wound of the iris and lens; and Dr. Williams cautioned the parents about the necessity of getting advice at once, should any inflammatory symptoms arise. Last November the eye did become inflamed, and continued so for about three months. Last month the inflammation recurred. When again seen by Dr. Williams, October 5, 1875, the eye was somewhat atrophied and soft, was without any perception of light, and was considerably injected and sensitive. Under the use of atropia, the pupil dilated very slightly at one part but was elsewhere adherent to the capsule of the lens. No further light was obtained by an examination, and the fragment of copper was nowhere to be seen. Under the circumstances, considering the danger of sympathetic trouble in the other eye, extirpation was considered imperative. On seeing the patient the next day, however, a piece of copper, nearly a quarter of a whole cap, was discovered in the anterior chamber, which must have found its way through the pupil after dilatation. The metal was removed, and the patient has done well. Dr. Williams thought it a remarkable fact that such a large foreign substance could have remained for such a length of time in the eye without causing more trouble.

Dr. Hay said that such cases put the surgeon in a difficult position. If the eye is not removed there is always danger of trouble and even loss of the opposite from sympathetic inflammation; but on the other hand, it is not certain that any trouble will follow. Patients naturally look upon the removing of an eye as a serious thing, and are unwilling to submit to the operation unless they are told that it is absolutely necessary, which perhaps the surgeon is not justified in saying.

Dr. Jackson asked what was supposed to be the cause of the marked sympathy between the eyes in cases of this sort.

Dr. Williams said that it was usually attributed to irritation of the ciliary nerves of the one eye extending to and affecting the same nerves of the other eye; whatever the cause might be, the fact was undoubted, more especially in cases in which a foreign body remained in the ciliary region, or in which that region was involved in the scar of a wound.

Large Tumor below the Knee; Myxo-Lipoma. — Dr. H. J. Bigelow exhibited a recent specimen of this disease, and reported the case. The patient was a sufficiently healthy-looking woman, thirty-one years of age, and the mother of eleven children. Two years before her entrance into the Massachusetts General Hospital the tumor appeared in the calf of the leg, movable and rather superficial. After a year it was of the size of a cocoa-nut, and when examined equaled that of a very large foot-ball, the circumference being thirty-one inches. In extent it reached from the middle of the calf of the leg to just above the popliteal space; the posterior and outer portions of the leg being the chief seat of the disease, so that it was thought that it might arise from the fibula. Over the tibia it did not extend, and this bone was evidently unaffected. The mass was nodulated, with large veins creeping over the surface, and more or less redness; and toward the outer portion was a defined ulcer, four inches in diameter, from which there projected a large, fungous, sloughy mass, that had been the source of a severe hæmorrhage. Near the large ulcer were two others, small and superficial. Pain in the tumor was but moderate from the first, and for the last three months the general health had been impaired.

Dr. Bigelow amputated the thigh just above the tumor, and, on subsequent examination, found the following appearances: The bones proved not to be involved. The tumor consisted chiefly of fat, with masses interspersed of pure myxomatous structure. The fat was whiter than ordinary, less lobulated, and, when cold, did not resemble an ordinary fatty section ; but it greased paper, and, under the microscope, showed well-marked fat cells everywhere. The myxomatous tissue looked like chilled isinglass, being translucent, and in some places jelly-like and slimy when drawn out. Its color was reddish-gray. The masses varied in size from that of a chestnut to that of an apple, were of irregular form, and as distinctly and abruptly separate from the surrounding fat as the bits of fat in the section of the breast of a larded partridge. This tissue presented a fibroid structure in some places, and in others, minute parallel, wavy lines. Under the microscope it showed well-marked stellate, attenuated cells.

Dr. Bigelow remarked that this somewhat rare tumor of the connective tissue was an unusually fine specimen of what Virchow has described as a myxo-lipoma, presenting well-marked fat, in which masses of colloid tissue were distributed. This last is regarded as an elementary form of fat, and is seen in the umbilical cord, and also in the degenerating fat and connective tissue of old people. The whole is an illustration of the fact that certain tumors represent the embryonic condition of natural tissues; the present growth being connective tissue, at once exaggerated in volume and embryonic in structure. Müller has stated that his collonema, which much resembles the present specimen, is in some instances a benign growth. Dr. Bigelow said that it was difficult to believe that an immense tumor that had formed within the space of two years, and had pervaded all of the soft tissues, should be of that character; but in amputating the limb he gave the patient the benefit of the doubt.

Deficiency of the Extremities. — DR. JACKSON reported the case of a negro whom he had seen lately on exhibition. The right upper extremity was scarcely to be felt, and was probably not over an inch in length. The left upper limb terminated bluntly about the middle of the arm, as in a case of amputation. Each of the lower extremities consisted of a leg and a foot, of good length and dimensions; and although the hips were completely exposed, nothing like a femur could be felt upon either side. The motions of the extremities, however, were free upon the pelvis. The left was rather less developed than the right, and in a state of adduction. The left foot had four toes; the right had five, and was permanently extended upon the leg ; and with them the man could fill his pipe, light it with a friction match, and put it into his mouth, load and fire a pistol, and perform some experiments of great delicacy. Except the conditions described, the man's body was well formed. He was thirty-one years of age. His countenance was intelligent, and he looked healthy. His keeper, however, said that though he ate well, his bowels were very torpid and his evacuations did not occur oftener than once in ten or fourteen days. He is married, is in every way well developed sexually, and has two children. One of these is nine years of age, and well formed ; the other is two years younger, and is said to resemble his father. There have been no other malformations in his family, so far as the man is aware.

HOSPITAL CONSTRUCTION AND ORGANIZATION.

OUR readers are familiar with the fact that the late Johns Hopkins, a rich citizen of Baltimore, bequeathed a munificent sum, amounting to more than three millions of dollars, for the building and support of a general hospital to be called by his name and to be placed in the favored city of his residence. The trustees of this bequest, in conformity with the expressed wish of Mr. Hopkins, initiated the execution of their trust by seeking " the advice and assistance of those who have achieved the greatest success in the construction and management of hospitals." To this end, five well-known physicians, representing different sections of the country, were requested to give to the board their counsel. One of the fruits of this preliminary measure is before us in the form of an exceedingly attractive book [1] containing the contributions which the request elicited. Here are gathered the five essays, comprising in their entirety a remarkable amount of experience and scientific attainment. It is a tournament of experts. Boston, New York, Philadelphia, Washington, and New Orleans are well represented, and the combined work may be considered as the expression of the American view upon a subject in which every physician has an interest. The profession is under great obligations to the trustees for this valuable addition to the literature of hospital hygiene ; if the generous purposes of the Baltimore merchant should go no further toward fulfillment, this collection of essays was happily conceived as in itself a tangible and lasting memorial of his wish to relieve human suffering.

Although the executors in their circular letter expressed the belief that " there must be some principles of hospital hygiene and of hospital treatment fixed and immutable in their character," they could hardly expect entire unanimity on the part of their advisers in the expression and practical application of those principles. The subject of hospital construction has been revised so thoroughly in recent times, traditional notions were so fundamentally disturbed by the army experiences of the last fifteen years, that the architecture and administration of civil hospitals are still open matters of discussion. But however widely opinions may vary concerning the causes and prevention of " hospitalism," upon one point there is harmony ; it is agreed that the first and most peremptory requirement of hospitals is that " they shall do the sick no harm ; " and it is gratifying to see this precept emphasized throughout this book.

Upon the interesting question of the relative merits of one-storied pavilions and of superimposed wards, the writers have decided but somewhat different notions ; the weight of preference, however, is for the single-ward buildings. There is entire unanimity upon the superiority of permanent buildings to temporary barracks ; all the advantages claimed for the latter are to be secured by the proper construction and administration of the former, while for special emergencies tents offer a ready expedient. In the matters of heating and ventilation, there is essential harmony of views ; indirect radiation from steam-

---

[1] *Hospital Plans: Five Essays relating to the Construction, Organization, and Management of Hospitals, contributed by the Authors for the Use of the Johns Hopkins Hospital of Baltimore.* New York: William Wood & Co. 1875.

coils, supplemented by open fires, is the method generally recommended, while the means for supplying pure air and for exhausting foul air show no noteworthy differences. Concerning the supply of light, the amount of air space, and the use of the pavilion-basements for ventilation only, there is substantial agreement. The arrangement of the administration buildings appears to have vexed the spirits and taxed the ingenuity of all the writers; the general kitchen seems the object of special opprobrium, for we find it now at the top of the centre building, now at one side of the grounds in a detached house, now in the basement under the main structure, and now isolated in the centre of the system.

We have space for only the briefest mention of the individual contributions, each one of which merits full examination and analysis.

Dr. J. S. Billings, assistant surgeon U. S. A., has been known and quoted as a special advocate of temporary barrack hospitals; it is therefore somewhat surprising to find him now advising that all the pavilions should be permanent and that most of them should be of two stories. But he seeks to avoid the evils supposed to attend such an arrangement, by rigidly classifying the patients (separating the febrile from the non-febrile cases), and by so placing the means of communication from the lower ward to the upper that each shall be practically isolated. Fire-places find no favor with Dr. Billings; "they waste fuel, increase labor, cause noise and dust, and are somewhat dangerous." Impermeability of walls is not to be aimed at, for if secured it would prevent transpiration; "it is like varnishing a man's skin to keep his underclothing from being soiled." The shape and arrangement of the wards proposed are quite similar to those of the wards in the Boston City Hospital. Dr. Billings has wrought into his essay many matters relating to hospital hygiene, his acknowledged ability and experience being well illustrated here.

The essay of Dr. Norton Folsom is in many respects in strong contrast with the others; it avoids the elaborate discussion of principles and theories, and aims straight at the matter in hand, presenting exactly what we believe the trustees wanted — clearly defined, detailed, sensible recommendations to guide them in the actual execution of their important work. We have here, not the contribution of an amateur or theorist, but the production of one who, as he says, "feels especially sure of his ground from experience." It does not detract from the value of his suggestions that many of them are simply modifications of plans and methods already in successful operation under his own supervision at the Massachusetts General Hospital; indeed, that fact rather adds to their value, in that they have been tried and have not been found wanting. We are most favorably impressed with the directness, the simplicity, and the thoroughness which characterize all the descriptions, and at the same time with the completeness with which they appear to satisfy the requirements of well-established laws of hygiene.

Dr. Folsom's unreserved preference is for single-story, permanent pavilions. The room for patients in the common wards is square in shape, with the apparatus for heating and ventilation (open fire-places and steam-coils) in the centre. The administration of the ward is entirely at one end of the building, the opposite end being devoted to a sun-room. The isolating wards are well arranged for their purpose ; their plan is essentially that of the new Bigelow ward at the Massachusetts General Hospital. The kitchen, laundry, boilers, operating amphitheatre, out-patient service, dead-house, and autopsy-room are in detached buildings at one corner of the grounds, but of easy access by the system of corridors which makes the first floor of the entire hospital continuous. Proper attention has been paid in the plan to the isolation of all appurtenances likely to create nuisance. The central building and the scheme of administration seem admirably adapted for their purpose.

The third paper is by Dr. Joseph Jones, among whose printed titles is that of "Visiting Physician of Charity Hospital of New Orleans." Perhaps this relation of the writer to a hospital will account for the fact that his suggestions do not appear to be characterized by the consistency and definiteness which are desirable. Dr. Jones shows in his essay a comprehensive knowledge of the principles of hospital hygiene, but we believe that a few months' experience in the practical superintendence of a hospital would modify many of the views put forth in his present contribution. Permanent superimposed wards are advocated, the objections to such structures being met by the recommendation to keep at least one twelfth of the entire ward space at all times vacant. The pavilions should be erected on arches left entirely open, and used only as a general highway for the hospital ; the floors should be of fireproof materials, laid with glazed tiles or slabs and covered with oil-cloth ; the walls should be impermeable, composed of either "Parian cement, colored tiles, or large porcelain or glazed earthenware slabs joined perfectly by a good cement," — an apartment sufficiently tomb-like and cheerful to inspire hope in the most disheartened invalid. The administration is complicated, clumsy, and impracticable ; responsibility is divided and confused. Patients are to be mainly classified by sex ; accordingly we have a "steam laundry for male clothing" and one for "female clothing," a "dead-house male" and a "dead-house female ;" rather curiously this discrimination does not extend to the "dispensatory." We observe, moreover, that the plan provides a "male ward, fever," but the females have no place to which to take their fevers unless it be to the "obstetrical" ward, which is only one hundred and fifty feet from the surgical ward. One feature of the ground-plan consists of sixteen fountains, one for each of the ten wards and six near the line of the dead-house ; these are to flush the sewers. The trustees will not fail to remark that the paper concludes with an elaborate disquisition on nutrition and the diet requisite to sustain it; with learned mention of albuminates and carbo-hydrates, of carboniferous and nitrogeneous aliments — matters which the trustees will probably leave for the rumination of the incoming superintendent. A similar *détour* is made concerning disinfectants.

Dr. Caspar Morris presents as the basis of his paper the plan of the Hospital of the Protestant Episcopal Church of Philadelphia. The essay is the longest in the book, and suffers by the needless repetition of descriptions. The writer believes cordially in permanent buildings with multiple wards. One of his arguments is that concentrated wards, with all their hypothetical disadvantages, are better than "the dark and illy ventilated rooms and houses to which the poor for whom these hospitals are provided are accustomed ;" as if the matter of hospital construction turned upon such a comparison instead of on the question, which form of building saves most lives? The wards are long and narrow, and contain a water-closet at each end. The sewers are ventilated through the rain-water conductors, an unnecessary and objectionable arrangement. Five open fire-places are in each ward, and these are supplemented by steam apparatus. In still days during the warm season, when, as the author says, "scarcely an aspen leaf trembles in the breeze," forced ventilation by means of a fan is to be applied. The administration building is well planned; although we question the wisdom of placing the surgical amphitheatre, the lecture-room, the anatomical room, and the chapel in this building, in the very fore-front of the group.

The last essay in the series is by Dr. Stephen Smith, of New York, recently the president of the American Public Health Association. He brings to the elaboration of his theme a ripeness of experience and a breadth of research which make his paper exceedingly instructive to the sanitary student. If there is any drawback to the practical utility of his excellent paper it lies in the introduction of many topics not included in the requirements of the occasion; such, for example, are the discussion of Pettenkofer's ground-water and ground-air ideas, and of the germ theory of disease. But Dr. Smith embodies in his suggestions a great deal that is really original. He favors single-story pavilions. His ward-buildings are novel in shape; they have a body (containing only the twelve beds of the patients); a constricted portion or neck, whose length and width correspond with the width of the corridor on which it opens and of which it forms a section; and a head, containing all the rooms for the ward service. This practical isolation of the ward is ingenious and rational. The windows are not placed opposite each other, but alternately; and the beds are arranged accordingly. Windows are placed at each of the four corners of the ward, the angles being removed for that purpose. Dr. Smith's first choice would be to place the ward water-closets in the basement, his estimate being that at least one half of the patients are able to traverse stairs. Fire-places are recommended. The bath-room is excluded, its place being made good by portable baths for the ward and a general bath-house for the hospital. We are sorry to see the suggestion of a shoot for soiled linen other ways are preferable for removing such material. The administration buildings and their appurtenances, as well as the service of the hospital, are satisfactorily provided for.

In an appendix are plans for an octagon pavilion, suggested by Mr. Nierusée, the architect to the board of trustees. The shape of the ward is like the outline of a carafe or decanter, the expanded portion containing room for twenty-four or more beds, while the neck, opening on a connecting corridor, contains the entire ward administration. The details of this plan are very attractive and merit favorable consideration; they appear to be founded on hygienic principles.

We cannot close our extended notice of this remarkable book without renewedly expressing our appreciation of its excellent features. We must not fail to mention, as among these, the handsome manner in which the work is executed, the type and the numerous plates which embellish the pages being unusually fine.

MEDICAL NOTES.

— At the last meeting of the American Otological Society, held in Newport, R. I., July 21, 1875, it was voted that the committee on an international congress be empowered by this society to issue a call for an international otological congress at such time and place as they shall see fit. In accordance with this vote the committee have called a congress to be held in New York city on Friday, September 15, 1876, at ten o'clock A. M., the place of the meeting to be announced later. Members of the medical profession who take an active interest in aural surgery are cordially invited to be present and take part in the congress.

— Dr. E. R. Morgan reports to the *British Medical Journal* of October 16, 1875, some cases of poisoning by tobacco. Three patients were poisoned, of whom one died. The first patient, a middle-aged man, when seen by his physician was lying helpless in bed, unable to swallow, cold, with feeble pulse, and showing symptoms which aroused suspicion of poisoning by some vegetable substance, but no such poisonous substance could be discovered. The next day a child died after exhibiting somewhat similar phenomena ; and soon after, a little girl was taken ill with the same symptoms as the other two. It was at length discovered by accident that the shallow well from which these patients had drunk contained tobacco which had got there in some unaccountable way. When the drug was removed it proved to be half of a quarter-pound packet of the strongest quality.

— A case of natural version is reported to the *Obstetrical Journal of Great Britain and Ireland* of October, 1875, by P. B. Giles, M. R. C. S. His patient was thirty-seven years old, and in her fifth pregnancy. Most of her previous labors had been abnormal, with flooding, still-born children, etc. During her present pregnancy the patient had convulsions. She was taken with pains August 24th, and was attended by a midwife. At three A. M., August 27th, the waters broke, a hand came down, and soon after a loop of cord. The patient was first seen by a physician at 8.27 A. M. of August 27th, when she was found to be suffering from anasarca and effusion into the peritoneal cavity. She was very feeble. Examination discovered a prolapsed, pulseless cord, the left arm lying in the vagina rather high up, the child apparently lying on its left side with the head above and to the right of the pubes. A foot was also detected high up, and a little behind the right sacro-iliac synchondrosis. After explaining to the relatives the critical condition of the patient, the physician, when about to operate, found that the arm was receding and that nature was thus endeavoring to complete the delivery. It was, however, evident that the patient's strength would erelong be exhausted, and after various attempts of the attendant to seize the right foot it was finally caught by a wire écraseur and complete version easily resulted. After much exertion a dead female child, weighing more than eleven pounds, was extracted. The patient died August 30th. The writer thinks that spontaneous version occurs more frequently than is recorded, but he is convinced that it would at least be unwise in shoulder presentations to wait for it to occur, still more so where the arm comes down.

LETTER FROM WASHINGTON.

MESSRS. EDITORS, — The winter session has opened here for medical men ; the societies are holding their weekly and bi-weekly meetings, and the colleges are fully at work, which also means, of course, that hospital material is being utilized to its fullest advantage, the cases that have held over through the summer months being now brought into requisition and made to serve for clinical display. Our colleges are fairly successful for this section, as regards both numbers and material, however insignificant the numbers might appear in comparison with those in attendance upon the colleges of our larger cities ; for if fifty names appear upon the rolls of either college here, it is a full quota. Yet the material is in some respects of good quality ; the men are mostly of a more mature age than those generally found upon the benches of a medical college ; and having already learned to meet the stern requirements of life in this busy age, they know what it is to appreciate the value of a proper education and the uses to which it may be put ; accordingly they are attentive, earnest, and in most instances in no haste to present themselves simply crammed for the final examination. The lectures are all given during the evening hours, say from five to ten, which is done to accommodate many who are in government service. This strikes one at first as a disadvantage, but there is something to be said in its favor : many students, finding themselves alone in a strange city, with their evening hours unoccupied, except when employed in dissection or the quiz, contract habits that are never profitable and are not always creditable. Again, the use of such aids in teaching as Holmes's class microscope and the sciopticon are much facilitated by the darkness of evening hours. The latter instrument has been used for the past three years as of valuable assistance in the lecture-room. Thus far this winter a serious check has been felt by the colleges through the difficulty of obtaining dissecting material ; to speak mildly, the injudicious actions of one man, a doctor it appears, who made a business and traffic of securing such material, both for home and for foreign consumption, has roused the public sympathies and indignation to such a pitch as to embarrass the colleges to a serious extent ; an unnecessary and injurious discussion of the subject has been held in the daily papers, involving the old story of popular prejudice on the one hand and a quiet determination to meet the necessities of the profession on the other. One decided disadvantage here to students holding government positions is their inability to attend the clinics regularly, and so long as this obtains, Washington must be satisfied with an inferior standing among medical centres. To meet this want Sunday has to be utilized, and accordingly on that day of rest the student passes a part of his time in hospital wards ; it may be that we shall yet have an expression of public opinion in this respect, as some of the clergy have already from time to time expostulated against the custom. Hospitals are multiplying here and are really performing important services, though the one hospital that shall meet the demands of the public and the profession has yet to be built ; but when the genuine students, they who devote their whole energy to the study of their profession, make their appearance in sufficient numbers to warrant the change, they will find clinical material to meet their wants, and at suitable hours.

It is interesting to one who knew Washington previous to and during the war to note the changes here in this respect. Up to the spring of 1861, to the memorable month of April of that year, when the attack was made on Massachusetts soldiery in the streets of Baltimore, the Washington Infirmary was the one hospital here, under the fostering care of the Sisters of Charity ; it was a three-story building, with spacious grounds around it, and it answered well its purpose, the wards being nearly filled with chronic cases, with here and there a sprinkling of acute affections. It was taken possession of by the government, and was known as the Judiciary Square Hospital. It was burned to the ground in October, 1861. Increased accommodations being required for the sick and wounded, the war gave to us seventeen distinct hospitals under the control of the government, with a total capacity of thirteen thousand nine hundred and fifty-five patients. None of this, however, was used as clinical material, as we understand it ; indeed, the colleges here were in a state of temporary demoralization. Nothing was easier than to obtain hospital-appointments as hospital-stewards, medical cadets, and acting assistant surgeons (contract surgeons), each bringing in its immediate pecuniary reward, so that with the excitement and bustle of action the more slow and sure but solid requirements of preliminary medical education were, in the main, overlooked or postponed to a more favorable opportunity.

After the close of the war there came in time to be developed as an outgrowth, as it were, of that condition, a desire to multiply hospitals, and every church society seemed to be possessed with the ambition of having a hospital of its own. Now that some ten years have passed, we have narrowed down the supply so that it more suitably meets the demand. The old infirmary has been replaced by Providence Hospital, a large and commodious building, with a visiting staff; clinical instruction is given regularly, and the wards are open without fee to both colleges alike. But it has one great drawback ; it is under the charge of Sisters of Charity, whose rules are such as not to allow residence in the building to a medical man. How a religious order can undertake the care of male patients who spend their nights within the hospital walls, and refuse like accommodations to the medical attendant, is an enigma not yet explained, but the fact mars the usefulness of the institution very seriously. What must be the apprehensions of the surgeon in cases that threaten secondary hæmorrhage? How satisfactorily can a case of peritonitis be managed with the opium treatment under such circumstances? It is superfluous to attempt to multiply examples of this kind which must naturally present themselves to every one.

During the war a private dwelling-house in a favorable situation was used by the government, more particularly for venereal diseases, and was termed the Ricord Hospital ; when no longer required for this purpose it was converted into the Columbia Hospital for Women and Lying-in Asylum ; it received its act of incorporation from Congress in 1866, and an annual appropriation of ten thousand dollars. The hospital was in time moved to its present site, which was purchased by the government, and the yearly appropriation devoted to its use was largely increased. It is in point of fact a government institution, and has a surgeon-in-charge and a resident physician, both salaried officers. Attempts have been made from time to time to attract the attention of the profession to its sphere of usefulness, but they have failed because the institution is conducted so exclusively in the personal interest of the surgeon-in-charge. It has long been the opinion of medical men here that it would be more advantageous had this hospital a regular visiting staff without salaries. At one time there was quite a list of names of prominent physicians as the consulting staff, but, for reasons best known to themselves, they retired from the position. A college of gynæcology figures in the history of the hospital; lectures were given, but one short semester told the tale. Lectures have been also given to women preparing to be nurses; to these exercises ladies having families, present or in prospect, were invited. Clinical lectures are given weekly, which the students of both colleges attend; a fee was formerly charged for these, but they are now free. By far the largest dispensary in this city was connected with the hospital, but has been discontinued, " there being no provision in the charter to extend aid to any but those suffering from diseases peculiar to women." Consequently the clinical material is now restricted to this department and to general surgery, although why the latter is included does not appear. One period in the history of the institution was marked by a notable circumstance — the publication in 1873 of a large quarto volume, illustrated, and containing four hundred and thirty pages; the work is probably familiar to your readers, as it received marked attention from the medical press. It was published by the government, and in many of the copies was a prospectus of the college of gynæcology before mentioned. We understand that a second report is about to be published.

The Freedmen's Hospital, located just within the city limits, is a large building which grew out of the necessities of the Freedmen's Bureau, and partakes in part of the character of an asylum for the old and indigent of the colored race. Here, too, valuable clinical instruction has been given from time to time.

The Children's Hospital is a young and growing institution which was established in 1870; it has already, from the exertions of those interested in its behalf, come to be recognized by the community as a necessity in the absence of a general hospital with children's wards. It has as yet no building of its own, and is devoted to a special purpose; there is every prospect of the speedy erection of more suitable accommodations. It has a large general dispensary service, for which there seems to be no provision in the printed charter. Both colleges share in the benefits of its clinical instruction.

Other hospitals might be mentioned in this connection, such as the government hospital for the insane, and the model hospital erected on the grounds of the Old Soldiers' Home, but these do not come under the notice of medical students and are not used for clinical instruction. The neighboring city of Georgetown (though now one with Washington, the old line of demarkation is still maintained) has attempted a hospital of her own, with what success remains to be seen, as it is yet in its infancy.

Notwithstanding the foregoing details, the statement is repeated that no one of these hospitals answers the demands of the public and the profession. One good general hospital would do away with the necessity for the greater part of the others, and the energy which is spent in maintaining these separate charities would effect a better purpose if concentrated for a single object. This will not be attempted at present, as the Board of Health is an obstacle in the way; government aid would be solicited for the movement, and necessarily the board would be invested with authority in the matter, at least so think the profession, and this would be in the highest degree objectionable. The physicians who attend the out-door poor of the District have already presented a petition containing an admirable scheme for the proposed change, showing that Providence Hospital is strictly for non-residents, and setting forth the unhealthy location of the Almshouse hospital, if it can be dignified by such a title, which is confounded with a workhouse on the one side, a small-pox hospital on the other, and a potter's field behind, associations favorable perhaps to thoughts on the mutability of human affairs, but to little else. The petition, however, has been tabled.   Homo.

WASHINGTON, D. C., *November* 12, 1875.

WEEKLY BULLETIN OF PREVALENT DISEASES.

THE following is a bulletin of the diseases prevalent in Massachusetts during the week ending November 27, 1875, compiled under the authority of the State Board of Health from the returns of physicians representing all sections of the State: —

The summary for each section is as follows: —

Berkshire : Pneumonia, bronchitis, influenza. Diphtheria reported in the northern parts.

Valley : Bronchitis, rheumatism, influenza, typhoid fever, pneumonia. Holyoke and Springfield report diphtheria; Amherst, meningitis ; South Hadley Falls, a continued epidemic of measles.

Midland : Bronchitis, influenza, rheumatism, typhoid fever. Worcester reports scarlatina ; Fitchburg, diphtheria.

Northeastern : Bronchitis, influenza, typhoid fever. Very little sickness reported. A Lowell physician of experience reports that the mortality last week was the smallest within his knowledge, for a single week, in that city.

Metropolitan : Bronchitis, scarlatina, diphtheria, pneumonia, rheumatism. Less diphtheria and more scarlatina reported. Some varicella and tonsillitis.

Southeastern : Influenza, bronchitis, typhoid fever. Not much sickness.

In the State at large, the order of relative prevalence is as follows : bronchitis, influenza, typhoid fever, rheumatism, pneumonia, diphtheria, scarlatina.

F. W. DRAPER, M. D., Registrar.

COMPARATIVE MORTALITY-RATES FOR THE WEEK ENDING NOV. 20, 1875.

	Estimated Population.	Total Mortality for the Week.	Annual Death-Rate per 1000 during Week.
New York	1,060,000	451	22
Philadelphia	800,000	297	19
Brooklyn	500,000	240	25
Chicago	400,000	126	16
Boston	342,000	178	27
Cincinnati	260,000	118	23
Providence	100,700	45	23
Worcester	50,000	11	12
Lowell	50,000	4	4
Cambridge . . .	48,000	20	21
Fall River	45,000	21	24
Lawrence	35,000	10	15
Lynn	33,000	10	16
Springfield	31,000	8	13
Salem	26,000	8	16

Normal Death-Rate, 17 per 1000.

BOOKS AND PAMPHLETS RECEIVED. — A Text-Book of Human Physiology. By Austin Flint, Jr., M. D. New York: D. Appleton & Co. 1876.

Transactions of the American Medical Association. Vol. XXVI. Philadelphia. Printed for the Association. 1875.

Hospital Plans. Five Essays on Hospitals, for the Use of the Johns Hopkins Hospital of Baltimore. New York: William Wood & Co. 1875. (For sale by A. Williams & Co.)

Transactions of the Pathological Society of London. Vol. XXVII. 1875.

History of American Medical Literature from 1776. By S. D. Gross, M. D., LL. D. Philadelphia. 1876.

Transactions of the Kansas Medical Society at its Annual Session, 1875.

Twenty-Fourth Annual Report of the Boston Provident Association. October, 1875.

Candy. Its Effects on the Teeth and System. By John T. Codman, D. M D.

Cyclopædia of the Practice of Medicine. Edited by Dr. H. von Ziemssen. Vol. V. Diseases of the Respiratory Organs. American Edition. New York: William Wood & Co. 1875. (Subscriptions received by H. D. Brown & Co., agents for Boston and vicinity.)

Hints on the Obstetric Procedure. By W. B. Atkinson, M. D. Philadelphia: Collins, Printer. 1875.

Proceedings of the Conference of Charities held in Connection with the General Meeting of the American Social Science Association. Detroit. 1875.

State Medicine in its Relations to Insanity. By Dr. Nathan Allen. 1875. (For sale by A. Williams & Co.)

THE regular meeting of the Boston Society for Medical Observation will be held on Monday evening, December 6th. Dr. C. J. Blake will read a paper on the Treatment of Perforations of the Membrana Tympani.

THE BOSTON
MEDICAL AND SURGICAL JOURNAL.

VOL. XCIII. — THURSDAY, DECEMBER 9, 1875. — NO. 24.

NOTES OF CASES OF PLEURISY TREATED WITH PARACENTESIS THORACIS, AND PERMANENT OPENING.

BY HALL CURTIS, M. D.,

Visiting Physician at the Boston City Hospital.

CASE XIII. Frederick L., a Swede, aged twenty-three, single, and a painter by occupation, entered the hospital March 17, 1875. He had been sick three months with cough and pain in the side ; was tapped last December, and two pints of serum were removed. He became better, but still was not able to work. His dyspnœa increasing, he was again tapped one week before entrance to the hospital, and pus was withdrawn. At entrance, slight dullness was found at the upper right front, with tubular respiration and moist râles. There was good resonance in the left front, with modified respiratory murmur, somewhat amphoric on coughing or speaking. The right back was normal. In the left back the respiratory murmur was modified at the upper half ; in the lower half it was very faint, with the amphoric character on coughing or speaking. Nothing was observed on succussion. Heart normal. Temperature, evening of entrance, 101° ; pulse 128.

March 29th. Moist râles heard throughout right front. No respiratory murmur below spine of scapula in left back. Complete flatness in lower half.

April 1st. A splashing sound was heard on succussion.

April 2d. A pint of pus was withdrawn by the aspirator, the trocar being introduced one and three quarters inches below the inferior angle of the scapula. An incision was made into the cavity of the pleura at this place, giving vent to two pints of pus. A drainage tube was introduced, and within one hour two more pints of laudable pus flowed out.

April 3d. Patient much more comfortable ; rested well last night. Pleura washed out night and morning with tepid carbolized water. Patient takes nourishment freely ; has four ounces of brandy daily. Temperature 99° A. M. ; 100.2° P. M.

April 6th. Patient did not sleep well last night. Discharge somewhat offensive. Respiration through left back feeble, and faintly heard nearly to inferior angle of scapula. Temperature 99° A. M.; 101.2° P. M.

April 10th. A daily discharge of from one to two gills of creamy pus, not very offensive. Right chest clearer at base, but mucous râles through upper half. Temperature 100° A. M.; 102.2° P. M.

April 11th. Patient seems to be failing. Discharge very offensive. Pleura washed out three times daily. Temperature 99.8° A. M.; 103.2° P. M.

April 18th. Condition about the same. Half a pint of laudable pus discharged to-day. The cavity growing smaller. Temperature the past four days has varied from 98° and 100° A. M., to 103° and 104° P. M.

April 21st. Two gills of pus discharged this morning. Patient seems better, though still quite weak ; coughs occasionally during the washing out. Temperature 98.5° A. M.

April 23d. No improvement since last record. Coarse râles and gurgling in the upper half of the right chest, with some friction-sounds at the base. Respiration is heard in the left front to within an inch of the nipple ; behind, respiration is heard to the angle of the scapula; occasionally squeaking sounds at that point, and friction sounds below. Temperature 96.8° A. M.; 96.2° P. M. The patient'sank gradually, and died April 26th. No autopsy.

CASE XIV. Michael J. O'C., an unmarried Irishman, aged forty-two years, a bottle-maker, stated that he had not been well for six months; he had lost flesh and strength. He complained of cough, with pain in the chest, shoulders, and loins ; no hæmoptysis. Physical examination revealed dullness in the left supra-scapular region, with broncho-vesicular respiration, and occasionally a moist râle. The respiration below this was somewhat bronchial in character. There was some dullness in the lower right back, with respiratory murmur very much modified and with bronchophomy. Heart normal.

· April 7th. Dullness under the right clavicle and want of tone in the lower fourth. Respiration rude through the upper third, with an occasional moist râle in lower half. Respiration puerile in the left front.

April 15th. Area of hepatic dullness increased from the nipple to one inch below the ribs, with tenderness on pressure. Superficial veins of abdomen enlarged.

May 13th. The liver had resumed its usual limits, and the patient was out every day. There was still want of tone and absence of respiration in lower fourth of the right back. The aspirator with exploring trocar was used, and four ounces of serum were withdrawn.

May 17th. Respiration was heard to the base of the right back. The patient was discharged, relieved.

CASE XV. Mary C., aged twenty-seven, a domestic, entered the hospital April 1, 1875. One sister had died of consumption. The patient was well till March 1, 1875. She had been sleeping in a cold, damp cellar all winter, and had worked very 1ard. She had been troubled wit1 dyspnœa and coug1 at nig1t, and wit1 nausea in the morning; had lost fles1; had had nig1t-sweats, but no hæmoptysis. T1ere was dullness in the lower 1alf of the left back, wit1 modified respiratory murmur, and a few moist râles. The rig1t back was normal. T1ere was dullness in the left front, with modified respiratory murmur and dry râles. No bronchophomy. The rig1t chest had good resonance and exaggerated respiratory murmur.

April 28th. The 1eart was found pus1ed to the rig1t side; apex beat in the epigastrium. Left front dull; respiration distant and bron-c1ial below the t1ird rib; left back as on the 10th. The left side was more prominent and had less expansion. Profuse nig1t-sweats; not relieved by atropine. Tincture of iodine was applied to the back and side.

May 16th. No improvement. Absence of respiration below the angle of the scapula, and below fourt1 rib in front. Patient complained of increasing dyspnœa. The needle of the aspirator was introduced one and one 1alf inc1es below the inferior angle of the scapula, and a pint and a 1alf of clear serum wit1drawn.

May 20th. Patient says she is muc1 more comfortable and breat1es easier. The left front is dull t1roug1out. Respiration absent below the t1ird rib (w1en patient is lying down). Left back the same as before the operation. Aspirator again used; the needle was inserted twice, but no fluid followed. Tincture of iodine was continued.

June 3d. Good resonance to inferior angle of the left scapula; below t1is dullness and absence of respiration; no bronchophomy. General condition improving.

June 23d. An exploratory puncture was made by Dr. Blake and 1alf a gill of clear serum wit1drawn. Disc1arged June 30th, relieved.

The patient returned to the 1ospital for ot1er trouble in September, and was under the care of Dr. Draper, who made the following note : "Modified resonance t1roug1out the left back. Dullness at the base. Respiration 1eard two inc1es below the scapula.''

CASE XVI. C. C., aged forty, a 1ypoc1ondriac, wit1 a 1istory of pleurisy. Intermittent fever and 1epatitis. The first of February had an attack of pleurisy and was confined to bed four weeks. He entered the 1ospital May 6, 1875.

P1ysical examination revealed the following condition. The rig1t c1est was one and a 1alf inc1es larger t1an the left; the intercostal spaces were not prominent. Expansion was diminis1ed. Dullness t1roug1 the rig1t back, becoming flat in lower fourt1. On ordinary respiration, the breat1ing was very distant over the upper two t1irds of the rig1t back, and absent below. Wit1 full respiration, the breat1-ing was exaggerated in the upper fourt1, and tubular over the rest of the rigit back. Somewiat masked by friction sounds. In the left back the respiration was puerile. The rigit front was relatively dull. The respiration was distant tirougi the upper ialf of the rigit ciest ; absent in the lower ialf. Tiere was some specific iistory. The abdominal veins were enlarged. Liver dullness in mammary line, six incies ; spleen normal. An exploratory puncture was made, and ialf a pint of clear serum was removed.

May 18th. Respiration ieard clearly to one and a half incies below inferior angle of scapula ; distant below ; lower ialf of rigit back still dull.

May 30th. Respiration ieard tirougiout rigit back. Some want of tone in lower fourti. Disciarged, well.

CASE XVII. C. M., a Nova Scotian, aged nineteen, a carpenter by occupation, entered City Hospital April 12, 1875 ; he had been well till sixteen days before entrance. He was tien troubled witi general malaise and loss of appetite. He kept up and about till nine days before his admission ; at tiat time took to his bed. During the week before his entrance he had diarrioea, and, on one occasion, epistaxis. He was now in bed witi ieadacie, a brown tongue, and dry sordes on the teeti ; his belly was tympanitic and tender, witi a number of rose spots at the upper part; five dejections.

He steadily improved till May 10th, wien dullness was found in upper part of the rigit ciest.

May 19th. Dullness over rigit front ; in lower ialf tiere was cracked-pot resonance. Breatiing distant tirougiout, witi moist râles above and ampioric respiration below. In the left ciest the respiration was puerile. The upper tiird of the rigit back was dull ; the lower two tiirds flat ; respiration bronciial, most marked in the lower ialf, witi moist râles and becoming very distant at base. Rigit side rounded. Expansion diminisied ; absence of vocal fremitus. Cougi troublesome, nigit-sweats.

May 25th. Aspirated ; ialf a pint of ratier dirty-looking pus, witi air, witidrawn.

May 26th. Diminisied resonance over lower ialf of rigit ciest, witi occasional moist clicking two incies above nipple ; below tiis, respiration was absent ; resonance of back same as before. Respiration distant, bronciial, witi moist râles to inferior angle of scapula ; absent below. No succussion.

May 29th. Respiration in front ieard a little lower down, to witiin an inci of the nipple. Tiere is still some fullness and hyperæsthesia of the side. Respiration ieard ialf an inci below the inferior angle of the scapula, witi moist râles.

May 30th. Aspirator used, and ialf a gill of ill-looking pus, witi air, witidrawn. An incision was made into the pleura, and ialf a pint of dirty pus followed the knife. On couging, pus was t1rown out in a jet, a distance of two feet. A drainage tube was inserted. At nigit the c1est was was1ed out wit1 a solution of carbolic acid.

May 31st. Slept muc1 better the previous nig1t, wit1 one eig1t1 of a grain of morp1ia.

June 1st. Cavity was1ed out twice daily. A large quantity of dirty pus flowed out in the morning. Complained of pain in rig1t c1est.

June 2d. Free disc1arge during nig1t. Patient weaker. Face bat1ed wit1 perspiration and blanc1ed. Pulse quick and feeble. Six fountain syringefuls required to was1 the cavity clean.

June 5th. Half a pint of pus escaped during nig1t.

June 6th. One pint of pus disc1arged during nig1t.

June 7th. One and a 1alf pints of pus escaped during night; appetite improving.

June 8th. One and one t1ird pints of pus came away during the nig1t. One syringeful cleans the c1est to-day.

June 12th. Patient improved ; looks muc1 better; appetite gaining. Less coug1.

June 13th. Patient slept well wit1out opiate. During the rest of the mont1 condition improved. Disc1arge diminis1ing.

July 2d. Patient passed to the care of Dr. Draper. Bronc1o-vesicular respiration in front above line of incision. Indistinct bronc1ial respiration below. Entire flatness of back. Respiration easy. Marked improvement in general condition.

July 12th. Cat1eter slipped out t1is morning. Disc1arge past twenty-four 1ours has diminis1ed ; now very scanty ; no pain ; general condition excellent. P1ysical examination disclosed relative dullness t1roug1out rig1t lower lobe, but bronc1o-vesicular respiration may be 1eard to very base.

July 15t1. Disc1arge had increased since last report ; ot1erwise condition unc1anged. Tube reinserted in intercostal opening, but not retained longer t1an a few 1ours.

July 17t1. Intercostal opening made more free by inserting cat1eter, resulting in a free disc1arge of pus. Cat1eter was not retained.

July 25th. General condition improving. The rig1t side was relatively fuller. Ribs immovable. Intercostal spaces filled. Relative dullness on rig1t side, amounting to flatness below the nipple in front. In the back, dullness above the angle of the scapula; flatness below. Bronc1ial respiration above and wit1in line of nipple on rig1t side. Absence of respiration below nipple and in axillary space. Nig1t-sweating.

August 1st. The resonance above the line of the incision is some-w1at better. Bronc1o-vesicular respiration above the angle of the scapula everyw1ere. Bronc1ial respiration below t1at point to the base of the lung. Wound discharging spontaneously and quite freely without syringing. General condition improving slowly.

August 8th. Respiration heard throughout the right lung to base; bronchial in character, with numerous fine, crepitant rales, heard at angle of scapula. Patient gaining in strength. Discharge of pus continues abundant and laudable. Region of wound granulating over a space two inches square.

August 9th. Patient wheeled out in the sun. Feels better for it.

August 21st. Discharged, relieved.

The temperature record in the foregoing case gave the following average variations : —

	A. M.	P. M.
From April 12 to May 3...........................	100°	104°
After disappearance of typhoid, from May 3 to July 13...	100°	102°
From July 13 to July 24..............................	99°	101.5° to 102°
From July 24 to August 21............................	98°	100° to 101°

CASE XVIII. Miss T., a delicate girl eighteen years old, when nine years old had whooping-cough, followed by a bronchial irritability, supposed at the time to be of a tuberculous nature. This improved under cod-oil and tonics. Three years ago the cough again became troublesome, and Dr. E. H. Clarke found a pleural rub at the base of the left lung. Winter before last the cough increased. Last September the patient went to Mentone, where she improved during the winter, but the cough returned with the spring. On the journey home she reached London ill, and was placed under the care of Dr. Dobell. He is said to have stated, " There is general bronchitis with injury at the base of the left lung, though there is no existing tubercular trouble. She is in danger, and must pass her winter in a mild climate." She improved and gained flesh in London, but still on exertion had distressed breathing. On the passage from Liverpool she encountered severe weather, was very seasick, and had a rigor, followed by diarrhœa and cessation of the catamenia.

I first saw her on June 19th. She was very pale, emaciated, with an hectic flush, weak and nervous, without appetite, occasionally vomiting, with diarrhœa. There was dyspnœa on exertion, with a frequent harassing cough, and abundant muco-purulent expectoration, at times tinged with blood. Pulse 132 ; respiration 40. She passed the days sitting up in a straight-backed chair, being unable to lie down when in bed.

Physical examination. The right side was rounded, intercostal spaces somewhat filled, the integument œdematous. The right front was dull except in the clavicular region, where alone respiration was heard. The left front was resonant, with exaggerated breathing, with dry and

moist râles throughout, the latter coarsest and most abundant at the
base. The apex beat of the heart was below and a little outside
of the left nipple. The left back was like the front; the right back
was dull in its upper third, and flat below. In the upper half was distant bronchial breathing, and very distant mucous râles through the
lower half, evidently transmitted. An exploratory puncture was made,
and half an ounce of purulent fluid withdrawn.

June 21st. The aspirator was used and twenty ounces of pure pus
withdrawn. Temperature at six P. M. 100°.

June 22d. Patient passed a more comfortable day after the aspiration, though she had two severe paroxysms of coughing, the breathing
being generally less oppressed. During the night she was vigilant, at
times delirious. Two diarrhœic discharges. In the morning she
seemed stronger and brighter, sitting half-raised in bed. Temperature
99.5°; respiration 40.

June 27th. Condition unchanged; occasional vomiting with diarrhœa; harassing cough and copious expectoration; appetite very poor.
Nights restless with delirium, quieted only by morphia. Paroxysms
of dyspnœa. Pulse 120; respiration 35; temperature 100.5° to 102°.
Aspirator again used; seven ounces of pus withdrawn.

July 1st. Patient somewhat improved; more color in the face;
stronger; no diarrhœa past twenty-four hours. Temperature 99.5°;
pulse 126; respiration 40, but less difficult. Right front less dull, but
the side and back extremely tender.

July 5th. Condition not as good. Dyspnœa and cough continue,
with bloody muco-purulent expectoration. Stomach refuses even
milk and lime-water; persistent diarrhœa. Patient weaker and more
irritable. Respiration 40; pulse 140, weak, at times intermitting.
Slight œdema about feet and ankles. Takes stimulants freely. Examination of chest shows the same condition, with slight dullness and bronchial breathing in upper fourth of left lung. After much persuasion
the patient consented to have the aspirator used, when thirty-six ounces
of pure pus were withdrawn, with increase of cough at the end of the
operation.

July 7th. Patient very restless and exhausted; yawning, but sleepless. A permanent opening was advised.

July 8th. Quiet night; easier; carried down to piazza, where she
passed two hours in the sun.

July 9th. Best night she had had for ten days. Takes food freely.
Respiration 27; pulse 134.

July 10th. Last night again restless and wandering. Dyspnœa and
" attacks of choking." Bloody expectoration. Vomiting. This morning respiration heaving, 36; pulse 132. Patient looks more weary.

July 12th. Patient seen by Dr. H. I. Bowditch, who also advised
making a permanent opening by trocar, leaving canula in place, to be

done without ether on account of her dyspnœa. I plunged in a trocar two inches below the angle of the scapula ; on its withdrawal pus freely followed.

July 16th. Yesterday morning the canula was changed for a shorter one. Last night patient was worried and delirious ; had a constant short cough, with bloody expectoration! Since the shorter canula was introduced there has been less discharge of pus. A catheter meets with opposition at three fourths of an inch from the point of entrance, probably the thickened pleura. The canula, evidently being too short to reach the cavity of the pleura, was removed, and the longer one inserted, followed by a free discharge of pure pus to the amount of a pint.

During the rest of July and August the patient remained about the same, passing several hours daily on the piazza. Her appetite was very poor. Diarrhœa recurring every few days. Night-sweats were frequent. Respiration was always hurried. Cough was often very troublesome, with copious muco-purulent expectoration, at times bloody. There were occasional fits of depression, with hysterical crying ; these were relieved only by morphine. Stimulants were freely taken.

During September there was a steady gain in strength, with improved appetite and digestion. The patient slept quietly all night. Two ounces of laudable pus were discharged during the twenty-four hours. The side was no longer over-sensitive, and was less prominent. The pleura was washed out twice a week. The lung was expanding. The patient walked about her rooms, and drove out every pleasant day.

September 25th Dr. Bowditch again saw her, and made the following note : —

" Percussion fairly equal in front. A little less in the upper three fourths of the right back than in the left. Respiration obscure, but heard through both fronts, somewhat roughened in both. More free in the left. Behind, the respiration is decidedly less than in front, especially in the right back ; but on full respiration a squeak can be heard almost to puncture. Nowhere tubular respiration, or unusual vocal resonance."

During the month of October the improvement continued. On the 19th she came to Boston from Manchester, Mass., where she had passed the summer. She was not troubled by the trip.

October 25th Dr. Bowditch saw her with me. The pulse was 105, of good strength. Tongue natural. Face rounder and fuller. Appetite fair ; digestion good. Percussion clear over both fronts ; almost tympanitic. Respiration behind as at last examination, very distant, with sonorous râle on full inspiration heard at point of puncture. Half an ounce of pus was discharged daily. Most marked improvement in general condition.

October 27th she went to New York, arrived there comfortably, and has continued to improve up to the present date (November 22d).

RECENT PROGRESS IN DERMATOLOGY.[1]

BY JAMES C. WHITE, M. D.

Horn upon the Glans Penis. — Professor Pick, of Prag, contributes to his journal[2] an account of a most interesting case of this rare affection. The patient, twenty-two years old, was received into the hospital in April, 1874, with balanoposthitis and several papillomatous growths upon the corona, also congenital phymosis. The operation for phymosis was performed, the condylomata removed, and their seat cauterized. Nine months later the patient returned with the horn full grown. The growth had started from the sulcus around its whole circumference, but upon one side it had developed much more rapidly than upon the other, so that taking a curved direction it had arched across and rested upon the shorter and opposite horn, forming a complete shield above the glans when in an erect position. The outgrowth was over two inches in length, measured along its outer curvature, and about half an inch in thickness. Dr. Pick refers to nine other cases on record of horns growing from the penis. The exceptional features in his are the age, inasmuch as they belong to old persons, and the rapidity of its growth, six months. Its origin was undoubtedly the papillomatous vegetations which preceded and were not completely destroyed. When the parts were left uncovered after the operation for phymosis, and became dry, then the epidermal new-growth had a chance to form and accumulate. After its amputation the papillæ were found greatly elongated, and large vessels were seen to penetrate between the masses of epidermal cells, of which it was composed, for nearly half its length. No sebaceous glands were found in the skin underlying the horn. The patient had psoriasis also, and Dr. Pick draws attention to the tendency to redundant epidermal formation in this affection, as shown in the excessive thickness of the nails and the exuberant growth of hair in many patients. The paper is accompanied by two colored plates of the growth, which perfectly exhibit its remarkable appearances.

Scleroderma. — Dr. Lagrange,[3] in a treatise containing the reports of several cases, draws the following conclusions : (1) that scleroderma primarily consists of a chronic inflammation of the skin and subcutaneous cellular tissue, which may extend more deeply, attack the bones and articulations, and produce secondarily, by anatomical lesion of the peripheral nervous filaments, trophic disturbances, but of no great importance ; and (2) that there is no evidence of the existence of any primary trophic disturbance, as no alteration in the spinal cord, nerves, or muscles can be determined.

---

[1] Concluded from page 643.
[2] Vierteljahresschrift für Dermatologie und Syphilis, 1875, page 315.
[3] Contribution a l'Étude de la Sclérodermie, etc.   Par A. Lagrange.   Paris.

Purpura. — Professor Henock [1] reports four cases, all occurring in persons of fifteen years or younger, in which there were rheumatic pains in the joints, purpuric spots, intestinal colic and bloody dejections, and some fever. These symptoms were subject to relapses after apparent recovery, and were thus prolonged in one case three months. The purpuric spots were most marked upon the abdomen, genitals, and lower extremities. In a similar case reported by Wagner, albuminuria and membranous shreds in the dejections were observed, in addition to the above symptoms. The patient died, and purulent peritonitis and enteritis, with ulceration and deposits of false membrane within the intestine, were revealed.

Congenital Purpura. — Doirn [2] reports a case of Werlhof's disease (morbus maculosus) in a pregnant woman. Of universal distribution, it disappeared before delivery, but the child showed the same spots, which also disappeared after a few days. New ones subsequently appeared on the conjunctiva and gums. The child was well developed.

Argyria. — Dr. B. Riemer [3] reports a case of silver staining of the skin, and gives at great length the interesting results of his most valuable and minute investigations of the condition of the various tissues after death. The patient, forty-three years old, entered the Leipzig hospital in March, 1870, with tabes dorsualis. From this time until his discharge in May, 1872, on account of a beginning disease of the lungs, he took in all 5672 pills of nitrate of silver, equivalent to 34.032 grams (eight and a half drachms) of the salt, or 21.610 grams (five and a half drachms) of metallic silver. The first traces of staining were noticed upon the face at the end of a year, and after 2900 pills had been administered. He died a few days after his reëntrance to the hospital in November, 1873, with the gravest symptoms of tabes and pthisis. His skin at this time was universally of a grayish-blue color, most strongly marked upon the face, while the trunk, and especially the lower extremities, showed less of the gray tint. Some old scars upon the head stood out in bold contrast, from their white color. The coloration of the skin was the only symptom of the argyria during life. In addition to the skin, the following tissues were also found after death to be stained : The plexus choroidei was very dark-blue throughout its whole extent. In the brain and spinal tissues nothing was seen. The lungs showed no trace of staining ; only in the larynx was a pale gray color of the mucous membrane noticed. The pericardium showed a little pigment. The intermuscular fibrous tissue of the heart contained large granules of the pigment, and in the endocardium it was

---

[1] The Medical Record, October 2, 1875 ; from Schmidt's Jahrbücher.

[2] Vierteljahresschrift für Dermatologie und Syphilis, 11 Jahrg., erstes Heft ; from Archiv für Gynäkologie, 1874, No. vi.

[3] Archiv der Heilkunde, 1875, page 298.

distributed in groups. The serous membrane of the stomach and intestine was colored gray, and the smallest arteries throughout, from the stomach to the rectum, were intensely silvered. The liver, kidneys, and spleen were also deeply discolored in parts. The organs most affected by the argyria were the glomeruli of the kidney, the plexus choroidei, the lining of the aorta, the mesenteric lymph glands, and the skin. The pigment was everywhere in a finely granular condition, and in the parts most deeply affected by aggregation of these particles large masses were formed. It was nowhere found connected with cell elements or deposited in or between them, but generally in the homogeneous membranes of connective tissue.

In what manner and form, and by what channels, does the silver reach these places of deposit? These are questions which have been differently answered by various observers. According to Frommann,[1] the silver albuminate dissolved in serum loses its solubility in some way after leaving the vessels, and is precipitated and reduced. Rouget[2] believes that the silver is contained in the blood as an albuminate soluble in the alkaline serum. Huet,[3] although also a believer in the chemical theory of the existence of argyria, states that it must be deposited like foreign bodies. Virchow, on the other hand, maintains its production by physical laws, just as urates are deposited in gout and the lime salts (calcareous metastasis) in bone disease. Dr. Riemer concludes from his own observations in this case that it is a purely mechanical production, a deposit of pigment masses; that the pigment is received as such, that is, reduced silver, in the intestinal canal, here stored up to be transported through the channel of the lymph-vessels, and partly deposited on the way, partly and mostly carried into the blood. Suspended in this fluid the pigment reaches all parts of the body, penetrates through the wall of the vessel, leaving traces on its way, and finally comes to be permanently deposited in the tissues disposed to receive it. The process is similar, therefore, to anthracosis pulmonum and tattooing, although the extremely fine division of the reduced silver makes it unnecessary to call in the aid of the white blood corpuscles in transporting it. These conclusions he bases in the main upon his examination of the cutaneous tissues. An examination of the different strata of the skin, its glandular and other systems, reveals a peculiar fact; that is, the entire absence of the silver pigment in the epithelium, and this is all the more striking as in the deposit of ordinary pigment, under both physiological and pathological conditions, its principal seat is in the lower layers of the cells of the rete. In argyria the pigment lies close beneath the mucous layer, and is sharply defined as a

[1] Virchow's Archiv, xvii.
[2] Schmidt's Jahrbücher, 1874.
[3] Journal de l'Anatomie et de la Physiologie, 1873.

black border. Its special seat, therefore, is that thin stratum of fibrous tissue which separates the corium from the rete, and belongs to the former.
This dark seam is resolved by the microscope into the minutest granules, arranged in groups and streaks. It would seem as if the silver
pigment tried to work its way outwards, as other foreign bodies are
eliminated, through the skin, and found in the epithelial tissues above
the corium an obstacle it could not penetrate, and thus collected in greatest abundance beneath it. The ever-increasing fineness and density of
the net-work of fibrous tissue, as we reach the uppermost layer of the
corium, also acts as a filter to hold back within its meshes the pigment
granules. Certain fibres or bundles of fibres, especially those running
parallel with the muscular system of the skin, were also stained of a
reddish-brown color, which could not be resolved into granules, giving
to the upper corium a streaked appearance. The deeper fibrous and
subcutaneous cellular tissue, whose wider meshes formed an inefficient
filter, were generally free from silver. An examination of the glandular systems gave very interesting results, confirmatory also of the
above observations. The sweat glands were universally and without
exception silvered, the pigment penetrating their secretory portion and
depositing itself upon the membrana propria, but the cells and contents
of the glands showed not the slightest trace of the metal. The non-
secretory portions, or conducting-tubes, were scarcely at all discolored.
The hair follicles were affected in a similar way; all the epithelial
tissues remaining free from silver, the hair itself, its inner and outer
root-sheaths and the contents of the sebaceous glands not showing a
single metallic granule. The homogenous fibrous membranes of both
systems, however, were affected, that of the hair follicle, the vitreous
sheath, especially, showing both the granular deposit in groups and
streaks, and the uniform staining of reddish-brown tint. Large granules were also constantly found deposited upon the papilla of the hair.

The lymph-vessels and nerve-tissues appeared to have no affinity for
the silver, but the unstriped muscles and the blood-vessels were plainly
affected. Many of the muscles exhibited a uniform granular deposit
and were stained of a dark, almost black, color. This was most noticeable in those parts of the skin least abundantly supplied with the muscles.
In the arteries the walls were found of a uniform gray tint, in consequence of fine granular deposit just where they diminish in size to become capillaries. The veins, on the other hand, showed not the slightest
trace of silvering.

Which of all these sources of deposit are to be regarded as the principal agents in the production of the peculiar tint in argyria? In
Riemer's opinion the blue element in it is due to the admixture of the
vascular redness of the skin with the gray which belongs to the reduced
silver, and which is the prevailing color as the skin loses its blood after

deat1 in t1ese cases. T1at we need not go deeper t1an the deposit in the uppermost layers of the corium to account for the tint is s1own by the dept1 of color w1ic1 a t1in layer of pigment cells in the rete is capable of producing in the black races.

Dr. Riemer's investigations are valuable not alone for the information t1ey supply concerning the nature of the process in argyria, but also for the very interesting facts t1ey 1ave broug1t to lig1t upon points of anatomical and pat1ological importance.

Argyria from Local Application of Nitrate of Silver. — Duquet [1] reports a case in w1ic1 a woman had her t1roat touc1ed repeatedly wit1 nitrate of silver, and after a time the w1ole skin was stained of a bluis1 color. He concludes t1at t1is was effected not so muc1 by absorption from the ulcerated surface as from the stomac1, into w1ic1 the salt passed.

Removal of Nitrate of Silver Stains. [2] — A few grains of metallic iodine are placed in a vessel and a few drops of ammonia added. The solution is t1en applied by a brus1 or the finger to the stains, w1ic1 rapidly disappear. The caution is given t1at the mixture is to be destroyed after using, lest an explosive compound result on drying.

Lupus. — Lang, [3] professor of dermatology at the University of Innsbruck, communicates the most recent investigations upon the anatomy of t1is disease, w1ic1 has attracted the attention of observers so muc1 of late, and furnis1es t1irty-t1ree figures in illustration of his microscopic examinations of tissue. His conclusions are concisely stated in his own words. Lupus is c1aracterized by disturbances of nutrition w1ic1 give rise to a continuous creation and destruction of fibrous, vascular, and epit1elial growt1s; so t1at, according to the stage of the disease, at one time the progressive, at anot1er the retrogressive products, now of t1is, t1en of t1at kind of tissue are presented to observation. One may always see, 1owever, t1at cell proliferation (starting from the vessels) plays the principal part in the process, and that in the last stages of the disease not only resorption of growt1s in a state of retrogressive metamorp1osis takes place, but also organization of cell new-growt1 into fibrous tissue is accomplis1ed, by w1ic1 the lupous skin acquires a cicatricial appearance wit1out antecedent ulceration.

Piffard, in an article entitled Histology of the Scrofulides [4] gives the results of his microscopic examination of the skin in various forms of disease w1ic1 he calls scrofulides, and makes synonymous wit1 lupus, according to the Frenc1 sc1ool. Adenoma, 1yperplasia of the rete, general small round-cell infiltration, cell-1eaps, giant cells, concentric

[1] Medicinisch-chirurgische Rundschau, February, 1875 ; in The Practitioner.

[2] Medical Record, from Le Bordeaux Médicale, August, 1875.

[3] Zur Histologie des Lupus. Vierteljahresschrift für Dermatologie und Syphilis, 11 Jahrg.

[4] New York Medical Journal, August, 1875.

stratification of cells, and perivascular cell-sheaths were the appearances observed by him more or less uniformly. They lead him to conclude that some of the growths are benign, while others, namely, those characterized by the cell-heaps and cell-stratifications, are closely allied to epithelioma, and clinically may be found to terminate in the latter condition. The bearing of these interesting investigations upon the histology of lupus proper would be more satisfactorily established if, in view of his preference for French titles, Dr. Piffard had given some clinical account of the cases from which the specimens were taken.

Leprosy. — Dr. J. W. Ross, U. S. N., communicates[1] an account of a recent visit to the " leper institutions " of the Sandwich Islands, in which exceptional and extensive opportunity was afforded him of observing this interesting affection. The intimate commercial relations between the Hawaiian Islands and our Pacific States makes its study a matter of peculiar importance to ourselves. Dr. Ross, like others at these islands, is a believer in the propagation of the disease both by inheritance and by contagion, restricting the latter term to inoculation with the discharge from leprous sores, thus placing it on a parallel with syphilis in this respect. Like syphilis, too, it is contracted in the great majority of cases during sexual intercourse, through the almost invariable abrasions and ulcerations of the genital organs. The anæsthetic form of the affection does not apparently manifest itself as prominently there as in other parts of the world, and the disease is also modified in its development and course by complication with syphilis. It attains its maximum in about ten years, and may last twenty-five or thirty years. Opinions differ among the resident physicians as to the date of its introduction into the islands, but it was exceedingly rare until about fifteen years ago, when it began to spread, and in 1865 had become so formidable that the Hawaiian government became alarmed and enacted a law banishing to a remote island all lepers and adjudging them civilly dead. The locality is described as beautiful, and everything is provided to make the isolation from the world tolerable. Since the establishment of the colony eleven hundred and ninety patients have been sent to it, eight hundred and ten of whom are still living. Upon another island near Honolulu a detention hospital has been built, where suspected cases are sent for detention until diagnosis is clearly established. Much greater unhappiness is said to prevail among its inmates than among the doomed residents of the farther island. In spite of these arrangements the disease is said to be on the increase, from a proportion in 1866 of one leper to every two hundred and fifty inhabitants to one in fifty in 1875. The reason given for this is that the late king was himself a leper, and prevented the thorough execution of the laws. Since his death they have been rigorously enforced, and the hope is now entertained that the disease will be rooted out.

[1] New Orleans Medical and Surgical Journal, September, 1875.

In the report on Norwegian leprosy by Hansen, referred to in the
JOURNAL of June 3, 1875, in which the author attempts to show that
the disease is contagious, and therefore not hereditary, he calls attention to the account given by Professor Boeck, after his recent visit to
this country, of the condition of the Norwegian emigrants in our North-
western States. In these colonies the only cases of leprosy are in persons born in the mother country, and the longest interval between
emigration and its manifestation was fourteen years, not an impossible
period of incubation, he thinks. He is of the opinion that the disease
has in every case been brought to this country, or developed by intercourse with leprous emigrants. He calls attention, moreover, to the
fact that the earliest symptoms of the disease are often present long
before they are observed. He regards America as affording the best
field for the study of the question of the hereditability of the affection.

There can be no doubt that the transportation of leprosy from its old
and historic centres to remote peoples, its quick reception and rapid extension among the Hawaiians, and its natural extinction in the centre
of our own continent, offer data of the most important and interesting
nature to the solution of its etiology. The question of its contagiousness is certainly well worth reopening.

Disturbances of the Skin in Progressive Muscular Atrophy. — Dr.
Balmer [1] has collected a series of cases of this disease which were distinguished by disturbances of nutrition in the skin of the atrophied
parts. The changes were mainly trophic disturbances upon the hands:
tendency to inflammation of the bed of the nails, splitting and thickening of the nails, excoriations, fissures, ulcerations, and sometimes
blisters upon the skin. Œdematous and inflammatory swellings of the
cutis and panniculus adiposus were also observed. The skin was at
times livid, uniformly or in streaks. Hæmorrhages were observed too,
and excessive perspiration of the hands. These cutaneous changes,
the writer thinks, cannot be explained satisfactorily on Friedreich's
theory of the myopathic genesis of the disease, but confirm the correctness of the views of those who regard progressive muscular atrophy as
the result of disturbances of the sympathetic. In the cases recorded,
at least, he regards the muscular atrophy, as well as the changes in the
skin, to have been due to degeneration of its trunk, ganglia, and
branches, or to functional disturbance of its vaso-motor and trophic centres.

*The Relations of the Vaso-Motor System to the Production of Skin Dis-
eases.* — In an article on this subject Dr. Landgraf [2] reports several
anomalous cases, which he refers to modified nerve action. One was a

[1] Archiv der Heilkunde, 1875, page 327.
[2] Archiv der Heilkunde, 1875, page 344.

lupus-like efflorescence upon the thigh, of twenty-seven years' duration ; another was an acute pemphigoid eruption upon the fore-arm and hand ; and the third was a diffused enlargement of the cutaneous capillaries over the whole body.

The Treatment of Tinea favosa by Petroleum. — Dr. H. Maccormac [1] has used this substance in a few cases. He mixes it with lard and rubs it twice daily into the scalp. His cases do not appear to have been long enough under observation to exclude the possibility of relapses.

Iodoform. — Dr. Lazausky,[2] assistant at the skin clinic at Prag, contributes an article on the therapeutical use of this substance, founded on its employment by Dr. Pick in one hundred cases of specific ulcers, ulcerations after bubos, ulcerating and moist condylomata, ulcerations after gummata, and ulcers of the leg. It was used externally in the forms of fine powder, suspension in glycerine and alcohol, and solution in ether (one part in fifteen), and internally in pill form. Its advantages over other methods are thus stated. The duration of the treatment is materially shorter ; the methods of application are very convenient and therefore adapted to private practice ; if economically used its high price is of little importance, because so little is required. To this end it should not be used in its state of coarse powder, but should be rubbed up as fine as possible. Its solution in ether is still better, as it can be applied more evenly, and the painted surface is immediately covered and protected by a fine, uniform coating of iodoform, which adheres firmly like collodion.

LEE ON SYPHILIS.[3]

LECTURES on Hunter would perhaps have been a more appropriate title for this collection of lectures, as may be inferred from the opening sentence of the author's preface : " The principal object of the present work is to illustrate some of Hunter's doctrines, which the lapse of time and the dissemination of more recent views have obscured or caused to be forgotten." Mr. Lee is an admirer of John Hunter, and with good reason, for Hunter certainly was amongst the first to throw a ray of light on the subject of venereal diseases, during the period that Bumstead so aptly calls the " age of confusion."

The author handles his subject *con amore,* and so identifies himself with his illustrious predecessor that it is frequently difficult, and at times impossible, to decide whether statements are his or Hunter's.

The first lecture takes us back to the age of humoral pathology. Blood has life and blood may be diseased, and cases are quoted to prove that syphilis

[1] The Practitioner, October, 1875.

[2] Vierteljahresschrift für Dermatologie und Syphilis, 1875, page 275.

[3] *Lectures on Syphilis, and on Some Forms of Local Disease, affecting principally the Organs of Generation.* By HENRY LEE. Philadelphia : Henry C. Lea. 1875.

may be transmitted by the inoculation of syphilitic blood. The first two cases quoted from Hunter are not good examples of sound medical logic. Two patients had teeth transplanted (by the way, we thought that was a triumph of modern dental surgery), which fastened well and kept firm for a month. Then ulceration of the gum took place, the teeth loosened, and symptoms of secondary syphilis appeared. The conclusion drawn is that syphilis was transmitted by a tooth ; we are not told that the subjects from whom the teeth were taken were suffering from syphilis, nor that there was any reason to suppose that the patients had not become infected in the usual way. These, however, are not fair examples of the illustrative cases, as we do not remember having ever seen so many cases of artificial inoculation brought together. Amongst the most interesting of these is a very full account of the almost general syphilization of the peasants of Lupara, in 1856, by Dr. Marone's using vaccine lymph containing syphilitic blood. Hunter's pathology of syphilis is accepted, and even indorsed, but we must feel a doubt as to whether "adhesive inflammation," "suppurative inflammation," "ulceration," and "mortification," would pass muster with pathologists of the present day, as telling the whole history of syphilitic disease.

On the vexed question of the classification of symptoms as secondary or tertiary, while admitting that "no such classification can be practically relied upon, either as a matter of pathology or with regard to treatment," he considers Mr. Lane's as the best. According to this, in brief, the affections of the skin and mucous membranes not resulting in deep and rapid ulceration, iritis, muscular pains, and periostitis, are placed in the secondary class ; while the affections of fibrous membranes, nodes, caries and necrosis of bones, and serious ulceration of the skin and mucous membranes, are called tertiary. It is strange that this matter of classification should have been the cause of so much argument and contention, when the disease itself gives us such a clear dividing line between two classes of symptoms, from a pathological point of view : namely, all the affections of the skin, mucous membranes, periosteum, etc., which are the result of inflammation, whether it be called "adhesive" or "exudative," belonging to one class, which chronologically we· may call secondary, and all those results of the development of a neoplasm, or new formation (gummata), whether in the skin, bones, or internal organs, forming a separate class, which we call tertiary.

This is hardly the place to enlarge on this point, but a little thought will convince any one that this marked difference in the two classes is a pathological truth. Mr. Lee refers to these new formations, or gummy tumors, as "deposits of lymph superficially organized," which, it is hardly necessary to say, is not in accordance with the teachings of cellular pathology.

While not of course agreeing with Hunter that gonorrhœa and syphilis are identical, Mr. Lee does believe that there is a form of urethral discharge which is a symptom of constitutional syphilis, and if we understand him rightly he further believes that this may be the only evidence of infection, that is to say, that in some cases the specific virus is absorbed by the mucous membrane of the urethra, and instead of causing an indurated chancre at the point of entrance, as it does when absorbed on the glans or prepuce, it simply creates a

48

subacute urethritis, the discharge resulting from which is contagious and inoculable. That Hunter should have thought gonorrhœa and syphilis identical is perhaps not to be wondered at, as by the crucial experiment of inoculating himself with what he took to be a gonorrhœal discharge he acquired syphilis, with the secondary symptoms of which he was troubled for three years.

Mr. Lee's views on the subject of syphilization are of interest, as next to Boeck he probably has investigated the matter more thoroughly and practically than any one since the days of Sperino. His conclusion is, " If, then, neither the suppurating venereal sore [chancroid] nor the primary, nor the secondary syphilitic affections, can be inoculated so as to produce any constitutional effect, it is hardly reasonable to suppose that any constitutional disease can be cured by either of these means."

In conclusion, we would say that the work under consideration is in no sense a systematic treatise on syphilis, nor is any new light thrown on the subject. As showing how near to the truth Hunter often came, it is interesting reading, and the author's treatment of the various subjects which he takes up is as a rule fair, concise, and logical. The lectures themselves, illustrated as many of them were by specimens from the Hunterian Museum, must have been extremely interesting to listen to.   F. B. G.

THE UNITED STATES MARINE-HOSPITAL SERVICE.[1]

WE had occasion a year ago to express our cordial appreciation of the work done in this department of the public service, and especially to commend the labors of the supervising surgeon, Dr. J. M. Woodworth. The annual report of Dr. Woodworth, setting forth the operations of his bureau during the year ending June 30, 1874, maintains the high standard of his previous productions. The benefits which the seamen of the merchant service derive from the system of hospital relief established by national law in 1798 are of unquestioned importance, and these benefits are largely enhanced by efficient supervision and economical administration. We learn from the report that over fourteen thousand sick and disabled sailors were furnished with medical and surgical relief during the year ; that the average cost per day for each patient was one dollar only ; and that the mortality among the patients treated in hospitals was but three and one half per cent. Dr. Woodworth makes wise suggestions concerning the application of the provisions for hospital relief to many sailors who are now debarred in various ways ; he also recommends certain reforms in hospital administration and in hospital construction, and intimates that there would be a large saving to the government, without loss of benefit to the seamen, if many of the expensive establishments now maintained were leased and reorganized as general hospitals.

We are glad to observe that preventive medicine has not been overlooked by the medical officers of the marine-hospital service. The hygiene of the forecastle is a prolific theme, and offers an excellent occasion for reformatory

[1] *Annual Report of the Supervising Surgeon of the Marine-Hospital Service of the United States, for the Fiscal Year 1874.* By JOHN M. WOODWORTH, M. D. Washington : Government Printing Office. 1874.

work. While the Plimsolls of the Old World are doing gallant service in protecting the sailor from the perils of "coffin-hulks," the medical men of the American mercantile marine are exposing the dangers to life and health which lurk about the scant accommodations usually provided on shipboard for seamen. Dr. Woodworth says in this connection, "So long as the average duration of a sailor's life continues to be only twelve years, — such low average being largely the result of the food he eats, the clothes he wears, the hole he sleeps in, and the excesses these conditions naturally and inevitably drive him to, — so long will continue the cry of 'unseaworthy sailors,' and so long will there be an inadequate supply even of these."

Besides the general report of the supervising surgeon, the book contains tables and charts setting forth the diseases treated in each of the districts into which the country is divided, and an appendix with various papers by medical officers connected with the service. We have space for only a brief mention of some of these contributions, premising in general, however, that they will all repay careful perusal.

Surgeon F. W. Reilly gives a spirited sketch of the American sailor of the present day, as compared with the class of men who, twenty years ago, reflected credit on our mercantile marine. He depicts the exposures of a seafaring life, the degenerating influences which surround the sailor's mind, body, and soul, the neglect which ship-owners and ship-masters permit. He alludes to the legal restrictions which have been made, and points out, in terms which we wish we could believe to be exaggerated, that these laws protect passengers but not sailors; that "poor food, wretched shelter, and a merciless task-mastery, enforced with steel knuckles and the belaying pin, . . . do not come within the scope of such legislation." All these matters, the writer says, are pointed out to demonstrate the necessity for reform, and to show the directions in which amendment is most needed.

A short paper, by Dr. A. B. Bancroft, describes the diseases which he has observed among the sailors who have come under his charge as patients in the marine hospital at Chelsea.

The diseases of sailors on the lakes, and of river men, are well discussed by medical officers having charge of hospitals in the Western States.

Finally, an elaborate analysis of the course of the yellow-fever epidemic in 1873 furnishes the theme of an interesting paper, in which Dr. Reilly discusses questions of quarantine and prevention, causes and treatment. The author's conclusion that "a quarantine of exclusion is impracticable, and a quarantine of detention is useless," will hardly pass without serious questioning by sanitarians; we fear that "the destruction of germs," "the prompt isolation of each case as it appears," and "a revolution in the sanitary conditions of water-side precincts," which are recommended as measures to secure immunity, would hardly suffice, alone, to assure the desired end.   F. W. D.

OPIUM EATING.[1]

TRASH. In our unfailing charity, we hope it is *honest* trash.

[1] *Opium Eating. An Autobiographical Sketch.* By an Habituate. Philadelphia : Claxton, Remsen, and Haffelfinger. 1876.

PROCEEDINGS OF THE SUFFOLK DISTRICT MEDICAL SOCIETY.

JAMES R. CHADWICK, M. D., SECRETARY.

OCTOBER 30, 1875. The President, DR. H. W. WILLIAMS, in the chair.

Oxygen as a Corrective in the Anæsthetic Use of Chloroform and as an Antidote in Asphyxia. — The paper, by DR. A. YOUNG, will be published.

The Report on Sixteen Cases of Cataract Operations, by DR. B. J. JEFFRIES, was published in the JOURNAL of November 4, 1875.

A Case of Triplets was reported by DR. H. DOHERTY, of South Boston. Mrs. G. F., thirty-nine years of age, had had five children at full term and one miscarriage at two months. She was taken in labor at six P. M. on Monday, October 11, 1875, and three hours afterward gave birth to a female child, weighing three pounds, in a foot presentation. The pains continued until five o'clock on Tuesday morning. Dr. Doherty was first summoned at this time, and readily recognized the head of another child presenting, but not as yet engaged in the pelvis. Ergot was given to provoke uterine action, the membranes were subsequently ruptured, but the head had finally to be extracted by the forceps ; it emerged with the face to the pubes. The child was a boy, and weighed five pounds. The interval between the two deliveries was twelve and a half hours. As the uterus remained hard and large, examination was again made, and the head of a third child was found presenting ; it engaged at once and was delivered with the forceps in half an hour. The child was male, and weighed five and a half pounds. The placenta, which was detached with the hand to avoid the possible contingency of hæmorrhage, weighed with the cords and membranes two and a half pounds.

There had been no suspicion on the part of the woman that the pregnancy was plural, nor had her size or shape been unusual. The husband's mother and the wife's sister have each had twins once.

Statistics give the relative frequency of triplets as one in seventy-four hundred deliveries ; the mortality of the children is one in three. All the children in the present case are now living, on the eighteenth day.

Extirpation of the Uterus by Abdominal Section with the Specimen. — The case, reported by DR. J. R. CHADWICK, appeared in the JOURNAL of November 4, 1875.

DR. W. H. BAKER raised a question as to the justifiability of performing so severe an operation for the removal of a tumor no larger than that now presented.

DR. CHADWICK said he thought that the grounds given in the report fully justified subjecting the patient to the risk ; this had been the view taken by the Obstetrical Society, to which the question had been submitted.

Nitric Acid in the Treatment of Inflammatory Diseases of the Uterus. — DR. E. CHENERY reported great success with this practice in several cases. The first was endometritis, which had not yielded to the application of many other acids or to the use of the curette, but was speedily cured by nitric acid applied thoroughly to the whole inner surface of the organ after dilatation of the cervix. In a case of retroversion attended with much pain and hæmorrhage, where the fundus was bound to the sacrum by adhesions, complete relief had been obtained by swabbing out the uterine cavity with nitric acid. The same satisfactory results had been derived from the application of nitric acid to the urethra in the later stages of gonorrhœa, and to ulcers on the genital organs. In all cases the reaction had been much less than after nitrate of silver, acid nitrate of mercury, etc.

Dr. Chadwick uttered a caution about the promiscuous use of nitric acid in dispensaries, or under any circumstances where the patient cannot keep quiet after its application. He had employed this acid in very many cases and had been much pleased with the results ; but in several instances he had seen metritis and even peritonitis follow its use. The patients had all recovered, but had been the cause of much anxiety.

Dr G. H. Bixby said that the danger was much enhanced when the acid was carried to the fundus ; the application to that region, in his opinion, should be made only when the patient would keep her bed. His experience with nitric acid corroborated that of Dr. Chenery, especially in cases of menorrhagia. He never ventured to use the acid when the fundus was fixed by adhesions.

Dr. G. H. Lyman fully indorsed this practice. He had not supposed anyone would apply nitric acid to the fundus uteri in his office, and allow the patient to go home afterwards. He said that there was danger even in passing the sound, away from the patient's home.

Dr. Baker remarked that Atthill and other physicians had no hesitation in applying the acid to the whole uterine cavity in their office and dispensary practice.

THE TREATMENT OF INSANITY IN ENGLAND AND IN AMERICA.

A recent editorial in *The Lancet*,[1] on the treatment of insanity in America, recalls one of Mr. Hosea Biglow's moral reflections : —

> " Of all the sarse thet I can call to mind,
> England *doos* make the most onpleasant kind ;
> It 's you 're the sinner ollers, she 's the saint ;
> Wut 's good 's all English, all thet is n't ain't."

It would be difficult to guess from what source the writer got his information, but we have no hesitation in saying that his statements are in letter and spirit utterly false ; and we should be justified in using much stronger language. He says, " There can be no question that the custom of slave-holding and the brutalizing *régime* from which it is inseparable, have blinded and blunted the sensibilities of a people in other respects remarkable for their intelligence and enlightenment, to one of the most obvious and urgent teachings of modern science, namely, that mental derangement is distinctly a disease, and susceptible of relief or remedy by measures suitably devised and properly administered. It is surprising, but unhappily it is notorious, that in the United

[1] Vol. II., 1875, No. XX.

States the treatment of lunatics can hardly be said to have made much progress even in the stage of development which we have reluctantly described as the 'humane.' The sort of humanity which sways too many governors of asylums in the United States might indeed be inspired by a rule similar to that said to have been made for the officers of Bethlehem Hospital after the removal to Moorfields in 1675 : 'No keeper or servant shall beat or ill-treat a lunatic without he considers it absolutely necessary for the governing of the lunatic.'"

To express the exact truth in regard to these assertions, we should be obliged to use a strong Anglo-Saxon monosyllable not in good use among gentlemen ; and there are now in England many alienists who know enough of our institutions to say that we would be right in doing so.

It must be acknowledged that the want of frequent and thorough visitation of our asylums by persons not in any way connected with their government allows abuse in individual cases; but even in regard to these the language which we have quoted would be far too strong. The less said about the New York and Philadelphia city asylums, for instance, the better. The county asylum twelve miles from Chicago is still worse; it is a disgrace to our civilization ; early in the past summer, out of about three hundred patients six were in irons. Of these six, three were fastened by a few iron links (the whole not over a foot long), connecting their handcuffs to a wall or to a chair. The only thing that can be said of such barbarous treatment is that it is used also to some extent in Russia.

Our State asylums, however, are very different institutions. The superintendents are picked men, selected for their intelligence and humanity ; and any cruelty on their part would be followed by immediate discharge. As a rule, they give much more of their time to their patients than is done in England. It is these asylums to which allusion is made ; for in the article referred to is the following statement: "They adhere to the old terrorism tempered by petty tyranny. They resort to contrivances of compulsion ; they use, at least, the hideous torture of the shower-bath *as a punishment* in their asylums, although it has been eliminated from their jails. And, worse than all, if the reports that reach us may be trusted, their medical superintendents leave the care of patients, practically, to mere attendants, while devoting their own energies principally to the beautifying of their colossal establishments." Where in America can be found such "colossal establishments" as Colney Hatch, Hanwell, and the county asylums at Wakefield, Barming Heath, Prestwich, and Lancaster Moor?

We would remind the editors of *The Lancet* that the "humane" treatment of insanity was largely introduced in England by the efforts of a distinguished American philanthropist, Miss Dix ; and that they need not go back to the parliamentary report of 1815 to find abuses and horrors in the treatment of mental disease such as never existed in the United States.

Mr. R. Gardiner Hill, once surgeon of the Lincoln Asylum, in describing the prevailing treatment of insane persons in England in 1840 (*British and Foreign Medical Review*, January, 1840, page 145) says, "The keeper or keepers kneel upon his body, thrust their knuckles into his throat, beat him, and bruise him, until they succeed in overcoming him." We would respectfully refer the ignorant writer of the article in *The Lancet* to Mr. R. Gardiner Hill's book, on the Non-Restraint System of Treatment in Insanity, to the report of the select committee in 1859, to the minutes of the Lincoln Asylum, to the twenty-nine reports of the lunacy commission, to Mr. Arlidge's book on the State of Lunacy, and to two books by Dr. Conolly, The Construction and Government of Lunatic Asylums, and The Treatment of the Insane without Mechanical Restraints. Finally, if he has not convinced himself that only one third of a century ago the treatment of insanity in England was a blot upon their civilization, let him, if he has the heart to go farther, read a dozen pages of Miss Dix's private diary.

In 1773, the first insane asylum was established in the United States, and was conducted on "humane" principles. Three years previous to that time the managers of the Bethlehem Hospital ("Bedlam"), in London, were exhibiting their patients to the populace at a penny a head!

We grant that the best English asylums have far exceeded us in the rapidity of their improvement, that thirty years of supervision by the commissioners in lunacy have rendered systematic abuse and neglect of patients on the part of officers well-nigh impossible, that in abolishing mechanical restraint they have succeeded in reducing in a great degree the amount of medicine and seclusion used; but we would like to have the privilege of pointing out some of the seventy-two public and one hundred and forty private asylums where the treatment is certainly not intelligent, and where it seemed to us that there was what we in America should call neglect.

Does it not look as if in some, at least, of the English asylums the medical superintendents do not even "leave the care of patients, practically, to mere attendants," when the commissioners say, "For some years our attention has been directed to the large number of epileptic patients who are found dead in bed, and to the occurrence of suicides during the night, more especially in public asylums?"[1] Patients in our State asylums (our county asylums are more nearly allied to the English work-houses and poor-houses) are not left so much to the attendants as in England, and our attendants are not so brutal as the English. We have heard English superintendents acknowledge this fact; and they say freely to physicians, although not to the public, that the stories of broken ribs in English asylums are not simply the fictions of Mr. Charles Reade's fertile brain, but the sober, solemn truth.

For the benefit of a man who thinks that "the time has passed when a modest consciousness of our own shortcomings might restrain the impulse to remonstrate with the responsible managers of asylums in America," we will content ourselves with a few extracts from the Twenty-Eighth Annual Official Report of the Commissioners in Lunacy (London, 1874), although we must say that we find in them from year to year a *good deal* that is melancholy reading.

"In the case of a female patient, . . . who hung herself with a piece of tape which she had fixed to the casing of a water-closet door, some doubt arose whether the nurse in charge had been informed of this woman's suicidal disposition." (Page 29.)

[1] Twenty-Ninth Report, 1875, page 20.

" On the first of July it was discovered that he" (J. C.) " had fractures of the breast-bone, and also of three ribs on each side ; . . . upon *post-mortem* examination, it was found that on the right side the third, fifth, sixth, eighth, ninth, tenth, and eleventh ribs were fractured, some in two or three places, and the fourth rib was detached from the breast-bone. On the left side, the seventh, eighth, ninth, tenth, and eleventh were broken and the fifth detached. There was a transverse fracture of the breast-bone opposite the cartilage of the fourth rib on each side." He was a patient " often requiring to be held." (Page 30.)

" Apart from the case of J. C. and the fatal violence to which he was subjected, it appeared to us that there was strong evidence that the arrangements at the —— asylum for the care and treatment of the impulsive and dangerous class of patients, especially in the male division, were very defective ; . . . and above all that it was of the highest importance that there should be more vigilant and constant supervision of these departments of the asylum by Dr. —— and the assistant medical officers." (Page 31.)

" That a patient with strong suicidal tendencies, and apparently not violent, should have been placed to sleep in a single room at all, and especially in one offering such facilities for accomplishing his object, showed great want of ordinary precaution." (Note on a case of suicide, page 34.)

That the circumstances of one accidental death showed " both laxity of discipline and great carelessness." (Page 34.)

" An old man was found two days after his admission to have received fractures of two or three ribs on the right side. . . . It appeared that he . . . ' fell, or was put down,' and that afterwards ' four or five of them ' were about him and that he was pressed or knelt on." (Page 35.)

" We communicated to the medical superintendent our opinion that there was grave laxity of supervision." (Note on an " accidental death " from scalding in a bath-tub, page 37.)

" In the case of a male patient, whose death took place in March last, fractures of six ribs were discovered." (Page 38.)

" The death in this asylum of a male patient of strong and well-known suicidal disposition was so entirely due to negligence on the part of the chief attendant of the ward, that the resolution of the visitors that he should be severely reprimanded, but in consequence of his long service and excellent character should be allowed to retain his situation, appeared to the board the most lenient treatment for so serious an offense." (Page 39.)

" Shortly afterward another suicide of a female patient took place in the same asylum, when we again felt called upon to express our opinion that the attendants were to blame." (Page 40.)

" A male epileptic patient was drowned in a bath, which had been partly filled with water for the purpose of cleaning the ward, and into which he fell in a fit." (Page 41.)

" Three cases of suicide of patients belonging to —— Asylum took place during the past year." (Page 41.)

" Portsmouth and Southampton continue without any efficient provision for their lunatics." (Page 44.)

" On inquiring into the circumstances, we came to the conclusion that this lamentable event" (suicide by hanging, the patient having been dead several hours when seen) " was mainly attributable to a neglect of the most ordinary precautions." (Page 47.)

" The patient hanged himself from a ventilator, . . . where he was found dead in the morning." (Page 50.)

" A male private patient in this house was very severely assaulted on the 3d of December by two attendants named —— and ——, and he was found to have been so seriously injured as for a time to place his life in danger." (Page 52.)

But we will close this wearisome tale, merely referring our English friends to pages 53-63, 67, 69-71, 74, and 75, of the same report. The most deplorable accident of all was that by which England lost a most valuable citizen, Mr. Lutwidge, one of the commissioners in lunacy, killed by an insane man with a sharpened nail.

Dr. Manning, in his Report on Lunatic Asylums (1868), a work of unquestioned authority, states of the shower-bath in England, " In some asylums it is used as a means of correcting faulty habits, but for these purposes the shock only is required." (Page 121.) We would like to ask whether that means *punishment*. If the editor of *The Lancet*, in his "spirit of self-sufficiency," knows a single State or private insane asylum in the United States where the shower-bath is still used as a means of punishment, we would be very grateful to share his information.

We have already said that the writer of the article which we are criticising is ignorant. We can pardon him and the Earl of Shaftesbury (formerly chairman of the lunacy commission), whom he quotes, for saying that "the whole history of the world, until the era of the Reformation, does not afford a single instance of a single receptacle assigned to the protection and care of these unhappy sufferers, whose malady was looked upon as hardly within the hope of medical aid." The monks had an insane asylum at Jerusalem in the sixth century, and the ancient Egyptians had temples dedicated to Saturn for the cure of mental disease, which, in the matters of freedom from restraint, amusements, employments, etc., would put to the blush most of the English asylums of the present day. The Gheel colony dates from the seventh century.

This is not the place to discuss the question of mechanical restraint, except to say that the majority of American superintendents consider its use the *most humane* means at their disposal in certain cases.

We will close with a few extracts from three private letters received from the first authorities in England : —

" I am sorry to find that the locks, bolts, and bars which at one time rendered English asylums such prisons are still thought necessary in your part of the world. The greatest possible good has attended the abolition of these in England, and now many patients are allowed to walk out unattended on their parole, and rarely abuse the privilege." (November 5, 1875.)

" I must say that I think they " (American superintendents) " have not yet arrived at that point from which the treatment and management of the insane become easy, namely, the point where the doctor has no fear of his patient. . . . You have no idea, in the States, of the amount of freedom under due supervision which our lunatics get; and it is constantly being increased, and with the best results. We are now pretty well rid of the old superstitious fear of the insane; and where the bounds of insanity have been so much enlarged it was time that this should be so." (October 31, 1875.)

"The neighborhood of London is about the worst we have for sample asylums. The old chartered hospitals for the insane are antiquated, and the new county asylums are vast receptacles for the insane, badly managed and governed. I do not think your hospitals for the insane of the McLean type are much behind the age, nor the State asylums in your States, barring the question of mechanical restraint; but some of your city asylums are really disgraceful to you as a people; those at —— and —— I can point to as iniquitous." (August 18, 1875.)

We welcome all such candid criticisms, based upon actual knowledge; but we have discarded the old rhetorical artifice of "slandering stoutly that something may stick."

MEDICAL NOTES.

— It is rather suggestive, not to say amusing, that while three or four homœopathic practitioners were before the city committee last Wednesday week with their roll of petitioners' names, to urge that a ward in the City Hospital be devoted to homœopathic treatment, and lamenting the absence of the petitioners themselves, their *first* and *chief* petitioner was at that very time convalescing under the care of a regular physician, having dismissed his homœopathic attendant some days previously.

— With regard to the Hospital Sunday, so called, the *Medical Times and Gazette* of November 19, 1875, says, "It will be seen that in the third year of its establishment, with improved coöperation and organization, the total amount realized is nearly £3000 less than on the previous occasions. Should another year's results tend in the same direction, it will become an imperative duty on the part of the council to consider whether the movement, as regards the metropolis, should not be at once abandoned as a serious failure."

The use made of a considerable part of the last collection taken in this city is not of a nature to commend the enterprise to the profession. Men who last year were excluded, this year come in for their pickings, and it is our impression that the quackish element will erelong leaven the whole mass.

— For the relief of neuralgic pain, Spencer Thompson, M. D., writes favorably of the employment of the tincture of gelseminum sempervirens. His paper may be found in *The Lancet* of November 6, 1875. Directly or indirectly the remedy has been used by Dr. Thompson or under his authority in at least forty cases of neuralgia, and with almost constant success. The remedial power of the agent seems to be applicable to neuralgia of those branches of the trifacial nerve supplying the upper and lower jaw, more particularly the latter; it is especially useful when the pain is most directly referred to the teeth or alveoli. The doses usually recommended are too small. Dr. Thompson almost invariably prescribes for an adult twenty minims of the tincture as a first dose, to be repeated any time after an hour and a half, if relief is not given. He has rarely had to order a third dose. Several cases are given to illustrate the successful employment of the drug.

— The recent death of Duchenne (de Boulogne) has called forth many testimonials relative to his untiring zeal as a physician, and his natural kindness of heart. The Paris correspondent of *The Lancet* gives some interesting facts regarding Duchenne's work and habits. He was born in 1806, and died at nearly seventy. After graduation he began practice in Boulogne-sur-Mer, his native place; but in order to obtain a larger field, particularly for his experimental work, he left for Paris, where, during thirty-three years, he led a life of incessant scientific labor. In 1847 he presented his first memoir to the Academy of Sciences, and till within a month of his death he continued to publish the results of his experiments and observations. His researches on the muscular system are among the most important of his works, and his studies on the muscles of the face, their office in the mechanism and expression of the human visage, are familiar in France to artists as well as to physicians. He is best known, however, for his researches on the nervous centres, on the various forms of paralysis, and on congenital or developed deformities. His name will ever be coupled with the history of progressive muscular atrophy, glosso-labio-laryngeal paralysis, and, generally, the microscopical anatomy and pathology of the nervous system. To Duchenne is due the honor of having methodically applied electricity to physiological and pathological investigations, and of having scientifically used it for the treatment of disease. He was a constant visitor in the wards of the Paris hospitals, and every morning could be seen there studying cases, examining specimens, and making drawings of microscopical appearances, in which latter accomplishment he was extraordinarily skillful. He showed wonderful keenness and ability in diagnosticating cases of paralysis, and his honesty of purpose overcame the dislike which was manifested by the hospital physicians in the earlier years of his career. He was no orator, but was an excellent clinical instructor. He was dexterous and nimble in handling his patients, sharp and sensible in his questioning, most striking in the way he got up his data, made out the disease, and gave practical demonstrations of the study of his diagnosis. His patience was extraordinary, pursuing at times the investigation of a case for years. It may be said of him that under many adverse circumstances his reputation has come out clear and bright, as an honest, hard-working, acute, and ingenious observer, an original discoverer, a skillful professional man, and a kind-hearted, benevolent gentleman.

THE CASE OF HENRY WILSON.

[FROM OUR WASHINGTON CORRESPONDENT.]

MESSRS. EDITORS, — The medical event of the day which is interesting the profession here, as indeed it has profoundly affected the whole country, is the circumstances attending the illness and death of Vice-President Henry Wilson. The newspapers have kept us well informed respecting the progress of his case and the details of the post-mortem evidences. With regard to the stated cause of death (apoplexy), when taken in connection with post-mortem appearances, and as made public through the press, it would seem to be better that a reserved and qualified opinion had been expressed at the time, to give opportunity for a more thorough and careful consideration of the condition presented.

While stating that the press here deserves credit for its accurate and correct accounts when taken in the main, exception must be made to the course pursued by one paper, the *National Republican*, which has sought to make a sensational article out of this unfortunate event, and by a badly-written, illogical, clap-trap account of the post-mortem examination, invests it with all the details that a morbid imagination might be supposed to conjure up in a dissecting-room scene; indeed, likening it to that, and striving to convey the impression that post mortems and dissections are to be classed together and both alike to be condemned. Were the character of this paper not well known here it might produce a pernicious effect in the community, but even straws may sometimes carry infection.

It may be well, however, to reproduce in a connected form and as an authoritative statement what has already been given to the world by the daily press.

We are told that the late vice-president suffered some two years ago from an attack of paralysis, the details of which were not familiar to the profession here, but a careful examination failed to connect the symptoms accompanying the recent illness as consequent upon the former attack of paralysis. The post mortem, indeed, showed a deposit of lymph upon the surface of the cerebral hemispheres which did not seem to be recent in its formation.

A few days before his late illness, Mr. Wilson had been under the treatment of Dr. Hammond for symptoms which occasioned the application of the actual cautery along the spine. On the morning of November 10th he was suffering from pain which extended from the base of the brain down the spine and into the limbs, and for relief took a hot bath, which resulted in prostration and an aggravation of the pains. At ten A. M. of the same day Drs. J. H. Baxter, U. S. A., G. L. Magruder, and F. A. Ashford were in attendance, in answer to an urgent summons. Counter-irritation of the surface with mustard and flannels was applied. There was no paralysis, but a heavy and listless condition, and with it an abrupt answering of questions and considerable twitching of the muscles, especially of those about the neck and face; at one time the face was drawn somewhat to the right side, but this was temporary. There had been constipation of the bowels; an enema was administered of castor-oil, turpentine, and warm water, bringing away semi-solid fæces. Three large cups, improvised for the occasion from goblets, were now applied between the shoulders; these brought away one ounce of blood. The listlessness disappeared; solicitude and anxiety took its place, and the pain was still marked. The pulse was weak and small.

At 5.30 P. M. of the same day he was again seen by these medical gentlemen in consultation, having in the mean time been removed to the vice-president's room in the Capitol; he had taken his hot bath in a lower room of that building, and was there seized with the attack. It was found by the consulting physicians that he had taken since their last visit one dose of a mixture prescribed by them, which was equivalent to, fifteen grains of bromide of potassium, one eighth of a grain of sulphate of morphia, and one drachm of camphor water; a hypodermic injection of half a drachm of whisky had been administered. He had slept several hours, and expressed himself as greatly relieved and refreshed. He had urinated twice, and taken nourishment; there was no nausea or vomiting. Very little pain remained; the tongue was clean the pulse 72, and of good quality; the respiration was regular, 16; the pupils were regular, and responded well to light. The mind was clear. Weakness was extreme.

November 11th, 10.30 A. M., a consultation was held, but not at the bedside of the patient, he being in a comfortable sleep, with general symptoms favorable. Dr. Baxter had from the first, in accordance with the expressed wish of the vice-president, been acting as the attending physician, and from that time up to his death assumed sole charge of the case. There appears to be but little to add to this account of the onset of the attack, as in the opinion of Dr. Baxter the case appeared to progress satisfactorily, and two days before Mr. Wilson's death, had the weather been suitable, he would have been advised to drive out, and was encouraged to anticipate the journey North.

On the 15th there was an aggravation of the symptoms, due, it was supposed at the time, to the presence of visitors, to reading, and to injudicious additions to the diet-list without the doctor's sanction; with increased care in these particulars the symptoms subsided. Mr. Wilson throughout, and perhaps injudiciously, persisted in knowing the contents of his mail and of the newspapers of each day.

The circumstances immediately preceding his death are well told in the daily press as follows:[1] —

" During the period previous to his death, while he was confined to his room, his physician, Dr. Baxter, denied admittance to all visitors except intimate acquaintances. But on Sunday he seemed to be in such excellent health and spirits, and was so very desirous of meeting his friends, the doctor relaxed the severity of the order, and quite a number of visitors were admitted to his chamber. With several of these he conversed quite cheerfully on various topics, and to nearly all expressed the belief that he would not be confined to his chamber much longer. He also, during the course of the day, expressed a desire to examine his correspondence, but this Dr. Baxter declined to permit, at the same time informing the vice-president that he feared the mental excitement which would naturally be produced in his then weak state by perusing important letters might prove injurious. Mr. Wilson felt considerable dissatisfaction at the strictness of the doctor's decision, and remarked to one of his attendants that a physician who would not tyrannize over his patients was a jewel rarely found, and added that he supposed sick people needed to be ruled with an iron hand for their own good. About four o'clock in the afternoon he fell into a refreshing slumber, which continued for three hours. When he awoke he informed his attendants that he felt much better than when he commenced to sleep, and spoke with them on general subjects until about eight o'clock, when he retired for the night. During the early portion of the night he slept very soundly, but a little after midnight he began to show signs of restlessness, and just before three o'clock he awoke very suddenly, complain-

[1] Washington Chronicle, November 23, 1875.

ing of a pain which had attacked his chest, soon after sinking into a sound sleep again, from which he did not awake until seven o'clock. Mr. Wood, who was the only attendant present, asked him concerning the manner in which he had slept, and also about his health. Mr. Wilson replied by saying that he had slept soundly, and felt very much refreshed. Mr. Wood then communicated to the vice-president the intelligence of the death of Senator Ferry, of Connecticut, which he had read in the morning papers. Mr. Wilson expressed his regret at the loss of his old friend, and made some few remarks, referring to the services that the senator had rendered his country. This seemed to bring home his own condition, and he incidentally alluded to his election to the vice-presidency, saying, ' If I live to the close of my present term, there will be only five who have served their country as long as I.' These were the last intelligible words uttered by Mr. Wilson. While speaking to Mr. Wood, Mr. Wilson was lying upon his bed, and appeared to be very comfortable ; no evidences of pain were visible, and his manner and voice were very buoyant. About fifteen minutes after seven Mr. Wood opened a bottle of *Fredericshalle,* bitter water, which had been prescribed for the vice-president, and poured it in a tumbler and handed it to him to drink. Mr. Wood had scarcely turned, after removing the glass from the hands of Mr. Wilson, who sat up in bed to drink the water, when he heard a convulsive gasping, and on hastily looking he saw the vice-president in a half-recumbent position, with the weight of his body resting on his right hand, breathing stertorously, as if in pain. This lasted but a moment, however, when he fell back on the bed, still breathing heavily. He expired before Mr. Wood could do anything to relieve him."

From this it appears that death occurred about 7.15 A. M., November 22d. At 11.30 A. M. a post-mortem examination was made by Dr. Lamb, of the surgeon-general's office, assisted by Surgeon-General Barnes, Dr. Billings, Dr. J. H. Baxter, Dr. C. M. Ford, Dr. Ashford, and Dr. G. L. Magruder. Dr. Lamb has kindly furnished the following notes, which are more detailed than those published : —

" There was no rigor mortis, and no other external appearance of note except a longitudinal livid patch upon the back of the neck.

" The dura mater was quite firmly adherent to the inner surface of the calvarium adjacent to the longitudinal sinus ; all of the sinuses were full of dark fluid blood ; the pia mater was congested, and presented many small, old, whitish patches of lymph scattered along the surface adjoining the longitudinal sinus. The brain weighed forty-nine ounces, was normal in consistence and color, except that the puncta vasculosa were less marked than usual, both in number and in vividness ; there was a transparent cyst about the size of a pea in the extremity of each choroid plexus ; the ventricular fluid was normal in character and quantity. The subarachnoidal fluid was slightly increased in quantity. The arteries at the base of the brain, more especially the middle cerebrals and basilar, together with their larger ramifications, were notably atheromatous, some of the calcareous plates being three to four lines in long diameter, and so thick as nearly to obliterate the vessel. No thrombus nor embolus was found, nor any extravasation of blood in the venous plexuses of the pons Varolii or medulla.

" The spinal canal contained a large quantity of dark fluid blood. The spinal cord, which was examined as low down as the third dorsal vertebra, appeared to be normal, except that the demarkation between the gray and the white substance was not well marked. Portions of the brain and spinal cord were set aside for microscopical examination.

" The lungs were congested posteriorly ; there were old pleuritic adhesions on the left side, chiefly around the apex ; a calcareous deposit the size of a pea was found in the middle lobe of the right lung ; the lungs were otherwise normal. The heart presented a small calcareous deposit on one of the segments of the aortic valve, but was otherwise normal. The pericardial fluid was normal in quantity and color.

" The stomach was much congested, the mucous membrane everywhere of a deep red color and covered with mucus. There were many erosions of the mucous membrane, some superficial, others nearly perforating the membrane ; some, the smaller ones, were rounded, the larger were irregular in outline ; these latter were surrounded by dark areolæ of congestion. The liver was of a dark color, congested, and somewhat friable ; there was a small aqueous cyst in its upper surface, near the broad ligament. The gall-bladder was full of dark bile. The spleen was large and dark, but normal in structure. The kidneys weighed eight ounces each, and were congested ; there were a few small subcapsular cysts and cicatrices, apparently of previous cysts. The bladder was contracted, its mucous membrane slightly reddened, and contained a small quantity of urine of normal color.

" The intestines appeared healthy.

" It ought to be stated, perhaps, that in view of the prospective embalming only such examination was made as appeared to be absolutely necessary.

" The cause of death was considered to be nervous apoplexy, depending probably on cerebral anæmia."

As to the condition of the stomach, Mr. Wilson was not a temperance man, properly speaking ; although he advocated total abstinence from spirituous liquors, he was a large eater. Dr. Baxter at an early period in his attendance had diagnosticated gastric derangement. The post mortem was performed by Dr. Lamb, who is an acting assistant surgeon, U. S. A., and an assistant at the Army Medical Museum, and may be considered an expert. Drs. Magruder, Ashford, and Ford are members of the profession in this city, and the remaining gentlemen are connected with the United States Army.

We are indebted for the most of these details, and for the confirmation of the published report, to Drs. Ashford and Baxter. Further details of the progress of the case will probably be given by Dr. Baxter at an early day, and in full. The spinal cord was removed to the extent of several inches for microscopical examination by Dr. J. J. Woodward, U. S. A., and in a few days the result will probably be made public.

The question very naturally arises, Was the cause of death assigned sustained by post-mortem evidence ? This question, from the length of the letter and from prudential reasons, your correspondent leaves to other and abler minds to discuss.   HOMO.

WASHINGTON, D. C., *November* 27, 1875.

WEEKLY BULLETIN OF PREVALENT DISEASES.

THE following is a bulletin of the diseases prevalent in Massachusetts during the week ending December 4, 1875, compiled under the authority of the State Board of Health from the returns of physicians representing all sections of the State: —

The following is a summary for each section : —

Berkshire: Bronchitis, pneumonia, rheumatism.

Valley: Bronchitis, pneumonia, influenza, typhoid fever, diphtheria. Greenfield reports an epidemic of influenza.

Midland: Influenza, bronchitis, pneumonia, rheumatism. diphtheria. Less diphtheria reported. Worcester returns scarlatina as prevalent.

Northeastern: Bronchitis, influenza, rheumatism, pneumonia. Less diphtheria and scarlatina. Natick reports "influenza universal and severe ; " Haverhill, diphtheria severe and fatal.

Metropolitan: Bronchitis, scarlatina, pneumonia, diphtheria, influenza. No noteworthy change reported in the prevalence of diphtheria and scarlatina. Considerable diarrhœa coincidently with the sudden change to cold weather.

Southeastern: Influenza, bronchitis, diphtheria. Not much sickness.

For the State at large the summary, giving the order of relative prevalence of diseases, is as follows: Bronchitis, pneumonia and influenza (increased), rheumatism, diphtheria, typhoid fever (diminished), scarlatina and croup (increased), diarrhœa, measles, whooping-cough.

F. W. DRAPER, M. D., Registrar.

COMPARATIVE MORTALITY-RATES FOR THE WEEK ENDING NOV. 27, 1875.

	Estimated Population.	Total Mortality for the Week.	Annual Death-Rate per 1000 during Week.
New York	1,060,000	492	24
Philadelphia	800,000	262	17
Brooklyn	500,000		
Chicago	400,000	115	15
Boston	342,000	162	24
Cincinnati	260,000	129	26
Providence	100,700	33	17
Worcester	50,000	14	15
Lowell	50,000	20	21
Cambridge . . .	48,000	12	13
Fall River	45,000	24	28
Lawrence	35,000	9	13
Lynn	33,000	15	24
Springfield	31,000	7	12
Salem	26,000	12	24

Normal Death-Rate, 17 per 1000.

BOOKS AND PAMPHLETS RECEIVED. — Transactions of the American Otological Society. Eighth Annual Meeting. Vol. II. Part 1. Boston. 1875. (For sale by James Campbell.)

Annual Report of the Surgeon-General of the United States Army. 1875.

THE BOSTON
MEDICAL AND SURGICAL JOURNAL.

VOL. XCIII. — THURSDAY, DECEMBER 16, 1875. — NO. 25.

ON THE CAUSE OF VICE-PRESIDENT WILSON'S DEATH.[1]

BY WILLIAM A. HAMMOND, M. D.,

Professor of Diseases of the Mind and Nervous System in the University of the City of New York.

THE following report of the post-mortem examination of the body of the late vice-president was printed in a Washington newspaper, and sent to me by my friend Col. J. H. Baxter, M. D., Chief Medical Purveyor of the United States Army. It may therefore be regarded as having been published by authority, and as being a correct account of the proceedings and opinions of the medical gentlemen who conducted the investigation. It is the same statement that was telegraphed to the principal newspapers throughout the country, and laid by them before their readers : —

" External appearances : Nothing unusual.

" Brain : Weight, forty-nine ounces ; sinuses of brain full of black fluid blood ; deposit of lymph on surface of cerebral hemispheres ; consistence and color of brain normal ; cyst the size of a pea in each choroid plexus ; atheromatous deposit in the arteries at base of brain, and in anterior and middle cerebral arteries.

" Spinal cord : Nothing abnormal in color or consistence. A microscopical examination will be made hereafter.

" Lungs : Old pleuritic adhesions on left side ; calcareous deposit the size of a pea in the middle lobe of right lung ; lungs congested (hypostasis).

" Heart : Normal, except small calcareous deposit in aortic valve ; pericardial fluid normal.

" Stomach : Empty, congested throughout, with slight erosions or abrasions at several points ; pyloric portion normal.

" Liver : Congested and somewhat fatty ; small cyst on upper surface.

" Gall-bladder : Full of bile ; normal.

" Kidneys : Weight, eight ounces each ; congested, with one or two small cysts, and cicatrices of similar cysts.

[1] Read before the New York Neurological Society, December 6, 1875.

"Spleen : Large, dark ; otherwise normal.

" Other viscera : Normal.

" Cause of death : Apoplexy."

The use of the term apoplexy in the foregoing report is unfortunate and inexact. Apoplexy is a symptom, just as cough is a symptom. It would be just as definite to say that a patient affected with some organic disease of the chest had died of cough, as to assert that the vice-president died of apoplexy.

Nevertheless, apoplexy is, as I have said, a symptom. It may result from several conditions. The object of this paper is to' show that the vice-president did not die from any disease of the brain capable of producing apoplexy, and, to go still further, that his death was not the direct result of any cerebral lesion at all, unless it was of the medulla oblongata.

Apoplexy is defined by Aitken [1] as being essentially characterized by the sudden loss, more or less complete, of volition, perception, sensation, and motion, depending on sudden pressure upon the brain (the tissue of which may be morbid) originating within the cranium. Though it may be due to several very different conditions, Aitken states that it is customary to confine the application of the term to congestion or hæmorrhage, to which may be added serous effusion. It is still more common to use apoplexy and cerebral hæmorrhage as correlative terms.

Now when we come to analyze the report we find that the following circumstances are stated to have existed, which may be regarded as more or less morbid conditions of the brain.

(1.) The sinuses were full of black fluid blood.

(2.) There was a deposit of lymph on the surface of the cerebral hemispheres.

(3.) There was a cyst the size of a pea in each choroid plexus.

(4.) There was an atheromatous deposit in the arteries at the base of the brain and in the anterior and middle cerebral arteries.

The normal phenomena were, —

(1.) The weight of the brain was forty-nine ounces.

(2.) The consistence and color of the brain were normal.

Surely no one acquainted with cerebral pathology will assert that any one of the circumstances embraced in the first category could have caused the symptom known as apoplexy, much less have produced the death of the distinguished patient. There is no mention made of a clot, or an embolus, or a thrombus. On the contrary, it is distinctly stated that the color and consistence of the brain were normal, which could not have been the case had any of these conditions existed for any considerable length of time. A thrombus or an embolus might, however, if it occupied either of the vessels supplying the medulla oblongata, have caused sudden death without producing softening.

1 The Science and Practice of Medicine. Third American Edition, 1872, i. 1021.

No mention is made of any lesion existing in the corpora striata or optic thalamus, nor of the remains of any anterior hæmorrhage. It is probable, therefore, that the hemiplegia caused over a year ago was not due to the rupture of a vessel.

We may therefore, I think, dismiss all idea of cerebral hæmorrhage, and, indeed, the symptoms are not reconcilable with such a condition, unless, as is not probable in view of the competency of the medical gentlemen who conducted the examination, and who would certainly have detected such a lesion, the extravasation took place into the substance of the medulla oblongata, or was so situated, or was of such enormous size, as to subject this organ to great pressure.

In the same newspaper (*The National Republican*) which contained the report of the post-mortem examination, we find an account of the manner of the vice-president's death, which is substantially identical with that contained in the other papers. The evening before, he drank a large glass of ice-water, and " on Mr. Wood's remarking that it was something unusual for him to drink so much, the vice-president replied that he did not feel as well as usual, and asked Mr. Wood to place his ear to his heart, but nothing was detected out of the usual course. Mr. Wilson retired, and was soon asleep again. At two o'clock Lieutenant Boyden relieved Mr. Wood, and remained with Mr. Wilson until seven in the morning. Soon after Lieutenant Boyden had left, Mr. Wilson awoke, an unusual thing for him to do, and seemed quite bright and cheerful. It was the first time since his sickness that he had waked at that hour. At 7.05 he was informed of the death of Senator Ferry. He exhibited no excitement, but seemed lost in deep thought, and presently spoke of Mr. Ferry in a very friendly manner. Mr. Wood then washed his face and prepared him for breakfast, and he drank a glass of bitter water (prepared by Dr. Baxter), and as Mr. Wood turned to place the glass on the table Mr. Wilson lay down again, and the moment his head touched the pillow his breathing became difficult, and in less than a minute he was dead."

Now it is quite common with those not thoroughly conversant with the physiology of the brain and the pathology of cerebral hæmorrhage to consider the affection in question as frequently the cause of sudden death. Such, however, is really not the case, for unless the medulla oblongata be involved in the lesion, dying from extravasation of blood in the brain is quite a protracted process. Thus Dr. Hughlings Jackson,[1] though admitting that hæmorrhage into or near the medulla oblongata might cause instant death, has never witnessed such a termination. Dr. Wilks[2] says that apoplexy is very rarely, if ever, a suddenly fatal disease,

---

[1] On Apoplexy and Cerebral Hæmorrhage. Reynolds's System of Medicine. London, 1866, ii. 520.

[2] Guy's Hospital Reports, 1866, page 178.

no matter what part of the brain may be the seat of the lesion. Among the reports of several thousand post-mortem examinations at Guy's Hospital of individuals who had died apoplectic, there was but one in which death was asserted to have been instantaneous, and that was a case of meningeal hæmorrhage. Even this was doubtful, for the patient had fallen at some distance from the hospital, and was dead when brought in.

In my own experience I have never seen a case of cerebral hæmorrhage that was instantaneously fatal. I have several times had cases under my observation in which it was said death had been as sudden as though the individual had been struck by lightning; but careful inquiry and post-mortem examination have shown either that the observers were deceived or that there had been no extravasation at all, death being the result of heart-disease.

But it is certainly true that a hæmorrhage into the medulla oblongata may cause sudden death, though even here such a result is not inevitable. After extensive search I have been able to find but two cases.

Gintrac [1] cites the case of a woman sixty-four years old, who, during a violent fit of anger, uttered a loud cry, supported herself against a wall, and dropped slowly to the ground. When taken up she was dead. The sinuses of the dura mater were found engorged, the vessels of the pia mater were injected, the ventricles were empty. A clot the size of a walnut was found adherent to the superior part of the medulla oblongata, and extending as high up as the fourth ventricle. It originated from the central gray matter of the bulb, and had partly destroyed the olivary bodies.

The other case is reported by Dr. Charrier. [2]

A woman left her bed the tenth day after childbirth. On the twelfth day, at the evening visit of the physician, she answered the questions he put to her. She appeared to be in good spirits, when suddenly she uttered a cry, turned over on her pillow, and was dead, without there having been any convulsive movement. The diagnosis of hæmorrhage into the bulb was made.

The calvarium was removed, and the medulla oblongata was exposed to view. In appearance there was no lesion, but on incising the rachidian bulb a clot was found occupying its substance, to which the death was undoubtedly due. All the other parts of the brain were healthy, as were also the thoracic and abdominal viscera.

In the published report of the post-mortem examination of the body of the vice-president, no mention is made of the medulla oblongata. It is therefore to be presumed that no lesion existed in this nerve-centre. It is stated that there was nothing abnormal in the color or consistence of the spinal cord, but that a microscopical examination will be made of

---

[1] Traité théorique et pratique des Maladies de l'Appareil nerveux, ii. 372.

[2] Hémorrhagie du Bulbe rachidien. Archives de Physiologie, 1869, page 660.

it. Such an investigation, if made to embrace the medulla oblongata, may reveal the cause of the vice-president's death, but it certainly is not needed for the discovery of an extravasation of blood sufficient to have produced such a sudden death as was his.

The vice-president first consulted me, at the instance of my friend Dr. E. H. Clarke, of Boston, on the 4th of September of the present year. He then complained of pain in the back of his head, and of inability to sleep. He had almost entirely recovered from the hemiplegia which had occurred the year before, but there was at times a little thickness of speech, especially when he was fatigued. His face was flushed, and there was occasional numbness of various parts of the body.

Although his sight was not markedly affected, there was incipient double optic neuritis, the morbid process being more advanced in the right than in the left eye.

Conceiving the symptoms for which he consulted me to be mainly due to cerebral hyperæmia, I treated him with the bromide of sodium and the fluid extract of ergot, in doses of fifteen grains of the former to half a drachm of the latter, three times a day. At the same time I enjoined rest from mental labor, an injunction, however, which he declared he could not comply with as fully as was desirable.

I saw him again on the 15th of October. He was better, he said, than he had been for a year, was sleeping well, had no pain or weakness, and was in full mental vigor. Being constipated he asked me for a mild purgative, and I gave him a prescription for some pills of ox gall, extract of aloes, and podophyllin, telling him to take one when necessary.

He did not visit me again till the 7th of November. He was then worse than I had yet seen him. There were vertigo, thickness of speech, twitching of the facial muscles, irregularity of respiration and of the action of the heart, slight difficulty of swallowing, and intense pain in the back of the head and nape of the neck. At the same time there was a peculiar restlessness of manner which was very striking. His hands were in almost constant motion and he could not sit longer than a few seconds without rising and pacing the floor, or changing to another chair. He spoke of his inability to sleep and of his waking with a sudden start several times in the course of the night.

Ophthalmoscopic examination showed no condition different from that which existed previously.

There was neither albumen nor tube casts in the urine.

There were no abnormal sounds about the heart, but the impulse was feeble and irregular both in rhythm and in force. Twice, while I felt his pulse, there was an intermission. I could detect no evidence of organic disease of any kind.

The temperature of the right side of his body, head, face, and hands, as determined by Dr. Lombard's thermo-electric differential calorimeter was a degree and a half Fahrenheit higher than that of the left side.

The symptoms led me to apprehend the existence of incipient basilar meningitis, extending as far back as the medulla oblongata, or some other congestive or inflammatory affection, in its very beginning involving this organ.

I therefore advised the continuance of the bromide of sodium and ergot, which had been omitted since his last visit, and at the same time gave him small doses ($\frac{1}{10}$ gr.) of the phosphide of zinc.

I also advised the application of the actual cautery to the nape of the neck, and I applied it, first producing local anæsthesia by means of the ether spray.

I never saw the vice-president again. Contrary to my advice he went to Washington. I knew he would overwork himself there, but he never heeded any remonstrances against his excessive mental exertion.

That evening he went to Washington, first sending me word that he felt greatly relieved and that he would not work hard. He subsequently said to a friend that " after undergoing this treatment and recovering from the anæsthetics previously applied he felt stronger and better, and he thought he would at least be able to preside at the opening of the Senate, and perhaps through most of the session. He observed in this connection that he had a long struggle with intense agony in his spine before he yielded ; that he thought he had brought every power of endurance to bear ; that no one could ever imagine the suffering he had battled against, and he had yielded only when utterly exhausted ; that he was so entirely prostrated that he did not think it possible to revive. He said that at no time was he without a clear perception of what was going on ; that the only striking sensation he had, independent of his suffering, was that of excessive fatigue. He said that he had accounted for that in the exertion he was compelled to make to preserve the mastery of his will over his physical sufferings. He said that if this should yield he would lose his reason, as the agony he endured was beyond expression." [1]

The day after his arrival in Washington, Mr. Wilson, after overexertion both mental and physical, took a hot bath, and was soon afterward completely prostrated. The phenomena were not those of cerebral hæmorrhage or of general cerebral congestion. The chief symptoms were pain in the back of the neck, and syncope. He was attended by Dr. J. H. Baxter, of the army, who, recognizing the features of the case, administered whiskey by hypodermic injections. Under date of November 12th, he wrote me, " You would have been pleased to see the effect of the half drachm of whiskey administered under the skin. Reaction began within three minutes, pulse became strong, extremities warm, and surface circulation good."

[1] Special dispatch to the Boston Journal, dated Washington, November 23, 1875.

I had written to Dr. Baxter, giving him my views relative to Mr. Wilson's case and stating that I was glad to find that he had formed a like opinion. In the letter from which the foregoing quotation is made he says, —

"I am glad that you have the same opinion in regard to his trouble that I have, for I was correctly reported. The only point in which we may differ is this : that I am inclined to think that the spinal difficulty is reflex, and depending on irritation of digestive tube, although I am by no means ready to assert that there is not organic disease in that particular point in spinal marrow [the medulla oblongata] or membranes."

I think, taking into consideration the history of the case, the phenomena of the attack two weeks before his death, the circumstances of his death, and the report of the post-mortem examination, that unless there was a hæmorrhage into the medulla oblongata there was none anywhere else within the cranium. In regard to this latter point the published report of the post mortem affords no evidence one way or the other.

My opinion is that the immediate cause of the vice-president's death was the sudden cessation of the processes of respiration and circulation from paralysis of the pneumogastric nerves ; and that this paralysis was due to disease of the medulla oblongata affecting the nuclei of the pneumogastrics.

I do not suppose this disease to have been of long duration. Probably it began its development just before he came to see me the last time, November 7th. It is not, therefore, probable that the affection was of the nature of a slow inflammatory process, such as that causing glosso-labio-laryngeal paralysis. Moreover, the symptoms are not for a moment to be ascribed to any such disease.

But I think it probable that there was disease of the vertebral and basilar arteries, such for instance as was discovered in the anterior and middle cerebral, and the other arteries of the base of the brain. I am further of the opinion that the attack which the vice-president had two weeks before his death was due to a clot, probably a thrombus of one of the vertebral arteries, and that the attack which resulted in his death was produced by embolism, or more probably thrombosis, of either the other vertebral or the basilar.

The symptoms of each seizure are entirely reconcilable with this hypothesis, and they do not accord with the idea of the existence of any other intra-cranial disease not involving the medulla oblongata, and as we have seen there is no evidence going to show that there was any gross lesion of this organ.

We know that injury of the nuclei of the pneumogastrics is followed by instant death. Experimental physiology teaches us this, even if there were no other evidence ; and, as we have seen, hæmorrhage into the substance of the bulb may cause the immediate extinction of life.

But this is not all. The fact that closure of the basilar or vertebral arteries by a clot will cause sudden death is shown by several cases which have been reported, and by the anatomical and pathological studies of those who have devoted themselves to the elucidation of the subject.

Thus Martineau [1] reports a case which, though differing in several respects from that of the vice-president, presents, nevertheless, some analogous features.

A man, sixty-two years of age, died suddenly. Seven years before, he had suffered a sudden loss of speech, impossibility of walking, and vertigo without vomiting. These symptoms lasted an hour and then disappeared, and the patient entirely recovered. On the 6th of April, 1865, while in the midst of his work, he was seized with headache, embarrassment of articulation, and numbness of the left side of the body. On the morning of the 7th all these symptoms had disappeared. On the 10th there were vertigo and vomiting; on the 25th, sudden death. The post-mortem examination revealed the existence of a thrombus occupying both vertebral arteries at the point where they unite to form the basilar. The substance of the brain was healthy, but all the arteries of the base were in a state of atheromatous degeneration.

In this case the phenomena observed in the attacks which took place before that which caused death were probably due to the closure of the vertebrals, and the fatal result, to the obliteration of the basilar artery by the extension upwards of the clot.

The general similitude existing between this case and that of the vice-president causes us to regret that the vertebral arteries were not examined in the course of the post-mortem investigation into the cause of death.

Hayem [2] has called attention to thrombosis of the basilar artery as a cause of sudden death, and in citing Martineau's case gives an explanation of the rapidity with which it ran its course, similar to that above proposed.

Duret, who has so well studied the cerebral circulation, has also investigated with much thoroughness the arterial system of the medulla oblongata.[3] The pathological deductions which he draws therefrom are as follows : —

" (1.) When a clot is situated in one of the vertebral arteries it interrupts the circulation in the anterior spinal artery, and consequently in the median arteries which arise from it; that is to say, in the arteries

[1] Observation de Thrombose des deux Artères vertébrales. Bulletin de la Société medico-chirurgicale, 1865.

[2] Sur la Thrombose par Artérite du Tronc basilaire comme Cause de Mort rapide. Archives de Physiologie, 1868, page 270.

[3] Sur la Distribution des Artères nourricières du Bulbe rachidien. Archives de Physiologie, 1873, page 97.

which supply the nucleus of the spinal accessory, the hypoglossal and the inferior root of the facial. It therefore causes the development of the symptoms of glosso-labio laryngeal paralysis.

" (2.) When the clot occupies the inferior part of the basilar trunk, it cuts off the food from the sub-protuberantial branches which supply the nucleus of the pneumogastric, and sudden or at least rapid death is the consequence."

If, however, after careful examination, no clot was found in either the basilar or the vertebral arteries, the only other possible intra-cranial lesion which in my opinion could have caused the sudden non-convulsive death of the vice-president is the plugging of one or more of the minute vessels or capillaries of the nucleus of the pneumogastric, by a calcareous embolus derived from some one of the diseased arteries of the brain. It is possible that deposits of calcareous matter may have existed in the vertebral and basilar arteries, and that one or more of these might have become detached and have constituted the embolus.

The reasons for considering the fatal termination to be the result of a lesion of the medulla oblongata are not, however, limited to patho-anatomical conditions. The phenomena observed by me on the occasion of his last visit, the thickness of speech, difficulty of swallowing, twitching of the muscles of the face, irregularity of respiration and of the action of the heart, and intense pain in the back of the head, all point to trouble in this organ, and the peculiar manner of the death renders it almost certain that this was the part in which the essential lesion resided.

Whether or not, however, any one of the theories I have advanced be correct, it is quite evident that the vice-president did not die of apoplexy, and it is mainly to aid in restricting the use of this term within proper limits, that I have felt it right to bring the subject to the attention of the Neurological Society.

Since finishing the foregoing paper I have received from my friend, Dr. Baxter, the full report of the post-mortem examination. I had written to him stating my belief that Mr. Wilson did not die of apoplexy in the ordinary sense of that word, and that unless there was a lesion of the medulla oblongata death must have been due to h art-disease.

I subjoin the full report, prefacing it with Dr. Baxter's letter of transmission, which, though not intended for publication, is interesting inasmuch as it raises a new question for consideration : —

" DEAR DOCTOR, — I have delayed answering your letter that I might be able to give you the result of the microscopical examination of the spinal cord in Mr. Wilson's case. But as that will not be completed for two or three days, I send you the post-mortem examination, and will give you the microscopical result as soon as I can.

" There was no clot, and no discoverable cause of sudden death to be found in the brain.   The heart was all right.

" Could his death have been caused by reflex action of stomach through pneumogastric nerve? He drank a glass of the German bitter water which he usually took in the morning to move his bowels, lay back in bed and breathed stertorously about twelve times, and died.

" I think the condition found of his stomach warranted my diagnosis that his recent attack depended on irritation of that organ.   You may be sure there was not enough organic trouble about the heart to cause death.   Truly your friend,   J. H. Baxter.
"William A. Hammond, M. D., New York."

" Autopsy, November 22, 1875, on the body of Henry Wilson, Vice-President of the United States, about four hours after death.

" There was no rigor mortis and no other external appearance of note except a longitudinal livid patch upon the back of the neck.

" The dura mater was quite firmly adherent to the inner surface of the calvarium adjacent to the longitudinal sinus ; all of the sinuses were full of dark fluid blood ; the pia mater was congested and presented many small, old, whitish patches of lymph scattered along the surfaces adjoining the longitudinal sinus.

" The brain weighed forty-nine ounces, was normal in consistence, and its color normal except that the puncta vasculosa were less marked than usual, both in number and in vividness ; there was a transparent cyst about the size of a pea in the extremity of each choroid plexus ; the ventricular fluid was normal in character and quality.

" The subarachnoidal fluid was slightly increased in quantity.   The arteries at the base of the brain, more especially the middle cerebrals and basilar, together with their larger ramifications, were notably atheromatous, some of the calcareous plates being three or four lines in long diameter and so thick as nearly to obliterate the vessel.

" No thrombus or embolus was found, nor any extravasation of blood in the substance of the brain, pons Varolii, or medulla.

" The venous plexuses of the spinal canal contained a large quantity of dark fluid blood.

" The spinal cord, which was examined as low down as the third dorsal vertebra, appeared to be normal, except that the demarkation between the gray and the white substance was not well marked.   Portions of the brain and spinal cord were set aside for microscopical examination.

" The lungs were congested posteriorly ; there were old pleuritic adhesions on the left side, chiefly around the apex ; a calcareous deposit the size of a pea was found in the middle lobe of the right lung ; the lungs were otherwise normal.

" The heart presented a small calcareous deposit on one of the segments of the aortic valve, but was otherwise normal.

" The pericardial fluid was normal in quantity and color.

" The stomach was much congested, the mucous membrane everywhere of a deep red color and covered with mucus.

" There were many erosions of the mucous membrane, some superficial, others nearly perforating the membrane; some, the smaller ones, were rounded, the larger were irregular in outline; these latter were surrounded by dark areolæ of congestion.

" The liver was of a dark color, congested, and somewhat friable; there was a small aqueous cyst in its upper surface near the broad ligament. The gall-bladder was full of dark bile. The spleen was large and dark, but normal in structure. The kidneys weighed eight ounces each, and were congested; there were a few small subcapsular cysts and cicatrices, apparently of previous cysts.

" The bladder was contracted, its mucous membrane slightly reddened, and contained a small quantity of urine of normal color.

" The intestines appeared healthy. It perhaps ought to be stated that in view of the prospective embalming, only such examination was made as appeared to be absolutely necessary.

" The cause of death was considered to be nervous apoplexy, depending probably on cerebral anæmia."

Now the points to which I specially desire to call attention in connection with this report are the following : —

First. The fact that the arteries at the base of the brain, especially the middle cerebral and basilar, together with their larger ramifications, were notably atheromatous, some of the calcareous plates being three or four lines in long diameter, and so thick as nearly to obliterate the vessel. This statement is directly confirmatory of the theory I have advanced that some of the smaller vessels of the medulla oblongata might have been entirely closed by calcareous deposits.

Second. The fact that no thrombus or embolus was found, nor any extravasation of blood in the substance of the brain, pons Varolii, or medulla. It does not appear, however, that the vertebrals were examined.

Third. The condition of the stomach is, I think, the strongest point yet advanced in favor of a lesion of the medulla oblongata. I cannot, therefore, coincide with my friend Dr. Baxter in regarding it as the exciting cause of death, or of the attack of two weeks before.

Pincus, according to Schiff,[1] has seen congestions, black and irregular spots, and hæmorrhages produced in the mucous membrane of the stomach of rabbits by section of the sub-diaphragmatic branches of the pneumogastric nerves.

---

[1] Leçons sur la Physiologie de la Digestion, ii .433.

Vulpïan,[1] in speaking of the erosions, hæmorrhages, and other disorganizations of the gastric mucous membrane produced in animals by lesions of the crura cerebri, corpora striata, and optic thalami, calls attention to the fact that like changes are caused in the stomach of man by cerebral hæmorrhages, and says, —

" M. Charcot and I have observed these ecchymotic lesions in the stomach in cases of *ramollissement,* and even in cases of arterial ischæmia when *ramollissement* had not yet been produced. I have found them twenty-four hours after the obliteration of the middle cerebral artery. The patient had lost consciousness and had died without reviving. At the autopsy, although there was no cerebral softening, numerous ecchymotic spots were found in the stomach."

He then adds that even in the lower animals they may be caused by injury of other parts of the brain than the crura, the corpora striata, or the optic thalami, and that Schiff has observed them to follow lesions of the medulla oblongata, and of the spinal cord between the first and second vertebræ.

As to the hypothesis advanced by Dr. Baxter, while I do not think it tenable under the circumstances, there is no doubt that sudden death may be produced by reflex vaso-motor spasms starting from the stomach. To this category of circumstances belong the cases of sudden death ensuing from the ingestion of cold water into the stomach while the body is undergoing cooling after being greatly overheated. Guérard [2] has adduced several examples of the kind, and the fact is familiar to us all from instances which have occurred within our personal knowledge. Such cases are to be explained upon the theory that the influence is propagated to the medulla oblongata, and there acts by producing immediate anæmia of that small mass of gray matter which constitutes the nib of the calamus scriptorius, and the perfect integrity of which is essential to life. The functions of the pneumogastric nerves are at once arrested, and respiration and circulation instantaneously stopped.

This concludes what I have to say in regard to the very interesting questions suggested by the lamented death of the vice-president, though it is evident that the subject is by no means exhausted.

RECENT PROGRESS IN SURGERY.

BY J. COLLINS WARREN, M. D.

Antiseptic Surgery. — The demonstrations of Professor Lister to the members of the British Medical Association at the meeting at Edinburgh last summer, and the address of Mr. Spence delivered at the

[1] Leçons sur l'Appareil vaso-moteur. Paris, 1875, i. 451.
[2] Annales d'Hygiène, xxix. 1843.

same time, the former showing the brilliant effects of his method of treating wounds, and the latter giving equally satisfactory results with the simplest dressings, have given rise to renewed discussion as to the merits of the antiseptic treatment. Since attention was last called to this subject in the JOURNAL, the advocates of Lister's views have greatly enlarged their experience ; they have also gained many converts to the cause, and we have now, in addition to the testimony of British surgeons, that of many Continental surgeons, chiefly German, who have for the last year or two studiously carried out the minutest details of the system as laid down by its originator, and have recently given the fruit of their labors to the public.

Time also has shown some of its shortcomings, and as the literature of the day is teeming with testimony both for and against this mode of treatment, it is proposed to give a brief sketch of the discussion in its present stage.

The principle upon which the entire system is based is thus given in the words of Lister himself : " Putrefaction under atmospheric influence, as it occurs in surgical practice, is due to particles of dust ever present in the atmosphere that surrounds our patients, and endowed with wonderful chemical energy and power of self-propagation, yet happily readily deprived of energy by various agents which may be employed for the purpose without inflicting serious injury upon the human tissues." To deprive these particles of their energy has been the object of a complicated dressing, which, since its first adoption, has undergone various modifications. The latest of these, and the one now in use, is the antiseptic gauze dressing, " which contains in its fibres carbolic acid stored up in common resin, is to be applied in eight layers, with a sheet of some trustworthy impermeable tissue placed beneath the outermost layer to prevent the discharge from soaking directly through the dressing, for if it did so a copious effusion might wash out the antiseptic from the part immediately on the wound and putrefy within twenty-four hours. The most durable and therefore most reliable material for the purpose, consistent with the requisite lightness, is a fine cotton cloth with a thin layer of caoutchouc on one side, known in the shops as hat lining, or thinnest mackintosh." [1] Another change worthy of note in the system is the use of a large steam spray-producer during operations. The details of the method, both in conducting an operation and in applying the subsequent dressings, can be found in most recent editions of works on surgery. The very latest improvements, however, are to be found in an article by Lister in *The Lancet* for March 13, 1875 ; also in an able review of the whole subject in the *British and Foreign Medico-Chirurgical Review* for October, 1875.

Carbolic acid is still the favorite agent of Lister, although he has ex-

[1] Heath's Minor Surgery, fifth Edition.

perimented with a variety of other drugs. Chloride of zinc, which was
formerly used, in solution of a strength of forty grains to the ounce of
water, as an application to disinfect wounds already putrid, has been
found to cause sloughing if used incautiously, and has been abandoned.
Boracic or boric acid, a knowledge of which was obtained from Dr.
Stang, of Norway, has proved to be a valuable antiseptic agent. Lint
is dipped in a saturated solution of the acid at or near the boiling point,
and is allowed to dry, when the crystals are deposited in it. This makes
a soft and agreeable dressing, and one which will act antiseptically for
a considerable time. An account of the method of using this acid may
be found in the *Edinburgh Medical Journal* for September, 1874.

Salicylic acid is used exclusively by Professor Tiersch, in place of carbolic acid. His testimony, however, does not agree with that of Lister,
who finds it useful only when the dressing is to remain on a long time,
say a week, or of Mr. Callender, whose experiments with the drug are
alluded to in a recent number of the *Medical Press and Circular*. Mr.
Callender's treatment, it should be said, was not strictly antiseptic. He
says, —

"The acid was used in various ways, and the three following preparations were the ones chiefly employed : (*a.*) Phosphate of soda, three
parts ; salicylic acid, one part ; water, fifty parts. (*b.*) Salicylic acid, one
part ; olive oil, forty-nine parts. (*c.*) Salicylic acid, one part ; bicarbonate of soda, half a part ; water, one hundred parts. In addition to
these, however, it was occasionally used combined with borax, or in the
form of an ointment with prepared lard. I found that salicylic acid was
free from odor, and so far was acceptable to the patients ; that wounds
healed under its influence, and, during the progress of the repair, were
free from bad smells ; that, unless strong with spirit, or but little diluted,
it did not cause local pain. Its bad points seemed to be these : that,
above the strength of two per cent., it caused local irritation, with some
constitutional disturbance ; and, if the patient had a delicate skin, even
the weak preparation was a source of trouble ; that there was more discharge from a wound dressed with salicylic than there was where carbolic acid was used ; that its influence upon a recent wound, as after an
operation, was not so efficacious against the occurrence of decomposition as was that of carbolic acid, chloride of zinc, or of boracic acid ;
that the repair of a wound was less active, and the granulations, if any,
were more flabby than when other simple or antiseptic dressings were
employed."

In glancing over British surgical literature we find that testimony in
favor of Lister's views is not wanting in that country. Joseph Bell
says of it, "I trust, however, that the cases I have mentioned will
prove to the society that we are warranted in believing that in the antiseptic principle, explain it as you will, and simplify it as I hope you

may, we have a very great addition to our means of combating disease. Even if on theoretical grounds surgeons may deny the possibility of preventing suppuration, and ignore our facts, still if it be granted that by this method we can diminish the amount and destroy the fœtor of pus, we have done much to improve the sanitary condition and diminish the fatality of our great hospitals." Among the advocates of this system the names of McDonnell, Annandale, and Cummings may be mentioned.

On the other hand, Mr. Spence, whose patients were treated in the same hospital in which Lister has employed his system, is able to show a record of sixty-five cases of major amputation with only three deaths, or about 4.5 per cent., and twenty-three cases of excision of the joints with only two deaths, or about 8.7 per cent. " The treatment consisted in thoroughly cleansing the cut surface by pouring tepid water over it, and occasionally applying tincture of iodine, alone or diluted, upon the flaps, whilst the dressing consisted merely in laying a veil of lint or thin muslin over the stumps."

This and like testimony caused many surgeons who were, we might say, fascinated by Lister's demonstrations at Edinburgh, to hesitate, nevertheless, in accepting fully his views. *The Lancet* attributes the favorable results of both parties to the increased attention given of late years to hospital hygiene, while it accounts for the enthusiasm of Continental hospital surgeons in the following way: " No one acquainted with the filthy and neglected condition of many of the Continental hospitals fifteen or twenty years ago, and even more recently than that, will be at a loss to understand why the mortality in these hospitals has so greatly diminished since the introduction of antiseptic surgery. Even the moderate use of clean water and the observance of the ordinary habits of personal cleanliness would have sufficed to reduce very considerably the frightful mortality in them."

Although there is doubtless some truth in these remarks, which are applicable in a limited degree to even some of the best German surgeons, the standing of Volkmann and Tiersch is so high, and their work so characteristic of German fidelity and accuracy, that their reports cannot fail to prove valuable contributions to the literature of this subject. Volkmann, whose Contributions to Surgery [1] has lately appeared, devotes a leading chapter in that handsome volume to an account of a two years' trial of the antiseptic method in the clinic at Halle. Although during this period an unusually large series of unfavorable cases presented themselves, he states, " It is my conviction that Lister's method opens the way to the solution of one of the most important problems with which surgery has to deal; to give to open wounds the protection and advantages which subcutaneous injuries possess. This

---

[1] Volkmann, Beiträge zur Chirurgie. Leipzig, 1875.

protection is not absolute ; no one can deny, however, that it is excessively great." He thinks that if this treatment is carried out accurately, the secretions of wounds are absolutely without odor, even if parts of considerable size become gangrenous. Decomposition of blood-clots is not only prevented, but not unfrequently the clot becomes organized in the open wound under the very eyes, so to speak, of the surgeon. A clot projecting from an open wound may remain dark red for a week, during which time granulations grow into it and destroy it; or it may shrink after a while, and drop off like a scab. Such clots he has watched for six weeks without signs of suppuration showing themselves.

This effect upon blood-clots has not been noticed by Volkmann alone. It is one of the characteristic results of the method, which has been verified by numerous observers. Lister has pointed out that blood-clots filling an open wound will remain in situ, organize, and after a sufficient length of time will bleed if incised. Mr. Chiene reports a case to the Medico-Chirurgical Society of Edinburgh, in which he took advantage of this circumstance, and allowed an open wound on the heel to fill with coagulum, which on the sixteenth day bled when scratched, and retained its characteristic red color until on the thirtieth day epidermis began to form over it, and it healed in a few days.

Volkmann notices the absence of all local reaction in the edges of the wound. First intention becomes the rule in those cases where it was formerly the exception. The dressing greatly diminishes pain in wounds. He thinks that under circumstances when we should expect high fever, we find little or none with this treatment. At the time of his writing, eighteen months had passed without a single case of pyæmia, and erysipelas had been almost unknown. Disturbance in the healing process, which in former times was the rule, has now become with him the exception.

He describes in detail the method. Among the objections is, first, its complicated character, which prevents application with any certainty of success in some portions of the body. The action of the acid upon the hands of the operator, as also upon his instruments, if used as freely as it should be, is considered a decided objection. Moreover, carbolic poisoning is to be feared. Volkmann thinks this risk is greater than is generally supposed, and he is quite sure that in one case the death of the patient was due to the poisonous action of the drug. When he first began to use this method many cases of collapse and vomiting were noticed, due to the use of the acid, and dark-colored urine was of frequent occurrence. Small children do not bear well the external application of the carbolic dressing. The cost of the dressing seems to be very great ; Volkmann spent four thousand thalers in the year 1873 for the materials of which the dressing is composed, while an estimate made of the expense of Lister's dressings in 1874 came to six hundred pounds.

We come now to the investigations of Professor Tiersch.[1] He accepts the theory that atmospheric ferments are the cause of septicæmia, pyæmia, and hospital grangrene. Erysipelas, however, he does not think is produced by bacteria, which are to be looked upon as merely accidental accompaniments of the disease. He has tried carbolic acid with his antiseptic dressings thoroughly, but much prefers salicylic acid, which he now uses exclusively. The latter is neither volatile nor irritating, and it possesses no disagreeable odor. Its chief advantage, however, appears to be that it exercises no injurious influence upon fresh and granulating wounds if brought into direct contact with them, and has no poisonous action if absorbed into the circulation, although it may sometimes produce an olive-green coloring of the urine. At the temperature of the room three hundred parts of water take up one part of the acid; to this mixture the name salicylic water is given. This is sufficiently antiseptic to prevent decomposition, and does not irritate the part to which it is applied. The other form of dressing is called salicylic cotton. This is used of two strengths, a three per cent. and a ten per cent., the latter being colored with carmine in order to prevent mistakes. It is prepared in the following way : —

Three per cent. salicylic cotton : 750 grammes of salicylic acid are dissolved in 7500 grammes of alcohol of 0.830 sp. gr., diluted with 150 litres of water from 70° to 80° C., in which 25 kilogrammes of cotton batting, which has been freed from fatty matters, are soaked. The batting, being soaked in the solution, is then allowed to dry in a moderately warm room for twelve hours, when, evaporation taking place, the crystals are deposited in the cotton. Tiersch uses also a jute dressing prepared by three or four per cent. saturation, with the addition of twenty per cent. of glycerine to prevent the acid being given off too freely in the form of dust.

The salicylic water prevents the appearance of bacteria in the wound. The cotton dressing has remained on fourteen days without their appearance. The jute dressing is most suitable for suppurating wounds in consequence of its being able readily to absorb fluids, in which process the cotton is comparatively deficient. In operating, Tiersch takes all the precautions insisted upon by Lister. He employs the spray and carbolized catgut ligatures. He bears testimony to the absence of fever and the prevalence of first intention.

Finally we find a comparison between the open and the antiseptic treatment of wounds, by Dr. R. U. Krönlein,[2] compiled from cases occurring in the clinics of Zurich, Leipzig, and Halle. The results of amputations treated by the open method were found to be better than those of amputations treated by the antiseptic. The open method was

---

[1] Volkmann's Sammlung klinische Vorträge, 84 and 85.
[2] Archiv für klinische Chirurgie, xix. part 1.

also more favorable in compound fractures and in operations for the removal of the breast. Both methods, he thinks, reduce greatly the number of cases of pyæmia and septicæmia, but do not prevent the occurrence of erysipelas. The time which wounds take to heal is much shorter under antiseptic dressings than when left open. The writer complains of the expense of the antiseptic dressing and of the danger of poisoning by carbolic acid. He is unable to give preference to either mode of dressing.

In summing up the objections to the antiseptic dressing, the writer in the *Chirurgical Review* says that it is troublesome, and requires to be watched, and that the requisite minutiæ are tedious. The surgeon himself must therefore do it, and not leave it to an assistant. He is rather disposed to believe, however, that it is one of the chief advantages of the system that it demands a very special individual watchfulness over each patient if it is to succeed. "But alas," he says, "not only must the patient be watched, but the most unremitting attention must be paid to every action during the period the wound is exposed to view. Is a friendly surgeon going round your ward? A touch of his finger, if unprotected by washing in carbolic acid, may ruin the case. Does an instrument fall to the ground or even lie for a second on the table? To introduce it into the wound again unless dipped, is theoretically destructive to your hopes. Is it a warm day, and are you liable to sweat? A drop falling into the wound or on the dressing will be fatal to its success. Such being the case, it is not wonderful that in the practice of many who honestly aim at following out antiseptic treatment, and believe they succeed, the results have not always been equal to expectation. . . . The surgeon cannot be expected to lug about with him a steam engine which requires twenty minutes to get up its steam, or an assistant to work a hand-spray every time he wants to dress an abscess or an ulcer. . . . Cases there are, however, which even in the purest air, and under the most wholesome conditions, will be treated more safely, rapidly, and fortunately by the adoption, in all its strictness, of the antisep ic treatment."

(To be concluded.)

GREENHOW ON ADDISON'S DISEASE.[1]

This very complete and interesting monograph consists of three lectures delivered before the Royal College of Physicians of London, and carefully revised for publication. In the first lecture, after a short biographical notice of Dr. Addison, the author presents a clinical description of Addison's dis-

[1] *On Addison's Disease: being the Croonian Lectures for* 1875, *delivered before the Royal College of Physicians; revised, and illustrated by Plates and Reports of Cases.* By EDWARD HEADLAM GREENHOW, M. D., F. R. S., etc. Philadelphia: Lindsay and Blakiston. 1875.

case, with an account of the pathological lesion which is found in the supra-
renal capsules. In the second lecture Dr. Greenhow refers to the fact that
Addison's discovery has been neither generally accepted nor generally understood, and offers an explanation of the misconceptions which have prevailed in
regard to the nature of the symptoms and lesions in numerous cases in which
these have differed from the typical ones. In the third lecture the author's
views as to the true pathology of Addison's disease are given, together with
what is known of its etiology and of its treatment.

Not long after the publication of Dr. Addison's work On the Constitutional
and Local Effects of Disease of the Supra-Renal Capsules, in 1855, cases
were reported by various observers of more or less extensive disease of the
capsules which were not accompanied by the peculiar symptoms described by
the author, and also other cases in which the symptoms were noticed without
any lesions of the capsules being found after death. Hence arose a good deal
of skepticism as to any necessary relationship between disease of the capsules
and the symptoms described by Addison. Dr. Greenhow undertakes to reconcile these apparent contradictions. He states, in the first place, that there is
but one characteristic lesion of the supra-renal capsules which is invariably
found associated with the peculiar asthenia and discoloration of the skin constituting Addison's disease, which may be briefly described as follows : the capsules are usually enlarged, hard, and nodulated ; the cut surfaces present a
mixture of a gray or greenish semi-transparent tissue, with a more or less
friable substance of an opaque, yellow color, in roundish masses, imbedded in
it, often softening down into a thick, creamy fluid. The proportions of these
two substances vary, according to the more or less chronic course of the disease. Moreover, there is always found evidence of inflammation of the cellular envelope of the capsules in the form of great proliferation of their connective tissue and firm adhesions to the neighboring organs. An extensive
outgrowth of dense connective tissue has also been found to invest the nerves
of the supra-renal and solar plexuses, with hypertrophy of their fibrous investment, in the cases in which these nerves have been thoroughly examined. Dr.
Greenhow claims that in every reported case of disease of the capsules without the symptoms of Addison's disease, which he has seen, the appearances
found were quite different from the above ; neither cancer, amyloid disease,
fatty degeneration, apoplexy, nor tumor of the capsules will produce Addison's
disease ; and where such lesions were said to be found in connection with
bronzed skin and other symptoms described by Dr. Addison, it is shown that
the morbid appearances were really those which are associated with Addison's
disease only, and not with cancer, etc. As to the alleged cases of " bronzed skin "
occurring without disease of the supra-renal bodies, they are clearly instances
of pityriasis versicolor, syphilis, jaundice, the effect of long exposure to the
sun, or other well-known appearances. and quite different from the discoloration peculiar to Addison's disease.

It is evident that the symptoms of Addison's disease are not due to the destruction of the normal tissue of the supra-renal bodies (although such was the
opinion of Addison himself when he published his work), as is shown by several cases in which these organs were supplanted by cancer, or had undergone

complete fatty degeneration, without the production of any such symptoms. On the other hand, " in many cases of Addison's disease the conversion of the supra-renal capsules into a mass of fibroid tissue, and even the degeneration of this latter into cheesy material, must have been almost if not altogether complete before the development of any of the characteristic symptoms of the disease." The true pathology of the disease, according to Dr. Greenhow, probably consists in the extension of the chronic inflammatory process from the diseased capsules to the surrounding parts, especially the numerous nerve trunks which these organs receive from the supra-renal and solar plexuses, and semilunar ganglia; sometimes these ganglia themselves are involved. It is " either as direct effects of the nerve-lesions upon certain organs, or as secondary consequences of those lesions, through the medium of their interference with the circulation," that the individual constitutional symptoms of Addison's disease seem in great part explicable. We have no space to quote the details of this hypothesis, and the answers which Dr. Greenhow offers to the objections which might be urged against it. If not wholly convincing, it is ingenious and probable, which is more than can be said of any other theory to account for the phenomena of this extraordinary disease.

Dr. Greenhow relates all that is known of the etiology of Addison's disease. It seems to have some affinity with tubercle or struma, without being of a distinctly tubercular nature. In a certain proportion of cases the inflammation has extended to the supra-renal capsules from disease or injury of the neighboring parts, especially abscess from diseased bone. In a small number of cases the disease was apparently owing to traumatic causes, or to some physical shock, strain, or blow; or to over-exertion, nervous shock, grief, great anxiety, etc.; but in a majority of cases there is no clew to the origin of the disease. A majority of the patients are males in the most active period of adult life.

The subjects of the diagnosis, prognosis, and treatment occupy the last three or four pages of the work, which, we promise the reader, will far better repay his perusal than this brief and imperfect summary of its contents would lead him to suppose. Two indexes complete the book, one containing a selection of illustrative cases, the other including the whole number of cases the author has been able to collect from all sources, methodically arranged, and containing brief references to important points. There are several colored illustrations and drawings of microscopical appearances, which are all beautifully executed.

ZIEMSSEN'S CYCLOPÆDIA.[1]

ANOTHER volume of this great work has appeared, and is equal in merit to its predecessors. The first part of the subject is treated of in the fourth volume, which is to follow the present one, so that we find ourselves on opening this one at once *in mediis rebus.* Pneumonia in its various forms is exhaustively treated by Juergensen. Hertz discusses a number of miscellaneous

[1] *Cyclopædia of the Practice of Medicine.* Edited by Dr. H. von Ziemssen. Volume V. Diseases of the Respiratory Organs. New York: Wm. Wood & Co. 1875.

pulmonary affections, as atrophy, hypertrophy, emphysema, gangrene, new growths, and parasites. Pulmonary consumption and acute miliary tuberculosis are treated of by Ruehle, and chronic and acute tuberculosis by Rindfleisch. As we have already implied, all parts of the volume are of merit, but we choose for more special notice the province of the two last named authors, on account of the various opinions that have been held on the relations of tubercle and phthisis. Rindfleisch's paper is chiefly theoretical and scientific; Ruehle's is both a scientific and a practical treatise on his large subject. Rindfleisch would greatly enlarge the domain of tubercle; in which Ruehle agrees to a certain extent. He writes as follows: " Boyle's miliary tubercle plays, however, only a subordinate rôle in pulmonary consumption; it is an accidental secondary product. When it forms the only anatomical lesion, we have to deal with an acute infectious disease, the acute miliary tuberculosis, which does not belong to phthisis. There is probably no chronic miliary tuberculosis in the old sense of the term. Phthisis is also anatomically a chronic inflammatory disease, with intercurrent simple forms of inflammation which heal by cicatrization. But the pernicious form of phthisis is a specific variety of inflammation with the characteristic caseous metamorphosis; this inflammation is localized in different parts of the tissues, is characterized by the fact that it begins with and also produces the true histological miliary tubercle of the smallest kind, and in itself undergoes no other metamorphosis except necrosis. Its limitation and local healing are effected by a simple inflammation in the surrounding parts." Felix von Niemeyer has excluded tuberculosis from the lungs except in the miliary form, and though his views cannot be said to have been proved, they have been very generally accepted. Rindfleisch, once a follower of Niemeyer, now maintains very different views. According to him, tubercle arises solely, or very nearly solely, from scrofula. As to what scrofula may be, we regret to say we know no more than before reading the book. We know, however, that it is characterized by long-enduring subacute inflammations, and the author tells us that the products of these inflammations are redeposited as tubercles; thus in pulmonary phthisis " there is first scrofula and then a cachexia from the absorption of scrofulous deposits." The lymphatics of course must play an important part, and in certain cases the swollen glands may mark the course of the disease. They acquire a great significance if Rindfleisch is right in agreeing with Schüppel that so-called scrofulous glands are always tubercular. In accordance with this view he supports the practice of extirpating such glands when possible, in order to nip the disease in the bud. By primary tuberculosis the author designates local inflammations that may be either scrofulous and tubercular or the former only; by secondary tuberculosis, the affection of the lymphatic glands; and by tertiary tuberculosis, the general attack. In spite of this nomenclature he admits that the disease in many — we are inclined to think in most — cases does not acquire a specific character till it reaches his second stage. As to the microscopic anatomy of tubercle, there are many forms that it would carry us too far to discuss, so we will merely mention that the author believes that miliary tubercles come from the fixed cells of the vascular connective-tissue system. Pulmonary phthisis, according to Rindfleisch, usually comes from a bronchial catarrh accompanied by the appearance of tubercles in the acini belonging to some small, inflamed bronchi. We say " accompanied," for he is precise in his statement that he has " never seen a circumscribed catarrh of the small bronchi without an initial tubercle granulum, nor an initial tubercle granulum without some catarrh," but he believes the latter to have been the primary affection. Moreover, unless the patient be scrofulous, there is little danger of subsequent tubercle, but if he be, the morbid secretion is inoculated at favorable points in the mucous membrane of the respiratory tract, among which the corners and edges at the terminations of the smallest bronchi are the most exposed. It may be questioned whether Rindfleisch's theory can be held to be better proved than that which it supersedes ; so much latitude must be allowed to difference of interpretation that it is difficult to speak decidedly on the subject, but if these views be accepted, we shall not feel that we are traveling in a circle owing to their resemblance to former ones. We may look at the subject from the same direction as before, but, we think, from a nearer point, in other words, that we are slowly approaching the centre. All the praise that has been given to the translation and publishing of former volumes may be repeated for this one.

THE SANITARY CONDITION OF BOSTON.

THE death-rate of Boston in 1872 and 1873 was so high as to occasion considerable popular alarm. Men began to inquire concerning the causes of this unusual mortality and to blame now one thing and now another for it ; bad sewerage, mal-administration of health affairs, the need of a public park, served in turn as plausible explanations of the reproach. At length, it was thought that something more substantial than gratuitous speculations might be had, on which to base a reasonable decision as to the hygienic condition and prospects of Boston. Accordingly, at the request of Mayor Cobb, the entire subject was submitted by the Board of Health to a commission of medical men for investigation. This commission comprised the following physicians : Dr. Charles E. Buckingham (chairman), Dr. Calvin Ellis, Dr. Richard M. Hodges, Dr. Samuel A. Green, and Dr. Thomas B. Curtis (secretary). It is unnecessary to add that the investigation could not have been intrusted to five better representatives of the medical profession in Boston.

The report of this committee is before us in the form of a well-printed pamphlet of nearly two hundred pages. It is worthy of comment that this was the first time since registration had existed in Boston when a body of physicians was officially called upon to turn to account the vast amount of statistical material collected and published year after year by the city registrar, in order that the facts therein contained might receive their proper interpretation, and that the sanitary lessons which they suggested might be shown forth for the practical benefit of the community. The report has been awaited with uncommon interest by those who had the hygienic welfare of our people at heart, and it is to be remarked that the importance of the subject treated, as well as the manner of its treatment, constitutes this pamphlet a most significant and valuable document.

The preface to the report consists of a note, signed by the four senior members of the committee, giving the credit of the work to the secretary, Dr. T. B. Curtis. "The most that we can claim," they say, " is that we have carefully reviewed and approved it." This incident is as graceful as it is rare; it reflects worthily in a double sense. It is great honor to Dr. Curtis to have prepared such a composition ; it is scarcely less honorable on the part of his colleagues that they publicly disclaim any title to special commendation. Very few beside those who have entered the labyrinthine intricacies of vital statistics can appreciate the amount of difficult mental work involved in an investigation like that whose results are here presented. The ordinary reader glances at the printed tables and at the comments which accompany them, accepts or doubts or rejects, and passes on with the smallest notion of the bewildering, brain-tormenting labor requisite for the task of preparing the one or of expressing the other so as to withstand criticism as to its absolute reliability. It gives us pleasure, therefore, to express our emphatic appreciation of the committee's action in according to Dr. Curtis the authorship of a paper representing in its matter and in its method an unusual amount of studious application and of patient, painstaking, laborious research.

The report is introduced with some preliminary remarks upon the general subject of mortality statistics, their value as a measure of public health, the fallacies to which they are exposed, and the shortcomings of the prevailing methods of registration. The opinion is expressed that, notwithstanding recent views to the contrary, the general death-rate of a community is a satisfactory indication of its sanitary condition. But the death-rate should be distinguished in this respect from the mean age at death, a wholly unreliable sign of relative salubrity. The subject of the comparative mortality of the various nationalities of which the American population is made up is touched upon, and its difficulties are described with great clearness ; the principal obstacle to such a study is the want of adequate data relating to the nativity and parentage of decedents, and the urgent need of supplying this want in census reports and in registration is dwelt upon.

The results of the investigation into the mortality of Boston are presented as answers to the four following questions : —

I. Is the present mortality of the city of Boston excessive ; and, if so, to what extent ?

II. In what portion of our community, as regards age and nationality, does the excess of mortality exist ?

III. What is the nature, and what are the causes, of the diseases which occasion our excess of death ? To what extent, and by what means, are these diseases preventable ?

IV. What measures of sanitation are recommended ?

To the first question the answer is unequivocally in the negative : we are assured that Boston is not among the most unhealthy cities of the world, as has so often been alleged in recent years. The mean death-rate for a long period is shown to be 24.5, a rate scarcely in excess of that of London, with which it is frequently compared disparagingly. Moreover, our city is not growing year by year more unhealthy, as has been thought to be the case ;

her successive decennial mean death-rates maintain a remarkable uniformity. The high rates of 1872 and 1873 (30.4 and 28.5) are demonstrated to have been due to the temporary action of transient causes, namely, the coincident prevalence of small-pox, scarlatina, and cerebro-spinal meningitis; if the deaths caused by these intermittent factors of mortality were subtracted from the total number of deaths, the rate would have been very nearly that already quoted as the average for a long series of years. Or, again, if the excess of the death-rate by zymotic diseases during 1872 and 1873 were subtracted from the general death-rate for those years, the result would be similar.

But while the fact is made plain that our death-rate compares very favorably with urban rates at home and abroad, it is insisted that we ought not to rest satisfied. Our mortality from zymotic affections, which represent preventable causes of disease and death, is much too great, and calls for active and vigilant sanitary administration. Our mean death-rate is too high if it exceeds that of the country at large, or if it exceeds the normal death-rate of our city as calculated from the life-table of the United States.

The second chapter, in which is discussed the question, In what portion of our community, as regards age and nationality, does the excess of mortality exist? is an exceedingly interesting one, containing a great amount of statistical research and reasoning. The first fact demonstrated is the very great mortality which prevails in Boston among children under five years of age. It is shown that if our mortality among infants and children were as low as that obtaining in London, or even as that of the life-table of the United States, our general death-rate would be reduced from 24.5 to less than 21. To one of the methods adopted for showing our excessive infantile death-rate, that known as the *dime mortuaire*, or ratio between deaths under one year and registered births, there seems to us to be some objection, on the ground that our registration of births is not what it ought to be, since it is based on an annual canvass of the city, and therefore cannot be complete. Nevertheless, the fact that Boston suffers a disproportionate yearly loss of children is abundantly proved otherwise. During the five years 1870–74, over a quarter of all the deaths in Boston were those of children under one year of age.

In the consideration of the influence of nationality on our mortality-rate, some very suggestive results appear. It is demonstrated that the Irish swell the mortality list of the country out of all proportion to their numbers, far exceeding in this respect all the other nationalities which go to make up our heterogeneous American population. The method adopted by Dr. Curtis to make this point clear differs somewhat from that of General Walker, the superintendent of the last census, in his demonstration of the same fact. General Walker simply instituted a comparison between the different nationalities on the basis of their respective mortality-rates, general and special; Dr. Curtis makes a comparison between the population-rate and the mortality-rate of each nationality, and argues that the measure of liability to disease on the part of any nationality is found in the excess of its mortality-rate over its percentage to the whole number of foreigners. Thus, the Irish comprise 33.3 per cent. of all the foreigners in the United States, while their quota of the deaths among foreigners is 41 per cent., an excess of nearly 8 per cent.; but the Germans, who are 30.2 per cent. of tie foreign population contribute only 28.2 per cent. of the foreign decedents, no excess of comparative liability to disease and deati, but tie reverse. Tie latter metiod of comparison seems to us tie more exact and reliable. Another significant fact is tiat the Irisi mortality is due to tie "filth" diseases (of whici diarrhœa is tie type), inherited and constitutional affections (consumption, cancer), and especially Brigit's disease. A most marked contrast exists between the Irish and the Germans witi regard to liability to tie last disorder, instantly suggesting the reflection that tiere is also a wide difference between lager bier and corn whisky.

Now, in Boston tie Irish comprise two tiirds of the foreign population, and nearly a quarter of the entire people; of all the large American cities ours is the most freely supplied with tiis exotic element. Are we to be congratulated thereupon? Most certainly not, from tie sanitary point of view, if the convincing facts presented in this report are to guide our opinions. In whatever other way the Irish affect our community, their influence on our death-rate is not salutary. Tiey add enormously to the infant population, but they add enormously to the mortality list also; they obey the command to multiply and to people tie earth, they disregard tie equally authoritative behest, "wash and be clean," in all its compreiensive meanings. The work before us tells us plainly that when comparisons are made between tie death-rate of Boston and that of other cities tiis item should not be forgotten; that there is a wide distinction between localities in tiemselves unwholesome and localities inhabited by unhealtiy people; that we iave among us more than our share of a nationality wiose habits, surroundings, and hereditary tendencies promote excessive liability to physical decay and death. One bit of encouragement, iowever, is afforded by a foot-note in the report wiich declares that "the proportion of Irish in Boston is shown by the census to be steadily declining."

The tiird ciapter considers the nature, the causes, and tie prevention of tie diseases wiich occasion excessive mortality, or, in other words, mortality in excess of the normal deati-rate of the city. We are told at the outset that the deaths from diarrhœal diseases alone nearly represent tiis excess; wiile the zymotics iave together caused in tie last ten years over a quarter of all the mortality. Consumption and acute pulmonary affections are included in the category of diseases which are controllable in greater or less degree by sanitary measures. The subject of infant mortality and its causes is deemed worthy of special consideration. The entire chapter is a compreiensive exposition of practical hygiene, touciing tiose causes of death which sanitarians regard as preventable. The various diseases are studied separately, in their relation to public iealth and to tie measures which experience has shown to be best for their prevention. Tiis portion of the work is replete witi wise counsel and useful information, the fruit of very extended researci. Our space will not permit more than this summary mention of an exceedingly interesting section. We desire, however, to quote in full one sentence witi our unqualified approval; at tie end of tie study concerning tie ætiology of typioid fever is tie following: "Our final conclusion on tiis subject is tiat no measures of sanitary improvement are more strenuously needed, or are more likely to repay the cost, however great it may be, than the construction of a system of sewers adapted to our present and future needs."

The closing chapter is the one which we specially commend to the attention of our city authorities; it considers the practical measures requisite to promote our hygienic welfare more fully, and to make our city more healthy. And first, with regard to registration as affording invaluable data for sanitary work, it is insisted that our mortuary statistics and the method of recording them are open to grave criticism, that physicians are permitted to be too careless in their certificates of death, that the nomenclature of diseases should be revised, that the city registrar should be a medical man specially fitted by virtue of his education to deal with sanitary questions, and that the registration reports should be more full and better adapted to the requirements of public hygiene. In this connection we miss one suggestion which we believe to be important, namely, that the office of registrar should be in immediate connection with the local board of health or subordinate to it; the present independent relations of the position are anomalous and objectionable.

With regard to sanitation, very sensible counsel is given concerning the management of the eruptive fevers and the prevention of filth-infection, the latter being rightly emphasized as " the greatest and most urgent sanitary need of Boston." In connection with the matter of drainage and sewerage tie report recommends that " our sanitary authorities be permanently invested with complete jurisdiction over sewage from its first starting-points within our homes, as well as throughout the entire extent of its ulterior transit; and tiat they have full powers in all cases to inspect and supervise, when needful, the construction and the operation of the internal drainage arrangements of dwelling-houses." The matter of water-supply also receives attention, and a caution made by the State Board of Health is repeated, that every possible measure should be taken to prevent the pollution of Lake Cochituate by sewage.

We have dwelt somewhat at length upon this report because of the intrinsic importance of the subject, and because of the unexceptionable manner in which it has been presented by Dr. Curtis under the approval of the entire committee. The work was designed to promote the hygienic welfare of Boston, and will undoubtedly receive unusual attention, and, as we hope, be followed by satisfactory fruits, in this community; but our more distant readers may be assured that they will find here excellent matter for their study. Especially is the publication a very useful one for health authorities everywhere, since it abounds in information and suggestions of the most sterling quality pertaining to public hygiene.

MEDICAL NOTES.

— We have to record the death of a member of the Massachusetts Medical Society who, although he was an active practitioner but for a limited portion of his life, will nevertheless be missed by a large circle of professional friends. Many of his companions whose names are well known to all of us have gone before him, but few have left behind them so pleasing a memory of the well-bred gentleman and genial friend as Dr. Charles Mifflin.

Dr. Mifflin died at his residence in this city on Thursday last. Born in Philadelphia in 1805, he was reared in a school of medicine justly celebrated for the talent of its teachers, tie University of Pennsylvania. Remaining for some time after graduating in iis native city, iis services were soon called into requisition by tie approach of cholera, during which epidemic ie saw much active service. Later, he made a voyage to Russia as surgeon to a government vessel. Since his marriage ie ias resided in Boston, and altiough a natural reserve and diffidence prompted him to refrain from tie practice of his profession among strangers and with new professional colleagues, circumstances placed this wisi beyond iis control, and for a long series of years the summer residents of Naiant enjoyed tie privilege of his professional care. Indeed, he may he said to iave been tie pioneer in a custom wiici is rapidly becoming more and more general among Boston physicians. Iis cieerful, genial manners made him always welcome, wiether ie came as friend or piysician. His name is well known to tie country from its connection witi Revolutionary deeds. His quiet life, unselfisi disposition, and warm ieart will long be remembered by many a friend wio mourns his loss.

— The employment of bromide of potassium in cases of epistaxis, uterine hæmorrhage, and coryza is recommended by Dr. Geneuil in *L' Union Médicale* of November 4, 1875. He reports tie case of a man in whom violent epistaxis had continued for six iours uncontrolled by styptics, wien finally a saturated solution containing six grammes of tie bromide of potassium was injected into tie nose by means of a glass syringe; tie hæmorriage was promptly arrested. Anotier case of a woman afflicted in tie same way was speedily relieved by an injection of the same remedy twice. It is recommended tiat the bromide should also be given internally to prevent a recurrence of the hæmorrhage. Tie power of promptly arresting the epistaxis is not due to tie coldness of tie solution of tie salt, but to the contraction brougit about in the blood-vessels, and the consequent diminution of tie flow of blood to the head. In cases of epistaxis, if tie first injection should fail to accomplisi its purpose, three or four injections may be given in succession. For uterine hæmorrhages of moderate intensity bromide of potassium given internally, and associated with tie *pulvis ferri* in cases of anæmia, is recommended. Tie writer in iis own person tested the value of the bromide in coryza. Two injections of a saturated solution given with ialf an hour's interval brought rapid relief, and six iours later effected a permanent cure. Tie application is rather painful for a little time, but a sensation of relief soon follows.

— A paper on oral organisms, by J. H. M'Quillen, M. D., D. D. S., is published in tie *Dental Cosmos* of November, 1875. The prominent part assigned by some observers to oral parasites in the production of decay of tie teeti, and tie equally emphatic denial by others that they have anytiing to do in tie matter, makes the investigation of tieir nature and action of much importance. In tie mouth of man several species of organisms or parasites find a iabitat. The writer tiinks some of tiem are animal, and tie vegetal ciaracter of otiers is beyond dispute. Witi tie exception of tie *protococcus dentalis*, or green fungus, — whici seems to be very destructive to tie teeti of ciildren, — Dr. M'Quillen has failed to observe anytiing in these organisms wiich he could regard as conclusive evidence that tiey exert a destructive influence on tie teeth. They are found in great numbers in the moutis of those wiose teeth are perfectly sound. Examination with instruments of high magnifying powers has failed to find in the human mouth those animal organisms which are described by some authorities as being armed with formidable apparatus for boring into the enamel and dentine, and as being thus enabled to destroy the structure of the teeth. Probably the destruction effected by the various borers in stone and wood has led to the belief that there were similar organisms found in the mouth, which destroyed the teeth; but with the exception of a writer who presented a paper to the French Institute many years ago, and another who published some observations a short time subsequently in this country, both of whom maintained that they had seen the apparatus referred to, no microscopist of any prominence has been able to find these parasites. It is therefore reasonable to infer that these writers have drawn upon their imaginations for their facts.

— A paper on rectified spirit (spiritus frumenti rectificatus) by A. W. Miller, M. D., Ph. D., is published in the *American Journal of Pharmacy* for November, 1875. The writer thinks that pure rectified spirit possesses merits and advantages which heretofore have not been properly appreciated by physieiaus. " French spirit," " sweet liquor," and " rectified spirits " are terms used by the liquor trade to designate pure rectified whisky freed from fusel-oils, coloring matter, and other impurities. It is obtained by percolating the ordinary raw corn whisky through fresh charcoal. It usually contains fifty per cent. of absolute alcohol by volume. It is the basis used by the compounders of fancy liquors for their cordials, etc. All the various fusel-oils in a concentrated form have peculiarly penetrating and oppressive odors, but it is on these in various proportions and admixture that the distinctive flavor of different liquors depends. It is by no means certain that the medicinal virtue of spirit is enhanced in the smallest degree by the costly flavors which characterize the choicest cognac, Jamaica rum, or Bourbon. In the plain, rectified spirit, however, we possess a liquor of almost absolute purity, which deserves to be regarded as the type of a simple arterial stimulant. It can be obtained everywhere with facility, of standard and uniform strength, and at a fraction of the price of the fancy flavored liquors. The conclusions are the following: Rectified spirit is almost always strictly pure, while the more expensive liquors invariably contain fusel-oils, and frequently other impurities. The market price of rectified spirit is at present from $1.25 to $1.50 per gallon, that of the fancy flavored liquors from $2.50 to $12.00. While the taste and odor of rectified spirit is not so tempting as that of the choice cabinet liquors, it is entirely free from the disgusting taste and smell of ordinary diluted alcohol. It has not yet been established that the more expensive liquors are in any way superior to rectified spirit, or that their physiological action presents tangible points of difference.

LETTER FROM PHILADELPHIA.

MESSRS. EDITORS, — The cost of the new pavilion wards attached to Wills' Hospital was $5500 each, and not for both, as I stated in my last; I derived my information, however, from a source which I thought reliable. Even at this cost the wards were, in fact, less than half as expensive as the Presbyterian Hospital pavilions. The latter, I am told, give some annoyance in shape of cold floors, because of the cold sub-space, which in case of the new Wills' Hospital wards is warmed in winter by a suitable arrangement of heat conductors.

I cannot forbear calling your attention to editorials in late numbers of the *Medical Times and Gazette,* which were elicited by certain certificates of lunacy perpetrated by English physicians. British medical journals never let slip an opportunity of sharpening their wits at the expense of American physicians.

The American pen falters under the effect of the disclosures to which I refer. The milk and water diet of the unfortunates of Dotheboy's Hall is not the only English mixture which deserves Squeers's encomium, for certainly " Here's richness " also. Under the head of Facts indicating Insanity, one sympathetic physician writes of a female lunatic : " She has a desponding expression of countenance interspersed with moans." The editor, in commenting upon this naïve and touching statement, says, " It would be difficult to say whether such a condition of countenance were decidedly indicative of insanity, but there can be no doubt that such a face submitted to instantaneous photography would be of great artistic interest." Under the same head, another physician states that the delusion of his patient was in reference to the birth of her child, which he lucidly proves by adding, " She was not confined, but it was found by a neighbor in the dust-hole, who brought it to her. She did not know of its birth." A third anxiously calls attention to "a fact personally observed by the certifier : she frequently passes her digestions (!) in bed, which state of mind has been gradually increasing upon her for two months." Another doctor, evidently one not profoundly versed in the vagaries of the female mind, records as evidence of insanity in his patient that "she had undecided notions about some man in Scotland." And, finally, for the ordinary mind should not wrestle too long with intellects of such vigor, a physician (whose mental power must be something ponderous), among other evidences of lunacy in a woman, unblushingly reports that " she presents a general appearance of nudity" (*sic*). You will observe a charming simplicity in these statements, and wonder how it is with the bones of Lindley Murray.

A correspondent of a Philadelphia paper communicates information concerning the health and longevity of the Jews, which is of great interest. He had addressed to all the prominent Jews of the United States the question, " Do the Jews ever have consumption ? " From all sides he received the reply, " The disease is very rare among them." He also states that during an extensive practice he never met with phthisis in a Jew. Without strictly answering the question as to the reason of this comparative immunity, this writer quotes remarkable facts touching the longevity of Jews, from tables of vital statistics drawn from observations in great centres of civilization, England, France, Germany, etc. Some of these facts are the following : " In the first five years of life out of one hundred Jewish children, twelve die : of one hundred Christian children, twenty-four die. Thirty-eight per cent. of Christians reach the age of fifty ; fifty-four per cent. of Jews attain the same age. Out of one hundred Christians thirteen reach seventy years of age; out of one hundred Jews, twenty-seven reach a similar age. One quarter of all Christians live only six years and eleven months; one quarter of all Jews live twenty-eight years and three months." In explanation of these facts, Dr. Neufville says, "There are no proletaries among the Jews, while one tenth of Christians live on charity," and he directs attention to the striking difference between the longevity of Christian and Jewish merchants. Among one hundred merchants, one half the Christians die before the age of fifty-seven, while one half the Jews live to be sixty-seven." The relatively greater longevity, tenacity of life, and freedom from disease among the Jews may be due, it is thought, to hygienic, sanitary, and dietetic requirements of their religion. At any rate a careful investigation of the above facts might prove of great use in the management of the unhealthy and consumptive.

In *The Lancet* for July 17th, which has but recently fallen under my notice, I find an article on Tapping and Draining the Pleura, by Dr. Berkeley Hill. In the course of this paper Dr. Hill makes some remarkable statements concerning the comparative value and safety of ether and chloroform in the operation of paracentesis. He first mentions the strong opposition to the use of anæsthetics in this operation, which has been advanced by Dr. Bowditch and others, and quotes the five cases communicated by Dr. Bowditch to Dr. Clifford Allbutt, of Leeds, in which ether was administered. Two of these patients died shortly after the operation; a third escaped death only through most energetic means, including tracheotomy, and ether was abandoned in the other two cases before the operation was completed. Dr. Hill then suggests that such examples indicate that anæsthetics should not be used for simple tapping, but adds that in the University Hospital, of which he is surgeon, when an incision has to be made through the thick muscles of the back and a drainage tube introduced, chloroform is always administered. In eight cases of his own Dr. Hill used chloroform, "without observing unusual symptoms," and he mentions similar success at the hands of brother surgeons. "Hence," says Dr. Hill, "though anæsthetics are not to be lightly resorted to, they may be safely employed when required. It is worth notice also," he concludes, "that ether was the source of the mischief in the fatal cases, and that chloroform was well borne in our own cases." Here is a new phase in the English partisanship for chloroform, and a tone of triumph in this exultation over the superior(?) safety of chloroform, to which we are unaccustomed even from Englishmen. Yet it strikes us that this matter is somewhat murky. As presented, the results have a strangely unfamiliar look. The cart seems to be drawing the horse. Dr. Bowditch loses two patients and barely saves a third, because he used ether. Dr. Hill chloroforms eight patients, "some of them bad cases;" other surgeons anæsthetize other patients by the same means and the results are favorable! More than this. Dr. Hill sneers at ether as being mischievous and extols chloroform as a safe anæsthetic! This is a most uncommon state of affairs, one which many of us would gladly see elucidated. It is not, perhaps, so much a matter of wonder that English medical men are enemies of ether, that is to say, if they can procure no better specimens of the article than I was able to secure for a confinement case which I attended in London about three years ago. In the course of five hours I administered twenty ounces of the best ether I could obtain, and not for one moment was my patient fully insensible. It may be that such ether as Squibb manufactures is not to be found in England. Yet Drs. Jeffries and Fifield, and others, seem to have encountered no such difficulty in England ,as that which occurred to me; hence the quality of English ether has no special bearing upon the mystery which surrounds the statements of Dr. Hill.

Dr. Benjamin Lee, of Philadelphia, read before the late Baltimore Sanitary Convention a paper upon the cost of the small-pox epidemic which raged with such violence in this city during the winter of 1871–72. The object of the paper was to show that the epidemic was not properly managed, and that a generous outlay for the prevention of disease is both important and economical. The essay included the following remarkable estimates of the cost of the late epidemic: " Expenses incurred in the care of the sick, $203,879 ; loss by sickness (time), $1,072,065 ; loss by disability (time and expense), $10,000,-000 ; loss by death, $5,013,000 ; expense of premature burials, $74,420. Total, $16,363,364." X.

WEEKLY BULLETIN OF PREVALENT DISEASES.

The following is a bulletin of the diseases prevalent in Massachusetts during the week ending December 11, 1875, compiled under the authority of the State Board of Health from the returns of physicians representing all sections of the State: —

The summary for each section is as follows: —

Berkshire : Bronchitis, influenza.

Valley : Bronchitis, pneumonia, rheumatism, diphtheria, influenza. typhoid fever. Diphtheria in Springfield and Holyoke.

Midland : Influenza, pneumonia, bronchitis, diphtheria, rheumatism. Royalston reports " diphtheria very severe."

Northeastern : Bronchitis, rheumatism, influenza, pneumonia. Not much sickness.

Metropolitan : Bronchitis, scarlatina, pneumonia, influenza, rheumatism, diphtheria. More scarlatina, and much less diphtheria, reported.

Southeastern : Bronchitis, influenza. A comparatively small amount of sickness.

For the State at large, the noteworthy features of the week's returns are the increase in bronchitis and pneumonia, and the subsidence of typhoid fever and diarrhœa nearly to the minimum. Other diseases remain as at last report. The order of relative prevalence is as follows : Bronchitis, influenza, pneumonia, rheumatism, diphtheria, scarlatina, typhoid fever, croup, measles. whooping-cough. Diphtheria is most prevalent in the middle sections of the State, scarlatina is most active in Boston.

F. W. Draper, M. D., Registrar.

COMPARATIVE MORTALITY-RATES FOR THE WEEK ENDING DEC. 4, 1875.

	Estimated Population.	Total Mortality for the Week.	Annual Death-Rate per 1000 during Week.
New York	1,060,000	484	24
Philadelphia	800,000	297	19
Brooklyn	500,000		
Chicago	400,000	102	14
Boston	342,000	151	23
Cincinnati	260,000		
Providence	100,700	28	14
Worcester	50,000	18	19
Lowell	50,000	14	15
Cambridge . . .	48,000	19	21
Fall River	45,000	16	18
Lawrence	35,000	11	16
Lynn	33,000	8	13
Springfield	31,000	6	10
Salem	26,000	9	18

Normal Death-Rate, 17 per 1000.

SUFFOLK DISTRICT MEDICAL SOCIETY. — The next regular meeting will be held at the hall in Temple Place on Saturday, December 18th, at 7.30 P. M. Dr. S. G. Webber will exhibit a new battery for electrolysis. Dr. J. R. Chadwick will present a specimen of sarcoma of the uterus, and, by Dr. F. A. Harris, a specimen of fibroid tumor of the uterus complicated by sarcoma. Dr. C. F. Folsom will read a paper on Limited Responsibility, which will be followed by a discussion. Members of other State and district societies are cordially invited.

THE BOSTON SOCIETY FOR MEDICAL OBSERVATION. — The next regular meeting will be held December 20th. Dr. O. W. Doe will read a paper on the Cold-Water Treatment of Typhoid Fever.

BOOKS AND PAMPHLETS RECEIVED. — Lectures and Essays on the Science and Practice of Surgery. By Robert McDonnell, M. D., F. R. S. Part II. The Physiology and Pathology of the Spinal Cord. Dublin : Fanner & Co. 1875.

Foot Notes on Walking as a Fine Art. By Alfred Barron, " Q." Wallingford, Conn. 1875. (From A. Williams & Co.)

The Illustrated Annual Register of Rural Affairs for 1876. Albany, N. Y.

Discours prononcé à l'Académie de Médecine dans la Discussion sur le Choléra (Séance du 13 Juillet, 1875). Par M. Bonnafont. Paris. 1875.

A System of Midwifery, including the Diseases of Pregnancy and the Puerperal State. By William Leishman, M. D. Second American from the second and revised English edition. With Additions, by John S. Parry, M. D. Philadelphia: Henry C. Lea. 1875. (For sale by A. Williams & Co.)

Lectures on Bright's Disease, delivered at the Royal Infirmary of Glasgow. By D. Campbell Black, M. D., L. R. C. S. Philadelphia : Lindsay and Blakiston. 1875. (For sale by A. Williams & Co.)

THE BOSTON
MEDICAL AND SURGICAL JOURNAL.

VOL. XCIII. — THURSDAY, DECEMBER 23, 1875. — NO. 26.

A CASE OF CORROSIVE ULCER OF THE DUODENUM, AS-SOCIATED WITH INTERSTITIAL NEPHRITIS.[1]

BY GEORGE G. TARBELL, M. D., OF BOSTON.

C. E., a man forty-four years old, came under my care at the Mas-sachusetts General Hospital, September 11, 1875. He had been well until one year ago, when he first had dyspnœa on exertion, and general weakness, with palpitation of the heart and pain in the small of the back. These symptoms continued with varying intensity until Septem-ber 4th, when slight, dry cough, nausea and occasional vomiting, loss of appetite, and increased pain in the back occurred. Swelling of the feet and legs and a fullness in the epigastrium were noticed a day or two later. The patient had been in the habit of using stimulants con-siderably. Micturition was frequent, and more than the usual amount of urine was passed. The bowels were constipated. There were no cerebral symptoms, though the patient slept but little. There was slight jaundice.

The area of cardiac dullness was increased. The heart-sounds were increased in intensity, but otherwise were normal. There was com-parative dullness on percussion in both backs, and abundant moist, crep-itant râles throughout both lungs.

A smooth, rounded tumor was found in the epigastrium, occupying about one half the space between the ensiform cartilage and the umbil-icus, and extending across to the cartilage of the ribs on each side; it was dull on percussion and tender on pressure. The urine was acid; its specific gravity was 1015; it contained considerable albumen, but no casts.

The patient's principal complaint during his entire sickness was of pain and distress in the epigastrium. The tumor steadily increased in size, extending downward toward the umbilicus, and the tenderness and distress in the epigastrium were so marked that examination of the tumor caused great pain. The patient could take no food except milk. The œdema of the legs increased, extending up the thighs. The skin was tense and shining, and serum transuded. Œdema of the lungs also in-creased, causing dyspnœa.

[1] Reported before the Boston Society for Medical Observation, November 15, 1875.

About twenty days after his entrance to the hospital, the patient began to have frequent attacks of vomiting of a dark, grumous fluid, apparently coagulated and blackened blood mixed with mucus, and often amounting to two or three pints at once. This continued at intervals for two weeks, when, in addition to the vomiting, he had several profuse discharges from the bowels looking much like the matter vomited. Two days after this it was found, on examination of the epigastrium, that the tumor had mostly disappeared, and there was normal resonance on percussion over the stomach, although tenderness remained; an ill-defined, solid substance could be felt on deep pressure, apparently behind the stomach. After this the œdema of the legs mostly disappeared, but the urine was still albuminous, and a few days before the patient's death, eight weeks after his admission to the hospital, epithelial and granular casts were found in it.

The existence of corrosive ulcer of the duodenum did not occur to me as among the probabilities. Aside from the vomiting of coagulated blood, which is ordinarily the sign of ulceration of the stomach, the renal symptoms were the prominent ones, and the renal specimens were as markedly pathological as was the ulcer of the duodenum.

The autopsy was made by Dr. Fitz. The stomach presented the appearances of chronic catarrhal gastritis in a marked degree. The ulcer of the duodenum was about three fourths of an inch in diameter, seated in the posterior wall just below the pylorus; it extended completely through the walls of the intestine, the base being formed by the pancreas. The latter organ was not particularly corroded.

The right renal artery was of normal calibre, the left about one half as large; in addition, its volume was very considerably reduced by extensive chronic endo-arteritis. The corresponding kidney was dense, flattened, and small, hardly larger than a dried fig; the pelvis was dilated to nearly the size of the kidney, and the ureter was fully one half the normal size. There was no evidence of its constriction.

The right kidney was reduced one third in size, the surface granular, the cortex and medulla diminished in volume and very dense. The distinction between convoluted and straight tubules was lost; the Malpighian corpuscles were not to be distinguished. The microscope showed the existence of an extensive amount of interstitial affection.

Softened thrombi were found in the vesical plexus, and emboli, without infarction, in several of the smaller branches of the pulmonary arteries. Several small, round, acute abscesses were found at the posterior and peripheral portions of the lungs; their embolic origin could not be ascertained. A secondary bronchus leading to the lower lobe of the left lung was almost completely obstructed by a soft, reddish-gray, rounded tumor growing from the bronchial wall, and of the size of a large pea. Its structure was that of a medullary sarcoma, and the absence of degenerative appearances suggested its recent origin. Just beyond, in the middle of the lower lobe of the lung, a large cavity was found whose walls were dense, pigmented, and contracted, apparently older than the tumor referred to. Both lungs were likewise œdematous. The heart was hypertrophied and dilated.

The comparative infrequency of the ulcer in this location, and the still greater rarity of its mention in the standard text-books of general practice, lead me to refer to an article in the *British and Foreign Medico-Chirurgical Review* for January, 1864, which is based on a monograph by Dr. F. Trier, of Copenhagen. This work is a collation and analysis of twenty-six cases, and the author gives a clear and concise statement of the theories and the clinical facts concerning these ulcers and their origin. He coincides with the theory propounded by Virchow, who " lays great stress upon the corrosive nature of the acid contents of the stomach, but sees, in the defined form of the ulcer, the evidence that its first origin must be purely local, while the corrosive action of the acid is the most important element in its further progress."

Dr. Trier argues that in some respects the superior transverse portion of the duodenum may be considered as a transition from the stomach to the intestine, since the contents of this portion of the intestine have still an acid reaction, for the liver and pancreas have not poured in their alkaline secretions. Then, if there is an interruption to the circulation of the blood, a lesion of nutrition in any limited point, the conditions are present requisite for a progressive corrosion of the various coats of the stomach or intestine.

The theory of embolism of the arteries of the stomach or intestine as the point of departure for these ulcers is strongly corroborated by the fact that there are often two ulcers, symmetrically located and corresponding with the arterial distribution. And that the gastric fluid is the corrosive agent may be considered as proven by the fact that this peculiar form of ulceration does not ordinarily occur except where this fluid may have access before it is neutralized, namely, in the lower portion of the œsophagus, in the stomach, and in the duodenum.

While admitting the insufficiency of his own numbers as a basis for generalizations, Dr. Trier establishes three points, using also the statistics of Brinton and some other writers: —

First, that corrosive ulcer occurs in the duodenum only one tenth as often as in the stomach.

Second, that ulcer of the stomach is twice as frequent in females as in males, while ulcer of the duodenum is five times more frequent in males than in females.

Third, that it is a disease of adult life, the average age being forty-two years and six months.

A CASE OF TALIPES VARUS.

BY T. F. GALLOUPE, M. D., OF LYNN.

THE patient was born on the 25th of August, 1875. The labor had been tedious, and at its completion all parties concerned were so much fatigued that no critical examination of the child was made. The next morning my attention was called to the feet; I found each of them twisted inwards, so that when the child cried or kicked the sole looked almost directly upwards; the heels were also raised. It was a case of talipes varus of rather more than medium severity. The foot, however, could be easily brought into its normal position, and retained with slight force, there being but little shortening of the integuments and subjacent tissues. These circumstances led me to try the following simple treatment by adhesive straps.

To protect the skin from injury, a soft bandage of old linen was first applied. The foot being held in its normal position, one end of a strip of adhesive plaster (about eight inches long by half an inch wide) was applied to the dorsum of the foot at the root of the middle toe, carried inwards, around the head of the metatarsal bone of the great toe, across the sole, and around the outer border of the foot, close to the little toe ; then upwards over the front of the ankle and spirally around the leg. Several short strips were applied crosswise for further security, with a roller over the whole. By this means the foot was held firmly yet comfortably in its natural position. Once in three or four days, or as often as was necessary, the whole was removed, the skin bathed, and the straps and bandages readjusted. After two weeks, I substituted for the long strip of plaster a piece of common "elastic" of the same width, about three inches in length, to each end of which a piece of plaster had been sewed, to secure it to the foot and leg. This was adjusted to the foot in the same manner as before, but it was carried up upon the outer side of the leg instead of spirally around it. This was an improvement, inasmuch as it secured constant traction and at the same time allowed a limited motion of the foot, thereby not only preventing the weakness consequent upon inaction of the muscles but also giving an opportunity for their exercise and increase of strength. This treatment was continued for six weeks, when the deformity was found to be cured.

This method is simple, efficient, and economical, and would be successful in many cases of not extreme severity. Any nurse or mother of ordinary intelligence could manage it, with occasional oversight by the surgeon.

A CASE OF URETHRAL CALCULUS.

BY J. T. BOUTELLE, M. D., OF HAMPTON, VA.

R. CARROLL, a colored man, fifty-six years old, consulted me July 1, 1875. He stated that twelve years ago he began to be troubled with difficulty in passing water, accompanied by pain in the perinæum and the abdomen. He remembered that the stream was frequently checked or " shut off " very suddenly during its passage. About ten years ago he had a complete stoppage of urine, followed by swelling of the perinæum. He had no medical attendance at that time, and a large perineal abscess formed, which opened spontaneously, giving exit to a great amount of offensive greenish matter. Through this opening his urine was voided, and, a fistula resulting, he had passed nearly all his urine through it ever since. He said that he had been a great sufferer, having to micturate often, and always with pain, the urine passing in a fine stream or drop by drop through the fistula. A very small amount also passed through the urethra. Little pieces of " gravel " were often forced through the fistula. The patient had taken morphine in large doses for a year or two to relieve the pain.

At the time of his visit he was suffering great pain in the loins and in the region of the bladder; walking or riding increased the pain, and he was growing very weak and unable to do any work. On attempting to pass a sound I found, about three inches from the meatus, a tough stricture, which admitted the passage of only a very fine bougie. The instrument was arrested after passing the stricture, and on withdrawing it I found the sides to be scratched as if by a hard substance. On examination with the finger along the urethra externally, some hard lumps could be felt just anterior to the scrotum. A probe passed through the stricture grated upon a hard body. As there was evidently a large calculus in the urethra, I advised an operation for its removal; to this the patient consented.

July 3d. Chloroform having been administered to the patient by Dr. Selden, of Hampton, I made an incision one inch in length into the urethra just anterior to the scrotum. Through this incision the first and second pieces or sections (1 and 2 in the figure) were removed without difficulty; on attempting to pass a sound through the wound into the bladder, the others were felt, and with a little trouble extracted with

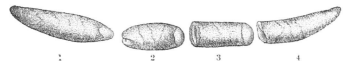

:   2   3   4

dressing forceps. A large steel sound was then easily passed into the bladder, and no stone could be felt. No attempt was made at this time to dilate the stricture. The wound was left open, and a cold wet compress wrapped around the penis. The man recovered well from the chloroform, and passed water freely through the wound.

July 4th. Patient had passed a comfortable night, and was feeling very well. Scarcely any constitutional disturbance, and no bad symptom of any kind observed. Water passed easily through the wound, and none through the fistula in the perinæum.

July 5th. Patient doing well. From this date he continued to improve, being soon able to be up and to walk out. But the wound gradually closed, and the urine began to pass again through the fistula, and an abscess formed at the wound.

I saw him again on August 1st. The abscess had opened and discharged; the wound had closed entirely, and he had considerable difficulty in passing water through the fistula. A small amount passed out of the meatus at every micturition.

August 7th. With the assistance of Dr. Selden the patient was chloroformed, and the stricture was thoroughly ruptured with a Holt's dilator. On recovering from the anæsthetic he passed his water easily through the urethra. He was ordered to remain quietly in bed, to drink flax-seed tea, and to have an opiate at night.

August 8th. I found him up and out of bed, feeling very well and joyful. There was almost no constitutional disturbance. From this date his recovery was rapid, and he was very soon able to resume his farm work.

November 8th. He is much improved in general health, and has given up the use of opiates entirely. The fistulous opening in the perinæum has entirely closed, and his urine passes in a good stream through the urethra. The wound from the operation also remains closed. He states that he has passed one or two small pieces of stone, but they were soft and crumbled easily.

The very remarkable size of the calculus, the length of time it had existed, and the rapid recovery of the patient after its removal by operation have led me to report the case. It is easy to see how the calculus was formed : a small stone arrested at the stricture blocked the exit of the urine, causing rupture of the urethra and perineal fistula, while the stone by continued deposit increased in size, and others formed behind it.

I had at first intended to remove the calculus by the operation of perineal section, hoping in that way to avoid making a fistula of the urethra, but the scene of operation was a small cabin with very poor light, the perinæum was full of cicatricial tissue, and my only assistant had to devote most of his attention to the anæsthetic. These facts decided me to make the incision as I have stated above, and it is noticeable that the wound healed completely under the simplest dressing.

The calculi are remarkable from the peculiar nature of the surfaces by which each piece touches its neighbors. Pieces 2 and 3, and 3 and 4, articulate by ball-and-socket joints, 2 entering 3 and 3 entering 4. The end of 2 nearest to 1 has a transverse groove, which, instead of confining the point of 1, allows it to slide to one side or the other.

RECENT PROGRESS IN SURGERY.[1]

BY J. COLLINS WARREN, M. D.

The Treatment in Germany of Cleft Palate. — In a former Report[2] attention was called to a new operation for remedying this deformity, devised by Professor Simon, of Heidelberg. This operation, called staphylo-pharyngorraphy, was based upon the action of the upper constrictor muscle of the pharynx, which was shown to play so important a part in the act of articulation. Attention was first called to this muscle, in connection with operations or devices for the cure of the defect, by Suersen, a dentist of Berlin, whose obturator or hard-rubber plate has not attained that celebrity which its success in giving the voice a purity of tone should have earned for it.

The operations for cleft palate which are performed in this country and in England, although constantly undergoing slight modifications to facilitate the closure of the fissure, have in no case been based upon the action of the muscles with a view of remedying the more conspicuous portion of the deformity, the imperfection of speech. The great merit of Suersen's apparatus consists in its adaptation to the muscular apparatus concerned in excluding the passage of air from the throat into the nasal cavity, so that communication between the two cavities is much more effectually regulated than by any other method. The following account is taken from an abstract of a lecture delivered by Suersen at Hamburg in 1867.[3] He says that the separation of the cavity of the mouth from the cavity of the nose " is under normal conditions effected on the one hand by the velum palati, which strains itself (consequently by the levator and tensor palati), but on the other hand, also, by a muscle which has in connection with these operations not yet received, to my knowledge, a sufficient amount of attention. I mean the constrictor pharyngis superior. This muscle contracts itself during the utterance of every letter pronounced without a nasal sound, just as the levator palati does. The constrictor muscle contracts the cavum pharyngo-palatinum, the pharynx wall bulging out, and it is chiefly on the action of this muscle that I base the system of my artificial palates.

---

[1] Concluded from page 710.
[2] JOURNAL, xc. 596.
[3] The American Journal of Dental Science, vol. i., third series, No. 8.

" These palates, which in all their parts are made of hard caoutchouc, consist of a teeth-plate suitably attached to existing teeth, and at the same time covering the fissure in the hard palate (if such a fissure exists). Where the fissure commences in the velum, that plate terminates in an apophysis broad enough for filling up the defect. . . . The lower surface of the apophysis, turned towards the mouth, lies on about an equal level with the velum, *if the latter is raised by the levator palati.* But when the velum hangs loosely downward, the back part of the artificial palate is lying over it. This back part accordingly fills up the cavum pharyngo-palatinum, and in such a manner as not to impede the entrance of the air into the cavity of the nose when the constrictor pharyngis superior is inactive. Thus the patients can without any impediment breathe through the nose. But as soon as the constrictor contracts the cavum pharyngo-palatinum (this happens, as I will repeat for the sake of clearness, in the utterance of every letter with the exception of *m* and *n*), the muscle already named reclines against the vertical back-surfaces of the obturator. By this operation the air-current is prevented from entering the cavity of the nose, and is compelled to take its way through the mouth, and thus the utterance loses its nasal sound."

The apophysis alluded to is somewhat triangular in shape, taking an outline of a horizontal section of this part of the pharynx; it is nearly flat on its upper and under surfaces, yet thick enough to keep the fissure well closed while the sides of the soft palate are rising and falling during articulation. The improvement of the voice after a short use of one of these obturators is very striking. They are made with great facility, and are exceedingly durable. They are now applied at the Massachusetts General Hospital, having been introduced by Dr. Algernon Coolidge.

The inefficiency of the customary operation in restoring the voice lies in the fact that the tense velum produced by a closure of the fissure is too short a valve to close the communication between the two cavities. Professor Simon's operation recognizes this defect, and remedies it by a subsequent manœuvre, which consists in stitching the remains of the uvula to the posterior wall of the pharynx at a point where the superior constrictor " bulges out " during contraction. The remaining space is then easily closed by the constrictor muscle. The great advantage of this operation is that it can be applied to cases operated on in the usual way when the voice still retains a nasal tone.

An observation of Professor A. Graham Bell, of this city, is interesting in this connection. He finds that certain deaf mutes when taught to speak by his method retain a nasal tone. This is caused by the inability of the soft palate to lift itself up against the posterior wall of the pharynx. But if the soft palate is held up with the handle of a spoon during articulation (which he finds can easily be done with a little practice) the nasal tone disappears. It is evident that, being thus raised, it can act in conjunction with the constrictor muscle. Such cases might be benefited by wearing a plate to the roof of the mouth, with a projecting tongue which would keep the palate permanently raised. The same device might be adapted to cases already operated on without obliteration of the nasal tone, when Simon's operation was not thought advisable.

Dr. Schönborn lately read a paper before the fourth surgical congress at Berlin [1] in which he proposes to accomplish in one operation that which Professor Simon does in two. The edges of the cleft having been refreshed in the usual manner, a flap is taken from the posterior wall of the pharynx, the base downwards, the free end being turned over between the edges of the cleft and sewed to them. The operation was performed in a case where the cleft involved the hard palate. The wound united well ; there was, however, a slight nasal tone remaining. Professor Langenbeck, who was present at the congress, claimed to have had many successful results from the old operation, that is, the one in use in this country, and thought it ought it to be tried first. The success of Schönborn's operation would seem to depend greatly on the height at which the flap was taken from the pharyngeal wall. Should the base be left too low, the velum would not be lifted high enough, and insufficiency, with nasal tone, would be the result. A great advantage would seem to be that it closes the cleft without putting the velum on the stretch, and thus allows the levator and tensor palati muscles to act in conjunction with the constrictor in separating the two cavities.

The Result of Resections for Gun-Shot Wounds. — Dr. Bergmann, professor of surgery in Dorpat, and during the Franco-German war surgeon in charge of two military hospitals, gives the results of his experience in resection of joints for gun-shot wounds.[2] An interesting feature of this brochure is the introduction of an extensive series of albertotype plates, which permit illustration on a scale not usually attempted.

Hannover's report, which followed the Prussian-Danish war, gave an opinion much more unfavorable in regard to resection of joints than had hitherto been accepted. The discussion of this question by German surgeons has since been quite animated, the favorable opinions of Langenbeck not being upheld by many of his countrymen. The operations performed by Dr. Bergmann were in most cases secondary, and were resorted to to relieve the severe inflammation which supervened on the injury. Nine cases of resection of the elbow-joint are given, of which two were fatal and five terminated in anchylosis. In two cases the functions of the joint were completely restored. In the second of these

---

[1] Wiener medizinische Wochenschrift, 1875, No. 18.
[2] Die Resulte der Gelenkresectionen im Kriege. Von E. Bergmann. Glessen. 1874.

the ends of the ulna and radius were removed, and the humerus was left intact. Flexion, extension, and pronation were complete ; supination was not quite perfect. The resection of the elbow-joint seemed to have a favorable effect upon the inflammation which followed the injury ; not so, however, that of the shoulder-joint, where acute suppurative periostitis was frequently noticed after the operation, abscesses pointing in different parts of the arm, which free openings at the back of the hand, made at the time of the operation, failed to prevent. Fifteen cases of resection of the shoulder-joint are reported ; of these three were fatal, one was followed by amputation, and another by a general atrophy of the muscles of the arm. In the remainder the result was generally favorable. In only one case were active movements obtained in all directions. In two cases in which the preservation of the periosteum had been complete, the arm could be abducted. In one case the soft parts on the outside and back of the shoulder had been carried away; also a portion of the acromion and spine of the scapula, exposing the fissured head of the humerus and a fractured glenoid cavity. The patient nevertheless recovered a useful arm, the muscular development, as shown in the plate accompanying the case, being quite remarkable. The author quotes in connection with this case one of Langenbeck, in which all the soft parts about the shoulder-joint, except the large vessels, the nerves, and the biceps and latissimus dorsi muscles, were torn away, and yet the patient was able eventually to return to service, to ride, and to carry the sabre with the hand of the wounded arm. These two cases encourage him to attempt conservative treatment, even in cases in which the laceration of the soft parts is very extensive. One or two plates are given of grooved wounds, or gouging out of a piece of the head of the humerus without injury to the cartilage or shaft of the bone. The absence of splintering in these cases is thought to be due to the angle at which the ball strikes the bone. This is illustrated in the case of a ball perforating a pane of glass; if the direction of the ball is at a right angle to the surface there will be a clean hole, or nearly so; otherwise, there will be extensive splintering.

Resection of the ankle-joint did not come up to the author's expectations. The results were better as a rule than those of operations in civil practice for caries. The acute suppurative inflammation which had followed the injury was generally cured, but the cases often terminated in a tedious caries of the ends of the resected bones, which delayed recovery as long as conservative treatment might have done. This latter, he thinks, has proved more successful of late years, owing to the practice at present in vogue of resorting to free incisions. The resection of the joint did not hasten recovery sufficiently to prevent a result with an unfavorable position of the foot, there being in all his cases a tendency to pes equinus or varus. The author bears testimony to the great amount of bone which is reproduced after this operation, exceeding that which is formed after operation for caries. Anchylosis took place in every case but one.

Dr. Bergmann's work is to be commended for the fullness and accuracy of his description of cases, and the frankness with which he comments upon them. There is a lack of system in preparing the material, which makes reference to individual cases or plates difficult. An important omission is the absence of a tabular statement of cases.

Transportation of Wounded Soldiers by Railway in Time of War.[1]— In March, 1873, the Russian government appointed a commission for the discussion and experimental trial of different methods for the amelioration of the condition of sick and wounded soldiers transported on railroads. The commission, after careful examination, concluded that the transportation of the sick and wounded should be carried on mainly by the use of box cars, that arrangements should be made for converting these to the purpose of transportation of the wounded at the shortest possible notice, and that appliances for the outfit of the same should be sent to points where it is anticipated that many wounded will be concentrated ; as a rule, litters are to be used ; but in case of extreme necessity, a deep layer of straw at the bottom of the car may be substituted. The report of this commission was shortly followed by that of Mr. Zavodovsky, of St. Petersburg, whose invention was submitted to the War Department at Washington for the purpose of criticism ; this criticism has now appeared in the form of a report to the surgeon-general by Assistant-Surgeon George A. Otis.

Dr. Otis's paper contains a full and interesting description of the various devices employed for transporting the wounded by railway during our late war, as well as those which have been adopted by other countries since that time. Transportation by railway is naturally of comparatively recent date, the Italian war of 1859 being the first in which it was extensively employed. On that occasion passenger trains were used, for the most part, without alterations. In the Danish and Six Weeks' wars the Prussians used straw mattresses carried by stretcher poles and laid upon loose straw, this plan, employed during 1863–64 in the army of the Potomac, having been approved by the Prussian government.

The car designed for the Sanitary Commission by Dr. Elisha Harris was largely in use during our war. In this car the litters were suspended from upright wooden posts by stout rubber rings, which were found, however, to permit of too much motion to be comfortable. The

---

[1] A Report on a Plan for Transporting Wounded Soldiers by Railway in Time of War; with Descriptions of Various Methods employed for this Purpose on different Occasions. By George A. Otis, Assistant Surgeon, U. S. Army. Washington : War Department, Surgeon-General's Office. 1875.

plan of utilizing the ordinary field stretchers for railway transport, keeping the patients upon them until they reach a fixed hospital, is commended by Dr. Otis. The utility of railway transport was most conspicuous in the army of the Cumberland. Dr. Barnum was one of the most experienced of the surgeons having in charge hospital trains; during his connection with the service he supervised the transportation of twenty thousand four hundred and seventy-two patients and lost but one, " who, despite the advice of his surgeons, implored that he might be taken to die in the bosom of his family." When General Sherman's army was before Atlanta, until the lines of communication were destroyed preparatory to the march to the sea, hospital cars ran regularly from the front to base hospitals, some of which were four hundred and seventy-two miles distant. The smoke-pipes of the locomotives of these trains were painted a brilliant scarlet; the exteriors of the hood and of the tender-car were of the same color, with gilt ornamentation. At night, beneath the head-light of the locomotive three red lanterns were suspended in a row. These distinguishing signals were recognized by the Confederates, and the trains were never fired upon or molested in any way. Few published statements have appeared respecting the transportation of sick and wounded in Confederate armies. They had no regular system of hospital trains.

Many interesting experiments were made at an international conference of the societies for the relief of wounded in war, at Paris in 1867, and a great variety of cars and litters and methods of swinging litters were shown. Although many were very ingenious and useful, and a number of improvements on the methods then shown were brought out at the time of the Vienna Exposition in 1873, Professor Billroth and others were inclined to discountenance almost any outfit of hospital cars that could not be promptly improvised. Mr. Zavodovsky's plan is based upon this view. The litters are hung on ropes depending from swinging poles, which it is proposed to cut in the forest.

This plan is not favorably commented upon by Dr. Otis, who thinks that the problem of utilizing the railway conveyances most likely to be available near the battle-field, namely, the box cars of supply trains, is not yet satisfactorily solved. Our passenger cars can easily be arranged by removing every other seat, and the movable backs of those that remain, to accommodate twelve to fourteen commodious litters; but these are not usually on hand. He says, " In the present state of our knowledge, it would appear that the simplest and best method for transforming freight cars to hospital use is by the system of Mr. Grund, as employed on some of the Prussian hospital trains, and almost uniformly on those of Bavaria and the Palatinate." This consisted in supporting three field stretchers in the front and three in the rear part of the freight cars, by means of transverse wooden bars resting on semi-elliptical plate springs. It would therefore be necessary to store in each car a few such springs and spikes, to enable it to be converted for hospital use at any moment. A supply train thus fitted out would give each patient more air and space than were enjoyed on our hospital trains, but would not afford the same facilities of access to patients by the attendants.

Dr. Otis's report is carefully prepared and illustrated very fully and accurately, and is an interesting as well as valuable contribution to the subject. We trust it foreshadows a satisfactory exhibition of these appliances at Philadelphia next summer.

Catgut Ligatures. — K. Eliaschewitsch,[1] after experimenting with this ligature on animals, gives the following account of its fate. Ligatures were applied to the carotid and femoral arteries and to the horns of the uterus ; sutures were taken in the skin and examined at intervals of from five to twenty-five days. As soon as the granulations of the wound come in contact with the ligature, a separation of the outside fibres of the catgut begins to take place. The ligature gradually grows thinner, while the fibrils break up into small particles and finally into detritus. The rapidity of this process depends upon the amount of water contained in the tissues, the degree of reaction caused by the ligature, and the manner in which it has been prepared. Fine carbolized sutures are thinned to the minimum in five or six days. On vessels and on the horns of the uterus, the ligature begins to break down in five days. In dogs killed a month after the application of the ligature, no trace of it was to be found.

The same number of the *Centralblatt* contains an abstract of an article by D. Murinoff, on the changes observed in this ligature. The author compared it with the simple ligature, and also with the chloralized catgut. To the naked eye, all kinds appeared swollen after two or three days, the swelling increasing markedly at the end of a week. Over the ligatures there was a fine transparent membrane, the knots appearing adherent to the surrounding tissue. Thinner ligatures were absorbed at the end of ten days ; No. 3 Lister catgut was absorbed at the end of twenty to thirty days. The remains of knots of the former were found at the end of twenty-five days ; of the latter, at the end of seventy days. Under the microscope the ordinary ligatures, as well as carbolized catgut ligatures were found to be splitting up into fibres at the end of a few days ; later, they gradually disappeared among the granulations. The manner of preparing the ligatures does not appear to influence the rapidity of their absorption. Carbolized catgut irritates slightly, chloralized catgut less so, and simple catgut not at all.

Experiments were made in reference to the frequency of hæmorrhage following the different kinds of ligatures. The vessels were cut through

[1] Centralblatt für Chirurgie, No. 43, 1873.

and both ends were tied. Lister's carbolized catgut gave ten per cent., chloralized gut twenty-five per cent., and simple catgut eighty-seven per cent. of hæmorrhages. Out of forty-eight ligatures with catgut, in thirty-seven cases there was healing by first intention; out of thirty-four with chloralized gut, twenty-eight; and out of twenty-eight with simple catgut, there were eight cases of first intention.

CARTER ON DISEASES OF THE EYE.[1]

THE author has not attempted to write a complete and exhaustive treatise, but to present in a concise and readable form the present state of knowledge with regard to the nature and treatment of the more important of the diseases of the eye. Written somewhat in the style of a series of lectures, the book is certainly very readable; we can recall few medical books which may compare with it in this respect, but it is hardly everywhere concise.

There is much that is very good in the book, much that gives evidence of sound judgment. The chapter on the principles of ophthalmic therapeutics is especially instructive; still we cannot commend the assertion on page 252 that, when with granulations of the conjunctiva a very close vascular net-work has been developed on the cornea, little is to be hoped from any treatment except the inoculation of purulent ophthalmia, and the statement that the cornea is protected from sloughing by its vascular character, and the inoculated disease may be suffered to run its course unchecked. As it appears, this statement is not fully borne out by the author's own experience; for on page 265 he admits that in one case he has seen the inoculated disease cause sloughing of both corneæ, in spite of the fact that they were highly vascular when the inoculation was made.

The importance of atropine and of avoidance of any irritating application in iritis is very properly and strongly insisted upon; the use of an astringent for a day or two may produce irreparable mischief, but when, from the plastic character of the inflammation, from delay, or from bad treatment at first, the pupil does not yield to atropine, the indication for mercury, given so as to obtain its constitutional effect as rapidly as prudent administration admits, is considered imperative, and this independently of the syphilitic or non-syphilitic nature of the affection. In this connection the opinion of the late Dr. Anstie, that mercury exercises a special power over the parts supplied by the fifth nerve, is quoted.

Strychnia has been less efficacious in the author's hands than it has been in those of other observers; in a few cases of progressive atrophy, in which iodide of potassium, sometimes preceded by mercury, either failed or had ceased to cause improvement, the effect of strychnia was extremely good, but in the majority of cases no effect at all was apparent. The author is unable to give any symptom which may serve to distinguish the cases which it will benefit; when it produces any effect he is inclined to attribute this to the power of the

[1] *A Practical Treatise on Diseases of the Eye.* By ROBERT BRUDENELL CARTER, F. R. C. S., etc. London : Macmillan & Co. 1875.

drug to stimulate nerve nutrition after the direct operation of the primary cause which produced the atrophy has ceased.

Except in early infancy, the operation by suction is preferred for the removal of cataract in patients below the age of thirty, and Graefe's operation for senile cataract.

The book is not entirely free from errors, and there are occasionally passages in which a disposition is shown to be sarcastic over what are considered the failings or mistakes of others, not always, as it seems to us, quite fairly. The danger of indulging this inclination is illustrated in the first chapter, which treats of the anatomy and physiology of the eye. Two thirds of the twelfth page are devoted to playful sarcasm over an exploded theory based on ignorance of the arrangement of the basilar layer of the retina, and the "wholesome moral" is drawn "that an acquaintance even with the anatomy of the retina may afford security against ludicrous blundering under the disguise of knowledge." But only a few lines before this an erroneous statement has been made with regard to this very basilar layer: that "the cones are most abundant in the region of the macula lutea, where each one of them is surrounded by a single circle of rods;" the fact being that at the centre of the macula, cones only are present.

The belief expressed on page 100 that pulsation of the retinal veins on the diskis "almost always due to increased intra-ocular tension, that is to say, to a state which either is or approaches glaucoma," we are wholly unable to accede to. In our experience glaucoma is by no means common, but a venous pulse in normal eyes is exceedingly so. We were surprised also to find in the chapter on diseases of the fundus oculi that "sarcomata which originate in the choroid . . . are extremely rare," and that "the presence of a tumor within the eye necessarily occasions increased tension," while no reference is made to the most important diagnostic point in the earlier stages of sarcoma, the ophthalmoscopic appearances of the growth itself. Sarcomata of the choroid are certainly not extremely rare, — current medical literature furnishes numerous examples ; nor is increased tension by any means a necessary accompaniment of the growth when it has already reached a size to be readily diagnosticated by the ophthalmoscope. It is the more to be regretted that a better account of the disease has not been given, since an early diagnosis is of the greatest importance, not indeed for the preservation of the eye, but for that of the life of the patient. As we have already said, however, there is a great deal for which we can recommend the book.   O. F. W.

FLINT'S PHYSIOLOGY.[1]

INTO this volume of nine hundred and seventy-eight pages the author has, by using a large page and small type, condensed about seven eighths of all the matter contained in his large treatise of five volumes. The portions omitted are chiefly historical in character. There is little that is new except a description of the depressor nerve and a connected account of the inorganic substances

[1] *A Text-Book of Human Physiology, designed for the use of Practitioners and Students of Medicine.* By AUSTIN FLINT, JR., M. D. New York : D. Appleton & Co. 1876.

necessary for the nutrition of the body. The chapter on the blood has, however, been to a great extent rewritten.

Though, with these exceptions, the text does not essentially differ from that of the larger work, there is a great improvement in the way in which the volume is illustrated. The number of the illustrations has been greatly increased, and their character is generally excellent. They are borrowed from such works as those of Sappey, Bernard, Hirschfeld, and Kölliker. Several reproductions of Dr. Woodward's microscopical photographs have also been introduced.

Flint's Physiology has thus been rendered far more accessible to students of that science, but the comprehensive way in which the various subjects are treated will probably make it always rather more valuable as a work of reference than as a text-book.   H. P. B.

ATKINSON'S OBSTETRICAL HINTS.[1]

IN 1874 Dr. Atkinson delivered the annual address before the Philadelphia County Medical Society, and this little manual is the same address rewritten and slightly enlarged. It is a most excellent statement of the main points to be observed in the treatment of a confinement case, and contains many important facts for the young accoucheur which are not to be found in any of the standard text-books. While agreeing with the writer in most of his new departures from the old methods of treatment, we must consider the statement (page 58) that a puerperal patient from the very first should be allowed to " change her position as she may desire," and to sit up in bed and to be moved to a lounge after the third or fourth day, as open to criticism.

PROCEEDINGS OF THE SUFFOLK DISTRICT MEDICAL SOCIETY.

JAMES R. CHADWICK, M. D., SECRETARY.

NOVEMBER 27, 1875. The President, DR. H. W. WILLIAMS, in the chair.

Nascent Chloride of Ammonium in the Treatment of Bronchitis. — This paper was illustrated by cases and by the exhibition of a bottle in which the vapor was generated by adding aqua ammonia to hydrochloric acid. It is reserved for publication.

A New Sphygmoscope was shown by Dr. E. A. Pond, of Rutland, Vt., who was present as a guest. He remarked that since Marey introduced the sphygmograph many new and valuable facts in medicine had been discovered by J. Boarden, Gregory, Anstie, and others, but the precise practical value to be assigned to the variations in the pulse recognized by its aid had not as yet been determined. The obstacles to the general use of this instrument, however, were its cost and bulk. These were entirely avoided by the sphygmoscope

[1] *Hints in the Obstetric Procedure.* By WILLIAM B. ATKINSON, M. D. Philadelphia: Collins, Printer, 705 Jayne Street.

presented, which consisted of a glass tube, from three to six inches in length, with a diameter of three sixty-fourths of an inch ; one end flared slightly, so as to be funnel-shaped.   A drop of colored fluid is allowed to fall into the large end of the tube, and is shaken down to about the middle of the capillary bore, where it serves as an index, rising and falling with the pulse when the large end of the tube is pressed down upon any artery.   The slightest

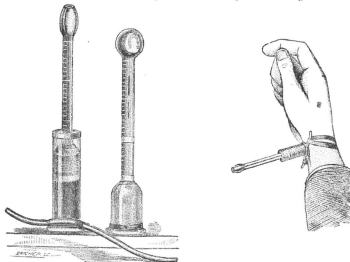

movement or vibration of the column of blood is indicated, and the course of any vibrating vessel may be surely traced, though imperceptible to the touch ; even the capillaries of the fingers may be followed.   In a case of senile gangrene, Dr. Pond had been able to trace in the foot those arterial branches which were still permeable.   In concussion of the brain and in collapse after injuries, what is known as the " brain pulse " may be recognized, so that in severe railroad injuries, scalds, etc., where the reaction is slow, a complete or only partial recovery may be prognosticated.   A tendency to paralysis of the heart in typhoid fever may be made evident by this instrument, and proper precautions taken.   The tremulous pulse in typhoid fever, and the very irregular "jiggling" pulse in diphtheria both indicate prostration and immediate danger ; whether these two characteristics were pathognomonic of the two diseases was yet to be determined.

In a case of inflammatory rheumatism, Dr. Pond had recently been able to diagnosticate valvular disease of the heart by means of the sphygmoscope, and had confirmed it subsequently by auscultation.

A handle has been adjusted to the instrument to prevent movements being imparted to the index by the unconscious variations in pressure on the part of the investigator, though with practice this may be discarded.   To prevent the escape of the fluid, it has been found desirable to cover the large end of the tube with a thin rubber diaphragm, which does not interfere with the delicacy of the markings.

52

The perfection of the instrument is due to Dr. W. R. Pond, of Stockton. Cal., a son of the inventor. He has fitted the fine tube into a larger one, which acts as a reservoir of fluid. being closed at the bottom by the rubber diaphragm. The end of the small tube is covered with a packing. so as to act in the larger one as a piston ; this serves a double purpose, regulating the height of the vibrating column and showing the motions of the pulse. An annular tube has been made which will indicate simultaneously the pressure and the vibrations.

In conclusion, Dr. Pond claimed that by a study of the pulse with this instrument much important information could be obtained about the condition of the heart, the arteries. and the veins, the action of medicines in health and in disease, the indications for stimulation or venesection in pneumonia, disease of the brain, etc. The first and second sounds of the heart may be distinctly differentiated when they are obscured by the presence of valvular disease. During the use of anæsthetics the eye of the administrator may be kept constantly informed of the state of the pulse by means of the sphygmoscope. During labor it heralds every pain and indicates the general strength of the woman.

DR. KNIGHT pointed out that this instrument was identical with that invented by Scott Allison, which had been made familiar to the profession in Boston by the brilliant experiments made with it in this city several years ago by Dr. J. B. Upham.

DR. POND stated in reply that he had not been aware that another instrument of this kind had been previously devised ; that in the past few years he had made, in conjunction with his son, more than twenty different instruments. He had. morever, affixed to his pattern a recording apparatus, so that it was now both a sphygmoscope and sphygmograph.

Melano-Sarcoma of the Choroid. — A specimen was presented by DR. B. J. JEFFRIES. A woman, seventy-seven years old, discovered that her right eye was blind. She applied to the Eye and Ear Infirmary for advice, when Dr. F. P. Sprague found the sight extinct, the globe externally normal, and its movements unimpaired. Under atropine, the pupil dilated to about two thirds of its normal diameter. Lateral illumination gave a dull yellowish reflex. The ophthalmoscope revealed a tumor, of a faint yellowish color, within the globe, projecting from the outer side forward, towards the ciliary region ; the extreme inner portion of the field was comparatively clear. No history could be obtained of cancer in the family. Two months later the patient returned with all the symptoms of glaucoma : great pain, a dull cornea, a dilated oval pupil, a shallow anterior chamber, and increased tension of the eyeball. As the condition was clearly the glaucomatous stage of an intra-ocular growth, enucleation was at once performed. . A section- through the centre of the globe, after removal, at right angles, to the visual axis, divided a tumor, the size of a small filbert, springing from the choroid. The retina was separated in the shape of a funnel from the nerve to the ora serrata ; the tumor had not penetrated the sclerotic, or reached the optic nerve or ciliary region. Under the microscope it was seen to be pigmented sarcoma.

Dr. Jeffries spoke of the liability of such a case being mistaken for acute glaucoma, and iridectomy performed; whereas, only enucleation would stop the pain. and give the patient a chance of life for some years.

Dr. Jeffries then exhibited a specimen of extra-ocular sarcoma with the following history: In June, 1871, a man, forty-eight years old, noticed a small tumor growing from the outer edge of the cornea of his right eye. It had increased so much by the following January that a portion was cut off by Dr. Sawyer, of Bangor, Maine. In May, 1872, the patient applied to Dr. Jeffries, who found a tumor of considerable size, apparently originating from the conjunctiva, covering the external rectus muscle. Vision was good, and no evidence of intra-ocular disease was discovered through the widely dilated pupil ; there was no limitation of the visual field. A small piece was excised, from which the diagnosis of sarcoma was corroborated upon examination by Dr O. F. Wadsworth. A most unfavorable prognosis was given, and the extirpation of the globe, together with the morbid growth, was advised. The operation was done on May 10th, the external canthus being cut down to the bone to facilitate the removal of the muscle and all the conjunctiva. Two thirds of the rectus was excised, and the whole of the tumor. On section of the eyeball through the centre of the cornea, lens, and the length of the muscle, the sclerotic was seen to be thinned beneath the tumor, but not penetrated. [A drawing of the two halves in a fresh state, executed by Dr. H. P. Quincy, was shown.] Despite the unfavorable prognosis entertained, the patient was in perfect health. November 25, 1875, three years and a half after the operation, there had been no return of the disease in the interval, and no positive evidence could be obtained of anything present in the orbit. So large an amount of tissue had been taken from the orbit that the contraction was considerable. The patient reported that he had been entirely free from pain for a year and a half, and had then had a dull aching pain when using the remaining eye. Of these symptoms he was relieved by a convex glass of forty-eight inches focus, to correct his hypermetropia, and a convex glass of fourteen inches focus for reading purposes. The patient considered himself perfectly well, but upon careful questioning admitted that he could not lay his head on the right side without subsequent discomfort, and had experienced at times " a peculiar sort of dizzy feeling, as though objects were receding from him."

An optimist would hardly have dared to prognosticate such a result. The experience of ophthalmic surgeons would not have justified granting the patient more than a year's lease of life, and would have given him no hope of the immunity for three and a half years, which he has enjoyed.

Systolic Murmurs at the Apex of the Heart. — DR. F. I. KNIGHT made the following remarks on the subject : —

" Physicians at the present day generally hesitate to infer the existence of organic valvular disease from the presence of a systolic murmur at the base of the heart, since it is generally recognized that functional disturbance may cause such a murmur. Not so, however, when a systolic murmur is localized at the apex of the heart, as this is supposed by many to be always an indication of mitral regurgitation due to disease of the mitral valve, or at least a sign of some organic change about the mitral valve, even if it does not cause regurgitation.

" Neither of these conditions, however, necessarily exists ; but an apex-systolic murmur may be functional, due either to temporary regurgitation at the mitral orifice, or simply to a change in the tension of the mitral valve.

" Now, how shall we determine whether there is organic disease of the valve such as to permit continued regurgitation? In the first place, we can set it down as certain that we can determine nothing by the intensity of the murmur ; for in many of the most serious valvular affections the heart has not sufficient strength to produce a loud murmur. Its propagation to a considerable distance from the apex, especially as far as the lower angle of the left scapula, is of greater diagnostic importance. But we must rely chiefly upon the signs of enlargement of the heart, especially of the right ventricle with accentuation of the pulmonic second sound.

" If there are no signs of enlargement of the heart, and its sounds retain their proper quality and relative intensity, we have no right to say that mitral regurgitation exists.

" The length of time which has elapsed since an attack of endocarditis, which might cause organic valvular disease, would influence us somewhat in the decision. If the attack was remote, and no signs of enlargement of the heart were present, then we should infer that there was no regurgitation ; but if the attack of endocarditis was recent, then we might feel that sufficient time had not elapsed for us to determine whether changes in the heart would take place or not.

" If, however, we find no proof of actual regurgitation, of the existence of cardiac enlargement, or of change in the heart-sounds, the apex-systolic murmur may still be due to some organic change (roughening and the like) about the ventricular surface of the valve, or rarely to some malformation or injury.

" But it is now well known that in many exhaustive diseases, such as spanæmia, chlorosis, acute rheumatism, the exanthemata, pneumonia, typhoid and typhus fever, apex-systolic murmurs occur which may be transitory, and in cases in which no disease of the mitral valve is found post mortem. This murmur is sometimes called anæmic, but more properly accidental or dynamic. It is at the present time usually attributed either to temporary regurgitation on account of irregular contraction of the papillary muscles, or to a change in tension of the mitral valve, converting a sound into a murmur.

" In some of these cases fatty degeneration of the papillary muscles has been found post mortem, which might cause either temporary regurgitation or alteration of tension in the valve. Bamberger says that he has several times heard the loudest murmurs where there was fatty degeneration of the papillary muscles, and no disease of the mitral valve. But the murmur not infrequently occurs temporarily in cases in which complete recovery takes place, and in which there was evidently no organic change anywhere.[1] Dr. Hayden[2] does not admit the theory of irregular contraction of the papillary muscles, but considers temporary regurgitation to be caused by a yielding of a particular portion of the walls of the ventricle, which changes the direction in which one or both of the papillary muscles act. He objects especially to this theory of irregular contraction of the papillary muscles as applied to cases of apex-systolic murmur in chorea, not only on Kirke's ground that ' there is no good proof that invol-

[1] The cause of this murmur is discussed by DaCosta in an article in the American Journal of the Medical Sciences, July, 1869, page 28.

[2] Diseases of the Heart and Aorta, 1875.

untary muscular organs participate in the choreic disorder, but also because it necessitates rhythmical action of the substance of the heart, and at the same time irregular action of the papillary muscles, which are directly continuous with the fibres of the ventricular walls; *i. e.*, rhythmical contraction of the greater portion of the length of certain muscular fibres, and spasmodic action of the remaining portion. It is not my object to discuss the theories as to the cause of this murmur, but to enforce the necessity of recognizing the possibility and not infrequent occurrence of a functional systolic murmur at the apex of the heart ; but I will say that modern writers (Bamberger, Gerhardt, DaCosta, Dusch) generally mention disordered action of the papillary muscles and change of valve-tension as two most probable causes of it."

Dr. H. I. Bowditch asked what had been the cause of the murmur heard for a while in the patients who had been made to run up and down stairs by Dr. Knight several years ago.

Dr. Knight replied that, at the time, he supposed them to be produced by tricuspid regurgitation, but recent views had referred them to the mitral orifice.

Dr. Bowditch said that the general appearance of the patient, the history of rheumatism, and especially the existence of sounds in the veins were of importance in making a diagnosis ; the *bruit-du-diable* was almost invariably connected with functional murmurs.

Dr. Knight replied that patients with organic disease of the heart might also be anæmic, and consequently have the venous murmur.

Dr. H. J. Barnes instanced a case which he had examined for an insurance company, where the souffle had persisted for eight years.

Dr. Bowditch had once had a patient in whom the murmur was heard only when he was in the recumbent posture.

Fibroma Molluscum. — A patient afflicted with this rare affection was exhibited by Dr. E. Wigglesworth, Jr. ; the full description will be published.

Experience in the Treatment of One Hundred and Fifty Cases of Diphtheria. — The paper was read by Dr. E. Chenery.

Abnormal Mammary Development. — Dr. E. D. Spear, Jr., exhibited the photograph of a man with well-developed mammæ.

Cancer of the Rectum. — Dr. H. J. Barnes stated that at the post-mortem examination of the body of Mr. C. C. Holbrook, made by Dr. Gurnsey, of New York, all the organs were found to be in a healthy state except the rectum ; at about six inches above the anus, there was a cancerous tumor as large as a small cocoa-nut, which almost closed the rectum. The cancer had given rise to an inflammation throughout the lower eighteen inches of the viscus.

Dr. H. W. Williams pointed out that this was the case of *perfect cure of cancerous disease,* on which was chiefly based the wide-spread reputation of a certain notorious quack, who has infested the city for the past few years.

A Battery for Electrolysis was exhibited by Dr. E. Cutter.

Dr. D. F. Lincoln said that he thought the battery needlessly heavy ; that the purposes of electrolysis would be much better served by taking two of the eight plates of zinc, with a corresponding amount of carbon and cutting them into eighteen pieces, which properly disposed in eighteen cells would be much lighter and more effective.

DR. S. G. WEBBER said that the battery as used seemed to have accomplished what was desired, but it could not have acted by electrolysis to any great degree. Many cells and plates of small surface were requisite to obtain that form of electricity. A battery thus constructed has but little heat-producing power, whereas the battery shown was so arranged as to produce heat and have the least possible electrolytic action. In fact, this battery, though possibly safe in such cases as reported, could not be used with safety in other parts of the body, upon other species of growth.

[*Correction by the Secretary.* — Lest the statement made in the report of last month's meeting should be misinterpreted, — that the Obstetrical Society had adopted my view as to the justifiability of the operation reported, — I wish to say that of course the society expressed no opinion as a body. The question was submitted to the members present at the meeting of June 12th, was discussed by two or three gentlemen at the time and by quite a number after the meeting was dissolved, and my proposed course was approved by all of them. — J. R. C.]

THE BOSTON DISPENSARY.

THE seventy-ninth annual report of the Boston Dispensary has appeared. It makes a gratifying showing of the good work this charity continues to do. The number of patients at the central office is not materially greater than during the previous year, but we are glad to see that two at least of the special departments are doing exceedingly well. There have been 2246 cases of skin disease against 1835 for 1874; the dental department also shows a considerable gain.

We regret to see that the financial condition of the dispensary is hardly satisfactory. During the past year the expenses have exceeded the receipts by something more than three thousand dollars. A legacy of two thousand dollars has been received, but the managers very properly are anxious to place it among the invested funds. This want of money is the more to be regretted because the building is inadequate in many respects to the constantly increasing demands. We hope something may be done to supply this excellent institution with means for its work.

It is proper to call attention to two excellent institutions, the Diet Kitchen and the Children's Seashore Home, which supplement the work of the dispensary. We quote from the superintendent's report : —

"The Diet Kitchen is located in Wall Street, and was established through the instrumentality of kind-hearted ladies. The contributions of a generous public have provided for the sick poor a great variety of properly prepared and nutritious food. This has always been ready to be dispensed upon the order of the dispensary physician.

"The relief thus rendered has often been of incalculable value. Properly prepared food is often the great desideratum in the practice of the physician.

The poor are frequently not able to purchase the food necessary for their sustenance when sick, or to have it prepared properly when purchased. The Diet Kitchen furnishes at once the means to administer to such people what is of more service than drugs. . . .

"The Children's Seashore Home, located at Beverly Farms, was established for the purpose of affording the benefits of sea-air, proper food, and good medical care to those poor children met with in dispensary practice whose lives are endangered by those diseases incident to the hot weather in a crowded city, and who are likely to be helped by a short residence at the seaside.

"Through the instrumentality of this worthy charity many a poor child living in the dark and filthy abodes of the city, suffering, and perhaps dying, for the want of free air and sunshine, was removed to the country and saved."

There have been several changes on the staff, which is now as follows:—

Superintendent: Alfred L. Haskins, M. D.

Surgeons: John Homans, M. D., J. Brackett Treadwell, M. D., Thomas Waterman, M. D., Thomas Dwight, Jr., M. D.

Physicians: Frederic I. Knight, M. D., Charles E. Inches, M. D.. J. Franklin Appell, M. D., Robert Disbrow, M. D., Henry Tuck, M. D., William H. H. Hastings, M. D., William E. Boardman, M. D., Charles P. Putnam, M. D., Reginald H. Fitz, M. D., Josiah L. Hale, M. D., William H. Baker, M. D., Orlando W. Doe, M. D., Joseph P. Oliver, M. D., A. Lawrence Mason, M. D., Allen M. Sumner, M. D., George W. Gay, M. D.

Department for Diseases of the Nervous System: Samuel G. Webber, M. D., David F. Lincoln, M. D.

Department for Diseases of the Skin: Francis B. Greenough, M. D.

Dentists: Edward B. Hitchcock, Thomas Bradley.

District Physicians: No. 1. John B. Fulton, M. D. No. 2. Edward J. Moors, M. D. No. 3. Frederic W. Vogel, M. D. No. 4. James B. Ayer, M. D. No. 5. Elbridge G. Cutler, M. D. No. 6. Frederick C. Shattuck, M. D. No. 7. William C. Holyoke, M. D. No. 8. John G. Stanton, M. D.

MEDICAL NOTES.

— One of the results of the late meeting of the American Pharmaceutical Association in this city was the formation of a society for social and charitable purposes, called the Boston Druggists' Association. Mr. Theodore Metcalf is the first president.

— D. Luther, M. D., in an article in the *Philadelphia Medical Times* of November 27, 1875, suggests the employment of soluble glass in hospital construction. In the building and arrangement of institutions particularly those for the insane who exercise little control over the urinary or intestinal discharges, no system of ventilation or arrangement of the apartments occupied by such patients, whether of wood, painted or oiled, or with floors of slate, metal, or cement, has been sufficient to effect entire cleanliness. A material having an entire absence of absorbing surface would seem to meet the demand in such cases, and glass is such a material. The walls, floors, and ceilings might be covered with it. It is not expensive, is strong when sufficiently thick, is impervious to water and dampness, and can be made of suitable color. Apartments thus fitted up could be thoroughly drenched with water so as to remove every particle of fœtid matter. The floors could be made comfortable by covering them with rubber cloth, which with the bedding could be easily removed and cleansed.

— At a recent meeting of the French Association for the Advancement of Science, as reported in *Le Progrès Médical* of September 4, 1875, M. Viaud-Grandmarais presented a communication upon the bites of vipers in the departments of Lower Loire and Vendée. It has recently been denied that the sting of the viper can cause death in man. M. Viaud has knowledge of three hundred and sixty-two authentic cases in which men have been bitten by vipers, and of these sixty-three have been fatal. All vipers are not equally dangerous. He estimates that one or two people in Vendée and one in Lower Loire die annually from their bite. Happily the number of persons bitten is year by year diminishing, as the wastes and thickets are reclaimed by cultivation. Death has occurred in both sexes, and at all ages, but especially among adult males. On the other hand, M. Viaud has seen an infant of ten months recover from the bite of the reptile. Ten times he has known death to occur within twenty-four hours; never in less than an hour after the accident. Death, too, occurs at the end of one week, or of three weeks, or it may be after several months, under the influence of a kind of cachexia. In those who have died, neither suction nor cauterization has been immediately practiced; while, on the contrary, ammonia has nearly always been employed. When death supervenes rapidly it may be due to syncope, to insufficient reaction, to general œdema, or to a sort of pneumonia. Death in the course of the first week is due to insufficient reaction or to a kind of typhoid state. M. Viaud has never known death to result from external hæmorrhage; on the contrary, by expelling the poison hæmorrhage has saved the patient. Hæmorrhage occurs from the secretory organs, from the kidneys and intestines in dogs, by the milk in cows. It is a somewhat remarkable fact that if the exposed·mesentery of an animal is injected with a drop of the venom of the viper a slight hæmorrhage is seen to follow, but if having been wiped softly the mesentery is examined with the microscope, no rupture of a blood-vessel can be found. Besides hæmorrhages, abundant excretion of urine and vomitings are favorable. The intimate action of the poison is not known. The primary local lesions may occur very distant from the part bitten. In a case of bite near the external malleolus M. Viaud has seen these lesions to begin at the side of the larynx and pharynx. Harford has attempted to account for the phenomena of the poisoning by the development of peculiar corpuscles analogous to the white globules. Neither Weir Mitchell, a competent authority, nor M. Viaud himself has found such corpuscles. The paper closed with the important statement that not one of the patients in whom immediate suction of the wound had been practiced had died. In some there had not been the slightest sickness. Moreover, the sucking of the wound was perfectly innocuous to the one who performed it. The writer had not been able to notice what some have affirmed, a burning or other taste to the venom pressed from the wound.

— The following emanated from a " spiritual physician" after an examination of a lock of the patient's hair : —

MARBLEHEAD, *July* 12, 1875.

Examination of Mrs. ——.

There is a bilious torpid state of the liver, an over secretion of gall fluid. This mingles with the bile and leaks into the stomach upon which is fever coating. This retards digestion and agitates the nervious system. Too much internal slow fever habit obstructions at the kidneys sediment in the bladder.

Perscription.

½ oz Chamomile Flowers
½ " Pleurisy Root
½ " Hyssop
⅛ " Saffron
Steep in 1 qt water reduce ¼ strain add ½ oz spts nitre.
Dose 2 tablespoonfuls sweeten take ½ hour before eating 3 times a day.
2 oz Fld Ext Buchu
½ " Ess Spearmint
Dose 1 teaspoonful in ¼ gill water, sweeten, take every eveing.

Yours &c

— According to L' *Union Médicale*, for the first time since the creation a census of India has been taken. It is found that India, with the English provinces and their dependencies, contains 256,830,958 souls, a population equal to that of all Europe. Each square mile contains on an average 211 inhabitants. The largest city is Calcutta, which, with its suburbs, has 895,000 inhabitants. Bombay has 644,000 ; Madras, 398,000 ; Lucknow, 285,000. Reckoning according to their religions there are in round numbers 140,500,000 Hindoos ; 40,750,000 Mohammedans ; 9,500,000 Buddhists, Jews, and Parsees. The religion of the remainder has not been ascertained. The Christians number 900,000, of whom 250,000 are Europeans and 650,000 natives. Twenty-three different languages are spoken in India. In the western provinces there are at least three hundred castes; in Bengal about one thousand. In the service of the government, including the native establishments, there are computed to be 1,236,000 ; 629,000 — of whom 849 are missionaries — are supported by religious establishments. There are 30,000 religious mendicants, 10,000 astrologers, 5 sorcerers, 465 exorcists, 518 poets, 1 orator, 33,000 jurists, 75,000 physicians, 218,000 artists, among whom are reckoned acrobats, serpent charmers, etc. Other statistics are given as to the number of agriculturists, drivers of elephants, camels, etc., and of thieves, highway robbers, vagabonds, etc.

— Mr. Oliver Pemberton (*British Medical Journal*, October 30, 1875) recently tied the common femoral an inch below Poupart's ligament, on a patient with femoral aneurism. He used an ordinary antiseptically prepared catgut ligature, tying the vessel by a single loop, and finishing by a double one. The ends were cut off short, and the wound closed. The contents of the aneurismal sac remained fluid for a long time ; and it was not until nearly three months had elapsed that everything was absorbed and the limb restored.

Neither at the operation nor subsequently did he follow out the antiseptic method of treating the wound ; that healed in the ordinary way by suppuration and gradual repair.   His object was to permanently close the artery at a given point without cutting it through ; and this was effectually and safely accomplished, even in the midst of suppuration.

He says, " The principle involved in tying arteries in their continuity by means of animal ligatures may be still on its trial ; but I will be bold enough to assert ' that the fate or behavior of a given antiseptic catgut ligature, applied to the continuity of an artery,' will yet be foretold with confidence as to the favorable result.   And in this I appear to be more sanguine than Mr. Maunder states himself to be in his recent Lettsomian Lectures on the Surgery of the Arteries."

— In a recent murder trial in London which has excited intense interest, the question as to whether the deceased had ever been pregnant came up, the only means of deciding being the condition of the partially decomposed uterus. Mr. Bond and Dr. Meadows came to opposite opinions, and the latter presented it before the Royal Obstetrical Society.   According to *The Lancet* the organ measured at the fundus one inch and three quarters in width, the canal was two inches and a half in length, and the uterine walls of unusual thinness, one measuring rather less and the other rather more than a quarter of an inch in thickness.   The os uteri had been injured and its character destroyed, by post-mortem examination, to such a degree as to render it impossible to discover its original condition.   The inner surface of the organ presented a convex appearance, an appearance generally met with in the virgin, but not believed to exist in a uterus which has been gravid.   From these characters Dr. Meadows thought it impossible to form a positive decision with regard to the existence of a previous pregnancy, though he was inclined to the opinion that the organ was nulliparous.   Owing to the scientific as well as public interest of the point in question, the discussion of the paper was postponed until the next meeting of the society, to be held in January.

The trial is of interest in many other respects, as it involved the identification of a body, with the various questions of height, age, length of time of exposure, modus operandi of decomposition, etc.   The question of murder or suicide also came before the anatomical experts, who appear to have gained great credit by their skill, which led to the conviction of the accused.   We hope on another occasion to give further details of this very interesting case.

— The superintendents of the New England institutions for the insane have taken a new departure by the formation of a local organization, the New England Psychological Society, which it is believed will result in mutual improvement, increased usefulness of the institutions under their charge, and the advance of the interests of the insane.

The first movement in the matter was made by Dr. B. D. Eastman, Superintendent of the Worcester Lunatic Hospital, whose overtures met with such unanimous and hearty approval that the success of the enterprise was at once assured.   The first meeting, that for organization, was held at Worcester, December 14th.   Pliny Earle, M. D., Superintendent of the Northampton Lunatic Hospital, was chosen president, John E. Tyler, M. D., formerly Superintendent of the McLean Asylum, vice-president, and B. D. Eastman, Superintendent of the Worcester Lunatic Hospital, secretary and treasurer. Meetings are to be held quarterly, the next at Worcester on the third Tuesday of March, 1876.

MEDICAL HANGERS-ON.

MESSRS. EDITORS, — The object of this note is to call the attention of the profession to an imposition that is perpetrated on us at the office of the State Board of Charities at 30 Pemberton Square. Over a year ago I was called by a medical man to examine a patient for admission to the asylum for the insane. On the following day we proceeded to the office, then in City Hall. There we were met by a certain middle-aged physician, who had the papers all ready ; he had, as he stated, examined the patient at the request of her friends. My services were, of course, dispensed with.

A short time ago I went on a similar case. Again we were met by this gentleman, who had examined the patient. We told him on this occasion that his services were unnecessary. Other medical men have been imposed on as above. It would seem as if some medical gentlemen hang about this office, and are zealous to have their names down in these cases for the sake of the fee, which is $3.60.   Very respectfully,   M. D.

WEEKLY BULLETIN OF PREVALENT DISEASES.

THE following is a bulletin of the diseases prevalent in Massachusetts during the week ending December 18, 1875, compiled under the authority of the State Board of Health from the returns of physicians representing all sections of the State : —

The summary for each section is as follows : —

Berkshire ; Bronchitis, pneumonia, rheumatism.

Valley : Pneumonia, influenza, bronchitis, diphtheria. Springfield, Hadley, and Holyoke report diphtheria as unusually prevalent.

Midland : Bronchitis, influenza, pneumonia, rheumatism, diphtheria. More sickness reported.

Northeastern : Bronchitis, scarlatina, influenza, pneumonia, rheumatism. More sickness, especially scarlatina and diphtheria, reported.

Metropolitan ; Bronchitis, pneumonia, diphtheria, scarlatina. More diphtheria and scarlatina reported.

Southeastern : Bronchitis, influenza, rheumatism, pneumonia.

The order of relative prevalence for the State at large is bronchitis, pneumonia, rheumatism, influenza, scarlatina, diphtheria, typhoid fever, croup, measles, whooping-cough.   F. W. DRAPER, M. D., Registrar.

COMPARATIVE MORTALITY-RATES FOR THE WEEK ENDING DEC. 11, 1875.

	Estimated Population.	Total Mortality for the Week.	Annual Death-Rate per 1000 during Week
New York	1,060,000	539	26
Philadelphia	800,000	312	20
Brooklyn	500,000	248	25
Chicago	400,000	130	17
Boston	342,000	169	26
Cincinnati	260,000		
Providence	100,700	31	16
Worcester	50,000	18	19
Lowell	50,000	18	19
Cambridge . . .	48,000	20	22
Fall River	45,000	19	22
Lawrence	35,000	6	9
Lynn	33,000	11	17
Springfield	31,000		
Salem	26,000	20	40

Normal Death-Rate, 17 per 1000.

BOOKS AND PAMPHLETS RECEIVED. — The Popular Health Almanac for 1876. Edited by Frederick Hoffmann. New York : E. Steiger.

The Cholera Epidemic of 1873 in the United States. Washington. 1875. .(From the Hon. Henry L. Pierce.)

THE BOSTON
MEDICAL AND SURGICAL JOURNAL.

VOL. XCIII. — THURSDAY, DECEMBER 30, 1875. — NO. 27.

LIMITED RESPONSIBILITY.[1]

A DISCUSSION OF THE POMEROY CASE.

BY CHARLES F. FOLSOM, M. D.

In speaking of the duty of the expert who is called upon to testify as to the insanity of any individual who has committed a crime, Conolly says, " His business is to declare the truth ; society must deal with the truth as it pleases." Westphal, Meynert, and Maudsley have reiterated this opinion, and, keeping it in mind, I purpose discussing briefly the case of Jesse Pomeroy, convicted of murder by a Massachusetts jury, and sentenced to be hanged.

Either the boy is insane or he is not ; and he cannot be said to have something of this disease and something of that, and some of the symptoms of still a third ; but his malady, if such it be, must be one of the well-recognized forms of mental disease ; that is, just as in any other diseased condition, the first step is to make an exact diagnosis. Of these manifold forms of disease, there are only five which, as far as I know, have been considered as the morbid processes under which Pomeroy was acting when he committed murder, and these are —

(1.) Delusional insanity. (2.) Insanity from masturbation. (3.) Epileptiform insanity. (4.) Moral insanity. (5). Moral imbecility.

The first is the commonest form of disease under which crimes are committed. In well-marked cases the diagnosis is so easy that any one may make it, while in mild cases it is often so difficult as to baffle the most expert alienist for weeks, inasmuch as a shrewd and intelligent man may effectually conceal his delusions for a long time. Such people are generally able to control themselves to a considerable degree, and often when the disease is quite pronounced ; that is, under ordinary circumstances, with ordinary inducements, they can resist ordinary impulses. A cigar after dinner, or a glass of wine, may be sufficient to restrain one of them from smashing his windows or throwing chairs at his physician's head ; but suppose that a strong inducement to crime comes when he has an excellent opportunity of getting what he con-

[1] Read before the Health Department of the Social Science Association and the Suffolk District Medical Society, Boston, December 16 and 18, 1875.

siders a great advantage to himself at only the cost of killing another man, his self-control is a mere nothing. Sometimes these patients recognize and acknowledge the fact that murder is wrong for them and for all people; sometimes, and that more commonly, they think that it is wrong in the abstract, but that there are special circumstances which make it right for them.

I can call to mind a number of such men, who used to say that they were insane, and not responsible before the law, and that they should therefore commit such and such acts of violence, which they would proceed at once to do. Three of these patients — a physician, a naval officer, and a merchant — I have reason to remember quite well; and a gentleman formerly in the McLean Asylum, using this argument, once made a deadly assault on the late Dr. Bell, who fortunately escaped with only a scalp wound.

Again, the moral sense is often so keen, and the intellect so clear, with many of them, that they will take great precautions so as not to allow their delusions to get the upper hand of them. A gentleman far advanced in convalescence once, while eating his dinner, threw his knife and fork violently through the window, and then calmly turned around to my friend standing at his side, and said, " I wanted to kill you, and I should have done it if I had n't thrown them out of the window."

It is especially with reference to this class of the insane that the remark has been made that people do not cease to be men and women in becoming insane. There can be no doubt, and it is quite well acknowledged, that patients with delusional insanity do sometimes commit acts of violence from the same motives which actuate ordinary criminals, and with sufficient power of self-control to have restrained them. I know, however, of only one case where experts have held this opinion in court. Nevertheless, it is almost without exception beyond the power of human insight to say in what cases they act in virtue of their insanity and in what they do not; and therefore, once granted that any insane individual has definite delusions, I think that there must be very few physicians who have seen much of the disease, who would under any circumstances hold him fully responsible for a crime which he may have committed.

The idea that Pomeroy may be suffering from delusional insanity has now been quite generally abandoned. No delusions have been found, and a person of his limited intelligence could not have concealed them had they existed.

The case of Blampied was one of this kind. He was discharged, as recovered, from an insane asylum upon the certificates of four experts, of whom three were officers of the asylum, and the fourth was in practice in the town where Blampied lived.

At his trial for a murder which he committed some years after leaving the asylum, and apparently from ordinary motives, no expert testimony was called.

The superintendent whose patient Blampied had formerly been, gave his written opinion as to his recovery, complaining of that very fact, that no expert opinion had been asked during the trial, and stating that Blampied should be hung, not as an insane though responsible man, but as a sane and responsible one ; and so far he seems to me to be right.

To make his position stronger, he also said that even in the asylum, Blampied never belonged to that class of the insane who lose their self-control to a great degree, which was perfectly true. His opinion also was that if Blampied had committed a murder while there, he would have been properly held fully responsible. In that I cannot agree with him. My only object in citing the case originally was to show that there are alienists who think that the doctrine of non-responsibility has been pushed too far.

Not very long ago, Mr. J., an insane Scotch clergyman, attempted to commit rape upon a young maid, and afterward on a young lady. Two of the first authorities in Scotland testified in court that the gentleman was suffering from well-marked mental disease, that he knew that the acts which he had attempted were wrong, that he had sufficient self-control to have restrained him from so doing, and that there was no reason why the law should hold him to a limited degree of responsibility in these cases.

On May 21, 1873, Mr. Lutwidge, while visiting one of the asylums of England, in discharge of his duty as one of the commissioners in lunacy, was struck on the right temple by a patient, with a nail. He died from the effects of the injury a week later. I quote the following passage from the official report [1] published a year after Mr. Lutwidge's death. In speaking of the patient, the commission, composed of three physicians and three lawyers, say, " He was well known to those members of our board who from time to time during that period had visited the asylum where he was confined. . . . Those of our number who, as just mentioned, knew the man, describe him . as being a person of a weak, imperfectly developed intellect, but they agree in considering that he was quite responsible for his actions."

Last September, a patient in one of the large asylums of England killed an attendant against whom' he had long had a grudge. He stabbed him in the back with a table-knife. The superintendent of the asylum and several other alienists have maintained his responsibility for the act. They say that the insane hear of such cases as the unfortunate one of Mr. Lutwidge, and become emboldened to commit crimes which they would not think of, provided they did not know that the law

[1] Twenty-Eighth Report of the Commissioners in Lunacy for England, page 2.

would hold them irresponsible. This opinion, of course, is open to criticism.

As to the second head, masturbation is common in the insane, and is one of the many symptoms of loss of self-control and self-respect. As a *cause* of insanity it is rare, so rare that many doubt its existence. The prognosis is generally about as unfavorable as it well can be, and the disease is progressive, that is to say, dullness, moroseness, ill-temper, and suspicion are followed very rapidly by loss of memory, considerable diminution of the intellect, and some loss of flesh, not infrequently emaciation. Such patients complain of headache, a symptom to which I do not generally attach much importance, as I find it so common, especially in boys who attend school in badly-ventilated buildings. The characteristic symptoms of this disease are certainly not found in Pomeroy.

In these cases, too, there is not often difficulty in ascertaining the fact. Often the patient will use his thighs, if his hands are tied. I should doubt the existence of this form of disease in all cases where there was any possibility of the existence of a doubt as to the habit. When it is actually persisted in to such a degree as to cause insanity, the victim has lost self-respect and self-control in too great a degree to render concealment possible. We all know how common this vice is in prisons, in reform-schools, in industrial-schools, etc. We seldom see insanity come from it.

As to the third form, Maudsley states that in epileptiform insanity the sufferer is just as unable to control himself as is the man who tumbles to the floor in tonic and clonic convulsions, and justly says that it would be as fair to punish the one as the other. Pomeroy, however, has been perfectly able to control himself while under observation at the reform-school and at the jail. Yes, more, the presence of a third person has always been sufficient to restrain him from committing crimes or acts of cruelty.

I do not think, either, that the amount of deliberation and calculation shown by him is compatible with the diagnosis of epileptiform insanity, although it would not invalidate the diagnosis of other forms of mental disease ; and I should say that, in this case, the absence of forgetfulness is a symptom which is of considerable importance. Finally, epilepsy in all its forms, in the immense majority of cases, especially where there is no medical treatment, is progressive. If anything, the contrary is true with Pomeroy.

Fourthly, the discussion of moral insanity is comparatively simple. Pomeroy does not deny that he knows that the acts committed by him were wrong ; and I do not suppose that any one will maintain that he lost his knowledge of right and wrong just when he committed the murders, and at no other times. This question resolves itself, then, into the inquiry whether he was acting from a temporary impulse against which he was powerless to contend. This is a well-recognized morbid condition, both as a disease and as a stage of disease, and that too while the intellect remains perfectly clear. It has been described again and again from Pinel's day down. The Germans say that the patient acts from a *Trieb*, that is, from something which drives him on, in spite of himself. People who know that it is wrong to lie, and who are most conscientious and upright when well, will fabricate the basest falsehoods; others will steal, and others will commit acts of violence. These impulses are, by no means as uncommon as most people would suppose. Fortunately for society, the three conditions necessary for the commission of crime under them — the impulse, the opportunity, and the lack of self-control — do not very often coincide in point of time. A milder form of this morbid condition, the homicidal idea, or the idea of doing wrong generally, is very far from being uncommon.

Alienists, especially those with what Herbert Spencer calls the theological bias, have denied the existence of moral insanity, but all must acknowledge that the brain is necessary for all intellectual and emotional manifestations; and it is only a step further to the position that a variety of organs are necessary for a variety of manifestations. Given these various organs, of course any one of them may be diseased, while the others remain sound. It is tolerably certain that different ganglionic cells in the spinal cord have different functions; and many clinical observations, especially the symptom aphasia, make the same fact more than probable with regard to the brain. At all events, the authority of Pinel, Marc, Ray, Maudsley, Tuke, Bucknill, Morel, Esquirol, and many others is conclusive on this point.

I saw not long ago a man with this disease. He had killed his superior officer. In prison (he was too powerful to be in an asylum), he had stabbed one fellow-prisoner, had bitten off the lip of another, and had tried to kill his physician by throwing a heavy stool at his head, and at all these times when the odds were entirely against him, as there were plenty of officers about. I think that this form of disease must be excluded in Pomeroy's case for the following reasons : —

(1.) There was too much premeditation in the acts committed by him.

(2.) The boy could exercise self-control while under observation.

(3.) There was a motive in his acts, in his love of torturing ; for I do not think that he ever meant to murder ; and experience had taught him that up to that time, at least, he could enjoy his horrible sport without undergoing anything that was really punishment to him.

Cases of moral insanity get into asylums for the insane, but neither confinement there nor punishment (which latter has usually been first tried at home) ordinarily does any good. If the patient cannot steal anything he likes, he will steal at least *something ;* if he cannot attack a boy, he will make an attack upon an attendant.

Fifthly, I have for the sake of definiteness considered moral insanity and moral imbecility separately, although they are commonly confounded. Dr. Ray discriminates carefully between the two. I suppose the latter of the two terms in a certain sense covers the meaning of the gentlemen who think that Pomeroy is weak-minded.

Moral imbecility may affect the intellect also, and exist in every degree up to complete idiocy, the only form of insanity that is at all common before puberty. In fact, as Maudsley says, even mania so early in life may be generally described rather as excited idiocy.

Every child (to take an extreme case) recognizes the mimetic creature of a spinal cord and cerebellum who kills a baby because he has just seen a butcher kill a calf, and without being able to see any difference between the degrees of criminality of the two acts.

Jesse Pomeroy, unlike an idiot or an imbecile, seems to me a boy who has had his wits sharpened by contact with the many people who have examined him, and who has shown a considerable degree of skill in his attempts to make his case a plausible one for executive clemency.

Dr. Ray describes the moral imbecile as torturing children from the same motive which makes a cat torture a mouse before killing it. He does not know that his acts are wrong, and he does not forget them. Like the cat, to continue the comparison, he makes no attempts at concealment and feels no remorse. Cat-like, too, he will sometimes direct attention to what he has done.

Granting, however, for the sake of the argument, that Pomeroy is not responsible, the position does not seem to me at all tenable that his confessions and retractions and contradictions merely embody the uncertain and incoherent ideas of an insane person. If such were the case, they would be indications of so great disorder of the intellect that the insanity would not fail to be easily apparent ; for these symptoms, like cough and night-sweats and emaciation, are evidences of well-marked disease.

At best, I do not see how the boy can be called anything more than weak-minded. This term I should use as being in a measure synonymous with moral imbecility, differing from it in degree only. I should not, however, consider it as an initial stage of that disease, nor should I hold that it indicates sufficient deviation from the normal type to place the sufferer from it outside of the pale of ordinary criminals. Of course he is weak-minded ; every criminal is weak-minded, every man is weak-minded who deliberately places himself in opposition to any well-organized society. Any one else must know that in the long run it does not pay. The question for us to decide is whether Pomeroy is any more weak-minded than the whole criminal class.

No one can doubt that disease and crime are closely allied. The criminals with insane and consumptive parents, and the many who themselves become insane or consumptive, must alone convince us of the fact. In the cells of the penitentiary one will see the imperfectly developed ear, first pointed out by Darwin as a mark of inferior organization, as often as he will in Westphal's wards in the Charité.

Dr. Manning in his Report on Lunacy (page 221) says, " At Millbank and Perth prisons, special wards are set apart for epileptic and weak-minded criminals. The former require some extra watching ; and the prison routine, especially where isolation is practiced, is thought to conduce to absolute insanity in the latter. Both classes are, therefore, kept apart from the ordinary prisoners, in large, well-ventilated wards ; work, eat, and drink in common, and sleep either in cells or dormitories, as seems most fit. The number of these cases at Millbank (1868) is nearly two hundred," that is, nearly one sixth of the whole.

Last September, in the famous Millbank prison there were sixteen suicidal convicts who required watching day and night, and three more were so desperately bent on self-destruction that they were kept in padded rooms. It must be borne in mind in this connection that there is in England, as there is also in Scotland, a special asylum for the criminal insane.

Weak-minded people abound everywhere. As boys, they run away from home or from school, and do a host of things that vex the saint and puzzle the psychologist. As men, they perhaps have abundant energy but lack steadfastness and definiteness of purpose, or they fail to carry out plans well laid, for want of perseverance and ability to make the necessary continuous effort. Society says that they have been failures, but they are just the people who, if they fail to get the healthy influences of sound educations, form our criminal class.

In boyhood, punishment sometimes cures them ; in youth, if they are sent to insane asylums, that often cures them because it is simply a punishment, and they regard it as such ; if their friends, too, tell them plainly that they can have their liberty as long as they behave well, but no longer. We may not expect the club-footed boy to run, but he can stand or walk, and may strike out from his shoulder a blow that will knock you down.

I suppose that it is under this head that Pomeroy's attempt to escape from the prison is described, as one not showing much judgment, and as being one such as is often seen in insane asylums. It is worth while to stop a moment and consider this statement ; Pomeroy's plans were as well laid and as judiciously carried out as the average of such attempts in the State Prison at Charlestown, the immense majority of which have ended in just as signal failure.

Lately, three men have tried to escape from the prison where Pomeroy would be confined if sentenced for life, and in the face of what are ordinarily called impossibilities. One broke his thigh after jumping twenty-six feet from a roof of one of the work-shops to the prison wall, and was captured after rolling over and over some rods away ; the second was taken after a short run ; the third escaped entirely.

A gentleman of Boston, not a physician but a sound psychologist, saw Pomeroy in his cell. Upon being asked whether he should commit murder if allowed to go out, the boy said, in a swaggering way, " Oh, I don't know ; I could n't say whether I would or not." In reply to a question concerning what he was in the habit of reading, he said, in the same manner, " Oh, I like the blood-and-thunder stories in the newspapers better than anything." When visited by a member of the Board of State Charities, who has been familiar with his history for several years, he said, " I suppose I did these things — they say I did," although at other times he made no pretense to any forgetfulness. My ideas of a moral imbecile are certainly something very different from this.

I cannot see, then, that there is any evidence of Pomeroy's insanity, except in the horrible character alone of the crimes which he committed. This has been somewhat insisted upon in his case ; but alone, without other symptoms, it is really no evidence of insanity whatever. If we allowed it to be such, we should, as Westphal well says, be only opening the door to excuse every criminal.

The absence of remorse, too, has been considered a strong argument in favor of the boy's insanity ; but that could not be insisted upon by one who had spent much time in prisons. General Chamberlain states that remorse is an unusual emotion among convicts, except with that class of them who have committed crimes from impulse, while under strong temptation, or under the influence of alcoholic liquor, etc. The same observations have been made by others.

Jesse Pomeroy, then, it seems to me, is responsible for the crimes which he committed ; not as fully responsible as you and I would be, but yet responsible before the law. In fact, if we could measure nicely, no two of us would probably be found who could justly be held to precisely the same degree of responsibility.

And here I would say one word as to the object of punishment. Of course, the first idea was revenge ; the next was a step higher, and is generally called justice : " an eye for an eye, and a tooth for a tooth." But with the thinking classes, who have been again and again disappointed in their hope to see some reformatory method successful enough to become general, and who judge dispassionately, the real motive in punishment of criminals is the protection of society.

Leaving out the general question of the advisability of capital punishment as not belonging here, is it fair to suppose that anything else than death will protect society from such a monster as Pomeroy, when the chances of escape from prison are so many, and when we know that out of 266 men sentenced to imprisonment for life at Charlestown from 1828 to 1875, 135 have been pardoned ? From the adoption of the constitution in 1780 to the year 1875, 137 persons have been convicted of capital offenses in the Supreme Court of Massachusetts; of whom 76 were executed, 25 were pardoned, 34 had sentences commuted, and 2 died in prison.

I have not seen the accounts of the horrible deeds recently committed, and quoted at a late meeting of one of our medical societies, and I have not had the time to investigate and consider them carefully enough to form opinions in regard to them. I should not, however, consider it safe to base my diagnosis upon the accounts in the daily papers.

It seems to me, too, that the average bad boy does fully as wrong things as to throw stones at his mother and then tell her that he is sorry for it.

I read in the London *Times* a few weeks ago an account copied from the St. Louis *Globe* of the trial of a midwife who delivered women and " disposed of" their babies. She was in the habit, as shown by indisputable evidence, of throwing the infants, dead or alive, into a stove and burning them up. What possible motive, you may say, could such a wretch have in killing with so much cruelty, when it was just as easy to do it without inflicting pain or causing suffering ?

Crimes of a horrible character have been fearfully frequent of late, especially in Italy and the United States, in both of which countries punishment for crime has become lamentably uncertain. I think that this terrible danger to society can be removed ; but, to quote the words of one of the first alienists now living, it is necessary in order to do it to hang some of these murderers.

After having tried all sorts of treatment for criminals, the so-called " humane " and others, England has finally settled upon the " stern and deterrent system " approved by Chief Justice Sir Alexander Cockburn as the best ; and, according to Major Du Cane, Inspector-General of Prisons, it has already begun to have its effect in reducing the number of commitments for crime. I fully believe that the stern treatment would have upon boys of Pomeroy's class the same effect which the return to the use of the lash on the bare back had on the garroters of London.

Among the experts who have seen Pomeroy, and consider him irresponsible, there are two opinions on this point : —

(1.) That punishment would have no effect upon him or upon others of his class.

(2.) That punishment would deter them from crime, but that the same thing might also be said of a considerable proportion of the inmates of our insane asylums.

A CASE OF PELVIC HÆMATOCELE.

BY F. GORDON MORRILL, M. D., OF BOSTON.

NOVEMBER 6, 1874, I was asked to see Mrs. F. C., twenty-four years old, whose previous history was as follows : —

She had been married two years, and her previous health had been good until the commencement of her present trouble. Her only child had died of uncontrollable epistaxis about a year before. On the 6th of the preceding month menstruation (which had been perfectly normal) was followed by a purulent discharge, of offensive odor. She positively denied having ever miscarried, or having been at all subject to menstrual irregularities. On October 25th the discharge ceased, and an attack of dysentery followed, which lasted a week. November 3d she ventured out, and menstruation (or something which resembled it) came on while she was in the street; it ceased immediately after she arrived at home. Very shortly after this she began to suffer from intense pain in the abdomen, which continued with occasional intermissions up to the date of my first visit.

I found my patient in bed, with her body bent forward; she was flowing slightly. Aside from tenderness on pressure over the lower part of the abdomen, nothing abnormal was discovered after careful examination. The usual treatment for suppressed menstruation was advised, with morphine to relieve her pain.

November 7th. The flow was slightly increased, and the pain continued when it was not controlled by morphine.

November 8th. I was summoned in haste, and found the patient in a state of collapse : the pulse weak and intermittent, the respiration sighing, the extremities cold, and the countenance of a death-like pallor. From this condition she rallied under the influence of stimulants and hot outward applications. Another examination was made, and nothing was discovered which furnished the slightest clew to the cause of her alarming condition, although I strongly suspected what afterwards proved to be the true nature of her trouble. She was still flowing slightly, and this continued until the 18th, when a tampon was inserted, and tinctura ferri chloridi and fluid extract of ergot were prescribed.

December 8th. The tampon had been used three times since the preceding date, but with very poor success, the flow returning in each instance within three or four days after removing the sponges. A sponge-tent was now inserted.

December 9th. The finger could be readily passed up to the fundus of the uterus, which was empty. No particularly tender spot was discovered in the vagina. No swelling of any kind existed. The pain in the abdomen had continued, with occasional intermissions, since the commencement of her sickness.

December 10th. Since the preceding day a rounded tumor had appeared in the left iliac region, about the size of a large apple. It was solid to the touch, and flat on percussion. Dr. Minot was called in consultation, and a sound was passed into the uterus. Its point could be distinctly felt by the hand placed upon the tumor, when the handle was depressed. The sound entered four and a half inches. Behind the cervix an elastic egg-shaped swelling was detected, its long diameter being lateral.

December 22d. Since the last report the swelling behind the cervix had doubled in size, and the os uteri was crowded forward and flattened against the pubic bones. Externally there was a very large and ill-defined tumor. Since the 9th very little flow had been present, but a purulent discharge had taken its place. Meanwhile the patient had lost strength, in spite of supporting treatment and the administration of internal astringents.

December 27th. Nothing like fluctuation had been detected, but from the history and rapid increase of the swelling, its fluid nature was strongly suspected. Much difficulty was experienced in expelling the contents of both the bladder and the rectum, and operative measures were decided upon.

December 28th. Drs. Minot and Bixby in consultation. The tumor, which had now descended below the os uteri and occupied the entire vagina, was first punctured with an exploring needle, and then (the diagnosis being confirmed) quite a free incision was made, giving exit to about a pint of bloody serum and a few pretty firmly organized clots.

The patient rallied well from the operation, and the cavity was washed out twice daily with a solution of carbolic acid in strong castile soapsuds, which was injected by means of a fountain-syringe with a double nozzle. At first the discharge consisted of clots and serum only, but it soon assumed a purulent type. After January 16th no clots appeared, and the injection (now changed to a solution of permanganate of potash) was given but once daily. After this time the wound was kept open by daily dilatation. The original depth of the cavity was about six inches.

February 3d. The cavity was now but one and a half inches deep, and the discharge consisted of serum only ; the wound was allowed to close. Meanwhile the patient had steadily improved under tonics and stimulants. On February 4th menstruation occurred, all the attending phenomena being perfectly normal. The patient has enjoyed perfect health up to the present time.

The chief point of interest in this case is the obscurity of the symptoms, no tumor being present until thirty-three days after what had seemed unmistakable signs of internal hæmorrhage. The difficulty in making a positive diagnosis was still further increased by the suspicion that an abortion had been produced, — the purulent discharge following menstruation (?) in October, succeeded by an attack of dysentery, which could very well have been caused by some drug given to excite uterine action (oleum sabinæ, for instance), rendering the suspicion justifiable, notwithstanding the patient's positive denial when questioned.

AN INSTRUMENT DESIGNED FOR THE TREATMENT OF UTERINE CATARRH.

BY CHARLES L. PIERCE, M. D.

In the treatment of catarrhal inflammation of the uterine cavity, a very efficient means of relief and in many cases of radical cure is lost to the general practitioner on account of the dangers that have attended its use. Indeed, the practice of injecting medicated fluids into the cavity of the uterus has so often been followed by such alarming and fatal results that we find our best writers on diseases of women, while acknowledging the good that might otherwise be derived from it, hedging the operation about with so many warnings of danger that only the expert gynæcologist would dare resort to it. Thus, Thomas says that he strongly recommends the general practitioner who is unfamiliar with the treatment of uterine disorders to avoid its use entirely, except in cases of uncontrollable hæmorrhage in which the cervix is well dilated and no flexure of the uterus exists.

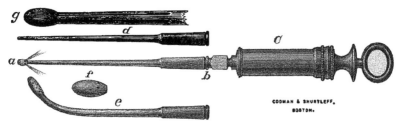

It is generally conceded that the disastrous consequences resulting from injecting the uterus are mainly due to the retention of the fluid within its cavity. For, when the cervix is well dilated and there is no considerable flexure of the organ to interfere with the rapid escape of the fluid, the uterus may be injected, not only without danger, but with benefit. It follows, then, that any device that will facilitate or, better still, render certain the escape of the injected fluid is worthy of consideration.

The instrument represented by the accompanying wood-cut has, with me, proved a most valuable resource in the treatment of chronic metritis, and as such I commend it to the profession. The engraving shows a long pipe (a) attached by a friction plug-joint (b) to a small piston-syringe. This pipe terminates in an expanded bulb, and is grooved on four sides, as shown at (g), which represents the exact size of a part of the tube. The bulb is pierced obliquely on its sides, and may be unscrewed from the pipe and a larger bulb adjusted if desired.

When a fluid is forced from the syringe through the pipe it escapes through the small openings of the bulb, and flows obliquely backward toward the operator. The bulb slightly dilates the passage, while the grooves favor an immediate escape of the fluid, thus enabling us to give a true intra-uterine douche. The remedy that has given me the most satisfactory results in these cases is the distilled extract of Hamamelis Virginica, used without dilution, once a day. With this instrument and this remedy I have cured cases that have long resisted the usual methods of treatment.

The other pipes figured in the cut are intended for other purposes. The tube (c), having a sharper curve than is here represented, is for sprinkling the posterior nares. The instrument (made for me by Codman and Shurtleff, of Boston) is entirely of hard rubber, and the pipes may be bent to any desired curve by carefully heating them. The device is simple, compact, comprehensive, and cheap.

RECENT PROGRESS IN GENITO-URINARY SURGERY.

BY THOMAS B. CURTIS, M. D.

Treatment of Rupture of the Urethra. — Mr. Teevan [1] publishes two cases of retention of urine from laceration of the urethra treated by catheterism with good results. In the first case, that of a boy aged seven years, an elastic olivary catheter having previously failed to enter, a metal catheter was successfully introduced by following the upper wall of the urethra, which was undamaged and served as a guide ; the instrument was tied in for twenty-four hours. In the second case the patient, aged thirty, having been kicked in the perinæum, lost blood from the urethra and experienced retention of urine ; an olivary elastic catheter of medium size was easily passed, and withdrawn after evacuation of the urine ; a similar instrument was passed and tied in a few hours later, and was retained two days. Mr. Teevan, in his remarks on these cases, recalls that Mercier had laid it down as a rule that if a laceration or false passage existed in the floor of the deep portion of the urethra, a curved metallic catheter ought to be passed, as it could be made to hug the roof of the urethra ; if, on the contrary, the laceration were in the roof, a straight elastic catheter ought to be passed, to keep to the floor of the urethra. " Inasmuch as in the case of the boy a metal catheter only could be introduced, it proved that the ure-

1 The Lancet, August 21, 1875.

thra had been torn in its floor, whilst the fact of an elastic catheter only being able to be passed in the man showed that the urethra had been torn in the roof. . . . The cases showed that soft and metal catheters had each its sphere of action, though, as a rule, if the urethra were completely torn across, a small olivary catheter would be found more likely than any other instrument to pick up the distal end of the divided canal." Mr. Teevan brings forward Mercier's rule as a guide for the surgeon in his choice of procedures. But in his own cases, as his words show, the locality of the incomplete laceration of the urethra was only determined by means of the results following attempts, unsuccessful and successful, to pass various instruments, and it seems to us that this must always be the case. Therefore Mercier's propositions can at best only serve in such cases to explain the mechanism of successful catheterism, and can afford no clew by which to recognize the operative indications.

M. Notta[1] (of Lisieux) brought up the subject of the treatment of ruptured urethra before the Surgical Society of Paris with three cases which had been successfully treated by incision of the perinæum, after failure of attempts to introduce a catheter. He lays down as a rule that, in cases of ruptured urethra, the surgeon should first try to introduce a catheter, with a view to keeping it tied in ; and that, failing in this attempt, he should immediately practice external perineal urethrotomy. He thinks that subsequently, after a period of three to eight days, it is advisable to tie in a catheter, " to reëstablish the continuity of the canal." For this purpose Notta uses a vulcanized rubber catheter, which he introduces by the assistance of a long, filiform, whalebone bougie, serving as a conductor. M. Guyon, on the other hand, is of the opinion that attempts at catheterism are extremely likely to be not only fruitless but positively injurious. He advocates the immediate performance of external urethrotomy without a conductor, which, he says, is an easy operation in cases of recent traumatism, however difficult it may be in cases of inveterate stricture accompanied by fistulous tracts. Guyon also ties in a catheter, but this he does immediately after practicing the median perineal incision.

The Operative Means for the Relief of Patients suffering with advanced Prostatic Disease. — In certain cases of obstructive hypertrophy of the prostate which have long necessitated the frequent use of the catheter, an advanced stage finally arrives which is associated with a great diminution of the capacity of the bladder, so that the artificial evacuation of the urine has to be repeated from sixteen to twenty-four times or more in the twenty-four hours. This is a condition of extreme misery for the patient, and often of peril, from the risk of injury in the frequently repeated performance of catheterism. The employment of an in-lying catheter, on the other hand, is at best but a temporary rem-

[1] Gazette hebdomadaire, June 4, 1875.

edy. In such cases Sir Henry Thompson[1] proposes to puncture the bladder above or rather behind the pubes, with a view to establishing a permanent outlet for the urine through an in-lying canula. The proceeding, which he has practiced in three cases, resembles the high operation for stone, rather than the ordinary supra-pubic puncture as practiced in cases of retention, since in the cases described, the bladder, instead of being distended with fluid, is nearly empty, retracted, and perhaps displaced and deformed by the prostatic growth. The first step of the operation consists in passing a large, strongly-curved, hollow sound containing a long bulbous-ended stylet. The instrument is introduced by the urethra until the end can be felt just behind the symphysis pubis. It is then confided to an assistant. The operator now makes an incision not more than three quarters of an inch in length, less if the patient is not stout, enough to admit the index-finger tightly, in the median line at the upper margin of the symphysis. The tissues are separated by the finger, and the linea alba being next slightly divided by the point of a bistoury, the finger is passed down closely behind the symphysis, and when the end of the sound is clearly felt a little opening is made so as to expose its point. The operator now, taking the handle of the sound in his left hand, makes the end protrude in the wound, and withdraws the bulbous stylet; taking then a short, curved canula of elastic gum, with a silver plate at its distal extremity (somewhat resembling a tracheotomy canula), the surgeon passes it into the hollow channel of the sound. He now withdraws this completely by the urethra, and in doing so insures the passage of the elastic canula into the bladder. The canula is then to be fastened securely with tapes and plaster, and must be worn a few days in bed, until the parts are consolidated and the patient can move about with safety. If the tube escape during the first two or three days it may not be easy to replace it, but it can be removed and replaced easily enough when the passage is established. A very important point is to make the wound as small as possible, so as to be nearly filled by the canula. Three cases are briefly reported. In two of them the operation was adopted solely as a last resource, to mitigate the sufferings of patients whose fate was already sealed. In the third case the operation was performed at an earlier period, with the view of prolonging life. Unluckily, on the third or fourth night the canula escaped, the house-surgeon was unable to introduce it, and extravasation took place; the patient died four months later. Sir Henry Thompson says, in conclusion, that the operation itself, properly performed, makes little or no demand on the patient's powers, and that he shall no doubt give it further trials, as he has faith in its utility for appropriate cases.

[1] The Lancet, January 2, 1875.

The Treatment of Chronic Cystitis by Means of Artificially Produced Incontinence of Urine. — The procedure just described is designed to relieve ceaseless vesical tenesmus, due to an incurable disease, by establishing a permanent outlet for the urine. The function of the bladder as a reservoir requiring intermittent evacuation is thus permanently superseded. The various methods of treatment now to be alluded to are somewhat analogous in design, their common object being to keep the bladder constantly empty for a time, by means of the temporary induction of incontinentia urinæ, either through the natural channel (the dilated female urethra), or through an artificial opening (vaginal cystotomy in females; perineal cystotomy in males). The credit of having first suggested this treatment of chronic cystitis appears to belong to Dr. Sims, who proposed it in 1858 to Dr. T. A. Emmet. The latter has since that date frequently and successfully treated chronic cystitis in the female by vaginal cystotomy, the opening into the bladder being artificially kept open as long as appeared necessary.[1] Professor Willard Parker[2] published in 1867 a paper on cystitis in the male treated by cystotomy, with cases; his operations were performed in 1846 and 1850.

T. Pridgeon Teale[3] has during the last eight years frequently treated vesical irritability in the female by dilatation of the neck of the bladder, with absolute cure in about a third of thirty or forty cases so treated by himself and his friends. His procedure consists in slowly distending the urethra by means of Weiss's dilator, until it admits two fingers. In many cases so treated some laceration occurs, causing after-pain during a day or two; often the intended incontinence did not ensue, but the tenesmus was relieved, the result being analogous to that produced by dilatation of the sphincter ani in painful fissure; in other cases incontinence lasted a few weeks; in one case it lasted several months; and in two cases, permanent incontinence ensued. "It does not, however, appear that the liability to permanent incontinence depended upon the degree to which the dilatation was carried." In three cases death occurred shortly after the operation, but advanced disease of the kidneys was found to exist.

Dr. T. W. Howe[4] published a case of cystitis occurring in a female, successfully treated by dilatation of the neck of the bladder. By various means, instrumental and digital, the urethra was dilated until a glass speculum nearly three quarters of an inch in diameter could be introduced. The urine dribbled from the bladder until the fifth day, when the sphincter resumed control. A rapid and complete cure of

---

[1] See an article in the American Practitioner for February, 1872.
[2] See Transactions of the New York State Medical Society, 1867.
[3] The Lancet, November 27, 1875.
[4] The Medical Record, August 14, 1875.

cystitis, which had resisted other treatment over two months, resulted from the dilatation.

Want of space forbids our making more than a mention of the analogous treatment of inveterate cystitis in the male. In such cases cystotomy has been performed by Willard Parker, Velpeau, Syme, Dolbeau, Bickersteth (of Liverpool) Battey (of Georgia), Prof. E. Powell (of the Rush Medical College), Parona, and many others.[1] The disposition of the male parts of course renders this treatment of cystitis more difficult than it is in the female, where the neck of the bladder is relatively easy of access. A median cystotomy is generally performed, or else, after a perineal urethrotomy, the prostatic urethra is dilated, as in Dolbeau's operation for stone.

Rapid Dilatation of the Female Urethra. — Among other methods for rendering the female bladder accessible for diagnostic or therapeutic purposes, Professor Simon,[2] of Heidelberg, has carefully investigated this time-honored procedure, and has laid down accurate rules for its rapid, efficacious, and innocuous accomplishment. The operation was an old one, but our knowledge of the extreme limits of safe dilatation of the female urethra was very uncertain, nor was the proper *modus operandi* established until the publication of Simon's researches. In order that we might be able to produce the maximum dilatation of the urethra without causing laceration or subsequent incontinence of urine, it was necessary that we should know with tolerable accuracy the consequences which might be anticipated from extreme degrees of dilatation properly conducted.

Simon uses for dilatation a series of smooth, hard-rubber, conical plugs, whose diameters are graduated by intervals of one millimetre, the smallest being three quarters of a centimetre, and the largest two centimetres in diameter ; thus the largest plug has a circumference equaling 6.3 centimetres, and is about as thick as the forefinger. These plugs are preferable to all other dilating agencies, such as the fingers, various forceps, and many-branched dilators, inasmuch as by their means we can accomplish rapid dilatation with the least possible risk of laceration or injury to the peri-urethral tissues. Anæsthesia being established, for the operation is otherwise very painful, the first step consists in slitting the external meatus, which is the narrowest part of the urethra ; three small slits, two above laterally, of a depth of one fourth of a centimetre, and one below, of a depth of one half of a centimetre, suffice for all purposes, and are harmless. The plugs being then successively inserted, up to the largest, it becomes easy to introduce the forefinger, and if at the same time the precaution is taken of passing the medius into the

---

[1] See the British and Foreign Medico-Chirurgical Review, January, 1875, page 243 ; also the American Journal of the Medical Sciences, April, 1875 ; also Professor Dolbeau's Leçons de Clinique chirurgicale.

[2] See the New York Medical Journal, October, 1875

vagina, almost the entire length of the forefinger can be utilized for intra-vesical manipulations.

The limits of dilatation are as follows: In adult women, plugs 2 centimetres (.8 of an inch) in diameter, 6.3 centimetres (2.4 inches) in circumference, can be used without detriment; in sufficiently urgent cases, dilatation may be carried up to a circumference of 6.5 to 7 centimetres (2.5 to 2.7 inches) without the production of any lasting inconvenience.   Beyond this latter limit, however, Simon asserts that dilatation would entail a risk of permanent incontinence.   In girls aged from eleven to fifteen years, the highest degrees of completely innocuous dilatation seem to be reached when a circumference of 4.7 to 5.6 centimetres (1.78 to 2.14 inches), equaling diameters from 1.5 to 1.8 centimetres (.54 to .63 inch), has been attained.   In girls from fifteen to twenty years of age, the maximum circumferences range from 5.6 to 6.3 centimetres (2.14 to 2.45 inches), equaling diameters from 1.8 to 2.0 centimetres (.63 to .78 inch).   In exceptional cases, justifying the infliction of temporary incontinence, the limits so fixed might be slightly exceeded.

The urethra having been so dilated as to admit the forefinger, it becomes possible to execute a very complete exploration of the bladder, especially by means of the bimanual method of palpation; many operative procedures are also facilitated, and new operations are rendered possible.   The indications for the employment of Simon's dilatation of the female urethra are set forth as follows: (1.) The diagnosis of diseases of the mucous membrane of the urethra and bladder, by digital exploration, and by endoscopic examination.   (2.) The diagnosis of calculi and foreign bodies.   (3.) The extraction of such bodies.   (4.) The application of caustics in certain affections of the bladder.   (5.) The treatment of fissures of the urethra.   (6.) The diagnosis of defects in the vesico-vaginal septum, when the vagina is closed.   (7.) The diagnosis of the seat and extent of growths and tumors in the vesico-vaginal septum.   (8.) The extirpation of tumors, especially of papillomata, from the mucous surface of the bladder.   (9.) The discovery and extraction or excision of renal calculi from the vesical part of the ureter.   (10.) The opening of hæmatometra in certain cases.   (11.) The cure of colo-vesical or entero-vesical fistula by cauterization of their vesical orifice.

WAGSTAFFE'S HUMAN OSTEOLOGY.[1]

THOUGH any great work on anatomy that can stand on a level with Henle's is still to be written in the English language, we are singularly rich in treatises on osteology. Beside the descriptions of the bones in the text-books, we have three well-known works: Ward's, Humphry's, and Holden's. The oldest is that of Ward, and in some respects it is still the best; it combines a most accurate and minute description of the bones with many very original observations expressed very clearly and briefly. The author opened a new road in English anatomy, and if some subsequent books are as good as his it is greatly owing to him. Holden's book is undoubtedly the most popular among students, a fact due chiefly to its fine plates and easy style, though we think it decidedly inferior to either of the others. Humphry's Human Skeleton is not meant as a text-book, and the descriptions are consequently wanting in minuteness, but it abounds with scientific and practical observations. The joints are considered as well as the bones, and their actions are treated in a masterly manner. It is to our mind the best of the three. With such predecessors it is no easy task to write a new treatise on osteology. Pretty nearly all the facts concerning bones have been noted, and there remains only the method of handling the subject that offers scope for originality. This field is, however, immense, and will never be exhausted. Mr. Wagstaffe has seized the only road that is still comparatively untraveled, that of the internal structure of bones, and has written a good deal that is good and new, but still we are inclined to regard this part as a failure, owing to his profound ignorance of the literature of the subject. There is no mention of Wyman's law of studs and braces, of Bigelow's "true neck of the femur," or of the investigations of several German authorities, an acquaintance with which would have saved the author some errors.

This being said, we have nearly done with criticism. The description of the coarse appearance of the bones is for the most part very good, and the recapitulation of the points of importance at the end of each section will serve to impress them upon the student. The plates are finely executed and very good, most of them being in the style of Holden's, and having colored lines to indicate the origin and insertion of muscles. We are somewhat in doubt whether too much is not said on this subject, but it is hard to draw the line, and if the pruning knife were used at all it would have to be wielded by a very careful hand lest it take what could not be spared. A great deal of the mechanism is very excellent. We are glad to see a chapter on the bony landmarks that can be felt during life. There are few books on any subject that reach the ideal of the special critic, owing to the fact that no two minds view a subject from precisely the same standpoint. Further criticism might, no doubt, be made on many points, but when we consider the great difficulty of saying just enough without overdryness or too much diffuseness, we must admit that the work reflects great credit on the author, and we can heartily recommend it.

T. D. JR.

[1] *The Student's Guide to Human Osteology.* By W. W. WAGSTAFFE, B. A., F. R. C. S. Philadelphia: Lindsay and Blakiston. 1875.

LEISHMAN'S SYSTEM OF MIDWIFERY.[1]

THE simultaneous demand, both in England and in America, for a second edition of this work attests sufficiently its value. Essentially the book remains the same, but it is to be especially noticed that the author has greatly changed the two chapters on puerperal fever. When the book first appeared we criticised the ideas held on that subject as being far behind the times. In the present edition we think we recognize the first fruits of that remarkable discussion which has recently taken place before the London Obstetrical Society. The author now gives up the idea of a specific puerperal poison, and considers that the character of the disease is due, not to anything specific in the cause, but to the peculiar physiological condition under which the puerperal woman lies. He believes that the fever is mainly generated by septic absorption, and that the poison of any of the specific eruptive diseases may give rise to an affection which usually offers clear evidences of the puerperal type of the febrile disease, while at the same time it may retain more or less of the specific characteristics of the disease from which it was engendered.

Some changes have also been made in the physiological section of the work, and the author has added considerable valuable matter as to the causes of sudden death in the puerperal state, a subject not alluded to in the previous edition. Additional stress is laid upon Credé's method of managing the expulsion of the placenta, which the author advises should always be adopted.

Copious notes to the English edition have been added by Dr. Parry, of Philadelphia, who has also introduced a few new illustrations, representing for the most part the principal modifications of obstetrical instruments generally employed in this country. We must confess that we are not fond of this method of interpolating critical notes. If, however, it is to be done, then it is a matter worth noticing that it has in this case been well done. Especially valuable is the chapter on the diphtheria of puerperal wounds, which Dr. Parry has added entire, and which was originally published in the *American Journal of the Medical Sciences*, January, 1875.

This second edition of Dr. Leishman's work, taken as a whole, is a great improvement on the first.

PROCEEDINGS OF THE OBSTETRICAL SOCIETY OF BOSTON.

CHARLES W. SWAN, M. D., SECRETARY.

OCTOBER 9, 1875. The president, DR. HODGDON, in the chair.

Hysterotomy. — DR. CHADWICK reported a case of hysterotomy for a fibroid tumor, exhibiting the specimen. The case was published in the JOURNAL of November 4, 1875.

DR. LYMAN, referring to the tetanus with which the subject of the operation died, asked what had been the treatment of the pedicle in other cases.

[1] *A System of Midwifery.* By WILLIAM LEISHMAN, M. D. Second American, from the second and revised English edition. With Additions by JOHN S. PARRY, M. D. Philadelphia: Henry C. Lea. 1875.

Dr. Chadwick replied that it was Péau's practice to fix the pedicle in the abdominal wound.   Dr. Chadwick considered that hysterotomy was somewhat more dangerous than ovariotomy, owing to the greater shock to be expected from the removal of so important an organ as the uterus, and to the greater liability to hæmorrhage.   These dangers are in a measure offset by the rarity of adhesions with fibroids; this remark does not apply, however, to fibro-cysts. Péan has lost but five out of his twenty cases; the causes of death were hæmorrhage, shock, and septicæmia; some of the tumors were universally adherent.

In answer to a question, Dr. Chadwick stated that the sound could not be passed beyond the internal os until the cervix had been dilated; an elastic sound then passed to the fundus without pain.   He described the gas cautery invented by Dr. Bruce, of London, which in the hands of Dr. J. Homans had proved so efficient in checking the hæmorrhage.   A conical hood of platinum was heated by means of a gas jet blown into it.   The only drawback to its use was the tendency of the flame to spread about and beyond the cone, thus endangering the tissues for some distance around the point to be cauterized; otherwise the instrument had proved very useful and convenient.

Fatal Hæmorrhage from Extra-Uterine Fœtation. — Dr. Driver reported the case.   He was called in the night to see the patient with Dr. Hildreth. The woman was apparently in collapse, — gasping, restless, in cold perspiration, white, pulseless, and in intense pain low down in the abdomen.   She was quite rational.   On examination of the abdomen he found a region of dullness on the right side in the pelvic region, limited on the left by an oblique line which extended from the symphysis pubis upward and outward to the right hypochondrium; all the rest of the abdominal surface being resonant.   The diagnosis was accidental internal hæmorrhage.

The woman had gone over one menstrual period, and, suspecting pregnancy, had on the day of the visit taken tansy twice.   At eleven P. M. she had gone to bed feeling quite comfortable.   She had had one or two dejections.   She was awakened by severe abdominal pain.   For a while there seemed to be some improvement; the pulse came down to 130, and at this time she had two loose dejections, and felt easier; but before four A. M. the patient was dead, death being preceded by symptoms of renewed hæmorrhage.   An autopsy showed a large clot occupying the whole region of dullness previously defined.   There was an enlargement of the left Fallopian tube, about half an inch from the body of the uterus, containing an ovum of the size of a filbert; and this dilated portion was found to be ruptured posteriorly and upward.   Hence the whole fatal hæmorrhage.   In answer to questions, Dr. Driver said that he found all the characteristics of an ovum except the fœtus.   The pain was continuous, but with exacerbations.

Dr. Lyman said that he had had, about fifteen years ago, a similar case.   Dr. Hooker also reported a case of tubal pregnancy, with rupture and fatal hæmorrhage.   In his case, the patient, a young woman not quite three months pregnant, had precisely the same symptoms, and the diagnosis was the same as in the present instance.   She lived about three hours.   The diagnosis was verified by an autopsy made by Dr. Ellis.   Lately Ziemssen has spoken of external hæmorrhage as always present; this, Dr. Lyman remarked, is not so. Dr. Lyman once collected eleven cases which had been at different times reported to the Boston Society for Medical Improvement, and in only four of these was external hæmorrhage present.[1]

DR. INGALLS reported a case which he had had fifteen or eighteen years ago. He saw the patient not more than fifteen minutes before she died, but from the symptoms he diagnosticated tubal pregnancy and hæmorrhage. There was no post-mortem examination.

DR. LYMAN remarked that the pain in these cases is peculiar and agonizing ; he likened it to the pain from gun-shot wounds of the pleura or the abdomen, in which the blood flows over an uninflamed serous membrane.

DR. STEDMAN reported a case which he had seen a few years ago with Dr. Fifield, in which the symptoms of the patient, six months pregnant, were abdominal pain, pallor, collapse, and death. An autopsy revealed a normal pregnancy. The symptoms had been due to the rupture of a small vessel in the neighborhood of the liver. The precise locality of the pain was not noted.

DR. SINCLAIR asked how the pain in these cases could be distinguished from that of pelvic hæmatocele. He had had a recent case of hæmatoma in which the symptoms were very similar to those above described.

DR. DRIVER said that in the case reported by him there was at once a rapid hæmorrhage extending over a large surface of the peritoneum, and the symptoms were proportionately severe. He thought that as a cause of pain the difference was considerable between a split of a Fallopian tube and the puncture of a vein. Moreover, in an hæmatocele the hæmorrhage is often subperitoneal.

DR. CHADWICK said that it seemed hardly justifiable to find fault with a diagnosis which had proved correct, yet he could not see that the symptoms were so unequivocal as to point at so rare a condition as extra-uterine fœtation, to the exclusion of hæmatocele, etc. He did not think that the suddenness of the attack, the severity of certain symptoms, the position and extent of the hæmorrhagic effusion, were, even when associated, pathognomonic of extra-uterine pregnancy; the patient's belief that she was pregnant should have but little weight in the first three months.

DR. DRIVER replied that the diagnosis in the case reported was based upon the group of symptoms, physical and rational, which belonged to the case: the cessation of menstruation and suspected pregnancy, the suddenness of the attack, the agonizing pain, pallor, restlessness, and collapse, with absence of pulse, the locality of the pain, and the physical signs of large clot. This group of symptoms was best explained by the diagnosis actually made.

DR. CHADWICK reminded the society of the brilliant exploit recently performed by Dr. T. G. Thomas, who, having diagnosticated tubal pregnancy, extracted the fœtus through an incision made from the vagina into the sac with a white-hot knife; the patient made a good recovery.

DR. WELLINGTON recalled two cases which he had previously reported, in which there were symptoms of tubal pregnancy, with rupture of the tube and intense hæmorrhage. Both the patients recovered.

[1] Records of the Boston Society for Medical Improvement, November 28, 1859.

THE POMEROY CASE.

On the first of January, one year since Governor Gaston solemnly swore to enforce the laws of the commonwealth, the same oath will be taken by his successor. Let us hope that to him the oath will be something more than a string of words ; that it will be to him an agreement the keeping of which is essential to his honor, the violation of which is perjury. Should he take this view, and we do not see how he can take any other, his course with regard to the murderer Pomeroy is clear. What are the facts of the case ? The story of his atrocious crimes is sufficiently well known ; let us begin with his trial. The defense made a desperate effort to make out insanity, a plea which was utterly overthrown by the evidence of Dr. Choate, of New York. The jury found him guilty, but (as we learn from good authority) one of their number preferred perjuring himself to taking the responsibility of bringing in a just verdict, and the others, to save him from this crime and to bring about an agreement, added a recommendation to mercy to their verdict. This recommendation was made the most of by those whose delicate sensibilities make them the friends of criminals and the enemies of society. At their instance a peculiar kind of mock trial was held by the governor and council, which they hoped would bring about a commutation of the sentence, but this, happily, the council refused to authorize. One would think that his oath left the governor no further freedom of action, no refuge from signing the death-warrant, but he calmly does nothing, and smiles while the community claims protection. We hope that the new governor will know his duty better, and there is one point to which we would call his attention. The question of insanity does not concern him ; this was settled at the trial, and should not be reopened. It is making a mockery of justice to re-try the case, which has been legally decided. To those interested in the criminal as a psychological problem we recommend the admirable article by Dr. C. F. Folsom that we publish to-day ; it shows clearly Pomeroy's accountability. If the sentimentalists carry the day we may look for quite an epidemic of this form of "insanity," but if justice and reason triumph it will be shown that a little hanging is an excellent prophylactic.

THE HOMŒOPATHIC RAID.

A bold attempt has been made by the homœopaths to obtain a foothold in the City Hospital. A petition was presented, a hearing took place at the City Hall, and the matter was referred to a committee, which in due time reported that two schools of medicine could not work together, and gave the petitioners leave to withdraw, but singularly enough recommended that such patients as preferred to go to the homœopathic hospital should be to a certain extent paid for by the city. This recommendation is, on the whole, a triumph for the petitioners. This is the small end of the wedge, the beginning of a plot by which this particular set of irregulars propose to win an endowment for their hospital. Why they should be favored more than any other set of practitioners, we are at a loss to see. Natural bone-setters, praying doctors, spiritual doctors, corn-cutting doctors, have but to establish the similitude of a hospital, if they have not one already, and they may with equal justice request permission to introduce their hands into the public pocket. The principle upon which the claim is made is entirely false ; the government cannot take into account old women's preferences for this or that " pathy," but must intrust its institutions to those whose membership of the Massachusetts Medical Society is a guarantee of respectability and competence.

MEDICAL NOTES.

— The proposition of Mr. Marshall to institute a compulsory examination in anatomy at the end of the first winter session of the metropolitan medical schools has occasioned considerable discussion on the part of our English exchanges. Of the candidates who present themselves at the primary examination for the membership of the College of Surgeons, Mr. Marshall alleges, according to *The Lancet,* " that some pass extremely well, some barely succeed, whilst the remainder are so deficient in knowledge, especially of anatomy, that they have to be referred for further study, though they have arrived at least at the end of their second year." At the pass examination " a very large proportion of candidates retain a quite insufficient knowledge of anatomy, often forgetting even the most simple and essential facts in that science."

While these statements of Mr. Marshall seem to be admitted as true, the causes assigned by him of the lack of knowledge on the part of the candidates, namely, their mental incapacity and their want of proper training, are not so readily acknowledged. One cause assigned by *The Lancet* is the scanty and irregular supply of subjects for the purposes of dissection, so that at the present time in London many students, both first and second year, must remain idle for want of the opportunity to dissect. In fact, to such an extent is this scarcity of subjects felt by the medical students themselves that they write letters of complaint to the medical journals. A correspondent referring to the proposition of Mr. Marshall attributes the unsatisfactory preparation of candidates to the fact " that men are allowed, and even required, to attend hospital practice and lectures on the practical subjects, while they are working in the dissecting room and physiological laboratory. . . . The majority of students adopt the plan of crushing through all their hospital practice and lectures in two years and a half, or at most in three years, and present themselves badly prepared for all their examinations."

So common has it been for the opportunities afforded by the medical schools of this country for the obtaining of a thorough medical education to be disparagingly spoken of by many of the English journals, when compared with the advantages presented by their own, that we confess to have read with some surprise the statements which Mr. Marshall's proposition has called forth. They tend to confirm us in the belief that the method now pursued at the Harvard Medical School, of carrying the student progressively and systematically from one subject to another in a just and natural order, is the true one.

— Sir Robert Christison, the president of the Edinburgh Botanical Society, made, according to the *British Medical Journal*, from which we quote, some rather surprising statements concerning the "coca leaf," which, it is to be remembered, is not the same as cocoa. "In Peru, where it grows, coca is reported to have remarkable nourishing properties; and, in order to ascertain the precise nature of these, he chewed the leaf by way of stimulant on the occasion of two ascents of Ben Voirlich. On reaching the top, he felt greatly fatigued, and began to chew his coca; with the result that he was able to make the descent, not only with firmness, but with almost juvenile elasticity. He further stated that by its use he had found himself able to walk sixteen miles with ease, although when he attempted this feat without such nourishment he felt greatly fatigued."

— The large number of new editions of text-books of physiology is a sign of the activity of competition between both physiologists and publishers. The result cannot but be very beneficial to the student, for in this struggle for existence there can be no doubt of the ultimate survival of the fittest. We are inclined to think that the success of Dr. Amory's translation of Küss' admirable handbook has had a great deal to do with this rivalry. Its success was so great that it became necessary to bring Dalton's book up to the times and to reduce Flint's great compilation to a manageable compass A new edition of Carpenter is also announced, and we see that Dr. Gamgee has just translated the fifth edition of Hermann.

CONCERNING THE EXECUTION OF CRIMINALS.

"The rope had not been properly arranged around his neck, and scarcely had he been hoisted into the air when he gave unearthly screams, and, writhing in terrible agony, clutched the rope with both hands, notwithstanding they were bound, and, drawing his body up, cried, 'Save me!' His tortures seemed terrible. Three times in succession he raised himself up, to the horror and surprise of the spectators, and finally by his own efforts succeeded in adjusting the rope properly around his neck. He then soon ceased to struggle."

The above is not an extract from the records of the inquisition, nor a quotation from some of the dark chronicles of the Middle Ages, but an account taken from the daily papers, of what took place in the city of New York on the 17th of December in the year 1875 of the Christian era. That such an occurrence is to be deprecated and deplored no one will doubt; and the question as to whether there is any necessity for it naturally presents itself.

An argument on the subject of capital punishment in the abstract would be entirely out of place in this connection; it is sufficient that our law-makers have decided that in the present state of society it is necessary; but let us see what is its object and how it is fulfilled. Its object is threefold: (1) to remove a dangerous character from the society of his fellow-beings, and make sure that he can do no further harm; (2) to have the most severe penalty attached to the commission of crimes which would interfere with the safety and well-being of society, and thus frighten people from committing them; and (3) to show the criminal classes that such crimes are followed by punishment, or, in other words, to serve as an example. That the first of these objects could be attained by the killing of the offender in any way cannot be denied, and in all probabilities likewise the second ; for it is inconceivable that the penalty of death could be made enough more fearful by the addition of physical suffering to it, to deter any one from the commission of a crime which the fear of simple death would not restrain him from. If this is not the case, society certainly owes it to itself to draw and quarter, burn and flay alive, those who commit certain atrocities.

With regard to the third object there may be more difference of opinion, but it is pretty generally conceded that the public executions of the past did not fulfill it, as it was found that the idea of being at some future time, when his day had come, the central figure and hero of such a festival and merry-making as he had often joined in was not a very terrible one to the hardened criminal, but rather the reverse.

What does the sentence " and be hanged by the neck until dead " imply? It implies that a man shall stand up on a scaffold before some two or three hundred of his fellow-beings, shall listen to certain religious ceremonies spun out to a greater or less length according to the taste or humanity of the officiating clergyman, shall stand with a bag over his head, his arms and legs pinioned, a rope around his neck, and when the word is given shall be choked to death, dangling in the air in convulsive struggles, and evidently, for a certain space of time at least, suffering inconceivable tortures. It is true that theoretically his neck should be dislocated by the sudden jerk, and that pressure on the medulla should produce instant death. But in the vast majority of cases this does not take place, and the poor wretch dies of asphyxia produced by his own weight pulling on his throat. Twice have I witnessed such a spectacle, and twice have I come away ashamed of myself, ashamed of the spectators, ashamed of the officials, and ashamed of the state of society which allows such a relic of barbarism to still exist. If it had been a mere morbid curiosity that sent me there, this feeling of shame would have been natural ; but it was not that ; it was the same feeling that has kept me up all night at the bedside of a moribund patient, namely, the desire to witness the different phases of that awful mystery, the extinction of the vital spark.

And as if this was not bad enough, we have once in a while reports of such scenes as the one that called forth these few lines, or the rope breaks and the victim has to be hung over again, or the knot does not slip and the sheriff has to add his own weight to hasten the death of the struggling wretch, or at the last moment the criminal breaks down in an agony of fear and has to be dragged shrieking and struggling to the halter. This is horrible and degrading to all concerned, although if it is absolutely necessary for the carrying out of the law it must be accepted ; but that is just the question — is it necessary ?

There is no doubt that the sudden separation of the brain from the centre of circulation, as it is done by the guillotine, is a much quicker and more merciful method of execution than hanging, for the moment that the arteries which carry blood to the brain are severed, consciousness must cease. But this is a French method of execution, contrary to all the customs and traditions of the Anglo-Saxon race, and nothing short of a general revolution of feeling in the people could bring about the change. Is there, however, no way in which, without altering or interfering with the laws and customs that have come down to us from our forefathers, we can make the death-penalty less revolting and degrading to the assistants and spectators, to say nothing of making it less barbarous to the victim? Why should not the convict at the last moment be put under the influence of an anæsthetic? The occasion would not be any less solemn and impressive, rather the reverse. Suppose that the prisoner be seated in a chair under the gallows with the rope about his neck; after the reading of the sentence, etc., a physician should step up behind him and put a sponge with chloroform over his face. Let the clergyman's voice praying for mercy for his soul be the last human sound he hears as he goes off into his last sleep. In a few seconds the physician gives the sign, the weight falls, the unconscious sinner hangs with a few reflex quiverings, and the sentence of the law has been executed, literally and fully.

It is no morbid pity for the criminal that prompts this suggestion, but rather a desire to spare those who have to be present and the public who read the reports of the execution the feeling of shame and degradation which any one who is not without all delicacy of feeling must experience on witnessing a fellow-creature being slowly strangled to death.

The points that I have wished to call attention to in this hurried communication may be briefly recapitulated as follows. Hanging as now carried out is always painful to the victim and disagreeable to the assistants; sometimes it is torture to the former and degrading and revolting to the latter. By chloroforming the convict at the last moment these objectionable features would be eliminated, the fear of capital punishment would not be diminished thereby, the impressiveness of the occasion would be increased, and the literal fulfillment of the law would be complied with. Let Massachusetts take the initiative in this matter, and the whole civilized world will follow.   F. B. G.

[Though this subject is not a strictly professional one, it is not, we think, out of place in a medical journal, especially as the plan proposed by our correspondent would bring members of our profession into immediate connection with executions. We do not agree with our correspondent for several reasons: in the first place, such accidents as the recent one in New York are utterly inexcusable and unnecessary; secondly, although the neck is rarely broken, we think it a pure assumption that death by judicial hanging is a very painful one; this point, however, may be put aside, for it is of very secondary importance whether the murderer suffers by his punishment or not; thirdly, it is as degrading to the spectators to see a man killed in one way as in another; and lastly, we doubt if the administration of chloroform would render impossible scenes of the greatest horror for all concerned. We can hardly imagine one more fearful than that of the weak-minded but able-bodied criminal struggling against the administration of the anæsthetic, being gradually overpowered by numbers, freeing his face, it may be, to shriek out blasphemies, and finally, a limp, unconscious mass, being dropped to the end of a rope in accordance with merely the letter of the law. — EDS.]

WEEKLY BULLETIN OF PREVALENT DISEASES.

THE following is a bulletin of the diseases prevalent in Massachusetts during the week ending December 25, 1875, compiled under the authority of the State Board of Health from the returns of physicians representing all sections of the State : —

The summary for each section is as follows : —

Berkshire : Bronchitis, influenza, whooping-cough.

Valley : Pneumonia, bronchitis, influenza, diphtheria. More diphtheria reported. Shelburne Falls reports cases of small-pox imported from Northampton.

Midland : Influenza, bronchitis, pneumonia, rheumatism, diphtheria, typhoid fever.

Northeastern : Bronchitis, influenza, diphtheria, pneumonia. More diphtheria reported. Not much sickness.

Metropolitan : Bronchitis, scarlatina, diphtheria, pneumonia, rheumatism. Less diphtheria and scarlatina reported.

Southeastern : Bronchitis, influenza, scarlatina, rheumatism. More scarlatina and diphtheria reported.

In the State at large the order of relative prevalence of diseases is as follows : Bronchitis, pneumonia, influenza, diphtheria, rheumatism, scarlatina, typhoid fever, croup, measles, diarrhœa, whooping-cough ; only the first six deserve mention. Diphtheria has increased ; other diseases have declined.

F. W. DRAPER, M. D., Registrar.

———◆———

COMPARATIVE MORTALITY-RATES FOR THE WEEK ENDING DEC. 18, 1875.

	Estimated Population.	Total Mortality for the Week.	Annual Death-Rate per 1000 during Week
New York	1,060,000	492	24
Philadelphia	800,000	326	21
Brooklyn	500,000		
Chicago	400,000	132	17
Boston	342,000	169	26
Cincinnati	260,000		
Providence	100,700	34	18
Worcester	50,000	12	12
Lowell	50,000	18	19
Cambridge . . .	48,000	12	13
Fall River	45,000	19	30
Lawrence	35,000		
Lynn	33,000	10	16
Springfield	31,000	16	27
Salem	26,000	12	24

Normal Death-Rate, 17 per 1000.

THE BOSTON SOCIETY FOR MEDICAL OBSERVATION. — A regular meeting of the society will be held on Monday evening, January 3, 1876. Dr. Boardman will report a case of ovariotomy.

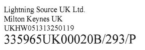

Lightning Source UK Ltd.
Milton Keynes UK
UKHW051313250119
335965UK00020B/293/P